ADOLESCENT
NUTRITION

ASSESSMENT AND MANAGEMENT

CHAPMAN & HALL SERIES IN CLINICAL NUTRITION

Ronni Chernoff, Ph.D., R.D.
Series Editor

Enteral Nutrition

Edited by:
Bradley C. Borlase, M.D., M.S.
Stacey J. Bell, MS., R.D., C.N.S.D.
George L. Blackburn, M.D., Ph.D.
R. Armour Forse, M.D., Ph.D.

Pediatric Enteral Nutition

Edited by:
Susan S. Baker, M.D., Ph.D.
Robert D. Baker, Jr., M.D., Ph.D.
Anne Davis, M.S., R.D., C.N.S.D.

Obesity: Pathophysiology, Psychology, and Treatment

Edited by:
George L. Blackburn, M.D., Ph.D.
Beatrice S. Kanders, Ed.D, M.P.H., R.D.

Adolescent Nutrition: Assessment and Management

Edited by:
Vaughn I. Rickert, Psy.D., F.S.A.M.

ADOLESCENT NUTRITION

ASSESSMENT AND MANAGEMENT

Edited by

Vaughn I. Rickert, Psy.D., F.S.A.M.

Division of Pediatric and Adolescent Gynecology
University of Texas, Medical Branch at Galveston

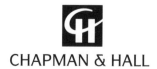

CHAPMAN & HALL

 THOMSON PUBLISHING

New York • Albany • Bonn • Boston • Cincinnati • Detroit • London • Madrid • Melbourne
Mexico City • Pacific Grove • Paris • San Francisco • Singapore • Tokyo • Toronto • Washington

Cover design: Andrea Meyer, emDASH inc.

Copyright © 1996 by Chapman & Hall

Printed in the United States of America

Chapman & Hall
115 Fifth Avenue
New York, NY 10003

Chapman & Hall
2-6 Boundary Row
London SE1 8HN
England

Thomas Nelson Australia
102 Dodds Street
South Melbourne, 3205
Victoria, Australia

Chapman & Hall GmbH
Postfach 100 263
D-69442 Weinheim
Germany

Nelson Canada
1120 Birchmount Road
Scarborough, Ontario
Canada M1K 5G4

International Thomson Publishing Asia
221 Henderson Road #05-10
Henderson Building
Singapore 0315

International Thomson Editores
Campos Eliseos 385, Piso 7
Col. Polanco
11560 Mexico D.F. Mexico

International Thomson Publishing–Japan
Hirakawacho-cho Kyowa Building, 3F
1-2-1 Hirakawacho-cho
Chiyoda-ku, 102 Tokyo
Japan

1 2 3 4 5 6 7 8 9 10 XXX 01 00 99 98 97 96 95

Library of Congress Cataloging-in-Publication Data

Adolescent nutrition : assessment and management / edited by Vaughn
  I. Rickert.
    p.   cm. -- (Chapman & Hall series in clinical nutrition)
    Includes bibliographical references and index.
    ISBN 0-412-05661-5
    1. Teenagers--Nutrition.   2. Teenagers--Diseases--Nutritional
  aspects.   I. Rickert, Vaughn I. II. Series.
  RJ235.A36 1995
  613. 2 ' 0835--dc20   95-7376
                                                                 CIP

To order this or any other Chapman & Hall book, please contact **International Thomson Publishing, 7625 Empire Drive, Florence, KY 41042.** Phone: (606) 525-6600 or 1-800-842-3636. Fax: (606) 525-7778. e-mail: order@chaphall.com.

For a complete listing of Chapman & Hall titles, send your request to **Chapman & Hall, Dept. BC, 115 Fifth Avenue, New York, NY 10003.**

To my sources of sustenance,

Cynthia, Jeffrey, Ryan, and Mason

Contents

Series Editor's Foreword

Often we speak of nutrition "through the life cycle" and we refer to infant nutrition, pediatrics, adult nutrition, pregnancy and lactation, and old age. There is a part of life that we would, perhaps, prefer to forget because it is not among our favorite period: adolescence! The teen years are, nevertheless, very important in growth and development. They are years when children are making the transition to adulthood, trying out responsibility, and learning about the world. During these years there are a great many nutritional issues that arise and to date we have had nowhere to go for answers. **Adolescent Nutrition: Assessment and Management** edited by Vaughn I. Rickert, Psy.D., addresses a wide spectrum of issues in adolescent nutrition with 30 chapters.

This book is divided into 7 parts, each of which examines a unique aspect of adolescent nutrition. The first part covers general issues: adolescent growth and development, exercise and fitness, contraception and weight, vegetarian and fad diets, and coronary heart disease prevention.

Psychological development in adolescent contributes to their perceptions of the body image and behaviors. The second part of this book discusses psychological development, behavior change and compliance, and body image. The concerns surrounding body image and behavior are very important during this period and should not be overlooked. The third part addresses the problems of eating disorders in this population including anorexia nervosa, bulimia nervosa, and obesity.

Topics that address the special needs of adolescents are included in part 4. These topics are important to provide comprehensive care to teens. One chapter deals with the competitive athlete; another discusses the special needs of the pregnant teenager. This part also contains chapters on adolescents who have genetic disorders, metabolic disturbances, and developmental disabilities. The nutritional management of young people with these problems is very important because of their unique nutritional requirements.

Approximately 31 million teens have at least one serious health problem and many have chronic diseases that require nutritional intervention. In part 5, the initiation of nutritional intervention starts with the nutritional assessment. In this part, the most common chronic illnesses are addressed. There are chapters on hypertension, diabetes, renal disease, inflammatory bowel disease, cystic fibrosis and other malabsorptive disorders, cancer, and acquired immunodeficiency syndrome (AIDS).

Teenagers sometimes have acute illnesses or chronic conditions that require surgical intervention. The nutritional aspects of presurgical preparation, organ transplantation, gastroplasty, and plastic and reconstructive surgery are discussed in part 6 of this book.

The last part explores some future directions for research in adolescent nutrition. There is also a chapter on building a nutrition team for the delivery of nutritional care to teenagers. Adolescents have many changes in their lives to cope with and having medical or nutritional problems adds many stresses to an already difficult period. The best that nutritional and health professionals can do is to be knowledgeable about their problems, guide them through difficult times, offer support, and work with them to successfully foster their transition into adulthood and its responsibilities. This book, edited by Dr. Vaughn I. Rickert, offers the most comprehensive approach to adolescent nutrition that is currently available. The authors are all experts in their fields and provide the best and most current information. This book is needed by every health professional who manages teenage patients. This is an outstanding addition to the **Chapman and Hall** *Series in Clinical Nutrition.*

Ronni Chernoff, Ph.D., R.D.
Series Editor, Chapman & Hall Series in Clinical Nutrition

Preface

This text, *Adolescent Nutrition: Assessment and Management* attempts to provide a comprehensive body of knowledge on the unique nutritional requirements and related needs of adolescents. The purpose was twofold. First, to provide a useful text for the training of dietitians who hope to provide care to adolescents. Second, to offer a clinically relevant reference to those already in practice who may find themselves ill-equipped to handle the particular nutritional needs of and the associated difficulties with managing, these challenging patients.

I have chosen authors from many areas, representing specialists in nutrition, pediatrics, adolescent medicine, nursing, and psychology. Most important, contributors were selected because they provide clinical care to adolescents. The format for the text is consistent, but sometimes presented difficulty. I hope that the introduction provided for each chapter will not be too cumbersome for those practitioners already familiar with a particular condition or disease state. Every attempt has been made to reduce the replication of information among chapters, but some remains because of the subject's importance to that individual chapter. The purpose of separating the assessment and management sections was to provide clarity to each of those components, but it is important to realize that these occur in tandem. Finally, instead of a summary section for each chapter, a case illustration was determined to be more helpful to integrate the salient nutritional assessment and management components, as well as the typical adolescent issues, that affect the provision of care.

The text is organized into seven parts. General issues affecting the nutritional care of adolescents is provided to review and highlight basic principals. In order to provide insight into psychological issues of this population, the second part deals with adolescent development, behavior change, and body image. It is felt that to effectively provide nutritional care to teens, dietitians must be familiar with the unique developmental issues that face this group, as well as strategies that may facilitate a good working relationship. Owing to the impact that eating disorders have on teens, especially females, the book's third part attempts to summarize relevant information for those dietitians who work with adolescents. Thus, the reader is referred to the many other texts that focus on each of these areas separately. Often, adolescents who have special needs because of developmental disabilities, metabolic disturbances, or genetic anomalies, as well as the competitive adolescent athlete, may be overlooked. The text's fourth part provides specific advice because these teens may be seen infrequently or overlooked by providers. The chapter on teen pregnancy covers both pre- and postpartum issues with great detail because of the tremendous importance of nutrition in pregnancy. The fifth part, "Chronic Disease," outlines the medical, nutritional, and psychological issues of various disease states. Although not all disease states are covered, I believe sufficient information can be gleaned that will aid the dietitian when dealing with a teen with any chronic disease. Organ transplantation, gastroplasty, and reconstructive surgery are presented in the next part. Particular care was given to overview preoperative nutritional status, as well as to provide useful information on the unique dietary factors of specific organ transplant or the youth undergoing plastic surgery. The use of vertical-banded gastroplasty and other surgical procedures to treat adolescent obesity is not commonplace. However, it was felt that surgical intervention does have a place in the treatment of adolescents who are morbidly obese. The book's final part is devoted to nutrition research, focusing on teens and building the nutritional team. Although primarily written for those in academic and teaching settings, the information does provide clinical pearls for those who may have an interest in research or those working in hospital settings where the use of multidisplinary teams is not the norm.

The completion of this text was dependent on a number of individuals. First and foremost, I wish to extend my sincere appreciation to all the contributors for their willingness to share their expertise in writing according to my constraints. The Series Editor, Dr. Ronni Chernoff, on numerous occasions provided guidance, support, and the needed advice to complete the scope of this text. The support of the Department of Pediatrics at the University of Arkansas for Medical Sciences was of great benefit, as was the guidance of Eleanor Riemer, Senior Editor at Chapman and Hall. Finally, I would like to acknowledge the ongoing support and understanding of my family throughout this endeavor.

Contributors

Lucy B. Adams, M.S.
Assistant Clinical Professor of
 Pediatrics
Division of Adolesent Medicine
University of California, San
 Francisco
400 Parnassus Avenue, AC-01, Box
 0374
San Francisco, CA 94143

Deborah Andrews, R.D.
Registered Dietitian
Department of Food and Nutrition
 Services
University of Colorado Health
 Science Center
The University Hospital

4200 E. 9th Avenue, Box A068
Denver, CO 80218

Dean L. Antonson, M.D.
Associate Professor of Pediatrics and
 Internal Medicine
Associate Director of Combined
 Section of Pediatric
 Gastroenterology and Nutrition
University of Nebraska Medical
 Center/Creighton University
 School of Medicine
Medical Director,
Eating Disorders Program
University of Nebraska Medical
 Center
600 South 42nd Street
Omaha, NE 68198

Martha R. Arden, M.D.
Assistant Professor of Pediatrics
Albert Einstein College of Medicine
Division of Adolescent Medicine
Center for Atherosclerosis Prevention
Schneider Children's Hospital
Long Island Jewish Medical Center
The Long Island Campus for the
    Albert Einstein College of Medicine
New Hyde Park, NY 11042

Joseph Cullen, M.D.
Assistant Professor
Department of Surgery
University of Iowa College of
    Medicine
University Hospitals and Clinics
Iowa City, IO 52242

Christopher Cunniff, M.D.
Associate Professor of Pediatrics
Section of Medical and Molecular
    Genetics
The University of Arizona College of
    Medicine
1501 North Campbell Avenue
Tucson, AZ 85724

Lawrence J. D'Angelo, M.D.,
    M.P.H., F.S.A.M.
Chairman,
Department of Adolescent and Young
    Adult Medicine
Children's National Medical Center
111 Michigan Avenue, N.W.
Washington, DC 20010-2970

Cornelius Doherty, M.D., F.A.C.S.
Assistant Professor
Department of Surgery
University of Iowa College of
    Medicine
University Hospitals and Clinics
Iowa City, IA 52242

Ann Erpenbeck, R.D.
Registered Dietitian
Department of Pediatrics
St. Joseph's Children's Hospital
3001 W. Dr. Martin Luther King Jr.
    Blvd.
P.O. Box 4227
Tampa, FL 33677-4227

Bruce G. Gordon, M.D.,
Assistant Professor of Pediatrics
Clinical Director, BMT Program
University of Nebraska Medical
    Center
600 South 42nd Street
Omaha, NE 68198

Estherann Grace, M.D., F.S.A.M.
Associate in Medicine
Division of Adolescent and Young
    Adult Medicine
Children's Hospital
300 Longwood Avenue
Boston, MA 02115
Assistant Clinical Professor of
    Pediatrics
Harvard Medical School

Jean E. Guest, R.D.
Clinical Dietitian
University of Nebraska Medical
    Center
600 South 42nd Street
Omaha, NE 68198

Ella Hasso Haddad, Dr.P.H., M.S.,
    R.D.
Associate Professor,
School of Public Health
Department of Nutrition
Loma Linda University
Loma Linda, CA 92350

Michael H. Hart, M.S., M.D.
Director,
Division of Pediatric
  Gastroenterology and Nutrition
Department of Pediatrics
Emory University School of
  Medicine
2040 Ridgewood Drive, N.E.
Atlanta, GA 30322

Leslie Heinberg, Ph.D.
Post-doctoral Fellow,
Department of Behavioral Medicine
Johns Hopkins University School of
  Medicine
Department of Psychiatry and
  Behavioral Sciences
600 North Wolfe Street, Meyer 218
Baltimore, MD 21287

Nancy A. Held, M.S., R.D., C.D.E.
Diabetes Nutrition Specialist
Department of Pediatric
  Endocrinology
Yale University School of Medicine
P.O. Box 208064
New Haven, CT 45229

Lori A. Higgins, R.D.
Registered Dietician
Division of Adolescent Medicine
University of Rochester Medical
  Center
601 Elmwood Avenue, Box 613
Rochester, NY 14642

Mark T. Houser, M.D.
Associate Professor and Associate
  Chairman
Department of Pediatrics
University of Nebraska Medical
  Center
600 South 42nd Street
Omaha, NE 68198

M. Susan Jay, M.D., F.S.A.M.
Professor of Pediatrics
Director,
Division of Adolescent Medicine
Loyola University Medical Center
2160 South First
Maywood, IL 60153

Patricia K. Johnston, Dr.P.H., M.S.,
  R.D.
Associate Dean,
School of Public Health
Professor and Chairman,
Department of Nutrition
Loma Linda University
Loma Linda, CA 92350

Theodore A. Kastner, M.D.
Director,
Center for Human Development
Morristown Memorial Hospital
100 Madison
Morristown, NJ 07960
Associate Professor of Clinical
  Pediatrics
Columbia University
College of Physicians and Surgeons

Shelley Kirk, M.S., R.D., L.D.,
  C.D.E.
Director of Nutrition
Division of Adolescent Medicine
Children's Hospital Medical Center
3300 Burnet Avenue
Cincinnati, OH 45229

Richard Koch, M.D.
Professor of Clinical Pediatrics
Division of Medical Genetics
University of Southern California
  School of Medicine
Children's Hospital, Los Angeles
PKU Program #73
4650 Sunset Blvd.
Los Angeles, CA 90027

Amy J. Kovar, M.S., R.D., C.S., L.D., C.N.S.P.
Nutrition Specialist
State of Maryland
Department of Health and Hygiene
201 West Preston Street
Baltimore, MD 21201

Karen J. Kozlowski, M.D.
Assistant Professor of Pediatrics, Obstetrics and Gynecology
University of Arkansas for Medical Sciences
Director, Young Women's Center
Arkansas Children's Hospital
800 Marshall Street
Little Rock, AR 72202

Richard E. Kreipe, M.D.
Associate Professor of Pediatrics
Chief,
Division of Adolescent Medicine
Unversity of Rochester Medical Center
601 Elmwood Avenue, Box 690
Rochester, NY 14642

Alan M. Lake, M.D.
Pediatric Consultants
10807 Falls Road, Suite 200
Lutherville, MD 21093
Associate Professor of Pediatrics
Johns Hopkins University School of Medicine

Jennifer M.H. Loggie, M.D.
Director,
Division of Clinical Pharmacology
Children's Hospital Medical Center
Children's Hospital Research Foundation
3300 Burnet Avnue
Cincinnati, OH 45229
Professor of Pediatrics
University of Cincinnati College of Medicine

David R. Mack, M.D.
Assistant Professor of Pediatrics
Pediatric Gastroenterology and Nutrition
University of Nebraska Medical Center
600 South 42nd Street
Omaha, NE 68198

Laurie Macleod, R.N.
Research Nurse
Advanced Surgical Institute
Center for Children at Medical City Dallas
7777 Forest Lane
Dallas, TX 75230

James F. Markowitz, M.D.
Associate Chief,
Division of Pediatric Gastroenterology and Nutrition
Associate Director,
The Center for Pediatric Ileitis and Colitis
Associate Professor of Pediatrics
North Shore University Hospital-Cornell University Medical College
300 Community Drive
Manahasset, NY 11030

Edward E. Mason, M.D., Ph.D., F.A.C.S.
Professor Emeritus
Department of Surgery
University of Iowa College of Medicine
University Hospitals and Clinics
Iowa City, IA 52242

Rose M. Mays, Ph.D., R.N.
Associate Professor
Indiana University School of Nursing
Section of Adolescent Medicine
James Whitcomb Riley Hospital for
  Children
702 Barnill Drive
Indianapolis, IN 46202

Barbara McCarty, R.D.
Director of Lifestyle Management
51 Osborne Avenue
New Haven, CT 06511

Laurel Mellin, M.A., R.D.
Associate Professor of Pediatrics,
  Family and Community Medicine
University of California, San
  Francisco School of Medicine
400 Parnassus Avenue, Box 900
San Francisco, CA 94143
Director,
Child and Adolescent Obesity Clinic
Founder, SHAPEDOWN Program

Carol N. Meredith, Ph.D.
Adjunct Assistant Professor
Division of Clinical Nutrition
School of Medicine
University of California - Davis
Davis, CA 95616

Polly Nelson, R. D.
Pediatric Renal Dietitian
University of California at Los
  Angeles Medical Center
10833 LaConte
Los Angeles, CA 90095

Donald P. Orr, M.D.
Professor of Pediatrics
Indiana University School of
  Medicine
Director,
Section of Adolescent Medicine

James Whitcomb Riley Hospital for
  Children
702 Barnill Drive
Indianapolis, IN 46202

Susan Porter-Levy, Psy.D.
Pediatric Psychologist
Advanced Surgical Institute
Center for Children at Medical City
  Dallas
7777 Forest Lane
Dallas, TX 75230
Adjunct Professor
University of North Texas

Heidi Puelzl-Quinn, M.S., R.D.
Director of Nutrition
Developmental Evaluation Center
Children's Hospital
300 Longwood
Boston, MA 02115

Vaughn I. Rickert, Psy.D.,
  F.S.A.M.
Associate Professor of Obstetrics and
  Gynecology
Division of Pediatric and Adolescent
  Gynecology
University of Texas Medical Branch
  at Galveston
301 University Boulevard
Galveston, TX 77555-0587

Cheryl L. Rock, Ph.D., R.D.
Assistant Professor
Program in Human Nutrition
School of Public Health
The University of Michigan
1420 Washington Heights
Room M5539, SPHII
Ann Arbor, MI 48109-2029

Ellen Rome, M.D., M.P.H.,
Head,
Section of Adolescent Medicine
Division of Pediatrics and Adolescent
   Medicine
Cleveland Clinic Foundation
9500 Euclid Avenue
Cleveland, OH 44195
Clinical Instructor,
Case Western Reserve University
   School of Medicine
Clinical Assistant Professor,
College of Medicine
Pennsylvania State University

Janet Schebendach, M.A., R.D.
Nutritionist
Division of Adolescent Medicine
Center for Atherosclerosis Prevention
Schneider Children's Hospital
Long Island Jewish Medical Center
The Long Island Campus for the
   Albert Einstein College of
   Medicine
New Hyde Park, NY 11042

Kathleen Selvaggi-Fadden, M.D.
Neurodevelopmental Pediatrician
Center for Human Development
Morristown Memorial Hospital
100 Madison
Morristown, NJ 07960
Assistant Clinical Professor of
   Pediatrics
Columbia University
College of Physicians and Surgeons

Edwin Simpser, M.D.
Physician-in-Charge
Pediatric Nutrition Service
Associate Attending
   Gastroenterologist
Assistant Professor of Pediatrics

North Shore University Hospital-
Cornell University Medical College
300 Community Drive
Manahasset, NY 11030

Bonnie Spear, M.S., R.D.
Assistant Professor of Pediatrics
Registered Dietitian
Division of Adolescent Medicine
University of Alabama, Birmingham
1600 Seventh Avenue South
Birmingham, AL 35233

Suzanne Nelson Steen, D.Sc., R.D.
Clinical Director,
Weight and Eating Disorders
   Program
Department of Psychiatry
The University of Pennsylvania
   School of Medicine
3600 Market Street, Suite 744
Philadelphia, PA 19104

Catherine Stevens-Simon, M.D.
Assistant Professor of Pediatrics
Division of Adolescent Medicine
University of Colorado Health
   Science Center
The Children's Hospital
1056 East 19th Street, Box B-025
Denver, CO 80218

Jean Stover, R. D.
Renal Dietitian
Outpatient Dialysis Unit
University of Pennsylvania Medical
   Center
4126 Walnut Street
Philadelphia, PA 19104

Cameron K. Tebbi, M.D.
Medical Director,
Division of Pediatric Hematology/
  Oncology
St. Joseph's Children's Hospital
3001 W. Dr. Martin Luther King Jr.
  Blvd.
P.O. Box 4227
Tampa, FL 33677-4227

J. Kevin Thompson, Ph.D.
Associate Professor
Department of Psychology BEH 339
University of South Florida
Tampa, FL 33620

Carleen Townsend-Akpan, M.S.N.,
  C.P.N.P., R.N.C.
Department of Adolescent and Young
  Adult Medicine
Children's National Medical Center
111 Michigan Avenue, N.W.
Washington, DC 20010

Isabel M. Vazquez, M.S., R.D.
Nutritionist,
MCHB Health Training Program
Division of Adolescent and Young
  Adult Medicine

Children's Hospital
300 Longwood Avenue
Boston, MA 02115

Georgia A. Walter, R.D.
Clinical Dietitian
University of Nebraska Medical
  Center
600 South 42nd Street
Omaha, NE 68198

Elizabeth R. Woods, M.D., M.P.H.
Director of Research,
Division of Adolescent and Young
  Adult Medicine
Associate in Medicine
Children's Hospital
300 Longwood Avenue
Boston, MA 02115
Assistant Professor of Pediatrics
Harvard Medical School

Katherine C. Wood, M.A.
Doctoral Candidate
Department of Psychology BEH 339
University of South Florida
Tampa, FL 33620

GENERAL ISSUES IN ADOLESCENT NUTRITION

Adolescent Growth and Development

Bonnie Spear, M.S., R.D.

INTRODUCTION

Adolescence is a time of dramatic change in the life of every human being. The relatively uniform growth of childhood is suddenly altered by an increase in the velocity of growth. This sudden spurt is also associated with hormonal, cognitive, and emotional changes. All these changes create special nutritional needs. Adolescence is considered an especially nutritionally vulnerable period of life for several reasons. First, there is a greater demand for nutrients and calories due to the dramatic increase in physical growth and development over a relatively brief period of time. Second is the change of lifestyle and food habits of adolescents that affect both nutrient intake and needs. Third are those adolescents with special nutrient needs such as those who participate in sports, become pregnant, diet excessively, or alcohol and drugs.

ASSESSMENT

Growth and Development

Adolescence is the only time following birth when the rate of growth actually increases.[1] Enormous variability exists in the timing of this change. Adolescents

3

of a given chronological age usually vary in their physiological development, and because of this variability among individuals, age is often a poor indicator of physiological maturity and nutritional needs.[2]

Adolescents of the same age often differ markedly in size and it is impossible to use age alone in evaluating pubertal growth status. An assessment of the degree of maturation of secondary sexual characteristics is useful to evaluate physical growth and in detecting certain diseases and disorders associated with adolescence. Sexual maturity ratings (SMR), often called Tanner stages,[2] are widely used to evaluate growth and developmental age during adolescence. These stages of growth correlate highly with other pubertal events.[2-7]

Sexual maturity ratings are based on the development of secondary sex characteristics and assigned on a scale of 1 (prepubertal) to 5 (adult). For males, this scale is based on the progression of genital and pubic hair development, and for females, it is based on the development of breast and pubic hair. Table 1.1 gives a description of each stage of development for boys and girls. Separate ratings should be established for each characteristic because variations in the stage of

Table 1.1   Sexual Maturity Ratings (SMR)

	BOYS		
SMR	Pubic Hair	Penis	Testes
1	None	Preadolescent	Preadolescent
2	Scanty, long, slightly pigmented	Slight enlargement	Enlarged scrotum, pink, texture altered
3	Darker, starts to curl	Penis longer	Larger
4	Resembles adult type, but less in quantity; coarse, curly	Larger, glans and breath increase in size	Larger, scrotum dark
5	Adult distribution, spread to medial surface of thighs	Adult	Adult

	GIRLS	
SMR	Pubic Hair	Breasts
1	Preadolescent	Preadolescent
2	Sparse, lightly pigmented, straight, medial border of labia	Breasts and papillae elevated as small mounds; areolar diameter increased
3	Darker, beginning to curl, increased amount	Breasts and areolae enlarged
4	Coarse, curly, abundant, but amount less than in adult	Areolae and papillae form secondary mounds
5	Adult feminine triangle spread to medial surface of thighs	Mature; nipple projects areolae part of general breast contour

Adapted from W. A. Daniel Jr., in *Adolescents in Health and Disease*, Mosby, St. Louis, MO, p. 22 (1977). Reprinted with permission.

maturity of each characteristic are not uncommon. Furthermore, although a mean value of the two ratings can be used as an approximate indicator of maturity many physical changes that occur during puberty have greater correlation with one of the individual ratings than with a mean value.[8,9]

Uses of Sexual Maturity Ratings

SMR 1, for all practical purposes, is an indicator of prepubertal development, in both males and females, whereas an SMR of 2 is assigned at the earliest visible signs of puberty. A SMR of 5 is generally considered to be evidence of adult growth, although height may continue to increase and other physical changes may occur after this rating has been made. Although great variability in growth is seen at any given chronological age, growth does proceed in a predictable sequential pattern, with only minor variations. This is illustrated in Figures 1.1 and 1.2. In girls, the first signs of pubertal change is the development of breast bud. If this has not appeared by age 13, puberty is considered to be delayed, although this is likely to represent a normal variant rather than an endocrine abnormality. Peak height velocity, the period of most rapid linear growth in girls, occurs after pubic hair development reaches SMR 2, and the menarche most often occurs after pubic hair and breast development reach SMR 4. Females manifest variability in age at onset and time required for completion of each stage of development. The first event to be noticed is breast budding at an average age of 10.6 yr, with an age range of 9–13 yr. Pubic hair usually develops later, but in one-third of all girls, pubic hair appears before breast development. The average time elapsed from breast budding to breast stage 3 is 1 yr. Average time elapsed before reaching adult breast development is 4 yr.[10] The average number of years from breast budding to menarche is 2.5 years (range 1.5–4 yr).

In boys, the first sign of puberty is enlargement of the testes, but sometimes this is difficult to evaluate. If minimal enlargement of the genitals has not occurred by age 14½, puberty is considered to be delayed, but is likely to be of constitutional etiology. Peak height velocity in boys occurs after pubic hair development reaches SMR 3; often, genital development has reached SMR 4. Individual differences also occur in the rapidity with which an individual completes a sequence once it has started. Average boys have 1 yr between genitalia stage 2 and genitalia stage 3 and 3 yr between genitalia stage 2 and genital stage 5, but others may progress from genitalia stage 2 to 5 in 2 yr.[10]

Height Attainment

During the pubertal process, teenagers attain approximately 15% of their final adult height and about 45% of the maximal skeletal mass.[1,11] Compared to girls, boys have a longer period of childhood growth before the adolescent growth

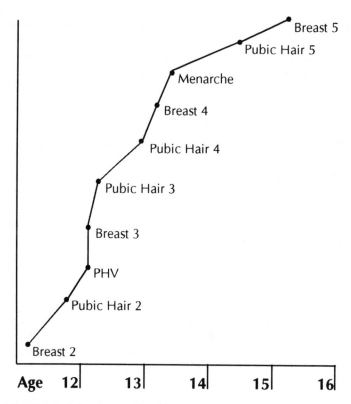

Figure 1-1.   Pubertal development in girls

A. W. Root, *J. Peds.*, 83, 1 (1973). Reprinted with permission.

spurt[5] and a higher peak velocity[3] (or maximum speed) in height growth, resulting in an average final height difference between males and females of 5 or more inches.[7,12] Using longitudinal data, Roche and Davila[13] reported that increases in height between menarche and adulthood were 1.7 in., 2.9 in., and 4.2 in. at the 10th, 50th, and 90th percentiles, respectively, with stature growth ceasing at a median of 4.8 yr after the onset of menarche. In females, growth in stature ceased at a median age of 17.3 yr and, in males, at a median age of 21.2 yr; however, there was great variability. The total increment in height achieved after menarche varied inversely with age of menarche. Girls who had early menses grew much more after menarche and for a longer period than girls with later menarche.

Weight Gain and Body Composition Changes

The rate of weight gain during adolescence parallels that of the height spurt. In males, peak height velocity coincides with peak weight velocity. In contrast,

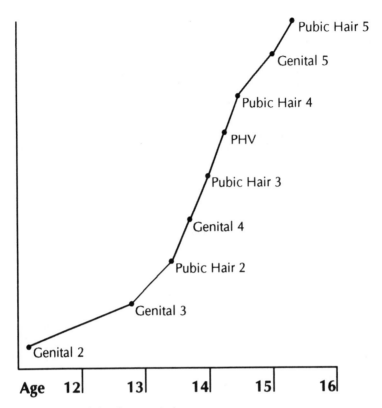

Figure 1-2.   Pubertal development in boys

A. W. Root, *J. Peds.*, 83, 1 (1973). Reprinted with permission.

peak weight velocity in females occurs 6–9 mo prior to height rate changes.[6] Weight gain during this period accounts for approximately 50% of the ideal adult weight.[1,11]

For both males and females, elevated androgen levels have a growth-promoting effect. However, the female sex hormones, estrogen and progesterone, promote the deposition of proportionately more fat than muscle tissue in girls.[3,5–7,14] Under the influence of testosterone, the anabolic androgens, boys gain proportionately more muscle mass than fat, experience increased linear growth to produce a heavier skeleton, and develop greater red blood cell mass than girls. Males have more lean body mass per unit height than females during pubescence.[15] Lean body mass significantly increases in boys, with muscle mass doubling between the ages of 10 and 17 yr of age.[16]

These changes in body composition have important implications for the nutritional needs of teenagers, particularly with regard to energy, iron, and protein for tissue synthesis. For example, increases in lean body mass increase iron requirement. Due to body composition differences, Hepner[17] reported that adolescent males who are at the 50th percentile for weight would require 19.1 mg of iron/lb weight gained, compared to 14.1 mg iron/lb weight gained for females at the 50th percentile for weight. Although blood volume, red blood cell counts, and hemoglobin levels increase in adolescent males throughout puberty, they remain fairly constant in females.[3,6,7] These measures affect the differential changes in body composition and nutrition requirement of males vs. females. Garn et al.[18] have shown that African Americans have approximately 1/100mL less hemoglobin than whites, which appears related to genetic not environmental factors.

Daniel[19] studied the association between hematocrit and physiological age and found that hematocrit values in males increased with increasing sexual maturity ratings and with advanced chronological age, although physiological age showed higher correlations. Little differences in hematocrits were reported for females, based on Tanner stages of development.

Genetic and Environmental Factors

Genetic and environmental factors interact in a complex system to affect growth and maturation during adolescence. There is a strong genetic component in the determination of height, weight, body shape, breast size, and rate of growth. Under stable environmental circumstances, genetic factors exert a major influence on puberty and growth.[3,14]

Growth and maturation have also exhibited secular trends. Successive generations in developed countries have generally been taller and attained puberty at progressively younger ages. For example, the average age of menarche decreased from 14 to 12.9 yr between 1900 and 1960. With no significant change in recent years, these trends are probably due to better nutrition and improved health.[3,6,14]

In addition to nutrition, the most important environmental factors affecting the onset of menarche include socioeconomic status, disease, and illness. Teenagers who are members of families that have a high socioeconomic status are taller than teens in families that have a low socioeconomic status.[1,20] The growth spurt occurs earlier and is often more marked among adolescents in developed countries. These differences are probably due, in large part to nutrition, health care, and related advantages of high socioeconomic status.[3,14]

Chronic disease affects 10–20% of youth from birth to 20 yr[21] and may contribute to growth retardation and delayed sexual maturation in children and adolescents.[3,14] In addition, chronic illness can significantly affect psychosocial development.[21] The impact on growth will depend on the nature, severity, age (chronological and physiologic) of onset, and duration of the disease or illness.[3,14]

Nutritional Requirements

Little specific experimental data exist on which to base the nutrient needs of adolescents. The Recommended Dietary Allowances (RDAs) for energy are based on the median energy intakes of adolescents followed in longitudinal growth studies.[22] The RDAs for protein in this group are calculated from growth rate and body composition data, if we assume protein utilization for growth is comparable with maintenance data among adults. Other nutrient recommendations are based on animal studies or adult or child allowances, with an allowance for adolescent growth. As noted earlier, because of wide variability in growth rates, physical activity, metabolic rates, physiological states, and adaptability, it is difficult to estimate specific nutrient requirements for adolescents. In addition, human studies involving youth are costly and permission to use them as subjects is often difficult to attain.

For practical reasons, the RDAs[22] for adolescents are categorized by chronological rather than maturational development. Thus, practitioners should use them with caution, particularly for individual assessments. For groups of teenagers, the RDAs can be used as general guidelines in evaluating the probability of populations at risk of consuming inadequate diets. It is important to remember that when comparing an individual's intake to the RDA, a safety factor is included. Thus, individual intakes below the RDA do not automatically mean that the intakes are deficient or the individual is not meeting their needs. An adolescent's nutritional status must be assessed on an individual basis, using information from clinical, biochemical, anthropometric, dietary, and psychosocial assessments.[23]

Energy.   The recommended dietary allowances for energy for teenagers of various chronological ages and for each sex are shown in Table 1.2. In contrast with other nutrients, the RDAs for energy *do not* include a safety factor for increased energy needs due to illness, trauma, or stress and should be considered to be only average needs. Actual needs for adolescents will vary with physical activity and stage of maturation.

Few studies have investigated the relationship between growth and calorie intake. Heald et al.[24] compiled data from previous studies of 2750 females and 2200 males between the ages of 7 and 20 yr. On average, males tended to increase their calorie intake steadily to approximately 3470 kcal/d at age 16 yr. From 16 to 19 yr the intake decreased to approximately 2900 kcal/d. In females, the rise in calories increase to age 12 with a peak calorie level of 2550/d, followed by a decline in calories to 18 yr with intakes averaging 2200 kcals/d. Calorie intake of girls at three different stages of development (prepubescent, rapidly growing, and postpubescent) was found by Wait et al.[25] to be related to stage of physiological development, not chronological age. These findings were confirmed by Daniel[26] who demonstrated that the highest caloric intakes occurred during the growth spurt (peak height velocity). Hampton et al.[27] reported the

Table 1.2   Recommend Energy and Protein Intakes

Age (yr)	Energy (kcal)		Protein	
	RDA (median)	kcal/cm (median)	RDA	g/cm
CHILDREN				
7–10	2000	15.2	28	0.21
MALES				
11–15	2500	15.9	45	0.29
15–18	3000	17.1	59	0.34
19–22	2900	16.4	58	0.33
FEMALES				
11–14	2200	14.0	46	0.29
15–18	2200	13.5	44	0.27
19–22	2200	13.4	46	0.28

Adapted from Food and Nutrition Board, National Academy of Science National Research Council, *Recommended Dietary Allowances*, 10th ed, Washington, DC, (1989).

great variations in daily caloric intake, but found more consistency from week to week. Wait et al[25] data support the thesis of calories per unit height as the best index in determining calorie needs. Wait and other researchers[1,28] suggest the use of kcal/cm as a rough predictor of energy needs. An estimated range for females 11–18 yr of age is 10–19 kcal/cm and for males 11–18 yr of age is 13 to 23 kcal/cm. Table 1.2 gives kcal/cm based on RDAs.

Protein.   During adolescence, protein needs like those for energy correlate more closely with the growth pattern than chronological age. Using the RDA for protein in relation to height is the most useful method of estimating need. The daily protein recommendations for adolescents are approximately 0.3 g/cm height, ranging from 0.29–0.32 g/cm height for males and 0.27–0.29 g/cm height for females.[1] Average intakes of protein are well above the RDAs for any age group. There is little evidence to show that insufficient protein intakes occur in the adolescent population. However, if energy intakes become insufficient for any reason (i.e., economic problems, chronic illness, or attempts to lose weight), dietary protein may be used to meet energy needs, but will be unavailable for new tissue synthesis or tissue repair. Thus, a reduction of growth rate and decrease in lean body mass may occur despite an apparent adequate protein intake. The current dieting patterns of adolescent females that result in restricted calorie intakes represent potential health problems when protein sources are used to meet energy needs. Protein metabolism is particularly sensitive to caloric restriction among adolescents during their growth spurt.[1]

Minerals. During adolescence, all mineral needs increase. Dietary surveys have consistently shown that calcium and iron are marginal in adolescents' diets.[29-33] These low intakes are often due to the popular food choices of adolescents, including convenience and fast foods[34-39] and sugar-containing snacks.[36,37]

Calcium. Due to accelerated muscular, skeletal, and endocrine development, calcium needs are greater during puberty and adolescence than in childhood or during the adult years. At the peak of the growth spurt, the daily deposition of calcium can be twice the average rates that occur during the other stages of adolescent development.[15]

The RDA for calcium increases from 800 mg during preadolescence to 1200 mg during adolescence.[22] The RDA is intended to cover the needs for the most rapidly growing adolescents, based on evidence that high bone mass achieved during adolescence and young adulthood decreases the risk of osteoporosis in old age.[38] Matkovic et al.[39] demonstrated that an average intake of 1500 mg was needed to attain maximal calcium retention in 14-year-old females. Based on retrospective data on college-age women, Anderson et al.[40] found that women with calcium intakes of less than 900 mg/d from milk products had lower bone mineral content and bone densities than women with calcium intakes greater than 900 mg/d. These data suggest that approximately 900 mg of calcium from milk products may be sufficient to promote optimal bone density in adult females. Data from Sandler et al.[41] also indicated that higher intakes of dairy products are associated with greater bone density. Women who reportedly consumed milk with each meal during childhood and adolescence have greater bone densities than those who reportedly drank less milk. More recently, Chan[42] found that among 164 children 2–16 yr of age, 70% of those less than 11 yr of age were at least consuming the recommended dietary allowance for calcium (800 mg/d). However, among adolescents, only 37% were consuming the recommended dietary allowances for calcium (1200 mg/d). These researchers did not find differences in bone mineral status between boys and girls when controlling for weight. Although intakes of calcium, phosphate, vitamin D, protein, and copper are important nutrients in bone mineralization, these data found dietary calcium intake responsible for the differences in bone mineral status among these children. Children ingesting more than 1000 mg of calcium daily had higher bone mineral content than those ingesting less. Leil et al.[43] studied the effects of race and body habitus on bone mineral density. He found that African Americans have a lower intake of dairy products and frequently consume less calcium. However, their genetically determined large bone and muscle mass makes them less susceptible to osteoporosis. Lloyd et al.[44] studied 94 girls with a mean age of 11.5 yr. All subjects averaged 960 mg/d dietary intake of calcium. Half received a calcium supplement of 354 mg/d of calcium citrate malate; the others received a placebo. Increasing daily calcium intakes from 80–110% of the RDA via supplementation resulted in significant increases in total body and spinal bond density in adolescent girls. The increase of 24 g of bone gain/yr among the supplemented group translates to an additional 1.3% of skeletal mass/yr during adolescent growth, which may provide protection against future osteoporotic fracture.

Surveys show that adolescent males are more likely than females to have adequate calcium intakes.[29,30] Thus, compared to males, teenager girls are at a greater risk of poor calcium status during this growth period. There is evidence to suggest that high soft drink consumption contributes to low calcium intake because adolescents may be substituting soft drinks for milk.[37]

Calcium metabolism is affected by protein and phosphorus intake. High protein intakes increase the urinary excretion of calcium.[45] A low calcium to phosphorus (Ca:P) ratio may have a negative effect on bone mineralization, as has been shown in adult women.[45–47] Pronounced bone loss in animals has been observed with excess phosphorus or insufficient calcium intakes.[45] Teenagers may have low Ca:P ratios, but additional research is needed to determine the effect of decreased intakes of milk in combination with increased intakes of soft drinks and processed foods high in phosphorus.[35] Although most adolescents have protein intakes that exceed the recommended allowance and may have low Ca:P ratios, it is unclear whether high protein and/or phosphorus intakes cause bone loss in adolescents.

Iron.   During adolescence, iron requirements are increased. Dallman[48] notes that among boys there is a sharp increase in the requirements for absorbed iron from approximately 1.0–2.5 mg/d. This increase reflects an expanding blood volume and rises in hemoglobin concentration that occur with sexual maturation in males. After the growth spurt and sexual maturation, there is a rapid decrease in growth and the need for iron. Consequently, there is an opportunity to replete iron stores that might have been developed during peak growth. In females, the growth spurt is not as great, but menstruation typically starts about 1 yr after peak growth. The requirement for absorbed iron reaches a maximum of approximately 1.5 mg/d at peak growth, but returns to a mean of approximately 1.3 mg/d in order to replace menstrual iron losses.

The study of adolescent growth during pregnancy by Harrison et al.[49] suggested that iron is required for skeletal growth. Among girls with marginal iron intake or those with increased iron losses, iron-deficiency anemia may result from growth demands. Conversely, iron deficiency may be a limiting factor for growth during adolescence.

Anemia due to iron deficiency in adolescence may also impair the immune response. For example, a study of children and adolescents found that the cell-mediated immune response and bactericidal capacity of leukocytes (in vitro methods) were significantly depressed in those with hemoglobin concentrations below 100 g/L.[50]

Dietary surveys indicate that iron intakes among female adolescents with normal dietary patterns were 12.5–14.2 mg/d and between 13.6 and 18.0 mg/d for males.[51] It has been estimated that the American diet contains about 6 mg of iron/1000 kcal.[34] Thus, adolescent females who typically have lower caloric intakes than males may have more difficulty in obtaining adequate levels of iron from their diets.

An important consideration in examining dietary iron is bioavailability. Viglietti and Skinner[52] found that the mean available dietary iron of adolescents was below the recommended levels. In fact, the calculated bioavailability of dietary iron was less than the 10% recommended in the RDA.[22] Higher levels of available iron were associated with high intakes of calories, animal foods, and ascorbic acid.

By using a ferritin model to assess the prevalence of impaired iron status in the Health and Nutrition Examination Survey II (NHANES II), the highest abnormal values were found among teenagers. Iron deficiency was found in 14.2% of the 15–18-year-old females and 12.1% of the 11–14-year-old males.[53] Iron deficiency is prevalent in adolescents of both gender and among teens of all races and socioeconomic levels.[29,54–55]

Teenage athletes may be at risk of iron deficiency due to the combination of red blood cell destruction, the increased need for red blood cell and tissue syntheses during the course of normal development, and poor dietary habits.[1,56] Furthermore, adolescent athletes may be particularly vulnerable to sports anemia. Sports anemia is defined as a condition of increased destruction of erythrocytes and a transient drop in hemoglobin as a result of an acute stress response to exercise and training.[51]

Zinc. Essential for healthy growth and sexual maturation in adolescents. There are no controlled studies on the adolescent requirements for zinc,[58] but growth retardation and hypogonadism in adolescents males with zinc deficiency have been reported.[57–59]

Thompson et al.[60] found that plasma zinc levels declined during pubertal development. This decline may reflect an increased zinc need during growth or a redistribution of plasma zinc due to hormonal changes. In contrast, Wagner et al.[61] found that males and females at Tanner stage 5 have higher serum zinc levels than those who are less mature. Another study suggested that low plasma zinc levels were found during the ages puberty was expected to occur.[62] However, these changes in zinc levels during puberty may reflect normal physiological changes during adolescence. Lower zinc levels could indicate adolescents are at risk of compromised zinc status due to increased needs for growth.[60-63]

In a study of the zinc and copper nutritional status of 59 adolescent females, the dietary zinc requirement was significantly related to the height of subjects. No correlation was found between dietary intakes of zinc and copper and the plasma levels of those nutrients. The authors concluded that because plasma levels were influenced by total meal composition and daily mineral intake variations, no direct relationship could be expected.[64] Others[65] studied the possible relationship of erythrocyte zinc to dietary zinc, physical maturity, and chronological age. They found no direct relationship between erythrocyte zinc and calculated zinc intakes.

Until future research enables us to make more precise recommendations for all vitamins and minerals, the consumption of a varied diet remains the best assurance of adequate and safe intakes.

Vitamins.   The need for vitamins is increased during adolescence even above that required during infancy and childhood. Due to the increased energy demands in adolescence, thiamin, riboflavin, and niacin are required in increased quantities for the release of energy from carbohydrates. With greater tissue synthesis, there is a heightened demand for vitamin B–6, folic acid, and vitamin B-12, which are required for normal DNA and RNA synthesis. There are also increased requirements for vitamin D (for rapid skeletal growth), and vitamins A, C, and E are needed for preservation of the structural and functional properties of new cells. Few satisfactory data are available to establish an adolescent-specific vitamin requirements. Thus, most of the RDAs have been extrapolated from other age groups. As with other nutrients, vitamin needs are most associated with the degree of maturity rather than chronologic age, due to the demands of growth.[66]

There are few reports of low serum vitamin C levels in teens.[34,67] However, vitamin C intake may be low among adolescents who habitually avoid fruits and vegetables and those who smoke cigarettes.[68] Also at risk may be teens who are dieting and poor adolescents.[67]

Inadequate folate status is relatively common among adolescents.[60-71] Survey findings found that 10 and 50% of adolescents had low serum folacin levels.[72] In Daniel et al.'s study,[73] 4.7% of the girls and 9.4% of the boys had below-normal plasma levels for folacin. Adolescents from low-income groups[69,73] and pregnant teens[74] may be most vulnerable with respect to poor folic acid status.

The Ten-State Nutrition Survey,[75] done in the late 1960s, demonstrated that vitamin A intakes in adolescents were often below recommended levels. Along with decreased intake, there were declines in the biochemical assessments, with 40% of Spanish American teenagers and 10% of African American and white teenagers having low plasma levels of vitamin A. Vahlquist et al.[76] found low retinol-binding protein (RBP) concentrations in children, even among well-nourished populations. A study of vitamin A in children[77] suggests that low RBP concentrations reflect low vitamin A consumption before puberty. Other data, largely in experimental animals, indicate that vitamin A is an essential nutrient for fertility and reproductive success.[78] Severe vitamin A deficiency is associated with sterility and amenorrhea, and in mild deficiency, fetal growth may be affected. The effect of vitamin A on the menstrual cycle in humans indicates the possible interactions of cyclic variation of vitamin A on reproductive health and fertility. There is, at present, no information to indicate what amount of vitamin A is required during adolescence for optimal sexual reproductive development.[78] In addition, studies by Brabin and Brabin[78] indicate that menstrual irregularities may be more frequent in women with low vitamin A stores or low serum RBP.

Factors Influencing Adolescent Nutrition Status and Eating Behavior

Adolescents are not only maturing physically, but also cognitively and psychosocially. They search for identity, strive for independence and acceptance and they are concerned about appearance. All these changes may greatly affect eating. Skipping meals, between-meal snacking, eating away from home—especially at franchised food stores—and following alternate dietary patterns, such as vegetarianism and dietary fads, characterize the food habits of adolescents. These habits are further influenced by family, peers, and the media.

Irregular meals.   Meal skipping and irregular eating patterns are common during adolescence. Breakfast and lunch appear to be the most frequently missed meals, but social activities and school programs may cause a teenager to miss an evening meal as well. Daniel[79] found that as many as 50% of adolescent boys and girls reported not eating breakfast. Although other studies[80] have shown 89% of surveyed adolescents believed breakfast was extremely important, only 60% ate it on a regular basis. Breakfast skipping appears more frequent among older adolescents. Not eating breakfast has been associated with a less than satisfactory consumption of nutrients.[81] This problem is especially important with females who tend to skip more meals than males.

Snacking.   A definite part of adolescents' food behavior. Between-meal snacking is often thought to be harmful because it reduces one's appetite for regular meals. In contrast, several studies have shown that snacks eaten by teenagers were not just empty calories, but did provide substantial proportions of recommended caloric intake as well as protein, riboflavin, and ascorbic acid.[2,82] Snacks are usually low in fiber, vitamin A, calcium, and iron. Snacking can have a positive effect on teenagers' nutrient intake, but adolescents must be taught to select appropriate snack foods.

Fast foods and the media.   The use of fast foods for meals or snacks is especially popular with busy adolescents. Through vending machines, self-service restaurants, convenience groceries, and franchised food restaurants, food is available almost 24 h/day. These fast foods tend to be low in iron, calcium, riboflavin, and vitamin A, and there are few sources of folic acid. Vitamin C is low unless French fries or fruit juice are consumed. Nearly all fast-foods are high in total and saturated fat, cholesterol, and sodium.[83] Most items from fastfood restaurants provide more than 50% of calories as fat, although menus are gradually offering a healthier choice of foods.

Television and magazines probably have more influence than any other form of mass media on adolescents' eating habits. It is estimated that by the time he or she reaches the teen years, the average teenager has viewed 100,000 food commercials, the majority being for products with high concentrations of fat and simple carbohydrates.[35] Kaufman[84] analyzed food-related messages on the 10 top ranked prime time television programs. Results showed 65% of food references promoted beverages (primarily alcohol) and sweets. The overall analyses of the program characters' food habits were (1) they frequently snacked on foods of low-nutrient density; (2) they ate hurriedly and while active; (3) they rarely ate balanced meals; and (4) food consumption was primarily used to meet emotional and/or social needs.

ASSESSMENT

Dietary Assessment

The assessment of diets among children of various ages is still a poorly developed area and requires attention, as accumulating evidence suggests that the origin of many diseases is in childhood.[85] Also, the development and evaluation of questionnaires for various ethnic groups require attention.[85]

When collecting dietary data on children, confidence about their responses is required. Children exist in multienvironments in their everyday lives (e.g., home, school, peers, media). These macroenvironments influence the format and type of data collection methods used to interview today's youth. Interviewers need to identify the influence of each environment on the child's eating patterns.[86] Age and respondent capability are important reasons for designing dietary interview methods. There is a fairly rapid increase in the capability of children to respond to eating behavior inquiries by 7–8 yr of age. By 10–12 yr of age, children can serve as their own respondents. Children 8–12 yr of age are often called on to respond to 24-h recalls, keep multiple-day food records, and asked frequency questions about how often they eat specific foods. The consensus of research is that students can accurately describe the foods they eat by using recall and record techniques, if proper probes and adequate instruction are provided.[86,87]

There are many methods for assessing dietary intakes but the two most commonly used are food frequency questionnaires (FFQ) and dietary recalls. The FFQ has advantages and limitations. It is easy and typically requires 15–30 min to complete. Thus, it is less expensive that dietary recall due to minimal use of the dietitian's time. Unfortunately, food listings are fixed on the FFQ and individuals with unusual or different diets would be unable to accurately describe their eating habits. In addition, because FFQs are highly structured and specific, those that elicit appropriate dietary information in one population may not be useful in a population with substantially different cultural or ethnic food habits. Numerous researchers have used the FFQs in individual nutrient analysis. When comparing FFQ data to dietary recall data, they found reliable results.[88–90]

The dietary recall is used by most nutritionists as a means of assessing nutrient intake. The dietary recall obtains accurate data on recent intakes. It also has the advantage of obtaining more precise portion sizes and food preparation techniques. However, an adequately completed diet recall usually takes between 20–40 min.

School-aged children present a unique population for dietary measurement. There are only limited studies reporting methodologies used to capture nutrient intake and/or food pattern in the preschool, school-aged, and teenage populations,[91–93] and reports have described some of the problems in the area.[94,95]

In clinical practice, a typical 24-h recall can be sufficient in eliciting dietary information for dietary instruction. This should be based on time of day rather than breakfast, lunch, or dinner. Since adolescents tend to eat throughout the day, targeting a meal-based assessment would likely miss a large portion of the food eaten on a daily basis. In addition, a short frequency list targeting high-risk foods for adolescents would be important to complete the assessment. For example, asking about high sodium foods (chips, luncheon meats, etc.), calcium sources (milk, cheese, yogurt, etc.), empty calorie foods (sodas, candy, cookies, etc.) would help to determine the accuracy of the 24-h recall. The majority of adolescents drink up to 50% of their calories, so a detailed history of beverage consumption would also be helpful.

Cultural and Ethnic Differences

Assessing food intake and communicating nutrition education messages to multicultural adolescents can be challenging. This is magnified by the rapid changes in the racial and ethnic composition of the U.S. population.

Specific foods mean different things in different cultures, but most cultural groups use food for similar purposes. People from virtually all cultures use food during celebrations. Many cultural groups use foods as medicine or to promote health. Nutrition educators must recognize the strong preferences that people have for the foods they eat and their special uses of food. A newly published book, *Celebrating Diversity: Approaching Families Through Their Food,*[96] is an excellent resource for nutrition professionals working with a culturally diverse population.

Communication is enhanced when nutrition education focuses on the individual's background and present situations without making assumptions. To be an effective counselor, one must learn to work within other values systems than their own. For example, adolescents of different cultural backgrounds may have differences in family structure, values, and interaction styles. Understanding these beliefs and backgrounds of the adolescent is essential to providing nutrition education and counseling that will be beneficial to the adolescent.

MANAGEMENT

Strategies for nutrition intervention may include education to improve a specific nutritional problem (i.e., high iron diet for anemia), improving food sources (i.e., increasing calcium), counseling, behavior modification to improve eating habits, or referral to other sources. Adolescents generally have many questions about their health and nutrition. Their questions should be answered in a direct and straightforward manner. They do not want to be treated as a child, lectured to, or ridiculed.

In a counseling sessions with adolescents, the nutritionist should listen attentively to their problems. They are very real to them and this information requires validation. Inform the adolescent of their nutritional needs and illustrate how well or poorly these needs are being met. Include the teen as an active participant in these sessions, i.e., work with adolescents to make changes they feel competent in making. Moreover, adolescents need to be taught that they have responsibility for their own health and nutrition status. Nutrition education/counseling should provide adolescents with the skills necessary for making appropriate changes and choices.

CASE ILLUSTRATION

Susan is a 13-year-old Caucasian female brought to the clinic by her mother. Mother states she is concerned because Susan has been complaining of being tired and having afternoon headaches. Susan states she has gained over 10 lb in the past year and wants to lose weight. Susan's height was 63 in. (75% percentile), weight 115 lb (75% percentile). Susan had grown 1½ in. over the last year and gained 10 lb. Menarche occurred at 12.5 yr (6 mo ago). Diet history revealed approximately 1500 kcal/d which consisted of 40 gm of protein and 80 gm of fat. Susan reported eating one meal and two snacks per day, usually skipping breakfast and lunch in attempts to lose weight. Susan was also not eating meat, thinking this was the way to lose weight. Snacks were unwisely chosen and often high in fat. Biochemical assessment found mild anemia, but other values were within normal limits.

Susan had realized weight gain, but did not appreciate her gain in height. In attempts to lose weight, she had reduced her protein intake below levels needed for continued growth and tissue repair and had increased her fat above the recommended 30% of calories. Her headaches may be attributed to the constant skipping of breakfast and lunch. The mild anemia is secondary to the low intakes of meat and low protein, as well as the beginning of menses.

The treatment plan for Susan included both education (normal growth and development) and food selection in addition to related counseling. Susan was instructed how to determine her appropriate weight for height and given basic information about growth and developmental parameters in adolescence. In order

Table 1.3 Iron Sources

Food	Iron (mg)
Heme sources (3-oz serving)	
Calves liver	5.3
Sirloin	2.9
Ground beef, lean	1.9
Pork tenderloin	1.3
Chicken, light meat	0.9
Chicken, dark meat	1.5
Tuna, light	2.7
Oysters (6)	5.6
Non heme sources	
Peanut butter (1 tbsp)	0.7
Legumes (½ cup)	1.3–3.0
Cooked cereal (½ cup)	0.7–1.3
Ready-to-eat cereal (¾ cup)	0.3–9.0
Whole wheat bread, (1 slice) enriched	0.6–0.8
Nuts, most kinds (2 tbsp)	1.0

Adapted from National Livestock and Meat Board, *Iron in Human Nutrition*, Chicago, Il, (1990). Reprinted with permission.

to improve the balance of her diet, carefully phrased information regarding her protein and fat selections were provided by the nutritionist. She was instructed on various food choices, as well as those designed to increase iron levels (see Table 1.3).

REFERENCES

1. E. J. Gong and F. P. Heald, in *Modern Nutrition in Health and Disease*, (M. E. Shils and V. R. Young, eds.), Lea & Febiger, PA, pp. 969–981 (1988).

2. J. M. Tanner, *J. Adol. Health Care*, **8**, 470 (1987).

3. H. Katchadourain, in *The Biology of Adolescence*, W. H. Freeman, San Francisco, CA, pp. 22–120 (1977).

4. J.T.Y. Shen, in *The Clinical Practice of Adolescent Medicine*, (J.T.Y. Shen, ed.), Appleton-Century-Crofts, NY, pp. 2–19 (1980).

5. L. S. Wright, in *Nutrition in Adolescence*, (L. K. Mahan and J. M. Rees, eds.), Times Mirror/Mosby, St. Louis, MO, pp. 1–20 (1984).

6. L. S. Neistein, in *Adolescent Health Care. A Practical Guide*, Urban & Schwarzenberg, Baltimore, MD, pp. 3–33 (1984).

7. G. B. Slap, *J. Adol. Health Care*, **7**, 13S (1986).

8. W. R. Harlin, G. P. Grillo, J. Comoni-Huntley, and P. E. Leavertson, *J. Peds.*, **95**, 293 (1979).

9. W. R. Harlin, E. A. Harlin, and G. P. Grillo, *J. Peds.*, **96**, 1074 (1980).

10. W. A. Daniel, in *Current Concepts*, Upjohn , Kalamazoo, MI, pp. 5–13 (1982).

11. S. M. Garn and B. Wagner, in *Adolescent Nutrition and Growth*, (F. P. Heald, ed.), Appleton-Century-Crofts, NY, pp. 139–161 (1969).

12. J. M. Tanner and P.S.W. Davies, *J. Peds.*, **101**, 317 (1985).

13. A. F. Roche and G. H. Davila, *Pediatrics*, **50**, 874 (1972).

14. D. Sinclair, in *Human Growth After Birth*, Oxford Univ. Press, Oxford, pp. 148–169 (1985).

15. G. B. Forbes, in *Textbook of Pediatric Nutrition*, (R. M. Suskind, ed.), Raven Press, NY, pp. 381–391 (1981).

16. D. B. Cheek, in *Control of the Onset of Puberty*, (M. M. Grumbach, G. D. Grave, and F. E. Mayer, eds.), John Wiley & Sons, NY, pp. 426–427 (1974).

17. R. Hepner, in *Nutrient Requirements in Adolescence*, (J. I. McKigney and H. N. Munro, eds.), The MIT Press, Cambridge, MA, pp. 87–91 (1976).

18. S. M. Garn, N. J. Smith and D. C. Clark, *Am. J. Clin. Nutr.*, **28**, 563 (1975).

19. W. A. Daniel, *Pediatrics*, **52**, 388 (1973).

20. J. R. Braisted, L. Mellin, E. J. Gong, C. E. Irwin, Jr., *J. Adol. Health Care*, **6**, 365, (1985).

21. D. M. Seigel, *JAMA*, **257**, 3396 (1987).

22. Food and Nutrition Board. National Research Council. *Recommended Dietary Allowances, X,* National Academy of Sciences, Washington, DC, (1989).

23. T. G. Jensen, D. M. Enlert, S. J. Dudrick, in *Nutrition Assessment. A Manual for Practitioners,* Appleton-Century-Crofts, Norwalk, CT, pp. 1–205 (1969).

24. F. P. Heald, P. S. Remmell, J. Mayer, in *Adolescent Nutrition and Growth*, (F. P. Heald, ed.), Appleton-Century-Croft, NY, pp. 235–250 (1969).

25. B. Wait, R. Blair, and L. J. Roberts, *Am. J. Clin. Nutr.*, **22**, 1383 (1969).

26. W. A. Daniel, in *Adolescent Nutrition*, (M. Winick, ed.), John Wiley & Sons, NY, pp. 19–24 (1982).

27. M. C. Hampton, R. I. Huenemann, L. R. Shapiro, B. W. Mitchell, *J. Am. Diet. Assoc.*, **50**, 385 (1967).

28. L. K. Mahan and R. H. Rosenbrough, in *Nutrition in Adolescence*, (L. K. Mahan and J. M. Rees, eds.), Times Mirror/Mosby, St. Louis, MO, pp. 40–76 (1984).

29. U. S. Dept. Health, Education and Welfare, in *Dietary Intake Findings: United States, 1971–1974,* DHEW pub. no. (HRA) 77–1647, series 11, no. 202, Health Resources Administration, National Center for Health Statistics, Hyattsville, MD, pp. 1–4, 25–36 (1977).

30. National Center for Health Statistics, in *Calorie and Selected Nutrient for Persons 1–74 Years of Age,* DHEW pub. no. (PHS) 79–1657, series 11, no. 209, U.S. Dept. of Health, Education and Welfare, Hyattsville, MD, pp. 1–88 (1979).

31. M. A. Wharton, *J. Am. Diet. Assoc.*, **42**, 306 (1963).

32. R. E. Hodges, in *Nutrient Requirements in Adolescence*, (J. I. McKigney and H. N. Munro, eds.), The MIT Press, Cambridge, MA, pp. 127–136 (1976).

33. U. S. Dept. Health Human Service, in *The Surgeon General's Report on Nutrition and Health*, General Printing Office, Washington, DC, (1988).

34. D. D. Marino and J. C. King, *Ped. Clin. North Amer.*, **27**, 125 (1980).

35. M. Story, in *Nutrition in Adolescence*, (L. K. Mahan and J. M. Rees, eds.), Times Mirror/Mosby, St. Louis, MO, pp. 77–103 (1984).

36. U. S. Dept. Agriculture, in *Human Nutrition Information Services*, General Printing Office, Washington, DC, pp. 1–435 (1977).

37. P. M. Guenther, *J. Am. Diet. Assoc.*, **86**, 493 (1986).

38. V. Matkovic, K. Kostial, I. Simonovic, R. Buzina, and A. Brodarec, *Am. J. Clin. Nutr.*, **32**, 540 (1979).

39. V. Matkovic, D. Fontana, O. Tominac, J. Lahman , and C. Chestnut, *J. Bone Mineral Res.*, **1**, (suppl.), 168 (1986).

40. J.J.B. Anderson, F. A. Tylavsky, J. M. Lacey, R. V. Talmage, and T. Taft, *Fed. Proc.*, **46**, 632 (1987).

41. R. B. Sandler, C. W. Slemenda, R. E. LaPorte, J. A. Cauley, M. M. Schramm, M. L. Barresi , and A. M. Kriska, *Am. J. Clin. Nutr.*, **42,** 270 (1985).

42. G. M. Chan, *AJDC*, **145**, 631 (1991).

43. Y. Liel, J. Edwards, J. Shary, K. M. Spicer, and L. Gordon, *J. Clin. Endocrinol. Metab.*, **66**, 1247 (1988).

44. T. Lloyd, M. B. Andon, N. Rollings, J. K. Martel, J. R. Landis, L. M. Demers, D. F. Eggli, K. Kieselhorst, and H. E. Kulin, *JAMA*, **270**, 841 (1993).

45. L. H. Allen, *Am. J. Clin. Nutr.*, **35**, 783 (1982).

46. R. P. Heaney, J. C. Gallagher, C. C. Johnston, R. Neer, A. M. Parfitt, and G. D. Whedon, *Am. J. Clin. Nutr.*, **36**, 986 (1982).

47. H. P. Heaney, R. R. Recker, and P. D. Saville, *Am. J. Clin. Nutr.*, **30**, 1603 (1977).

48. P. R. Dallman, *J. Int. Med.*, **226**, 367 (19890.

49. K. A. Harrison, A. F. Fleming, N. D. Briggs, and C. E. Rossiter, *Br. J. Obstet. Gyaecol.*, **5**, (suppl.), 32 (1985).

50. G. Srikantia, J. S. Prasad, C. Bhaskaram, and K.A.V.R. Krishnamachari, *Lancet*, **1,** 1307 (1976).

51. J. Bowering, A. M. Sanchez, and M. I. Irwin, *J. Nutr.*, **106**, 985 (1976).

52. G. C. Viglietti and J. D. Skinner, *J. Am. Diet. Assoc.*, **87**, 903 (1987).

53. Expert Scientific Working Group, *Am. J. Clin. Nutr.*, **42**, 1318 (1985).

54. U. S. Dept. Health, Education and Welfare, in *First Health and Nutrition Examination Survey. United States, 1971–1972: Dietary Intake and Biochemical* Findings, DHEW pub. no. (HRA) 74–1219–1, Health Resources Administration, National Center for Health Statistics, Rockville, MD, pp. 1–183 (1974).

55. R. Yip, C. Johnson, and P. R. Dallman, *Am. J. Clin. Nutr.*, **39**, 427 (1984).

56. Dietetic Practice Group, in *Sports Nutrition*, (J. B. Marcus, ed.), The American Dietetic Assoc., Chicago, IL, pp. 1–161 (1986).

57. Position of the American Dietetic Association, *J. Am. Diet. Assoc.*, **87**, 933 (1987).

58. J. A. Halsted, K. C. Smith, and M. I. Irwin, *J. Nutr.*, **104**, 345 (1974).

59. A. S. Prasad, A. R. Schulert, and A. Miale, Jr., *J. Lab. Clin. Nutr.*, **61**, 537 (1963).

60. P. Thompson, R. Roseborough, E. Russek, M. Jacobson, and P. B. Moser, *J. Am. Diet. Assoc.*, **6**, 892 (1986).

61. P. A. Wagner, L. B. Bailey, C. J. Christakis, and J. S. Dining, *Human Nutr.: Clin. Nutr.*, **39C**, 459 (1985).

62. G. P. Butrimovitz and C. Purdy, *Am. J. Clin. Nutr.*, **31**, 1409 (1978).

63. J. L. Greger, M. M. Higgins, R. P. Abernathy, A. Kirksey, M. B. DeCorso, and P. Baliger, *Am. J. Clin. Nutr.*, **31**, 269 (1978).

64. B. A. Sloan, C. C. Gibbons, and M. Hegsted, *Am. J. Clin. Nutr.*, **42**, 235 (1985).

65. T. A. Nicklas, G. C. Frank, L. S. Webber, S. A. Zingraf, J. L. Cresenta, L. C. Gatewood, and G. S. Berenson, *Am. J. Pub. Health*, **39**, 446 (1987).

66. B. A. Spear, *Seminars Adol. Med.*, **1**, 55 (1985).

67. U. S. Dept. Health Human Services/U.S. Dept. Agriculture in *Nutrtion Monitoring in the United* States, DREW pub. no. (PHS) 86–1255, Hyattsville, MD, pp. 1–356 (1986).

68. O. Pelletier, *Am. J. Clin. Nutr.*, **23**, 520 (1970).

69. L. B. Bailey, P. A. Wagner, G. J. Christakis, C. G. Davis, H. Appledorf, P. E. Araujo, E. Dorsey , and J. S. Dinning, *Am. J. Clin. Nutr.*, **35**, 1023 (1982).

70. A. J. Clark, S. Mossholder, and R. Gates, *Am. J. Clin. Nutr.*, **46**, 302 (1987).

71. L. A. Reiter, L. M. Boylan, and J. Driskell, *J. Am. Diet. Assoc.*, **87**, 1065 (1987).

72. M. S. Rodriques, *J. Nutr.*, **108**, 1983 (1978).

73. W. A. Daniel, E. G. Gaines, and D. L. Bennett, *Am. J. Clin. Nutr.*, **28**, 363 (1975).

74. M. S. VandeMark and A. C. Wright, *J. Am. Diet. Assoc.*, **61**, 511 (1972).

75. U. S. Dept. Health, Education and Welfare, in *Ten-State Nutrition Survey, 1968–1970*, DREW pub. no. 73–8133 ,Center for Disease Control, Atlanta, GA, (1973).

76. A. Vahlquist, L. Rask, P. A. Peterson, and T. Berg, *Scand. J. Clin. Lab. Invest.*, **35**, 569 (1975).

77. K. Hoppner, W. E. Phillips, T. K. Murray, and I. S. Campbell, *Can. Med. Assoc. J.*, **99**, 983 (1968).

78. L. Brabin and B. J. Brabin, *Am. J. Clin. Nutr.*, **55**, 955 (1992).

79. W. A. Daniel Jr., in *Adolescents in Health and Disease*, Mosby, St. Louis, MO, pp. 7–25 (1977).

80. L. K. Mahan and R. H. Rosebraugh, in *Nutrition in Adolescence*, (L. K. Mahan and J. M. Rees, eds.), Times Mirror/Mosby, St. Louis, MO, pp. 40–76 (1985).

81. K. J. Morgan, M. E. Zabik, and G. L. Stampley, *Nutr. Res.*, **6**, 635 (1986).

82. H. McCoy, *J. Nutr. Ed.*, **18**, 61 (1986).

83. Mass. Med. Soc. Comm. Nutr., *N. Engl. J. Med.*, **321**, 752 (1989).

84. L. Kaufman, *Nutr. J. Commun.*, **30**, 37 (1980).

85. W. C. Willet, *Am. J. Clin. Nutr.*, **59** (suppl.), 171S (1994).

86. G. C. Frank, *Am. J. Clin. Nutr.*, **59** (suppl.), 207S (1994).

87. S. B. Domel, T. Baronowski, H. Davis, S. B. Leonard, P. Riley, and J. Baronowski, *J. Am. Clin. Nut.*, **59** (suppl.), 218S (1994).

88. W. C. Willett, M. J. Stampfer, B. A. Underwood, F. E. Speizer, B. Rosner, and C. H. Hennekens, *Am. J. Clin. Nutr.*, **38**, 631 (1983).

89. L. Roidt, E. White, G. E. Goodman, P. W. Wahl, G. S. Omenn, B. Rollins, and J. M. Karkeck, *Am. J. Epi.*, **128**, 645 (1988).

90. W. C. Willett, L. Sampson, M. J. Stampfer, C. B. Rosner, J. Witschi, C. H. Hennekens, and F. E. Speizer, *Am. J. Epi.*, **122**, 51 (1985).

91. T. A. Nicklas, J. E. Forcier, L. S. Webber, and G. S. Berenson, *J. Am. Diet. Assoc.*, **91**, 711 (1991).

92. T. Baranowski, R. Dworkin, J. C. Henske, et al., *J. Am. Diet. Assoc.*, **86**, 1381 (1986).

93. G. C. Frank, R. A. Nicklas, L. S. Webber, C. Major, J. F. Miller, and G. S. Berenson, *Am. J. Diet. Assoc.*, **86**, 1381 (1986).

94. B. Haladay and A. Turner-Henson, *Nurs. Res.*, **38**, 248 (1989).

95. L. R. Fink, *Soc. Sci Med.*, **29**, 715 (1989).

96. D. C. Eliades and C. W. Suitor, in *Celebrating Diversity: Approaching Families Through Their Food*, National Center for Education in Maternal and Child Health, Arlington, VA, (1994).

97. National Live Stock and Meat Board, *Iron in Human Nutrition*, Chicago, IL, (1990).

Exercise and Fitness

Carol N. Meredith, Ph.D.

INTRODUCTION

If all you knew about the United States had been gleaned from movies and television programs, you would believe that this country's teenagers are strikingly lean, athletic, and fit. That is the American aesthetic ideal. The truth is that many American teenagers are not particularly fit, lead sedentary lives, and tend to be overweight. Adolescents spend many hours sitting, whether it is at a desk at school or in front of a TV set at home, as shown in Figure 2.1.[1,2] Table 2.1 outlines the circumstances that can hinder physical activity in adolescents and a shorter list of changes in the past 25 yr that have favored an increase in exercise.

A physically fit person can perform daily activities with vigor, has a lowered risk of health problems, and can enjoy sports and other athletic activities.[3] A physically fit person has greater flexibility, muscle endurance, muscle strength, aerobic power, speed, agility, balance, coordination, reaction speed and power, in addition to a leaner body.[4] The health benefits of physical fitness are associated with flexibility, low body fat, muscle strength, and aerobic power. From a public health perspective, these attributes are more important than athletic skill and should be emphasized in school and community programs.

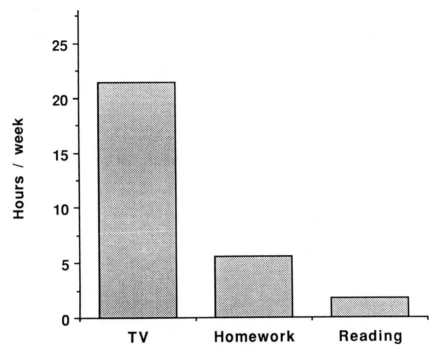

Figure 2-1.   Time devoted to sedentary activities out of school by the American eighth grader.

Adapted from National Center for Education Statistics, *A Profile of the American Eighth Grader NELS:88 Student Descriptive Summary*, U. S. Dept. Education, Washington, DC, p.48 (1990).

Adolescents are less active than children. Longitudinal studies of adolescents, carried out in Holland, show that the energy expenditure per unit of lean body weight declines from age 12–18 yr (Figure 2.2), with the greatest decline for vigorous activity.[5,6] In the United States, interviews found that between the ages of 12 and 16 yr, boys are 2.1 times more likely to be vigorously active than girls.[7] Participation in physical education classes declines from 98% at 10 yr of age to about 50% at age 17.[8]

A decrease in voluntary activity leads to lower physical fitness, with reduced strength, flexibility, aerobic power, and athletic skills (see Figure 2.3).[9] There is no scientific study proving that today's teenagers are less fit than their parents or grandparents were at the same age, but indirect evidence suggests that this may be true. Obesity is more prevalent among adolescents,[10] although data relating activity, food intake, and obesity in the United States are not entirely consistent. Adolescents who are poor or live in rural areas

Table 2.1   Present-Day Circumstances Impeding and Favoring Physical
Activity in Adolescents

IMPEDE

- Cutbacks on school physical education activities, due to budget problems
- Increase in sedentary entertainment (TV, video games, movies)
- Unsafe playgrounds and streets in inner cities, lack of nearby playground areas in rural areas
- Changing perception of socially acceptable forms of exercise (i.e., a teenager might run in public but might not skip rope)
- Smaller family sizes, making it difficult to put together sports team in a neighborhood
- Cheap motorized transportation (car, bus, subway)
- No sidewalks or safe walking areas in many suburbs and rural areas
- Few bicycle paths or lanes
- Expense of some sports, due to equipment or special facilities (ski, football, swimming, horse riding, ice-hockey)
- Fewer jobs demanding physical skills and labor, more jobs demanding intellectual skills
- Few extracurricular team sports for girls (such as Little League, PeeWee hockey)

FAVOR

- Title IX of the Education Amendments (1972), leading to increasing participation of females in sports
- Increased social acceptability of athletic and highly-trained women
- Increased popularity of less expensive sports (soccer, volleyball, bicycling)

have fewer opportunities to exercise properly, eat a healthy diet, and maintain healthy body weight. As poverty has become more common among young people in the United States, obesity and low physical fitness are more likely in these groups.[11]

Overweight adolescents may not be more sedentary than their normal-weight counterparts. Parents rate their obese offspring as less active than their nonobese siblings, but physical fitness per unit of fat-free mass is similar in both groups.[12] An objective measurement of daily energy expenditure, using the doubly labeled water technique, has shown that overweight and normal-weight sedentary adolescents expend a similar amount of calories per day.[13] On the other hand, highly active adolescents are not likely to be obese. Low physical activity may favor the development of obesity, but once excess weight is achieved, a larger lean body mass and the greater energetic cost of moving make total daily energy expenditure similar in the obese and lean adolescent.

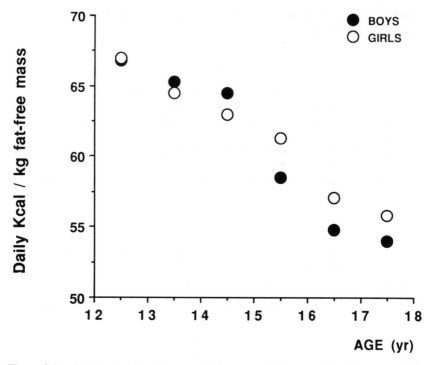

Figure 2-2.   Decline in daily energy expenditure per unit of lean weight in a longitudinal study of Dutch male and female adolescents.

Adapted from R. Verschurr and H. C. G. Kemper, *Child. Exer.*, **20**, 169 (1985).

ASSESSMENT

Body Composition

Adolescence is a time of rapid growth and dramatic changes in body composition, affecting the capacity for physical activity and the response to training. There is an increase in bone size and muscle mass, and changes in the size and distribution of body fat stores.

Muscle mass in boys sharply increases during puberty, both in absolute terms and as a proportion of body weight. At 13 yr of age among males, muscle makes up 46.2% of weight, and at 17 yr, it increases to 52.6%.[14] The increase in the muscle mass of females is less marked, reaching 42.5% of body weight by age 17. Muscle fiber size increases throughout adolescence,[15] in parallel to gains in muscle strength. In some sports, peak performance is typically achieved in late adolescence; the achievement of peak lean body mass at that age is an important part of athletic performance.

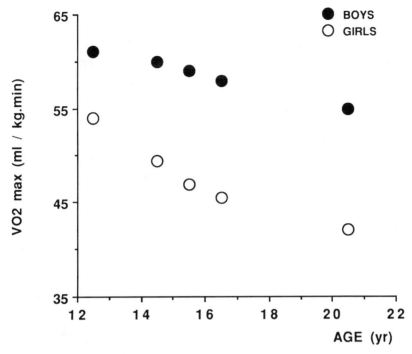

Figure 2-3.   Decline in aerobic power (VO_2 max) in a longitudinal study of Dutch male and female adolescents.

Adapted from H. C. G. Kemper, R. Verschuur, L. S. vanEssen, and R. van Aalst, *Child. Exer.*, **12**, 203 (1986).

Young girls get fatter during puberty. Subcutaneous fat increases, especially in the thighs and hips, a pattern dictated by the female sex hormones. This can lead to strenuous dieting, as plumpness is considered unattractive. Today's teenage girls probably grew up playing with Barbie dolls that portray the ideal of feminine beauty in the United States. The dolls have long slim legs and an unlikely 35–19–32 torso (determined by anthropometry by the author, if we assume the dolls represent women 5'8" to 5'10" in height).

Aerobic Power

There are no data of longitudinal changes in aerobic power in adolescents in the United States. Studies in Holland report that aerobic power (VO_2 max) in athletes peaks between 18 and 20 yr of age in boys and between 16 and 17 yr in girls, coinciding with the age of peak muscle mass. However, in the general population of Dutch adolescents, the aerobic power per unit of body mass tends to decline slightly in males and markedly in females.[9] After puberty in females, VO$_2$ max per unit of body weight may decline with increasing fatness, the tendency for lower hemoglobin, and a decrease in voluntary activity.[7,16,17] Children who are early maturers tend to be fatter and attain a lower adult VO$_2$ max.[18,19]

Fitness scores have been obtained in a cross-sectional study of 8800 Americans aged 10–18 yr.[8] Unfortunately, figures were not corrected for changes in weight, muscle mass or running efficiency that occur during adolescence.[20] These findings suggest that cardiorespiratory fitness (min to run 1 mile) tends to stay constant or increases between the ages of 12–18 yr, indicating that endurance per unit of lean body mass probably decreases or remains unchanged.

Strength

Muscle strength increases throughout adolescence, especially in males, as shown in Figure 2.4 for arm isometric strength.[21] The increase in lower limb

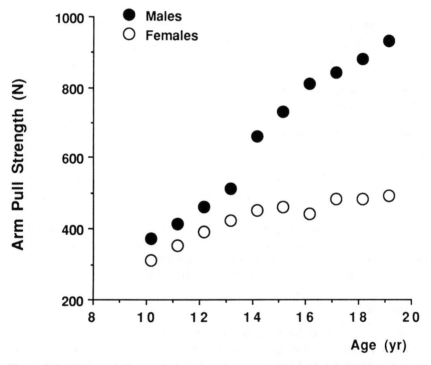

Figure 2-4.   Increase in isometric arm strength, measured by pull strength, in adolescent males and females.

Adapted from J. Alexander and G. E. Molnar, *Archives Phys. Med. Rehab.*, **54**, 424 (1973).

isokinetic strength is more similar in both sexes throughout adolescence (Figure 2.5).[22] Age and weight are the main predictors of static muscle force between 3.5 and 15 yr of age.[23] Measurements of static strength and isokinetic torque[22] show that boys rapidly increase their strength during puberty, after which it increases at a slower rate; in girls, the increase in strength during puberty is not different from prepubertal rates.[23,24] During childhood, girls have 92% of the handgrip static strength of boys, but this figure falls to 60% at 18 yr of age.[25] When strength measurements are corrected for weight and height, much of the gender difference disappears, while expressing strength as a function of lean body mass tends to eliminate gender differences completely.[26] Similarly, standardizing electrically evoked maximal force or voluntary maximal force for the size of muscle fibers (cross-sectional area) minimizes gender differences.[27]

Some determinants of muscle strength in adolescents are summarized in Table 2.2. Among males, strength increases with limb circumference and bone thickness; there is a negative relationship between strength and body fat.[28] As young

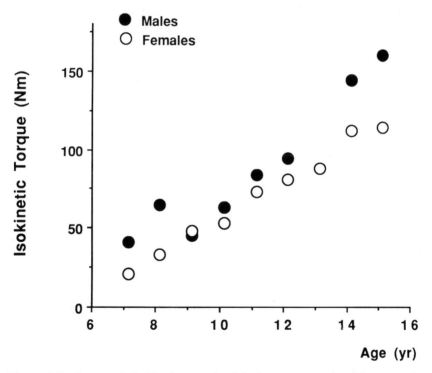

Figure 2-5.   Increase in isokinetic strength of the knee extensors in adolescent males and females.

Adapted from E. Backman, P. Odenrick, K. G. Henriksson, T. Ledin, *Scand. J. Rehab. Med.*, **21**, 105 (1989). Reprinted with permission.

Table 2.2 Determinants of Muscle Strength in Adolescents

	Indicators
Body size	Weight, height, body mass index, arm circumference, bicondylar diameter to humerus and femur, thigh volume, biacromial diameter
Skeletal muscle size	Body density, body potassium, body water, cross-sectional areas measured by CAT scan or other imaging techniques, fiber cross-section
Biomechanical efficiency	Height, length of limb segments, lever arm efficiency
Skill	Motor unit activation, psychological development, motivation, concentration, competitiveness
Endocrine system	Growth hormone, somatomedins, testosterone, thyroid hormone

boys grow taller, muscles can act mechanically more easily across one or more joints[24] and lean mass increases. The gain in muscle size, which is influenced by testosterone and other hormones, correlates with strength gain.[29] Strength also increases due to the maturation of the nervous system, as shown by motor unit activation of the muscles. Motor unit activation of the knee extensors is 77% in 10-year-old boys and increases to 95% in 16-year-old boys.[24]

MANAGEMENT

Aerobic Power, Exercise, and Strength

Trainability, or the capacity to increase VO_2 max, is greatest at the age of peak height increase.[20] Trainability is largely inherited, as shown by studies of identical twins.[30] As in older persons, adolescents with very low initial fitness tend to show the greatest improvement in aerobic power with training. The metabolic effects of aerobic training are important in adolescents as well as adults. In obese adolescents treated with a hypocaloric diet with or without exercise, blood pressure and HDL-cholesterol levels were reduced in the group that exercised, with no difference in body fat change.[31]

Tolerance to harsh environments increases after puberty. Sweat production increases, sweating starts at a lower core temperature, acclimation to exercise in the heat occurs faster, thirst threshold is lower, and core temperature increases less per unit of water loss.[32]

Tolerance for exercise in the cold increases after puberty. Adolescents can tolerate swimming in 20°C water for 30 min without a decline in core temperature, compared to only 18 min for prepubescent children.[33] Obese adolescents can tolerate swimming in cool water better than thin adolescents.

Pubescent children can increase their strength by 5–40% after static training[34] or dynamic training.[35] Voluntary strength increases due to neural adaptations that make it easier to activate motor units and to gains in muscle size. In boys, trainability and muscle hypertrophy due to training increase rapidly during puberty, in parallel with androgen levels. During and after puberty, boys respond to resistance training by increasing strength, limb size, and limb muscle area, whereas prepubescent children do not show muscle hypertrophy.[36]

Strength training in adolescents may have some cardiovascular benefits. Hypertensive adolescents who have lowered their systolic and diastolic blood pressure through endurance training can maintain or even further reduce blood pressure with strength training.[37] Strength training reduced systemic vascular resistance, but had no effect on aerobic power.

Strength training programs must be adapted for children and adolescents.[38] The adolescent must participate in planning the training regimen. Skills and techniques must be taught, with proper training of major opposing groups (i.e., extensors and flexors, adductors and abductors) and equipment that fits the adolescent's body size must be selected. Within an exercise session, the adolescent should exercise large muscle groups first. Initially, while the adolescent is acquiring the necessary skills and is not very fit, only single sets should be used; later, the volume of exercise should be gradually increased. There should be long rest periods between sets and exercises, especially when increasing the intensity of the exercise. Each set should include 8–10 repetitions, or even lighter sets at 12–15 RM. An RM, or repetition maximum, is the maximum amount of weight that can be lifted throughout the range of motion, a specified number of times. Strength should be part of a total conditioning program for the adolescent, with exercises for cardiovascular conditioning, flexibility, and skill development. Coaches should emphasize the need for warming up and cooling down, and provide variety, interest, and recreation during training.

Strength training has typically not been emphasized for adolescents, and especially not for girls, probably because of fear of injury. The reported risk of injury to the growth plate and other anatomical areas is very low if exercises are properly designed and supervised. Strength training may protect against injuries sustained in team sports, such as in football.[38] The most frequent injuries reported with resistance exercise are the patellofemoral joint and the lumbosacral area of the spine, usually due to inadequate exercise prescription, improper lifting technique, or unsafe training devices.[39] Blood pressure changes during resistance exercise in adolescents are not hazardous.[37,40]

Target Groups

It is unfortunate that most adolescents choose to decrease vigorous physical activity at a time that their bodies are better able to tolerate prolonged and intense exercise, even in harsh environments. All adolescents would benefit from programs designed to improve fitness, but there are some whose health and well-being improve dramatically with exercise interventions. This is the case among adolescents with conditions that favor a very sedentary existence, such as mental retardation, blindness, motor disabilities, and extreme obesity.

The most common cause of mental retardation in adolescents is Down syndrome. These adolescents tend to be short, obese, inactive, and physically unfit. Their inactivity may be due to poor motor skills, social isolation, and inadequate programs for exercise. However, training can increase their aerobic power to nearly normal values, produce good psychological effects, reduce subcutaneous fat, and increase strength.[41] Training must be sustained to maintain performance. In the United States, the creation of the "Special Olympics" in 1968 has drawn attention to the importance and feasibility of exercise programs for retarded children and adults.

Blind adolescents tend to be shorter, fatter, and have lower aerobic power than children with normal vision, especially girls.[42,43] This may be due to a lifetime of reduced physical activity, as sighted guides or special facilities are needed for the blind to exercise adequately. However, blind students attain nearly normal aerobic fitness after a training program.[42]

Adolescents with spina bifida, quadriplegia, or other disabilities that prevent walking tend to be fatter and less active than normal adolescents. The metabolic cost of crutch walking is very high.[44] Manual operation of a wheelchair has a metabolic cost that is similar to that of walking, but can be uncomfortably high on uneven surfaces, slopes, or carpeted floors. If the energy cost of mobility exceeds about 60% of a person's VO_2 max, it is impossible to sustain the effort for more than a few min at a time. Adolescents who are confined to wheelchairs need upper-body strength and sufficient aerobic fitness to allow them to propel a wheelchair independently, which can be achieved with circuit training; i.e., a program of strength training carried out at relatively low resistance and high speed that also leads to increased aerobic fitness.[45]

Although moderate obesity may limit an adolescent's physical activity, massive obesity almost ensures a sedentary way of life. In fact, some 10–30% of adolescents in the United States are obese.[10] Exercise helps them lose weight, but only on a long-term basis; it may be more useful in preventing additional fat gain. Obese adolescents who exercise and consume a hypocaloric diet can lower systolic blood pressure, lower heart rate, increase sensitivity to insulin, and lower insulin levels.[31,46] Obese adolescents tend to avoid sports and vigorous exercise. Some exercises can become hazardous. Jogging or running can injure the knees and ankles, and some obese adolescents may already have orthopedic problems that increase the pain and difficulty of movement. Obese adolescents run a greater risk of heat stress if they exercise in a warm environment. However, most hazards are probably social. Self-conscious adolescents who already feel "too fat" even if their weights are close to normal will not be willing to put on the bathing suit, gym tights, or shorts that are needed to participate in swimming, aerobics classes, or soccer. They may be readier to accept vigorous walking, skiing, or cycling. It is important for physicians, as well as teachers and dietitians, to know about effective exercise programs that are socially acceptable, available in the community, low cost, and safe for the overweight adolescent, while vigorous enough to produce a loss of body fat and improve fitness and health. As the main purpose of exercise should be weight loss, the total amount of exercise becomes more important than intensity. Walking long distances is safer and involves more energy expenditure than brief bouts of running.

Risks of Vigorous Activity and Training

Exercise enhances physical and mental health at all ages. However, very intense training or inappropriate exercise can be hazardous to health. The risks of vigorous endurance training in adolescence include dehydration and heat stress, poor bone health and stress fractures, other musculoskeletal injuries, eating disorders, and other psychosocial problems.

Dehydration and heat stress.   Before puberty, teenagers who are obese, not acclimated to heat, and physically untrained need more fluids to prevent heat illness. Heatstroke tends to occur in overweight young men in military training academies and football teams,[47] especially during the first or second day of training.[32] Unfortunately, some coaches are still not aware of the dangers of dehydration; not everyone knows that adolescents during exercise in the heat need to have free access to fluids and should be actively encouraged to consume them.

Injury to bones, joints and muscles.   Adolescents who are growing fast can easily get injured; safety is especially important in sports and physical exercise during early adolescence. The overgrowth of bony elements tightens the muscle-tendon units and soft tissue elements, decreasing joint flexibility.[16] Later, bones thicken and become more resistant, under the influence of sex steroids and adequate nutrition. Injuries are most common in boys during early adolescence, probably due to behavior and because they do not reach maximum muscle mass until some time after attaining peak height.[48] However, injuries related to specific activities are greater in girls. Overuse injuries in athletes, such as stress fractures and chondromalacia of the patella are two to three times more common in young female athletes than young male athletes.[16] For example, when young women were first accepted into military academies, 10% suffered stress fractures in the first year, compared to 1% of the men.[49] In cross-country running and track, the injury rate is three times higher in women than men.[50] Moreover, amenorrhea increases the susceptibility to stress fracture.[17] These figures suggest that coaches and trainers who work with young adolescents must be especially careful to avoid overtraining and hazardous maneuvers in sports.

Poor bone development. During adolescence, the skeleton can retain a larger proportion of dietary calcium; young girls gain more than a pound of calcium in their bones between 12 and 18 yr of age. Poor nutrition and an inappropriately delayed puberty in young athletes can prevent proper bone development, jeopardizing present and long-term bone health. Thin and active girls who have not started menstruating by the age of 14 yr may show low mineral density of the spine and femur[22,51,52] and risk scoliosis[53] and stress fractures.[17] Even among young women with normal menstrual cycles, the risk of bone injury due to overtraining is greater than for young men.[16,49] Cross-sectional studies suggest that the greatest bone density is achieved in young persons who are well nourished, consume a high-calcium diet, and are physically active,[54] especially in impact-loading sports involving running and jumping.[55]

Eating disorders. A survey of 494 girls between 16 and 18 showed that over 80% reported restricting their food intake in order to lose weight.[56] In a small proportion of adolescents, dieting can evolve into an eating disorder. Pathological attitudes to diet and eating tend to emerge in adolescence, especially in girls. About 90% of persons with eating disorders, including anorexia and bulimia, are female. Women who participate in sports or activities requiring a slender figure will go to great lengths to prevent fat gain. The prevalence of dieting and eating disorders is greatest in dancers, gymnasts, and ice skaters, who expend only moderate amounts of energy during training, compared to runners and rowers, whose sport has high energy demands.

Psychosocial problems. Adolescent athletes have special opportunities and problems. They tend to be motivated, disciplined, and hard-working. Athletic success can mean money from advertising, college scholarships, opportunities for travel. But intense training can also mean constant stress, isolation, and a poor education. For example, at tennis academies, adolescents may train 6 h a day, leaving no time for school and other activities.[57] These young athletes may end up taking some correspondence courses, but lose the opportunity to interact with their peers in class and acquire a solid base of knowledge. If they do not win gold medals or other prizes and have little academic education, they may reach young adulthood as a "might-have-beens," prepared only to coach others in their sport.

In women gymnasts, divers, dancers, and ice skaters, an additional stress is the need to "look cute" at a time when the body starts losing its slim, childlike proportions. Young athletes know that beauty makes them more marketable to companies seeking product endorsements and, in some sports, to judges evaluating performance. Efforts to acquire the right "look" for a sport can lead young women to dieting, purging, eating disorders, and amenorrhea, whereas young men are increasingly turning to anabolic steroids and other drugs to look leaner and more muscular.

The psychological health of young elite athletes depends on the values and stability of family and coach. Repeated competitions, knowledge that peak performance is usually attained at a young age, the financial costs of constant training, concerns with the threat of injury, periods spent away from home at competitions or training centers—all these are stressful for the elite adolescent athlete. More attention should be paid to the nutritional, educational, psychological, and physiological needs of young athletes to ensure future health and well-being and not just a brief moment of stardom.[58]

Physical Fitness Testing and Programs

Testing adolescents for physical fitness provides information that is useful to the adolescents themselves, parents, coaches, teachers, and scientists. It provides a basis for designing exercise programs or improving exercise habits, can help increase health awareness, and allows an evaluation of changes in fitness over the short or long term. From a public health viewpoint, it is important to relate the exercise habits and fitness of today's adolescents to the habits, fitness, chronic diseases, and mortality of tomorrow's adults. For example, poor performance of a 550-m run and situps in young boys has been associated with poor exercise habits in these same subjects once they reach adult yr.[59]

The reliability and validity of various test batteries have been reviewed recently by Safrit.[4] The field tests recommended by the American Alliance for Health, Physical Education, Recreation and Dance (AAHPERD) are shown in Table 2.3.[3] Although these tests are not as informative as a VO_2 max test or an accurate

Table 2.3 Field Tests for Physical Fitness Suggested by the American Alliance of Health, Physical Education and Dance

Field Test	Measurement of
Time to run or walk 1 mile	Aerobic capacity (approximate)
Sum of triceps and calf skinfolds, or of body mass index	Body composition (approximate)
Sit and reach test	Flexibility
Number of situps per minute	Muscular strength and endurance (approximate)
Number of pull-ups per minute	Muscular strength and endurance (approximate)

Adapted from American Alliance for Health, Physical Education, Recreation and Dance, *The AAHPERD Physical Best Program*, Reston VA (1988). Reprinted with permission from the American Alliance for Health, Physical Education, Recreation and Dance.

measurement of strength using a dynamometer or weight machine, they are useful for evaluating large groups of persons. Results can be compared to population norms or certain preselected levels of performance that are compatible with a low risk of disease and high functional capacity.

Encouraging exercise in young people promotes good attitudes towards a healthy way of life. Physical education classes in school are the logical place for teaching children to enjoy activities that involve moderate to vigorous exercise.[59] However, physical education in schools must be adapted to practices more consistent with health and fitness. Physical education classes are not synonymous with vigorous exercise that can be sustained once the student has graduated from school. Classes tend to devote only 20% of time to moderate or vigorous activity, and many of the skills taught are useful only for team sports (football, basketball, baseball) rather than activities that can be performed alone or in smaller groups (jogging, swimming, tennis).[60] Sports in the United States are usually linked to schools and colleges, unlike Europe and other places where teams may be formed as part of a neighborhood or club. Thus, young athletes who drop out of school or do not go to college have few opportunities to continue being active in sports and competitions.

Adolescents and children should engage in activity that requires moving large muscle groups, at a frequency ranging from 3 d a week to daily sessions, including 20–30 min of moderate to vigorous activity at a heart rate greater than 140 beats/min.[61] In school, classes should be taught by certified physical education teachers. Outside school hours, the combined efforts of schools, community organizations, and parents are needed to encourage exercise. Exercise activities should be designed to be appealing to adolescents and promote fitness and good long-term exercise habits.

CASE ILLUSTRATION

Tessa, a 15-year-old female who was 5'2" (158 cm) tall and weighed 176 lb (80 kg), was at the 90th percentile of weight for young adult women and had a body mass index (wt/ht^2) of 32.5. She was clearly overweight for her height and age. She had always tended to be chubby and most of her family were overweight. Tessa was unhappy about her looks, but beyond sporadic dieting she had not made any systematic effort to acquire a more appropriate weight and body composition.

After Thanksgiving, Tessa's father, who was also overweight, learned that his cholesterol levels were dangerously high. Tessa's grandfather and one uncle died before 60 of heart disease. The entire family decided it was time to try and "do something to lose weight."

Tessa's father asked the family to join him in adopting a low-fat, high-carbohydrate and high-fiber diet. Working with a dietitian, the family learned to identify high-fat foods and eliminate them from the household, and to snack only on fruits and vegetables, becoming semivegetarian. The dietitian was especially concerned about Tessa. As Tessa was a teenager and not a child, the dietitian met privately with her to discuss Tessa's choices for exercise and dietary changes. The dietitian wanted to encourage sustainable healthy habits rather than a crash diet that might harm Tessa's physical and psychological development. The dietitian, who knew the community and its resources very well, made the following recommendations, based on Tessa's schedule, age and preferences:

1. Eliminate the drive to school. The school was 2 miles away. By walking to school and back, Tessa added about 45 min of moderate aerobic exercise, 5 d/wk. Weekly increase in exercise time: 3.75 h.

2. Change after-school job. Tessa averaged about 5 h a day as a babysitter, involving mostly sitting in front of the TV set or playing indoors with children. Tessa confessed to a love of horses. She found a part-time job at the local stable, where she worked for an hour every week day, cleaning stalls and equipment, and helping children get ready for riding lessons. Work required strength for lifting and scrubbing, and involved some fast walking. Weekly increase in exercise time: 5 h.

3. Tessa joined a hiking club. Every Saturday, she and a group of teenagers spent about 6 h exploring the hills, either hiking or cross-country skiing. Activity involved aerobic exercise of moderate to hard intensity. Weekly increase in exercise time: 6 h.

Total increase in time spent doing exercise per week: almost 15 h. The activities chosen were acceptable to the dietitian, Tessa, and her family, because her activities:

1. Did not require expensive equipment or classes.
2. Did not require revealing or tight clothes (as might be the case with swimming or aerobics classes).
3. Allowed her to meet new people, especially young people.
4. Were not likely to cause injuries.
5. Could be sustained for many years.
6. Could be carried out with or without the assistance of her family.
7. Involved mainly aerobic exercise, which is more likely to improve health and facilitate energy output.
8. Did not rely on school physical education classes.

The dietitian explained to Tessa that her new "lifestyle" would not lead to a rapid loss of weight, but could help her feel better and fitter, and help her keep off whatever pounds she managed to lose through the change in the quality of her diet. "The effects will be noticeable after 6 months or a year, but not sooner," warned the dietitian. The dietitian was careful not to emphasize a reduction in food intake, because Tessa could still be growing and an obsession with food restriction at her age could lead to an eating disorder.

At the end of 6 mo, Tessa was able to walk to school briskly without feeling breathless or sweaty, had added some running to her weekend activities, and her weight was 160 lb.

This is a realistic program. Tessa will likely never be slim, but she gradually started acquiring the eating and exercise habits that are good for health, psychological well-being, and prevention of further weight gain, now and in the future.

REFERENCES

1. W. H. Dietz and S. L. Gortmaker, *Pediatrics*, **75**, 807 (1985).

2. National Center for Education Statistics, *A Profile of the American Eighth Grader NELS:88 Student Descriptive Summary*, U. S. Dept. Education, Washington, DC, p. 48 (1990).

3. American Alliance for Health, Physical Education, Recreation and Dance, *The AAHPERD Physical Best Program*, Reston, VA (1988).

4. M. J. Safrit, *Ped. Exer. Sci.*, **2**, 9 (1990).

5. R. Verschuur and H.C.G. Kemper, *Med. Sport Sci.*, **20**, 169 (1985).

6. R. Verschuur and H.C.G. Kemper, *Child. Exer.*, **11**, 194 (1985).

7. D. J. Aaron, A. M. Kriska, S. R. Dearwater, R. L. Anderson, T. L. Olsen, J. A. Cauley, and R. E. Laporte, *Med. Sci. Sports Exer.*, **25**, 847 (1993).

8. J. G. Ross and G. G. Gilbert, *J. Phys. Ed.*, **1**, 45 (1985).

9. H.C.G. Kemper, R. Verschuur, L. S. van Essen, and R. van Aalst, *Child. Exer.*, **12**, 203 (1986).

10. S. L. Gortmaker, W. H. Dietz, A. M. Sobol, and C. A. Wehler, *AJDC*, **141**, 535 (1987)

11. S. M. Garn and D. C. Clark, *Pediatrics* **57**, 443 (1976).

12. D. L. Elliot, L. Goldberg, K. Kuehl, and C. Hanna, *J. Peds.*, **114**, 957 (1989).

13. L. G. Bandini, D. A. Schoeller, and W. H. Dietz, *Pedr. Res,.* **27**, 198 (1990).

14. R. M. Malina, in *Human Growth: Postnatal Growth*, (F. Falkner and J. M. Tanner, eds.), Plenum Press, NY, p. 273 (1978).

15. E. Jansson and G. Hedberg, *Scand. J. Med. Sci. Sports*, **1**, 31 (1991).

16. L. J. Micheli and L. LaChabrier, in *Pediatric and Adolescent Sports Medicine*, (L. J. Micheli, ed.), Little, Brown, & Co., Boston, MA, p. 167 (1984).

17. G. W. Barrow and S. Saha, *Am. J. Sports Med.* **16**, 209 (1988).

18. S. M. Garn, M. LaVelle, K. R. Rosenberg, and V. M. Hawthorne, *Am. J. Clin. Nutr.*, **43**, 879 (1986).

19. H.C.G. Kemper, R. Verschuur, J. W. Ritmeester, *Child. Exer.*, **12**, 213 (1986).

20. O. Bar-Or, in *The Olympic Book of Sports Medicine*, (A. Dirix, H. G. Knuttgen, K. Tittel, eds.), Blackwell Scientific, NY, p. 269 (1988).

21. H. J. Montoye and D. E. Lamphiear, *Res. Quart.*, **48**, 109 (1977).

22. J. Alexander and G. E. Molnar, *Archives Phys. Med. Rehab.*, **54**, 424 (1973).

23. E. Backman, P. Odenrick, K. G. Henriksson, and T. Ledin, *Scand. J. Rehab. Med.*, **21**, 105 (1989).

24. C.J.R. Blimkie, in *Perspectives in Exercise Science and Sports Medicine:Youth, Exercise and Sport*, (C. V. Gisolfi and D. R. Lamb, eds.), Benchmark Press, Indianapolis, IN (1989).

25. A. V. Carron and D. A. Bailey, *Soc. Res. Child Develop.*, **39**, 1 (1974).

26. M. Miranda, M. Rivera, and W. R. Frontera, in *Proceedings of the IOC Second World Congress on Sports Sciences*, p. 265 (1991).

27. C.T.M. Davies, *Scand. J. Sports Sci.*, **7**, 11 (1985).

28. A.W.S. Watson and D. J. O'Donovan, *J. Appl. Physiol.*, **43**, 834 (1977).

29. G. B. Forbes, *Pediatrics*, **36**, 825 (1965).

30. D. Prudhomme, C. Bouchard, C. Leblanc, F. Landry, and E. Fontaine, *Med. Sci. Sports Exerc.*, **16**, 489 (1984).

31. M. D. Becque, V. L. Katch, A. P. Rocchini, C. R. Marks, and C. Moorehead, *Pediatrics*, **81**, 605 (1988).

32. O. Bar-Or, *Int. J. Sports Med.*, **1**, 53 (1980).

33. R. E. Sloan and W. R. Keatinge, *J. Appl. Physiol.*, **35**, 371 (1973).

34. B. Nielsen, K. Nielsen, M. Behrendt-Hensen, and A. Asmussen, in *Children and Exercise IX*, (K. Berg, B. O. Eriksson, eds.), Human Kinetics, Champaign, IL (1980).

35. R. D. Pfeiffer and R. S. Francis, *Phys. Sportsmed.*, **14**, 134 (1986).

36. J. Vrijens, *Med. Sport*, **11**, 152 (1978).

37. J. M. Hagberg, A. A. Ehsani, D. Goldring, A. Hernandez, D. R. Sinacore, and J. O. Holloszy, *J. Peds.*, **104**, 147 (1984).

38. W. J. Kraemer, A. C. Fry, P. N. Frykman, B. Conroy, and J. Hoffman, *Ped. Exer. Sci.*, **1**, 336 (1989).

39. T. A. Brady, B. R. Cahill, and L. M. Bodnar, *Am. J. Sports Med.*, **10**, 1 (1982).

40. K. Nau, R. Beekman, V. Katch, *Med. Sci. Sports Exer.*, **20**, S31 (1989).

41. J. Skrobak-Kaczynski and T. Vavik, *Child. Exer.*, **9**, 300 (1980).

42. R. J. Shephard, G. R. Ward, and M. Lee, *Child. Exer.*, **12**, 355 (1986).

43. S. Sundberg, *Acta Ped. Scand.*, **71**, 603 (1982).

44. J. C. Agre, T. W. Findley, C. McNally, R. Habeck, A. S. Leon, L. Stradel, R. Birkebak, and R. Schmalz, *Arch. Phys. Med. Rehab.*, **68**, 372 (1987).

45. D. G. O'Connell, R. C. Barnhart, and L. Parks, *Med. Sci. Sports Exer.*, **21**, 95 (1989).

46. A. P. Rocchini, V. Katch, J. Anderson, J. Hinderliter, D. Becque, M. Martin, and C. Marks, *Pediatrics*, **82**, 16 (1988).

47. C. Barcenas, H. Hoeffler, and J. T. Lie, *Am. Heart J.*, **92**, 237 (1976).

48. J. J. Wiley and W. M. McIntyre, *Curr. Concepts Bone Fragil.*, 159, (1986).

49. J. L. Anderson, *Phys. Sportsmed.* **7**, 72, (1979).

50. S. Petosa, *Phys. Sportsmed.*, **17**, 133 (1989).

51. K. H. Myburgh, L. K. Bachrach, B. Lewis, K. Kent, and R. Marcus, *Med. Sci. Sports Exerc.*, **25**, 1197 (1993).

52. B. L. Drinkwater, K. Nilson, C. H. Chesnut, Q. J. Bremner, S. Shainholtz, and M. B. Southworth, *N. Engl. J. Med.*, **311**, 277 (1984).

53. M. P. Warren, J. Brooks-Gunn, L. H. Hamilton, L. F. Warren, W. G. Hamilton, *N. Engl. J. Med.*, **314**, 1348 (1986).

54. B. Kanders, D. W. Dempster, and R. Lindsay, *J. Bone Min. Res.*, **3**, 145 (1988).

55. S. K. Grimston, N. D. Willows, and D. A. Hanley, *Med. Sci. Sports Exer.*, **25**, 1203 (1993).

56. L. M. Mellin, *Nutr. News*, **51**, 5 (1988).

57. W. B. Kibler, C. McQueen, and T. Uhl, *Clin. Sports Med.*, **7**, 403 (1988).

58. A. Smith, in *Eighth Annual Conference on Exercise Sciences and Sports Medicine in Puerto Rico* (1994).

59. B. A. Dennison, J. H. Straus, E. D. Mellits, and E. Charney, *Pediatrics*, **82**, 324 (1988).

60. O. Bar-Or, *Res. Quart. Exer. Sport*, **58**, 304 (1987).

61. B. G. Simons-Morton, G. S. Parcel, N. M. O'Hara, S. N. Blair, R. R. Pate, *Ann. Rev. Pub. Health*, 9, 403 (1988).

Contraception and Weight

Estherann Grace, M.D., F.S.A.M.
Karen J. Kozlowski, M.D.

INTRODUCTION

Adolescent sexual behavior and pregnancy are ongoing problems in the United States. The proportion of adolescents with sexual experience rises sharply with age. For example, by age 13 about 1% are sexually active, by age 15 yr 12%, and 58% are sexually experienced by 18.[1] As a result, one in eight women aged 15–19 yr in the United States becomes pregnant each year and one in 15 men fathers a child while he is a teenager.[2] Both pregnancy rates and birth rates among teens in the United States are very high when compared to those in other developed countries, but the rates of sexual activity are similar.[3,4]

Despite many contraceptive options, only 65% of teenage women surveyed in 1988 reported the use of a contraceptive at first intercourse. Of those using contraception, 73% indicated using a condom, 13% relied on withdrawal, and only 13% used the birth control pill.[5] There are multiple reasons why American adolescent women have failed to use contraceptives, including the belief that they cannot conceive or unplanned intercourse.[6] Moreover, adolescents are uncomfortable discussing sexual matters and often embarrassed to see a physician for this concern. As a result, adolescents typically wait 12 mo after onset of sexual activity before beginning contraception. Unfortunately, it is during this period after the initiation of sexual activity that 61% of all adolescent pregnancies occur.[7]

Essentially, the same contraceptive options are available for teenagers as for any reproductive-aged woman. Hormonal methods of contraception are most frequently prescribed for the sexually active adolescent woman, specifically, oral contraceptives pills, levonorgestrel implants (the Norplant system), and depo-medroxyprogesterone acetate (depo-Provera or DMPA). For sexually active women, the hormonal methods of contraception are the most effective reversible methods.

ASSESSMENT

Mechanism of Action, Metabolic, and Side-Effects

The three methods of hormonal contraception, oral contraceptive pills (OCPs), Norplant and depo-Provera, essentially have the same mechanism of action relative to providing contraception. The mechanism of action of combined oral contraceptives is through the combined actions of estrogen and progestin. Ovulation is inhibited by the suppression of follicle-stimulating hormone (FSH) and luteinizing hormone (LH), the cervical mucous is thickened and decreased, making it more difficult for sperm to penetrate, and the endometrium is rendered thin and atrophic, thereby preventing implantation. Premature luteolysis (degeneration of the corpus luteum) is an additional mechanism of contraceptive action. The progestin-only contraceptives, such as progesterone only oral contraceptives, depo-Provera injection, and Norplant implants, prevent pregnancy in the identical manner.

Combination oral contraceptive pills.   When we discuss the side-effects and metabolic effects of the various methods of hormonal contraception, the hormonal components must be considered. Combination oral contraceptives contain both an estrogen compound and a progestin compound. Only two estrogenic compounds, ethinyl estradiol and mestranol, are currently used in the United States. Ethinyl estradiol is pharmacologically active, whereas mestranol must be converted into ethinyl estradiol by the liver before it is pharmacologically active. The amount of estrogen in oral contraceptives varies from 20–50 μg. There are several progestogenic compounds available in pills: norethindrone, norethindrone acetate, ethynodiol diacetate, norgestrel, levonorgestrel, and the new progestins, desogestrel and norgestimate (see Table 3.1). In women taking oral contraceptives, the total estrogenic effect is the result of estrogen from the oral contraceptive and endogenous estrogen from the ovaries and adipose tissue. Progestins vary

Table 3.1 Contraceptives Available in the United States

Drug	Estrogen	μg	Progestin	mg
Ovral	Ethinyl estradiol	50	Norgestrel	0.5
Ovcon–50	Ethinyl estradiol	50	Norethindrone	1
Norinyl 1 + 50	Mestranol	50	Norethindrone	1
Ortho-Novum 1/50	Mestranol	50	Norethindrone	1
Demulen 1/35	Ethinyl estradiol	35	Ethynodiol diacetate	1
Norinyl 1 +35	Ethinyl estradiol	35	Norethindrone	1
Ortho-Novum 1/35	Ethinyl estradiol	35	Norethindrone	1
Ortho-cyclen	Ethinyl estradiol	35	Norgestimate	0.25
Ortho-TriCyclen	Ethinyl estradiol	35	Norethindrone	0.180 × 7 d
				0.215 × 7 d
				0.250 × 7 d
Brevicon	Ethinyl estradiol	35	Norethindrone	0.5
Modicon	Ethinyl estradiol	35	Norethindrone	0.5
Ovcon–35	Ethinyl estradiol	35	Norethindrone	0.4
Lo/Ovral	Ethinyl estradiol	30	Norgestrel	0.3
Loestrin 1.5/30	Ethinyl estradiol	30	Norethindrone acetate	1.5
Nordette	Ethinyl estradiol	30	Levonorgestre l	0.15
Desogen, Orthocept	Ethinyl estradiol	30	Nesogestrel	0.15
Loestrin 1/20	Ethinyl estradiol	20	Norethindrone acetate	1
Jenest 28	Ethinyl estradiol	35	Norethindrone	.5 × 7 d
				1.0 × 14 d
Ortho-Novum 7/7/7	Ethinyl estradiol	35	Norethindrone	.5 × 7 d
				.75 × 7 d
				1.0 × 7 d
TriNorinyl	Ethinyl estradiol	35	Norethindrone	.5 × 7 d
				1.0 × 9 d
				.5 × 5 d
Triphasil, TriLevlin	Estradiol	30	Levongestrel	.05 × 6 d
		40		.075 × 5 d
		30		.125 × 10 d
Ovrette			Norgestrel	0.075
Nor-Q.D., Micronor			Norethindrone	0.35

in both their inherit estrogenicity and antiestrogenic properties, as well as their androgenic effects. These features have an impact on the mechanism of action and metabolic effects and side-effects.

When taken perfectly, combined estrogen progesterone pills are very effective, with about 1 in 1000 women expected to become pregnant within the first yr. Failure rates during typical use are determined by the extent and type of imperfect use. Thus, in the United States about 3% of women become pregnant during the first year of contraceptive use.[8]

Pills are very safe for most women, including adolescents. In the United States, it is safer to use pills than to deliver a baby, unless a women is over 35 yr of age and smokes more than 35 cigarettes/d.[9] The risk of death from birth control pills is very low, and the statistics would be even lower if the heavy smokers over 35 yr of age did not take pills.[9] Most women can safely use pills throughout their reproductive yrs as long as they have no specific reason to avoid them. Age is not a reason to avoid pills, in very young teens or women toward the end of the reproductive life span. There are several noncontraceptive health benefits of oral contraceptive pills. Ovarian cancer risk is decreased by 40–80%. This protection begins with 1 yr of use, increases with the increasing duration of use, and persists 10–15 yr after oral contraceptives are stopped. Similarly, the risk of endometrial cancer is decreased by 40–60%, begins with one yr of use, increases with increasing duration of use, and persists 10–15 yrs after oral contraceptives are stopped. Oral contraceptive users have a decreased risk of pelvic inflammatory disease (salpingitis), decreased risk of benign breast disease (noncancerous tumors and cysts), fewer ectopic pregnancies, and increased bone density, thus offering protection from the development of osteoporosis. Beneficial menstrual cycle effects include more regular menses, decreased menstrual cramps and pain, decreased number of days of bleeding and the amount of blood loss, thereby decreasing a woman's likelihood of developing iron deficiency anemia. Functional ovarian cysts are less common in women using oral contraceptives due to the suppression of FSH and LH. In addition, some women note a reduction in premenstrual symptoms. Acne and hirsutism are often improved due to the lower serum testosterone levels seen with combination oral contraceptives.

When discussing the adverse complications of oral contraceptives, it must be remembered that the estrogenic, progestational, and androgenic effects of oral contraceptives affect a number of organs and tissues throughout the body. The exogenous hormones in birth control pills may stimulate a given end organ in a woman quite differently than do the endogenous hormones that she produced before using pills. A specific birth control pill may affect two different women quite differently.

In general, most women using the currently available pills that contain less than 50 µg of ethinyl estradiol or the equivalent do not experience estrogen-mediated side-effects. Side-effects that may be caused by the estrogen in pills are as follows: nausea, increased breast size (ductile and fatty tissue), stimulation of breast neoplasia, fluid retention, cyclic weight gain due to fluid retention, leukorrhea, cervical erosion or ectropia, thromboembolic complications, pulmonary emboli, cerebral vascular accidents, hepatocellular adenomas, hepatocellular cancer, rise in cholesterol concentration in gall bladder bile, growth of leiomyomata and telangiectasia. If one's goal is to minimize the risk of a specific effect that is usually estrogen-related, such as nausea or breast tenderness, it is wise to choose a pill with the lowest amount of ethinyl estradiol or lowest estrogenic effect.

The progestational component as well as the estrogen component of oral contraceptives may contribute to the development of the following adverse effects: breast tenderness, headaches, hypertension, myocardial infarction.

When considering androgenic effects, all low-dose combined pills tend to have a beneficial effect on oily skin, acne and hirsutism due to the suppression of the production of testosterone. The progestin component of oral contraceptives in some instances has androgenic as well as progestational effects and thus may be associated with the following adverse effects: increased appetite and weight gain, depression, fatigue, decreased libido, acne and oily skin, increased breast size (alveolar tissue) increased LDL cholesterol levels, decreased HDL cholesterol levels, diabetogenic effect, pruritis, and decreased carbohydrate tolerance. When attempting to minimize these androgenic effects such as hirsutism, oily skin, or weight gain, the new progestins (desogestrol and norgestimate) appear to be suitable options due to their low androgenic effects.

Progestin-only contraceptives. Progestin-only contraceptives may be administered via various routes: by mouth, injection, and implants, as well as intrauterine devices. There are several advantages that apply to all progestin-only contraceptives. Because they contain no estrogen, they do not cause the serious complications that have been attributed to estrogenic agents including thrombophlebitis and pulmonary embolism. Norplant, depo-Provera, and progestin-only pills offer several noncontraceptive benefits including scanty menses or no menses, decreased anemia, decreased menstrual cramps and pain, suppression of pain associated with ovulation (Mittelschmertz), decreased risk of developing endometrial cancer, decreased risk of developing ovarian cancer, decreased risk of developing pelvic inflammatory disease, and management of pain associated with endometriosis. The magnitude of these contraceptive benefits may vary and thus needs careful evaluation. The Norplant system consists of six capsules made of flexible, nonbiodegradable silastic rods, each containing 35 µg of levonorgestrel that is released at a slow steady rate. Until the 5-yr mark, the mean levels of levonorgestrel remain at about 0.40 ng/mL, well above the level of 0.25 ng/mL needed to suppress ovulation.[10] Body weight affects the circulating level of levonorgestrel. The greater the weight of the user, the lower the levonorgestrel concentration is at any time during Norplant use. Although there are no weight restrictions for Norplant users, heavier women (more than 70 kg) may experience slightly higher pregnancy rates in the fourth and fifth yrs of use compared to lighter women. Even in later years, however, pregnancy rates for heavier women using Norplant are lower than with oral contraceptives. These differences in pregnancy rates by weight are probably due to the dilution effect of larger body size on the low sustained serum levels of levonorgestrel.[11] Norplant is an extremely effective method of contraception. In studies conducted in 11 countries totaling over 12,000 women-years of use, the pregnancy rate was 0.2 pregnancies/ 100 women-years of use. All but one of the pregnancies that occurred during this evaluation was present at the time of implant insertion. When luteal phase insertions are excluded, the first-year pregnancy rate was 0.01/100 women-years.[12] Thus, it is recommended that Norplant be inserted within 7 d of onset of menstruation, or immediately postpartum or within 3 wk after a delivery. As Norplant provides effective reversible contraception that is free of failures due to compliance issues, it is especially convenient and reliable for adolescents and other reproductive-aged women who have failed other contraceptive methods requiring personal involvement for effectiveness. Because Norplant is a progestin-only method, it may be utilized by women who have contraindications for the use of estrogen-containing oral contraceptives. Because the serum levels of progestin remain low and no estrogen is administered, serious health effects have not occurred.[12]

There are some disadvantages associated with the use of the Norplant system. A minor surgical procedure is required to insert and remove the system. Women therefore cannot initiate or discontinue the method without the assistance of a clinician. As a result, initiation costs are higher than those of other forms of hormonal contraception. Other disadvantages include menstrual irregularity, weight gain, breast tenderness, visibility of implants, inflammation or infection at implant site, acne, galactorrhea, ovarian cysts, headache, depression and mood changes, and hyperpigmentation over the implants. Although these side-effects are minor in nature, they can cause patients to discontinue the method. Patients often find these side-effects tolerable after assurance that they do not represent any health hazard.[13] Many complaints respond to reassurance, whereas others can be treated with simple therapies. Menstrual irregularity was the most common side-effect reported by 80% of Norplant recipients.[14] Despite this, when properly counseled, a much lesser percentage of users describe this as bothersome, and despite the increase in the number of days of spotting and bleeding, hemoglobin concentrations rise in Norplant users due to a decrease in the average amount of menstrual blood loss.[15]

The sustained low dose of levonorgestrel delivered by the Norplant system in not associated with significant metabolic effects. Studies of carbohydrate metabolism,[16,17] liver function,[18,19] blood coagulation,[20] immunoglobulin levels,[16,21] serum cortisol levels[22] and blood chemistries,[16,19,23] have failed to detect changes outside of normal ranges. In terms of lipoproteins, minor changes are transient and with prolonged duration of use, lipoproteins returned to preinsertion levels. No major impact on lipoproteins can be demonstrated.[19,23] Just as the prolonged use of oral contraceptives has not seen to affect one's risk of athrosclerosis, similarly long-term exposure to the low dose of levonorgestrel in Norplant users is unlikely to affect their risk of athrosclerosis.

The advantages of Norplant in addition to those previously stated for oral progestin-only methods are that it is a safe, highly effective, continuous method of contraception requiring little user compliance or motivation and is rapidly reversible. Circulating levels of levonorgestrel are too low to measure within 48 h after removal of Norplant system. There are no long-term effects on future fertility and most women resume normal ovulatory cycles during the first month after removal.

Depo-Provera (DMPA) is an injectable contraceptive containing 150 mg of depo-medroxyprogesterone acetate/1cc. Injections are administered at 12-wk intervals. The failure rate is 0.3%. One reason the failure rate is so low is that each 150-mg injection actually provides more than 3 mo of protection.[24] There is a grace period of 2 wk, and up to 4 wk in some instances, during which a DMPA user can be late for her next shot, but still be at minimal risk of becoming pregnant. The major problems with DMPA are irregular menstrual bleeding, breast tenderness, weight gain, and depression. Weight gain and depression are not relieved until the drug clears the body, which is on the average 6–8 mo or more after the last injection. In terms of metabolic effects, there are no clinically significant changes in carbohydrate metabolism or coagulation factors.[25,26] High-density lipoprotein cholesterol levels fall significantly in women using DMPA.[27] In conjunction with the decrease in HDL cholesterol, increases in total cholesterol and LDL cholesterol have been documented.[25] Others have failed to demonstrate this, claiming that since there is not a metabolic first-pass effect in the liver with intramuscular DMPA, cholesterol levels are not adversely affected.[28,29] The clinical impact of these lipoprotein changes, if any, has yet to be elucidated. There is concern that the levels of estrogen in users of DMPA are lower compared to a normal menstrual cycle and, therefore, patients can lose bone density to some degree.[30] Decreased bone density was as likely to be found in thin as heavier women and was reversible when DMPA was stopped. Although other factors such as smoking were not controlled for in this study and the results of this one study should not prevent the use of DMPA, these data should caution one to assess osteoporosis and other effects of low estrogen in women using DMPA. There is no adverse impact on future fertility; however, the delay to conception averages 9 mo after the last injection. This delayed returned to normal fertility does not increase with an increase in the duration of DMPA use.

In addition to the benefits previously cited for all progestin-only contraceptives, DMPA has additional advantages and benefits. Amenorrhea is common with DMPA and viewed by many women as an advantage. During the first yr of use, 30–50% of women are amenorrheic and by the end of the second year, this number increases to 80%. There are no demonstrated interactions between DMPA and antibiotics or enzyme-inducing drugs, most important, the antiseizure medications.[24] The only drug that decreases DMPA effectiveness is aminoglutethimide. DMPA has been found to decrease the frequency of seizures probably due to the sedative property of progesterones.[31-33] Due to the fact that DMPA contains no estrogen and therefore there are no side-effects due to estrogen, it is often considered for patients with congenital heart disease, sickle cell anemia, a previous history of thromboembolism, and women over 30 who smoke or have other risk factors. In sickle cell disease, there is evidence that indicates the inhibition of invivo sickling in patients using DMPA with resultant hematologic improvement.[34] An additional advantage is that DMPA increases the quantity of milk in nursing mothers, which is in direct contrast to the effect seen with combination oral contraceptives. As the concentration of DMPA in breast milk is very small, no effects of DMPA on infant growth and development have been observed.[35] Other benefits associated with the use of DMPA include decreased risk of endometrial cancer, decreased risk of ovarian cancer,[36] and probably the same benefits associated with the progesterone effect of oral contraceptives, namely reduced menstrual blood loss and pain, less PID, less endometriosis, fewer uterine fibroids, and fewer ectopic pregnancies.

MANAGEMENT

Nausea can occur with combination oral contraceptives, but is very unlikely with progesterone-only methods of contraception (progestin-only contraceptive pills, Norplant, and DMPA). Nausea most often occurs during the first cycle of combination OCPs or the first few pills of each new package. With the low-dose pills, this is less of a problem. Vomiting rarely occurs. Nausea can often be controlled by taking the pills after eating a meal or snack, or at bedtime. If nausea occurs for the first time after several months of taking pills, pregnancy should be ruled out, as well as other causes of nausea including acute infections, hepatitis, gall bladder disease, or mononucleosis. When nausea persists as a problem, changing to a combination pill with less estrogen or a progesterone only form of contraception often dramatically decreases nausea, but may also lead to more spotting and breakthrough bleeding.

Weight changes, specifically weight gain, are cited as a side-effect with all methods of hormonal contraception. With combination OCPs, in most instances, weight change is minimal and often unrelated to pill use. Approximately as many women lose weight as gain it while taking combination OCPs. In some women, however, weight gain is caused by OCPs. In these patients, weight gain usually responds to dietary restriction, but for some patients, the weight gain is secondary to the anabolic effects of the sex steroids in OCPs, and discontinuation of the OCPs is the only way that weight loss can be achieved. This, however, must be rare with low-dose OCPs as the data in published studies fail to indicate a difference between users and nonusers.[11] When assessing weight change, a careful history should be obtained including the relationship of the weight gain to the initiation of OCPs, weight change on any other birth control pills, change in appetite, cyclical weight gain, symptoms of pregnancy, and patient recall of previous weights. Any changes in lifestyle that may be significant factors in weight gain should be sought including work, sleep and exercise habits, and signs of depression. When examining the patient, recording current weights and comparing them with previous weights in the chart are invaluable. One also should look for signs of edema, the amount and distribution of fat, uterine enlargement, and signs of pregnancy. In some cases, testing for pregnancy and 2 h postprandial glucose tests may be indicated. Both progestins, especially those with high androgenic activity, and estrogens can cause weight gain. Progestin-and/or androgen-induced weight may be due to increased appetite and increased food intake secondary to anabolic effects or altered carbohydrate metabolism that can cause hyperinsulinemia and is accompanied by symptoms of hypoglycemia.

Estrogen-induced weight gain is associated with an increase in subcutaneous fat especially in the breasts, hips, and thighs, and is not accompanied by an increase in appetite. Weight gain may also be associated with fluid retention due to either the estrogen or progesterone component of the OCP. This type of weight gain is usually cyclic and accompanied by other symptoms of fluid retention. One also must remember that if depression occurs, this may be accompanied by a concomitant increase in caloric intake. Weight gain usually responds to decreasing caloric intake or increasing exercise. Patients who have experienced weight gain should be informed that the use of OCPs is a possible cause. If the weight gain is accompanied by increased appetite and symptoms of hypoglycemia, an OCP with lower progestational and androgenic activity may be of benefit. A pill with decreased androgenic potency will often be beneficial if the patient has experienced an anabolic effect and persistent weight increase over time. In some cases, it may be necessary to discontinue pills. A diet designed for patients with hypoglycemia along with caloric reduction will reduce weight gain due to a progestational effect or from other causes. A decrease in the estrogen, progestin, or both is helpful in patients who have clearly experienced cyclic weight change. An OCP with lower estrogenic activity may be of benefit if the weight gain occurs mainly in the hips, breasts, and thighs, is cyclic, and /or is accompanied by bloating or edema.

Obese women can take combined OCPs. There is no need to prescribe a higher-dose pill in obese women. The protective effect of combined OCPs against endometrial cancer may be particularly desirable in overweight women whose risk of endometrial cancer is increased. In patients with a family history of diabetes or heart disease at a young age, one should strongly consider performing a lipid profile and a 2 h postprandial glucose test periodically. One of the new progestin OCPs as well as Ovcon 35, Modicon, or Brevicon may actually improve the lipid profile of a young obese woman who will be on OCPs for a number of years.

With progestin-only methods (progestin-only OCPs, Norplant, and DMPA), users may complain of weight gain or feeling bloated. Weight gain is probably due to increased appetite rather than fluid retention.[24] The World Health Organization monograph on injectable contraceptives states that a weight gain of 1 kg. (2.2 pounds) annually "is reported in nearly all women using injectable contraceptives."[24] Women using Norplant more frequently complained of weight gain rather than weight loss, but findings are variable. In central America, 75% of those whose weight changed lost weight, whereas in San Francisco, two-thirds of users gained weight. Over 5 yr of use, weight gain in Norplant averages about 5 lb which is close to the average weight gain for women in their early to mid-reproductive years. Weight changes ranging from weight loss to minimal to excessive weight gain of up to 40 lb have been reported. Assessment of weight change in Norplant users is often confounded by changes in exercise, diet, and aging. An increase in appetite can be attributed to the androgenic effect of levonorgestrel, but the low levels of levonorgestrel in Norplant are unlikely to have a significant clinical impact. Weight gain is clearly an unacceptable side-effect and contributes to user dissatisfaction and premature removal. Counseling for weight changes should include dietary review and focus on dietary changes and exercise changes as well as assessment for depression. Weight gain is less of a problem in women on progestin-only OCPs than those on combination OCPs.

Mastalgia can occur with any method of hormonal contraception. Once pregnancy has been ruled out as the cause, reassurance and therapy aimed at symptomatic relief are indicated. The symptoms often decrease with the increasing use of the hormonal contraception. Other treatments have included vitamin E, vitamin B-6, danazol, bromocriptine, and evening of primrose oil.

Acne, a common occurrence in adolescents, is improved regardless of which preparation of combination low-dose OCPs is used. Acne can be seen in Norplant users due to the androgenic activity of levonorgestrel. This is in contrast to combination oral contraceptives tha contain levonorgestrel where the estrogen effect produces a decrease in androgens. The acne usually responds to dietary changes, practice of good skin hygiene, and often the application of topical antibiotics.

Headaches, both true migraines and tension headaches, are common in women.[11] There have been no well-documented studies to determine the impact of oral contraceptives on migraine headaches. Patients report that headaches may be mild or severe, as well as better, worse, or indifferent while on the various forms of contraception. Because severe headaches may be an early warning of stroke, they need to be evaluated carefully. History should include questions about the age of onset of headaches, the severity and duration of the headaches, the relation to stress or sinusitis, location of the headache, cyclicity of the headache in relation to the menstrual cycle, associated jaw pain, and the relationship of headaches to taking the contraceptive. One must determine if the headaches are unilateral, throbbing, or associated with nausea, vomiting, dizziness, scotomata, or blurred vision, watering of the eyes, or loss of vision. Determine what medications have made the headaches better or worse. One must ask about alcohol use, caffeine intake, and history of drug use. A complete physical exam should be performed including checking the patient's blood pressure and performing a funduscopic exam. If the headache appears to be temporally related to beginning the use of OCPs, discontinue or change to a preparation with lower estrogenic or lower progestational activity and reevaluate after a cycle or two. If headaches are clearly worsened, one must definitely consider discontinuing pills. In some women, a relationship exists between their fluctuating hormonal levels during a menstrual cycle and their headaches, with the headaches characteristically coinciding with menses. In some of these women, headaches can be alleviated with either the use of low-dose OCPs or administration of a progestational agent.

In conclusion, oral contraceptives are associated with a collection of effects that yield an overall improvement of health. Similarly, progestin-only contraceptive methods have similar health improvements. In the adolescent, contraception is extremely safe. There is no evidence that the use of oral contraceptives in the pubertal sexually active girl impairs the growth or development of her reproductive system. Success of any contraception is dependent on appropriate education, counseling, and ongoing evaluation to assure compliance. When considering nutritional, metabolic, and other health factors, assessing risk factors prior to beginning contraception as well as ongoing during the contraceptive use will often minimize undesired effects and thus enhance patient compliance.

CASE ILLUSTRATION

Case 1

Kara is a 17-year-old adolescent with irregular periods who has started on birth control pills to regulate her flow. She has been sexually active for 1 yr using condoms. She has avoided the pill because of a fear of gaining weight. She has struggled to keep her weight in a healthy range by careful food choices and exercising 1–2 h/d at a health club. She consults the dietitian on how to avoid weight gain while on the pill for medical indications.

The initial evaluation of Kara by the dietitian determines if her weight and percent of body fat are appropriate for her height and body build. If they are, reassurance of the fallacy of the myth of mandatory weight gain and a follow-up visit in 3 mo of pill use should suffice. If at the follow-up visit, weight change has occurred, a careful review of appetite changes (increase vs. decrease), caloric intake, and exercise patterns is made and Kara is then advised to adjust her behavior to rectify the weight change. The pill provider should be consulted if the progesterone or estrogen content of the pill requires adjustment.

Case 2

Terry is an 18-year-old mother of a 3-year-old son. She is unhappy with the present method of birth control and desires the convenience of Norplant. She plans to start college in the fall and doesn't wish to become pregnant in the near future. At this time, she is 45 lb over her ideal body weight and has been sent to the dietitian for counseling by the provider prior to the insertion procedure. Terry has failed every weight-reduction plan she has ever tried. She simply can't give up her chips and candy bars.

The dietitian's goals in this case must be tailored to the patient's needs. Ideally, Terry would adhere to a weight-reduction caloric intake meal plan and increase the physical activity in her life. Realistically, this may be too much to expect. However, a comprehensive plan should be designed with Terry's lifestyle in mind. Granted her adherence may be doubtful, but she is still worth the effort. Knowing that weight gain is a possible consequence of Norplant, helping Terry achieve some weight loss prior to its insertion is a reasonable goal. Frequent visits to the dietitian for supportive counseling with frequent monitoring of intake have proved successful in some cases. The ultimate decision of whether a teen receives Norplant is usually made by the teen and the provider performing the procedure.

Case 3

Lisa is a 16-year-old with severe migraine headaches who has been advised not to take birth control pills. She is sexually active with a boyfriend who refuses to use condoms. She is requesting depo-Provera. She is a recovering bulimic and terrified of increasing her appetite and gaining weight. Her adolescent medicine provider has sent her to the dietitian for a consultation prior to starting the shots.

The medical indications for depo-Provera are appropriate. However, the nutritional complications of DMPA are likely to be problematic. It is clearly established in some women receiving DMPA that their appetites may increase and there is a subsequent weight gain. Should Lisa's appetite increase and she begins to eat voraciously, her bulimic purging behavior may well recur. She needs to know the risks prior to submitting to the shots. A calm supportive discussion with the dietitian of the possible side-effects of depo-Provera would it is hoped, booster Lisa's sense of control. She does need to be cautioned that once she receives the shot, while the contraceptive effect lasts for up to 16 wk, other effects may last for 6–8 mo until the drug completely clears the system.

Guiding the adolescent woman through her choices of hormonal contraceptives can be a daunting task for the clinician and teenager. Whatever the method chosen, the added counseling on the prevention of sexually transmitted disease, including HIV, is mandatory. No hormonal method should ever be prescribed in isolation, but always with the reminder of concomitant condom use.

REFERENCES

1. J. Trussell and B. Vaughan, in *Office of Population Research,* working paper no. 91–12, Princeton University Press, Princeton, NJ, (1991).

2. W. Marsigli, *Fam. Plan. Perspect.*, **19**, 240 (1987).

3. E. F. Jones, J. D. Forrest, N. Goldman, S. Henshaw, R. Lincoln, J. I. Rossoff, C. F. Westoff, and D. Wulf, *Fam. Plan. Perspect.*, **17**, 53 (1985).

4. C. F. Westoff, G. Calot, and A. D. Foster, *Int. Fam. Plan. Perspect.*, **9**, 45 (1983).

5. J. D. Forrest and S. Singh, *Fam. Plan. Perspect.*, **22**, 206 (1990).

6. M. Zelnik and J. F. Kantner, *Fam. Plan. Perspect.*, **11**, 289 (1979).

7. L. S. Zabin, J. F. Kantner, and M. Zelnik, *Fam. Plan. Perspect.*, **11**, 215 (1979).

8. J. Trussell, R. A. Hatcher, W. Cates, F. H. Stewart, and K. Kost, *Stud. Fam. Plan.*, **21**, 51 (1990).

9. F. H. Stewart, F. Guest, G. Stewart, and R. A. Hatcher, in *Understanding Your Body*, (F. Stewart, ed.), Bantam, NY, (1987).

10. H. B. Croxatto, S. Diaz, P. Miranda, K Elamsson, and E. D. Johansson, *Contraception*, **22**, 583 (1980).

11. L. Speroff and P. Darney, *A Clinical Guide for Contraception*, Williams & Wilkins, Baltimore MD, (1992).

12. I. Sivin, *Stud. Fam. Plan.*, **19**, 81 (1988).

13. P. D. Darney, E. Atkinson, S. T. Tanner, S. MacPherson, S. Hellerstein, and A. M. Alvarado, *Stud. Fam. Plan.*, **21**, 152 (1990).

14. M. L. Frank, A. N. Poindexter III, L. M. Cornin, C. A. Cox, L. Bateman, *Contraception*, **48**, L229 (1993).

15. O. Fakeye and S. Balogh, *Contraception*, **39**, 265 (1989).

16. H. B. Croxatto, S. Diaz, D. Robertson, and M. Pavez, *Contraception*, **27**, 281 (1983).

17. J. C. Konje, E. O. Otolotin, and O. A. Ladipo, *Contraception*, **44**, 163 (1991).

18. M. M. Shaaban, S. I. Elwan, M. M. El-Sharkawy, and A. S. Farghaly, *Contraception*, **30**, 407 (1984).

19. K. Singh, O. A. C. Viegas, D. Liew, P. Singh, and S. S. Ratnam., *Contraception*, **39**, 129 (1989).

20. M. M. Shaaban, S. I. Elwan, M. Y. El-Kabsh, S. A. Farghaly, and N. Thabet, *Contraception*, **30**, 421 (1984).

21. K. Abdulla, S. I. Elwan, H. S. Salem, and M. M. Shaaban, *Contraception*, **32**, 261 (1985).

22. M. Bayad, I. Ibrahim, M. Fayad, et al., *Contra. Del. Syst.*, **4**, 133 (1983).

23. M. M. Shaaban, S. I. Elwan, S. A. Abdalla, and H. A. Dawish, *Contraception*, **30**, 413 (1984).

24. World Health Organization, in *Injectable Contraceptives: Their Role in Family Planning*, World Health Organization, Geneva, Switzerland, (1990).

25. K. Fahmy, M. Khairy, G. Allam, F. Gobran, and M. Allush, *Contraception*, **44**, 431 (1991).

26. K. Fahmy, M. Abdel-Razik, M. Shaaraway, G. Al-Kholy, S. Saad, A. Wagdi, and M. Al-Azzony, *Contraception*, **44**, 419 (1991).

27. D. R. Mishell, in *Infertility, Contraception, and Reproductive Endocrinology*, (D. R. Mishell, V. Davajan, and R. A. Lobo, eds.), Blackwell, Cambridge, MA, (1991).

28. I. S. Fraser and E. A. Weisberg, *Med.J. Aust.*, **1** (suppl.), 3 (1981).

29. J. Garza-Flores, D. L. De la Cruz, V. Valles de Bourges, R. Sanchez-Nuncio, M. Martinez, J. L. Fuziwara, and G. Perez-Palacios, *Contraception*, **44**, 61 (1991).

30. T. Cundy, M. Evans, H. Roberts, D. Wattie, R. Ames, and I. R. Reid, *Br. Med. J.*, **303**, 13 (1991).

31. R. H. Mattson, J. A. Cramer, B. V. Caldwell, and B. C. Siconolfi, *Neurology*, **34**, 1255 (1984).

32. R. H. Mattson, J. A. Cramer, P. D. Darney, and F. Naftolin, *JAMA*, **256**, 238 (1986).

33. R. H. Mattson and R. N. Rebar, *Am. J. Obstet. Gynecol.*, **168**, 2027 (1993).

34. K. DeCeular, C. Gruber, R. Hayes, and G. R. Serjeant, *Lancet*, **31**, 229 (1982).

35. J. Jimenez, M. Ochoa, M. P. Soler, and P. Portales, *Contraception*, **30**, 5232 (1984).

36. WorldHealth Organization, *Contraception*, **28**, 1 (1983).

Vegetarian and Other Dietary Practices

CHAPTER

4

Patricia K. Johnston, Dr.P.H., M.S., R.D.
Ella Hasso Haddad, Dr.P.H., M.S., R.D.

INTRODUCTION

The period of adolescence is a time for defining attitudes, shaping personalities, expressing independence, to be accomplished concurrently with physiologic and psychologic maturation. It is often a time for making sometimes rebellious statements in both word and deed and adopting social causes. As in earlier periods of life, one of the ways in which independence is exhibited is through eating, or perhaps not eating.

Adolescence is also a time of particular vulnerability to societal and peer pressure, often reinforced through stereotypical media images. This may be evidenced by conformity in dress, behavior, attitudes, music, and in dietary practices and a variety of other areas. Teens are susceptible to spurious claims and may be caught up in popular fads. They often lack the knowledge and experience necessary to make adequate evaluations of such claims and may adopt ill-conceived diets. Combined with their often irregular eating patterns, these factors may lead to harmful dietary practices that may significantly impact adolescent nutritional status.

ASSESSMENT

Weight Concerns and Dieting Behavior

Abnormal eating patterns are common among adolescents and young adults. However, a recent report suggests that preoccupation with dieting begins much earlier.[1] The survey of 318 boys and girls in grades 3 through 6 found 45% of the children wanted to be thinner and 37% had already tried to lose weight. The percent of girls wanting to be thinner rose from 40% in grade 3 to nearly 79% in grade 6. Similarly, girls reporting they had tried to lose weight rose from 28% in third grade to 59.5% in the sixth grade. Boys reporting they wanted to be thinner increased from 31–41%, but there was no change in the approximate 31% of boys trying to lose weight. Nearly 70% of the children reported that their mothers had dieted at some time. Scores on a children's version of the Eating Attitude Test were within the anorexia nervosa range for 6.9% of the children, matching that reported in the literature for adolescents. The authors suggested that although anorectic eating attitudes may already be set, they are not acted out until adolescence.

Others have also suggested that concern with body image begins before the onset of adolescence.[2,3] Young children have been shown to be aware of their body shape and fatness.[4] As early as 5 yr of age children are apparently motivated to avoid obesity.[5] Thin figures were identified by school-age children as having more friends, being smarter, and being better-looking, than fat ones.[6] Overweight children are considered less likable.[7] Thus, the stage is set early in life for acting out a preoccupation with weight during adolescence.

Body image. The increase in adiposity naturally occurring in females in response to sexual maturation is generally viewed negatively by most girls.[8] As they progress through adolescence, dissatisfaction with their body image and desire for thinness increase.[9,10] Researchers found 90% of one adolescent population wanted to lose weight to improve physical appearance.[11] The aesthetic value placed by contemporary society on thinness may exacerbate the common adolescent dissatisfaction with a changing body configuration.[9] Nonetheless, it has been suggested that adolescent attempts to modify physical appearance and body shape are more than just a response to societal pressures; they are a continuation of earlier efforts to develop a stable body and self-image and to loosen parental ties.[9]

Societal expectations. Society's preference for thinness appears to play a role in adolescent expectations and dissatisfactions. Although the ideal body image of society "has nothing to do with the natural physiological or genetic growth and development of the individual . . . it results in putting presures on children to try to achieve the ideal."[12] The 1981 statement, "The pressure to be thin seems to be on the rise, and increasingly often parents, even physicians, condone and encourage excessive thinness," is unfortunately still true.[13] It is suggested that this overemphasis on thinness may predispose young women to excessive dieting.[14]

Fear of obesity.   Accompanying the pressure to be thin is the societal stigma of obesity.[15] Research has confirmed that adolescent obesity has important social and economic consequences in addition to health risks. A large cohort of adolescents was followed for 7 yr.[16] The researchers found that women who were overweight as adolescents completed fewer years of school, were less likely to be married, had lower household incomes, and had higher rates of poverty than women who had not been overweight as adolescents. These findings were independent of baseline socioeconomic status and aptitude-test scores and appear to represent society's discrimination against overweight persons.

Fear of obesity was recently described in adolescents with short stature and delayed puberty.[17] They did not not meet the inclusion criteria for severe eating disorders, such as anorexia nervosa and bulimia nervosa. Thus, they were considered to have an atypical eating disorder. Concern with obesity persisted in the families even after growth was reestablished in the patients without their becoming obese. Preoccupation with obesity also characterized a larger group of adolescents with nutritional dwarfing and their families.[18] More recently, 51% of underweight girls stated they were "extremely fearful" of being overweight.[19] This fear was expressed regardless of body weight or nutrition knowledge.

Nutritional knowledge among adolescents.   Researchers recently reported that girls had adequate nutrition knowledge, but it had no effect on their attitudes toward eating and fatness.[19] Earlier, adolescent girls who were dieting were reported to have greater nutrition knowedge than nondieting girls.[20] Others found nutrition knowledge could not distinguish students with and without dysfunctional eating attitudes and behaviors.[18]

In order to impact nutrition behavior among adolescents, it will be necessary to begin well before the adolescent years and to go beyond the mere provision of accurate nutrition knowedge. This is no small task in a society bombarded with often spurious nutrition claims, dieting advertisements, health concerns, and the stigmatization of being overweight. It has been reported that girls obtain information about proper weight from references and physicians, but information about weight control comes from family, friends, and magazines.[21] Still developing adolescents and their parents need to be assured that appropriate nutritional intake will result in normal growth without producing obesity.[18]

Dietary behavior.   It is not unexpected that the pervasive expectations of society toward thinness and the unacceptability of obesity would be acted out among adolescents. In addition, the medical evidence identifying high-fat diets as risk factors in chronic disease may influence dietary choices in some.[22] These considerations, as well as a strong desire on the part of some to avoid junk food, play major roles in determining food choices by many individuals, including adolescents and their parents.[18]

INCIDENCE.   Research suggests that dieting is the norm rather than the exception for adolescent females. In the mid-1960s, investigators found that 70–80% of older adolescent girls wanted to lose weight.[20,23] This level of dissatisfaction with weight status has not changed.[24] A recent study classified high school seniors as dieters if they said they had intentionally lost 5 lb or more through dieting.[25] Forty-one % of males and two-thirds of the females met this criterion. Especially disconcerting was the report that as many as 77% of normal-weight girls and 66% of slightly underweight girls wanted to lose weight.[26] Rosen and Gross[27] reported that 63% of high school girls were dieting the day of their survey, compared with only 16% of the boys. The excessive dieting in female adolescents is of particular concern because it may be antecedent to developing eating disorders.[28,29]

A large comprehensive investigation was conducted among Minnesota public school students in grades 7 through 12.[30] These investigators found that 61.9% of the females and 20.1% of the males reported dieting during the previous year. However, because repeated dieting is a risk factor for eating disorders and inappropriate eating behavior, the investigators chose chronic dieting as their main dependent variable. They classified adolescents as chronic dieters if they had been on a diet more than 10 times in the past year or they said they were "always dieting." Among the girls, 12% reported chronic dieting, whereas the figure was only 2.1% for the boys. The percentage of chronic dieters among the girls increased from 7.8% in grades 7 and 8 to 14.3% in grades 11 and 12. Chronic dieters were more likely than other students to report abnormal eating patterns and engage in unhealthful weight-loss methods.

DIETARY MANIPULATIONS AMONG DIETING ADOLESCENTS.   Dieting among adolescents takes many forms. Irregular eating patterns are typical of adolescents and meals are frequently skipped, most often breakfast and second, lunch. Unfortunately, the calories skipped at breakfast and lunch are more likely to be made up during the evening. Some adolescents consume qualitatively inadequate diets and some restrict calories of an otherwise nutritionally adequate diet. Others go to the extreme of fasting. Exercise, diet pills, and self-induced vomiting are other methods used by students to control weight.[31]

The report of 145 patients with nutritional dwarfing and their families is informative.[18] In addition to issues related to obesity, patients and their families were preoccupied with a healthy diet. They avoided dietary fat and reduced their intake of red meat, eggs, and shellfish and they used only low-fat varieties of dairy products. They rarely consumed high-energy junk foods; if anything, snacks were raw vegetables such as broccoli. They preferred high-fiber products and low-calorie foods. They usually skipped breakfast and had only a small lunch. Dinner was a "healthy meal" without excess fat. The patients consumed less food than other adolescents and their caloric intake was insufficient to meet their needs for growth. Their dietary restrictions resulted in low intakes of iron, zinc, calcium, and magnesium.

Although adults regularly frequent various diet and weight-loss centers, it is unlikely that teens use these programs for any length of time because their cost would generally be prohibitive. The literature gives little attention to adolescent use of commercial diet or weight-loss plans, other than SHAPEDOWN, a program specifically designed for overweight teens.[32]

Adolescents appear to follow their own idiosyncratic dietary patterns. However, they may be attracted to novel approaches to weight-loss, especially those promising rapid results, such as some of the commercial liquid diets. Surveys suggest self-imposed diets are followed for only a short time; thus, the risk of serious nutrient deficiencies is reduced.[33] However, chronic dieters are at increased risk of nutrient deficiencies, and because chronic dieting is common among adolescents nutritional adequacy must not be ignored.[34]

Consequences of adolescent dieting.   The adverse health effects of weight-loss may be greater in persons who are not overweight but who severely restrict caloric intake. There appears to be a greater proportional loss of lean body mass in such individuals.[31] Since adolescents frequently try to lose weight even though they are within the normal range, they may be at greater risk for such an outcome. Diet regimens characterized by very low-calorie intake or fasting may lead to rapid weight-loss, but it is primarily water and lean body mass. The body's response to starvation and the loss of lean body mass result in a decrease in basal metabolic rate. Because bingeing is a normal response to semistarvation, dieting may predispose the dieter to an on-going abnormal pattern of eating and consequent weight cycling.[35] Thus, dieting in the adolescent would appear to compound the tendency toward irregular eating behavior.

Chronic dieting among adolescents is associated with unhealthy eating and weight-control behaviors such as binge eating, self-induced vomiting, use of laxatives, diuretics, and ipecac.[30] Health hazards associated with adolescent attempts at weight control or reduction, in addition to an impact on growth, may include nutritional deficiencies, menstrual irregularities, weakness, fatigue, dizziness, depression, persistent irritability, constipation, poor concentration, and sleep difficulties.[18,31,36] Bad breath, loss of hair, and dry skin are frequent side effects of very-low-calorie diets. Increased risk of gall bladder disease is a more serious complication.[31] The immature individual who is still developing is particularly vulnerable to nutritional insults. The period of adolescence is one of increased anabolic needs and thus increased sensitivity to nutritional deficits.[37]

The ultimate nutritional impact depends on timing, duration, magnitude of caloric restriction, and quality of the diet, in addition to other factors. The consequences of inadequate nutritional intake accompanied by poverty are well recognized in the developing world. Less well described are the consequences of voluntarily inadequate dietary choices among adolescents in industrialized countries. Unfortunately, however, poor growth and delayed sexual development as a result of inadequate dietary intake are being recognized with increasing frequency and self-imposed malnutrition is a growing problem.[18] Permanent stunting as a result of compromised nutrient intake has been reported and as many as 39% of those with the atypical eating disorder described above do not achieve catch-up growth.[17,18]

The persistent emphasis of our society on thinness and its characterization of obesity as unacceptable may predispose adolescents, especially young women, to dietary behavior with long-term health consequences. Although the hazards of obesity are well recognized, weight control, especially in an adolescent, may be a more serious health hazard than often assumed.[36]

Vegetarian Dietary Practices Among Adolescents

Overview.   Although the literature contains numerous references to vegetarian preschool children, much less has been published about vegetarian adolescents.[38-40] Some of the studies described below include both adolescent and adult subjects and do not differentiate between the age groups in reporting results. They are included because of the importance of the topic under discussion and its relevance to adolescents.

Vegetarian diets in the context of ecologic, environmental, philosophic, and health concerns provide a ready focus for adolescents. Increasing attention has recently been given in both the popular and scientific literature to issues surrounding the use of animals as food, especially those relating to ecology, the environment, and animal rights.[41,42] The propensity of adolescents to adopt social causes and explore different philosophies may find expression in vegetarian dietary practices.

It has been noted that adolescents appear to be particularly attracted to vegetarian diets, perhaps because of their reaction to animal slaughter or their desire to be thin.[43] Vegetarians have lower average weight than omnivores and adolescents concerned with weight status may emphasize low-calorie vegetables and limit higher-fat animal products, thus adopting a de facto, if not planned vegetarian diet. Vegetarian diets are reported to be associated with lower risk of chronic disease, a factor that may make them attractive to some health-conscious adolescents. The adolescent who abruptly ceases to eat meat can cause considerable consternation within his or her family. The parents' concerned reaction may be just the response desired. Thus, adolescents may adopt vegetarian diets for a variety of reasons.

The varied rationales supporting vegetarian diets give rise to equally varied dietary practices. The term vegetarian, often used to include all types of diets emphasizing plant foods, is not precise enough to be informative about what is actually eaten. Various types of vegetarian diets are described in Table 4.1. It must be recognized, however, that there is great variability even within a particular category and nutritional adequacy depends on not what a diet is called, but the foods that are consumed.[44]

Relationship to anorexia nervosa. The use of vegetarian diets by anorexia nervosa patients to achieve weight-loss has been reported.[45] Huse and Lucas[46] found 15% of 96 patients with anorexia nervosa (mean age of 16.6 yr) were vegetarians and another 9% avoided red meat. No information was given as to the duration of these dietary practices. Others found vegetarian dietary practices to be associated with muscular weakness in two of 12 patients with complications of anorexia nervosa.[47] The weakness was also found in two patients who chronically induced vomiting, but not in patients with food restriction alone or with laxative abuse.

Table 4.1 Vegetarian Diets

Lacto-ovovegetarian	Includes grains, fruits, vegetables, legumes, nuts, seeds, milk, and eggs; excludes meat, poultry, and fish and other seafood.
Lactovegetarian	Includes grains, fruits, vegetables, legumes, nuts, seeds, and milk; excludes eggs, meat, poultry, and fish and other seafood.
Strict, total, or pure vegetarian	Includes grains, fruits, vegetables, legumes, nuts, and seeds; excludes all foods of animal origin.
Vegan	The term vegan is also used to describe total vegetarians. Originally, this term was used to describe persons who refrained from not only eating foods of animal origin, but also using animal products such as leather. The term is often used today to denote someone who excludes all animal products from his or her diet without implication regarding their use of other types of animal products.
Semivegetarian	Includes grains, fruits, vegetables, nuts, seeds, milk, and eggs; usually excludes red meat, but may include small amounts of fish or fowl on limited occasions.
Macrobiotic	Emphasizes whole grains and vegetables, including beans and sea vegetables (seaweeds). Uses only locally grown fruits. Foods of animal origin are limited to small amounts of white-meat fish once or twice a week. This diet may be similar to a vegan diet in its nutritional profile.

The motivation for vegetarian dietary practices among patients with anorexia nervosa appears to not be based on ecologic, environmental, or philosophic concerns. Rather, it is a convenient and socially acceptable way to reduce fat and energy intake.[48] It has also been suggested that avoidance of red meat is another means of striving for self-denial and control, behavior commonly found among patients with anorexia nervosa.[45] Finding vegetarians among anorexia nervosa patients does not necessarily mean that more vegetarians have this disorder, but that those concerned with their weight status use vegetarian diets to achieve their weight-loss goals.[40]

Menstrual function.

MENARCHE.   A 6-mo delay in menarche has been reported in lacto-ovovegetarian (LOV).[49] Further, mean height was lower in preadolescent school girls consuming a LOV diet or eating meat less than once per day compared to omnivore controls.[50,51] However, LOV girls were taller than their omnivore counterparts later in adolescence.[52] It was suggested that the lower height represents a delayed onset of the pubertal growth spurt.[53] This possible delay and later age at menarche appear to indicate a chronological delay in physical maturation that may be of benefit in adult life, particularly in relation to decreased risk of breast cancer.[53,54]

CAROTENEMIA.   Has been described in 10 otherwise healthy, anovulatory women aged 16–31 yr.[55] All were of normal height and weight. None of the women engaged in strenuous physical activity that could explain anovulation. All patients consumed a pure or predominantly vegetarian diet rich in raw vegetables, with no intake of red meat, but some chicken or fish consumed. As much as 0.45 kg (1 lb) of carrots was consumed by some per day, in addition to other vegetables and salads. Patients who were able to modify their diets showed a decrease in serum carotene levels and improved menstrual function.

Carotenemia had previously been reported in anorexia nervosa and menstrual irregularity.[56,57] More menstrual irregularities were recently reported among vegetarian premenopausal women compared to omnivores.[58] Several possible reasons for the difference were suggested. The nature of the relationship between vegetarian diets and/or high dietary carotene and menstrual dysfuntion is unclear, but merits further investigation, and dietary intake should be carefully evaluated in adolescents with menstrual irregularities.

Vegetarian diets among athletes.   Vegetarian or semivegetarian diets have been found among some women athletes experiencing amenorrhea.[59,60] Runners with normal menstrual cycles consumed five times more meat compared with amenorrheic runners; they also consumed significantly more fat. However, the total intake of animal protein was not different due to a larger use of dairy products by the amenorrheic group and both groups used similar amounts of

fish.[59] There were no differences in age, age at menarche, weekly training, and body fat.

Not all vegetarian women athletes are amenorrheic.[60] No significant differences in age at menarche, regularity of menstrual cycles, body weight, or fitness paramenters were found in a comparison of vegetarian and nonvegetarian women atheletes in Israel.[61] A somewhat surprising finding was that the nonvegetarian women had a significantly lower percent of body fat. Vegetarian, or near-vegetarian, diets may be used by athletes to achieve the high carbohydrate intake often recommended for certain types of athletic competition.[61,62]

Anthropometric parameters. The first reports describing the health status of vegetarian adolescents appeared some 40 yr ago. Fifteen male and 15 female vegetarian adolescents and their controls were included in the classic studies of Hardinge and Stare.[63] All subjects were LOV. No significant differences were observed in height or weight for either sex, nor were there differences in blood pressure. Hemoglobin levels were normal in male subjects and controls, but two LOV and three omnivorous females had hemoglobin levels below 12 g/100 mL.

More recently, 8000 children 6 through 18 yr attending Seventh-day Adventist (SDA) and public schools were studied.[64] Seventh-day Adventists are conservative Christians who do not drink alcoholic beverages or smoke. They tend to avoid caffeine-containing beverages and about half follow an LOV diet.[65] Blood pressure was not different in the SDA children compared to the public school children.[64]

Dietary intake and the relation of vegetarian diets to growth were also studied in these children.[40,50,52,53] SDA children were split evenly into three categories of meat consumption: vegetarian, less than once per week; low meat-consumer, once or more per week but less than once per day; medium/high meat-consumer, once or more per day. The vegetarians were virtually all LOV. Over 92% of the public school children had medium/high meat intakes; the remainder had low meat intakes with the exception of one who was a vegetarian.

Age-adjusted regression analysis found the SDA boys were slightly taller than public school boys, but there were no differences between the two groups of girls.[50] The mean height and weight for age for both sexes, in each school group, were at or above national norms. After controlling for height, both SDA boys and girls were leaner than the public school boys and girls. Further comparison of the SDA children by diet group found that the vegetarian girls and boys were both taller than their meat-consuming SDA classmates.[52] A reanalysis of these data using the methods of Tayter and Stanek to study preadolescent children 11–12 yr of age found the LOV girls to be slightly shorter than public school girls as noted previously, whereas there was no difference in height for boys.[51,53] Nonetheless, in later adolescence the LOV girls were taller than the omnivorous girls.[52] These results suggest that lacto-ovovegetarian diets can be compatible with adequate growth in children and adolescents and may be associated with lower weight for height and with lower risk of breast cancer in females in adult years.

   Intake and nutritional status.   Data on food and nutrient intake were also published.[40,50,52] When compared to the public school children, the SDA children as a whole consumed more fruits and vegetables and starchy foods. As would be expected, they consumed less meat and more vegetable protein products. They also consumed less junk foods and, perhaps surprisingly, fewer dairy products and eggs. Analysis showed similar differences in dietary intake between vegetarians and omnivores in SDA schools (Table 4.2).

   As expected from their higher intake of fruits, vegetables, and starchy foods, the vegetarians consumed a greater portion of calories as carbohydrates (Table 4.3). Their intake of calories as protein was similar to that of omnivores, whereas their percent of calories as fat was lower, largely due to decreased intake of saturated fat, which did not exceed 10% of total calories.

   Intake of selected nutrients among younger and older vegetarian and omnivorous SDA adolescents was also reported and is found in Tables 4.4 and 4.5 for males and females.[40] The fact that LOVs were leaner than omnivores may be reflected in their caloric intake that was lower than in the omnivores and also lower than recommendations, except in the 11–14-year-old LOV males. In contrast, the energy intake of omnivorous adolescents was greater than recommendations in both males and females. It was impossible to ascertain the impact of physical activity because these data were not available.

Table 4.2   Frequency of Use (times per month, mean ± SD) of Six Food Groups by SDA and Public School Children in Southern California

	Seventh-Day Adventist		Public School (n=895)
	Vegetarians (n=283)	Omnivores (n=587)	
Meat group	0.6 ± 1.3	40.9 ± 42.5	86.4 ± 56.0
Dairy products, eggs	75.8 ± 31.0	88.9 ± 39.5	92.4 ± 43.4
Fruit and vegetables	140.5 ± 64.6	111.6 ± 60.3	94.5 ± 58.9
Starchy foods	90.3 ± 37.8	81.3 ± 40.2	77.8 ± 45.5
Junk foods	51.7 ± 37.1	74.4 ± 48.4	95.6 ± 62.5
Vegetable protein products[b]	43.6 ± 33.1	27.7 ± 32.0	

*Differences between vegetarian and omnivorous SDA children and between vegetarian SDA children and public school children were highly significant, as were the differences between the entire group of SDA children and the public school children.

†Vegetable protein products were not included in the questionnaire given to public school children.

Adapted from J. Sabate, K. Lindsted, R. Harris, and P. Johnston, *AJDC*, **114**, 1159 (1990) and J. Sabate, K. Lindsted, R. Harris, and A. Sanchez, *Eur. J. Clin. Nutr.*, **45**, 51 (1991).

Table 4.3 Percentage of Calories from Macronutrients in Lacto-ovovegetarian and Omnivorous SDA Adolescents

	Males		Females	
	Vegetarians (*n*=73)	Omnivores (*n*=361)	Vegetarians (*n*=99)	Omnivores (*n*=337)
Protein	14	15*	14	15*
Carbohydrate	55	48†	57	49†
Fat	34	39†	32	39†
Saturated	10	15†	10	14†
Monounsaturated	9	11*	8	11†
Polyunsaturated	6	5*	6	5*

*Difference between vegetarian and omnivorous SDA adolescents, $p<0.05$.

†Difference between vegetarian and omnivorous SDA adolescents, $p<0.01$.

Adapted from P. K. Johnston, E. Haddad, and J. Sabate, in *Adol. Med.: State Art Rev.*, **3**, 417 (1992). Reprinted with permission.

Table 4.4 Dietary Intake of Selected Nutrients in Lacto-ovovegetarian and Omnivorous SDA Adolescent Males

	Ages 11–14		Ages 15–18	
	Vegetarians	Omnivores	Vegetarians	Omnivores
Energy (kcal)	2798 (921)	3256 (1228)*	2829 (1202)	3566 (1230)*
RDA	**2500**		**3000**	
Carbohydrate (g)	381 (120)	389 (167)	379 (165)	416 (163)*
Protein (g)	97 (51)	117 (52)*	9 6 (46)	136 (62)*
RDA	**45**		**59**	
Fat (g)	108 (49)	142 (62)*	113 (55)	156 (61)*
Cholesterol (mg)	300 (246)	440 (293)*	279 (205)	508 (617)*
		1866 (949)*		
Calcium (mg)	1597 (770)	1791 (917)	2040 (996)*	
RDA	**1200**		**1200**	
Iron (mg)	20 (14)	20 (12)	29 (19)	24 (13)
RDA	**12**		**12**	
Zinc (mg)	9.7 (7.3)	14 (8)*	10.3 (5.8)	16 (10)*
RDA	**15**		**15**	

*Difference between vegetarians and omnivores, $p <0.05$.

Adapted from P. K. Johnston, E. Haddad, and J. Sabate, in *Adol. Med.: State Art Rev.*, **3**, 417 (1992). Reprinted with permission.

Table 4.5   Dietary Intake of Selected Nutrients in Lacto-ovovegetarian and Omnivorous SDA Adolescent Females

	Ages 11–14		Ages 15–18	
	Vegetarians	Omnivores	Vegetarians	Omnivores
Energy (kcal)	2131 (738)	2563 (899)*	1654 (683)	2373 (927)*
RDA	**2200**		**2200**	
Carbohydrate (g)	301 (111)	308 (200)	227 (97)	284 (122)*
Protein (g)	70 (24)	94 (43)	53 (20)	85 (43)*
RDA	**46**		**44**	
Fat (g)	78 (35)	111 (45)*	65 (35)	104 (49)*
Cholesterol (mg)	165 (127)	322 (241)*	112 (131)	298 (227)*
Calcium (mg)	1327 (577)	1477 (879)*	862 (394)	1333 (828)*
RDA	**1200**		**1200**	
Iron (mg)	15 (9)	16 (11)	12 (15)	13 (7)
RDA	**15**		**15**	
Zinc (mg)	6.7 (3.3)	11 (8)*	4.9 (2.6)	10 (7)*
RDA	**12**		**12**	

Difference between vegetarians and omnivores, $p < 0.05$.

Adapted from P. K. Johnston, E. Haddad, and J. Sabate, in *Adol. Med.: State Art Rev.*,**3**, 417 (1992). Reprinted with permission.

Recommendations for protein intake were met by both males and females and both LOV and omnivorous females met recommendations for cholesterol intake. Cholesterol intake exceeded recommendations in omnivorous males, whereas intake by LOV males was consistent with recommendations.

Although the intake of macronutrients was in keeping with current recommendations, that of certain minerals was less than optimal among some. The 15–18-year-old vegetarian females consumed only 72% of the RDA for calcium. Reported calcium intake appeared quite high among the adolescent females compared to other more recent reports.[66]

The mean reported intake of iron by the older vegetarian adolescent females was 80% of the RDA. The mean iron intake reported by the omnivores was slightly higher at 86%; however, the mg of iron/1000 cal tended to be higher in the vegetarians (7.04 vs. 6.24 among 11–14-year-olds and 7.26 vs. 5.48 among 15–18-year-olds). Thus, the lower total iron intake by the vegetarians was influenced by their lower caloric intake.

Many studies report normal hemoglobin levels in vegetarians.[67] Some, however, report lower serum ferritin levels and thus lower iron stores.[68,69] Although iron stores can vary widely without any apparent impairment of body function, reduced stores are associated with the increased risk of iron deficiency.[67]

Reported zinc intake was low in the vegetarian adolescents, ranging from 40–

69% of the RDA, whereas the intake of omnivores ranged from 83–107% of the RDA (Tables 4.4 and 4.5). Others have suggested that the diets of some vegetarians may be deficient in quantity of zinc and concern has been expressed relative to its bioavailability from vegetarian diets.[70] Low zinc intake has been reported in vegan females who relied heavily on fruits, salads, and vegetables, all foods that are low in zinc.[71] Higher zinc intake has been reported among LOV adolescents compared to omnivores; however, hair zinc was significantly lower in the vegetarians.[72] Higher dietary fiber intake among the vegetarians was suggested as a reason for the difference in hair zinc. Others have reported that long-term vegetarian adults may adapt to the high-fiber, high-phytate sources of zinc.[73]

Cereals are the primary source of zinc in the diets of vegetarian adults, followed by legumes, nuts, eggs and soy products as secondary sources, and third by dairy products.[74] Flesh foods serve as the primary source for omnivorous adults, followed by cereals.

Because phytic acid (Phy) and dietary fiber are high in the main food sources of zinc in vegetarian diets and both independently inhibit the absorption and/or retention of zinc, it is thought to be less available from vegetarian diets.[74] Calcium appears to potentiate the inhibitory effect of phytate on zinc absorption via a Zn-Ca-Phy complex in the intestinal lumen, further reducing zinc availability, and a [Phy]/[Zn] or [Phy][Ca]/[Zn] ratio has been used to predict zinc bioavailability.[74]

Zinc status is of particular interest because of the role of zinc in growth and concern has been expressed relative to growth in children, especially those on restrictive vegetarian diets.[39,75,76] The low zinc intake reported by the LOV adolescent females (Table 4.5) appears to not have impacted their growth.[52] Whether this was because it was of short duration or the intake data did not represent actual intake or because they had adapted to a lower intake over time is not possible to ascertain.

Nutritional adequacy.   Although there are very few reports about the nutritional adequacy of vegetarian diets for adolescents, the literature has identified certain nutritional concerns associated with the more restrictive vegetarian diets, with special attention given to young children.[38,75] Since adolescence is also a period of growth and nutrient needs are high, it is anticipated that similar nutrient concerns might be present. Nutrients of concern for a particular individual will become apparent when the dietary intake is evaluated, but should not necessarily be extrapolated to other individuals.

ENERGY.   One of the reasons adolescents may be attracted to vegetarian diets is because they often have low caloric density, especially those that exclude all animal products. Because caloric needs are high during adolescence, special attention may need to be given to supplying adequate energy. Those foods that are good sources of energy, such as dried peas and beans, nuts and nut butters, dried fruits, whole grains and seeds, are also good sources for many of the vitamins and minerals. Added fat can supply additional energy; dairy products are also good energy sources for those who use them.

PROTEIN AND AMINO ACIDS.   Although protein adequacy remains a concern in many minds when vegetarain diets are discussed, this concern is generally unfounded.[77] Even with a lower protein intake than omnivores, vegetarians can easily consume enough to meet their needs. It becomes a legitimate concern when energy intake is low and food choices and variety are limited.

The requirement for protein is based on the need for the 20 different amino acids of which protein is made. Nine of these are essential and must be consumed in the diet. The remainder are synthesized by the body. Concern for the protein adequacy of vegetarian diets generally focuses on the differences in amino acid composition between plant and animal proteins. Animal foods such as milk, milk products, eggs, meat, fish, and poultry, contain a mix of amino acids very similar to the needs of the human body. Plant foods generally have limited amounts of one or more essential amino acids. Soy protein is an exception and contains the essential amino acids in a pattern similar to animal foods.

Many studies have shown that animals will not grow adequately when fed a single plant protein, however, appropriate combinations of plant foods produce normal growth.[78] The amino acid deficiencies of one plant food can be corrected by combination with another so-called complementary plant or animal food that contains adequate amounts of the amino acid in question.

Similar kinds of foods contain similar mixes of amino acids. The grains are limiting in lysine and the legumes (dried beans and peas) are limiting in methionine, but each contains adquate amounts of the limiting amino acid of the other to provide complementation. Thus, combinations of these two types of foods provide an appropriate mix of essential amino acids. Indigenous foods eaten around the world commonly contain such combinations: rice and dahl (lentils), corn tortillas and beans, rice and beans, black-eyed peas and cornbread, Boston brown bread and baked beans, peanut butter sandwich, etc.

A frequent concern is whether complementary proteins must be eaten within the same meal. Evidence suggests that this is not necessary.[77] It is known that rice and mungbeans, staples of the Philippine diet, can support growth when fed together, but not when fed alone. Recently it was shown that they can complement each other and support normal growth when fed to animals at alternate meals and at time intervals resembling the eating pattern of humans.[79] Animals grew no differently when the rice and mungbeans were fed at 5-h intervals from when they were fed together, and it did not matter which was fed first.

In addition to dietary sources, digestive enzymes and turnover of the gut mucosa contribute to the pool of essential amino acids available for absorption.

Thus, it is not necessary to combine specific foods within a given meal in order to achieve protein complementation.

Protein is widely distributed in most foods. It is recommended that we obtain 12–15% of our caloric intake from protein. Appendix A.1 shows the percentage of calories as protein found in various foods. The protein content of vegetables ranges from 5–48%, with the root vegetables, such as the yam, having the lowest percentage. Fruits also contain a low percentage of calories as protein. The percentage of calories as protein in grains ranges from 8–16% and in legumes from 22–30%. Meats and dairy products, commonly considered protein foods, contain 20–60% of calories as protein, depending on fat content. The largest percentage of calories in most types of meat and full-fat dairy products comes from fat rather than protein.

The calories and grams of protein in commonly eaten foods are shown in Appendix A.2. Six servings of grains or cereals; one of beans, peas, or nuts; and three of milk or dairy products add up to 60 g of protein, the highest recommended allowance for this age group. Vegans who avoid all animal foods must eat more legumes, nuts, and soy products to substitute for the protein obtained by most vegetarians from milk and other dairy products.

CALCIUM AND VITAMIN D.   The need for calcium and vitamin D to support the development of strong bones and teeth is well recognized. Growing evidence suggests calcium intake during and before adolescence is especially important for females in order to achieve peak bone mass and thus protect against osteoporosis later in life.[80] Evidence also suggests that calcium intakes at or above the RDA may be needed to ensure maximal skeletal calcium retention during the growing years.[81]

The RDA for both genders during adolescence is 1200 mg. This is greater than the average intake of adolescent females. Ingestion of carbonated beverages has increased in recent years, displacing milk as a beverage at mealtimes. An inverse relationship has been shown between soft drink consumption and calcium intake; the greater the soft drink consumption, the less likely teens were to consume adequate calcium.[82] Vegetarians may benefit by consuming fewer soft drinks than omnivorous adolescents. In addition, a large meat intake has been shown to increase urinary calcium excretion.[83] Thus, the lower intake of animal protein by vegetarians may also be an advantage. However, although calcium is found in all plant foods, few other than milk and dairy products have substantial amounts.[84] Recent studies suggest the high bioavailability of calcium from some dark green leafy vegetables, but it is unlikely that adolescents would consume 1–2 cups of cooked greens daily.[84–86] Thus, the total vegetarian adolescent, as well as those at other ages, may be at risk for low calcium intake. They are strongly urged to obtain an adequate calcium intake from a commercially available calcium-fortified milk alternate that is economical, low in fat, and acceptable. The calcium content of commonly eaten foods is found in the Appendix A.3.

Consideration should also be given to obtaining adequate vitamin D. Rickets have been reported among strict vegetarian children living in northern latitudes and low plasma 25-hydroxy vitamin D levels have been reported in a group of adult vegetarians.[87–89] It is especially important for vegetarians with lower exposure to sunlight and possible reduced dermal synthesis to consume vitamin-D-fortified food products. Ideally, the commercial milk alternate used as a calcium source would also be fortified with vitamin D and vitamin B-12.[40,84]

TRACE ELEMENTS.   As noted above, low iron stores have been reported in some vegetarians.[69,70] Nevertheless, the incidence of iron-deficiency anemia is not significantly different in vegetarians compared to omnivores.[67] Recent reports suggest that high blood iron levels are associated with the increased risk of heart disease and colon cancer.[90,91] Thus, the moderate intake associated with well-planned vegetarian diets may be another benefit.

Limited diets based on unleavened, unrefined cereals such as those often consumed in developing countries, are more likely to be associated with iron-deficiency anemia, whereas vegetarians consuming a variety of whole grains, legumes, nuts, and seeds, as well as good sources of vitamin C, should not experience any greater risk of iron deficiency than omnivores.[67] The darker-color varieties of legumes, such as lentils, kidney beans, and black beans, are particularly good plant sources of iron, as are whole-grain and enriched cereal products, leafy green vegetables, winter squash, sweet potatoes, and some fruits.[40] Vegetarian adolescents should be encouraged to include foods high in iron in each meal. Concurrent ingestion of good sources of vitamin C will enhace the uptake of iron and help to ensure adequate iron status.

Zinc intake among vegetarian adolescent females appears to be especially low compared to recommendations (Table 4.5). More than two-thirds of zinc in most American diets comes from animal foods. As noted, cereal products represent some of the richest plant sources of zinc; however, it may be less available due to the high-phytate and fiber content. The adequacy of zinc intake and status should be addressed in all adolescent females, but especially among vegetarians.[40] To be most useful, an evaluation of zinc status must go beyond merely comparing intake with RDAs and include laboratory assessment.[74] Good sources of iron and zinc are listed in Appendix A.4.

VITAMIN B-12.   This vitamin is of special interest to vegetarians, especially strict vegetarians or vegans, because the only practical food sources of this vitamin are those of animal origin. It is of special interest to nutritionists and clinicians because the effects of a deficiency may be irreversible.

Although dietary vitamin B-12 deficiency is extremely rare, it was recently reported in a 14-year-old female.[92] She had been a strict vegetarian for 8 yr, since she had witnessed the slaughter of a cow on her family's farm. She had very low serum B-12 levels and severe neurologic disturbances, but normal B-12 absorption was confirmed by xylose and Schilling tests. Based on these findings and her nutritional history, a diagnosis of dietary deficiency was made. Her parents had not realized the need for this vitamin and her physician was not aware of her diet; consequently, she had received no supplementation. She recovered completely after treatment and began to include some animal food products in her diet.

A number of cases of vitamin B-12 deficiency in infants have been reported in the literature. In contrast to adults, the deficiency developed rapidly in infants breast-fed by vegan mothers.[93,94] Recently, long-term follow-up was reported in several cases of dietary deficiency, as well as deficiency caused by pernicious anemia.[95] Of particular interest is a now 14-year-old male who experienced severe vitamin B-12 deficiency as a 9-month-old infant.[93,95] Although treatment with vitamin B-12 resulted in rapid clinical improvement, neurological recovery was incomplete at 18 mo of age.[93] Follow-up at 12 yr revealed borderline retardation.[95] He was "physically strong and healthy," but "clearly needs some assistance with his educational progress."[96]

These cases illustrate the importance of vitamin B-12 and the possible long-term adverse consequences of a deficiency. Although lacto-ovovegetarian and lactovegetarian diets generally provide adequate amounts of this vitamin, health providers should be alert to the possibility of deficiency in persons following a total vegetarian diet. Neurologic problems may develop before any hematologic evidence of a deficiency.[97,98] Vitamin B-12 status and intake should be investigated in any adolescent who presents with vague neurologic deficits.

There is some confusion about sources of vitamin B-12. The published vitamin B-12 content of foods may be in error because the analytical methods employed did not differentiate between the vitamin and its nonactive analogs.[97,98] Newer methods of analysis using a differential radioassay have shown that food yeasts, seaweed, spirulina, and fermented products such as tempeh may not contribute significant amounts of this vitamin.[97,98] It is imperative that vegetarian adolescents who eat no animal products identify and use a reliable source of this vitamin. Such sources include fortified food products and vitamin supplements.

Health benefits. Although nutritional concerns have been expressed in relation to vegetarian diets, health benefits have also been attributed to vegetarian dietary practices. They are discussed elsewhere.[38,78,99,100] Vegetarians have substantially lower risk of coronary heart disease and lower risk for obesity, as well as several types of cancer. There is evidence that risk is also lower for hypertension, noninsulin-dependent diabetes, and gallstones.

The food intake patterns of vegetarian adolescents reported in Table 4.2 conform more closely than do the patterns of the omnivores to current recommendations to consume more fruits, vegetables, and complex carbohydrates and less junk foods. Further, the distribution of calories among macronutrients in the vegetarian diets is also in keeping with current recommendations of the American Heart Association and others for the prevention of heart disease and is significantly different from the omnivorous diets (Table 4.3).

Vegetarian diets often contain lower total fat, saturated fat, and cholesterol; this may help prevent the development of atherosclerosis that is thought to begin or progress during adolescence. Although Hardinge[101] reported no significant difference in mean serum cholesterol levels between LOV and omnivorous adolescents, others have reported significantly lower levels in adolescents, in keeping with similar studies in adults.[102]

As noted earlier, the possible retarded onset of the growth spurt and delay in menarche may decrease the risk for breast cancer later in life. Thus, a variety of benefits have been suggested for those following vegetarian dietary practices.

MANAGEMENT

The Dieting Adolescent

The dieting adolescent may or may not actually need to lose weight, but in both instances guidance and support are needed. Adolescents may be attracted to the claims made by many commercial products and diet plans for rapid weight-loss. Helping the teen to understand that rapid weight-loss is ineffective in the long-term may be a challenge, but it is nonetheless important.[103] Similarly, chronic dieting is associated with poor outcome. The teen who engages in chronic dieting is likely to experience psychologic barriers to successful weight control and expectations of failure, as well as the physiologic adaptations to periodic limitation of food intake.[34] As noted earlier, weight cycling and, ultimately, weight gain are likely to result from crash diets and chronic dieting.[34]

Teens need to understand the disadvantages of these dieting behaviors and on the other hand, the benefits of healthful eating habits. Dietitians are particularly well equipped to explain the many possibilities of low-fat diets. The greater ease of maintaining normal weight on low-fat diets, as well as the short-and long-term benefits, need to be made clear.

Simplistic conclusions as to nutrient intake cannot be made on the basis of a teen saying she is following a certain commercial weight-loss program, regardless of how well designed or inadequate that program is thought to be. Nor is a simple evaluation of nutrient intake an adequate basis for intervention. Rather, an individualized assessment facilitated by a multidisciplinary team, and including evaluation of both physical status and personal attitude, is necesssary in order for intervention to be appropriately directed to the specific problem areas.[103,104] Useful tools to facilitate a comprehensive evaluation have been described.[103]

Dealing with dieting teens is not as simple as giving a supplement to provide the nutrients deficient in a particular diet. If optimal outcome is desired with the adolescent ultimately taking responsibility for his or her actions, the health professional must be willing to spend the time required to educate and inform, facilitate appropriate short- and long-term goal setting based on a particular situation, and provide strategies for dietary change.[103] Habits are formed over considerable periods of time and it should not be expected that they will be changed quickly. A year or more of intensive treatment may be necessary to facilitate major changes.[103] A comprehensive approach will include food management, exercise and fitness activities, and a psychosocial component providing motivational support, psychotherapy, and individual, family, and group counseling.[103] The dieting teen who is not overwieght is less in need of a weight eduction program than appropriate counseling to help them accept more realistic weight goals.[25]

The Vegetarian Adolescent

Counseling. It is important to recognize that dietary guidelines can be met satisfactorily in many different ways.[99] Further, unusual food patterns are not necessarily harmful.[105] Vegetarian diets may have usefulness for some and should not be considered inappropriate for adolescents. The dietary habits of the adolescent are likely to become the dietary habits of the adult and well-choosen vegetarian diets may provide a healthful foundation for adult eating. Like any diet, they should be well planned.

Vegetarian diets are highly variable and generalizations from the more restrictive to those with a broader intake of foods are not appropriate. As more foods are eliminated from the diet, it becomes increasingly difficult to achieve nutritional adequacy and greater care must be taken to do so.[40] Because the term *vegetarian* is often used rather loosely and the nutritional and medical consequences of a diet depend on not what it is called, but what is eaten, it is important to determine what foods are actually consumed and proscribed from the diet.[40] Careful inquiry and counseling is required.

Although it is always important to establish rapport in counseling, it is perhaps of even greater importance when dealing with vegetarian adolescents. The youthful vegetarian may have faced considerable controversy with parents and other family members. The parents themselves may have many questions and doubts as to the adequacy of the diet their child has suddenly adopted. There also may be disagreements over the philosophic, social, or ecologic rationale behind the new dietary practices.

Appropriate steps in counseling pregnant vegetarians have been outlined and are also applicable with adolescents.[44] A nonjudgmental, supportive environment, respect, and reinforcement of appropriate dietary behavior will help establish rapport and ensure a successful counseling outcome. Parents may need to be reassured that vegetarian diets can provide the nutrients needed to support health, and adolescents may need help in identifying acceptable foods to supply those nutrients.

Registered dietitians can be helpful in assessing dietary adequacy and identifying alternate sources of the various nutrients. Adaptability and creativity may be necessary to modify the usual dietary recommendations in order to meet nutritional needs primarily from plant foods.[40,44] Knowledge of food composition is helpful. Alternate sources of nutrients that may be limited when certain foods are excluded from the diet have been identified and are found in the Table 4.6.

Meal planning.   The same principles in planning vegetarian meals are used in planning omnivorous meals: using a variety of foods; meeting energy needs; limiting intake of nutrient-poor foods, fat, saturated, fat, and cholesterol.[40]

FOOD VARIETY.   The key to achieving an optimal nutrient intake is to eat a variety of foods. Although all foods contain nutrients, they vary in the kinds and amounts and no single food supplies all the nutrients in the amounts needed. Variety assures an adequate intake, especially of trace elements. Variety means selecting foods from each of the food groups every day. It also means selecting different kinds of food from within a particular food group from day to day, week to week, and season to season. And variety means preparing foods in

Table 4.6   Food Choices Providing All Key Elements using a Nonmeat Food Pattern

If you *exclude* these foods	Then you *limit* these nutrients	So *replace* with these foods
Meat	Protein, iron, energy, vitamin	Dairy foods grains, legumes
Fish	B-12, essential fatty acids, zinc	Fortified soy beverage
Poultry		
Milk, dairy foods	Protein, riboflavin, vitamins	Legumes, fortified soy beverage, dark green vegetables
Grains	Protein, iron, calcium, zinc	Legumes, dairy foods
Legumes	Protein, iron, zinc, calcium	Whole and fortified grains, dairy foods, dark green vegetables, nuts, miso, tofu

Adapted from C. M. Trahms, in *Nutrition in Infancy and Childhood*, (P. Pipes and C. M. Trahms, eds.), Mosby, St. Louis, MO, p. 265–287 (1993). Reprinted with permission.

different ways so the nutrients that may be diminished by one method of preparation will be obtained when another method is used.

MEETING ENERGY NEEDS.   Adequate energy intake is necessary to support the continuing growth and activity of adolescents. Providing enough energy will help to assure sufficient intake of the other nutrients. Many animal foods are high in fat and calorically dense, in contrast to plant foods that with few exceptions are lower in calories. Thus, the vegetarian may need to eat larger amounts of plant foods in order to obtain an adequate caloric intake.[40] Plant foods that are high in calories include avocados, olives, nuts, and seeds.

LIMITING FAT AND SUGAR.   Foods high in sugars, fats, and salt and low in vitamins and minerals are often preferred by adolescents and may be consumed in excessive amounts. Sodas, candy bars, cookies, and ice cream are common in adolescent diets, but supply few nutrients other than calories.

Although vegetarian diets tend to be lower in total fat, saturated fat, and cholesterol than omnivorous diets, this is not always true. Some less informed vegetarians remain concerned about protein and overemphasize cheese as a means of assuring adequate protein intake. This, along with large quantities of whole-milk dairy products and fried foods, may result in a vegetarian consuming large amounts of fat and cholesterol. Many of the foods popular among adolescents, such as pizza, French fries, potato chips, and Mexican dishes, are high in fat.[40] A more nutritionally adequate diet and better weight control will result if these foods are limited.

Food guide.   Although substantial evidence suggests vegetarian diets are associated with health benefits, knowledge related to planning a nutritionally adequate vegetarian diet may be lacking. This may be true especially for those who adopt vegetarian diets because of ecologic, environmental, or animal rights concerns. Those who adopt vegetarian or semivegetarian diets for weight control may be knowledgable about the caloric content of foods, but give very little attention to meeting other nutrient needs.

Vegetarian diets are sometimes thought to be difficult to plan. In some cases, little if any planning is undertaken and some vegetarians may simply eliminate animal food products without realizing the need to supply the nutrients, which as a consequence are missing.[92] Meeting nutrient needs on a vegetarian diet need not be complicated or difficult to accomplish.[84]

Food guides and menu patterns are helpful in planning meals; however, the dietary guides that include animal foods are not designed for vegetarian dietary patterns.[84] The development of a food guide system for vegetarians was recently described. The system was designed to be practical and reflect common food practices; it is comprehensive, flexible, and applicable to varied eating styles and situations.[84] It provides guidance for a nutritionally adequate diet that can help reduce the risk of disease. Foods with similar nutrient composition are grouped together and the recommended number of servings needed from the various groups is suggested. The food groups and serving sizes are found in Table 4.7. A description of the foods included and the nutrient contribution of the groups is found in Appendix A.5.

Vegetarian food guide patterns.   Daily dietary patterns were developed for LOV and total vegetarians at different energy levels.[84] They are found in Appendices A.6 and A.7. They illustrate a 2200-kcal pattern for adolescent females and a 2800-kcal pattern for adolescent males. Both the LOV and total vegetarian patterns provide less than 25% of kcal as fat and less than 10% of kcal as saturated fat. These levels of fat intake are achieved if low-fat or nonfat dairy, bakery, and plant protein food items are selected in the LOV diet and mainly lowfat or nonfat milk alternates and vegetable protein foods are selected in the total vegetarian diet.[84] Because of their important contribution to calcium nurtiture, green leafy vegetables are delineated as a separate group in the pattern for total vegetarians.

Nutrient analysis showed that the lacto-ovovegetarian pattern was adequate for all nutrients.[84] The total vegetarian pattern is adequate in most vitamins and minerals if ample amounts of whole grains, legumes, vegetables, and fruits are consumed. However, as would be expected, they are low in clacium and devoid of vitamin D and vitamin B-12 unless fortified foods and/or supplements are consumed.

Menu.   A sample LOV menu based on commonly available foods that are not highly fortified and require little preparation is found in Table 4.8.[40] The servings meet the RDAs for 15–18-year-old males and females, with the exception of zinc that is about 85% of the RDA. A total vegetarian menu can be developed by making appropriate substitutions or changes using appropriate soy products. Less familiar foods used by some vegans are found in Table 4.9.[40]

It is not surprising that the pressures and expectations of society find expression in the dietary practices of adolescents, nor is it surprising, given the issues found in contemporary society, that some adolescents adopt vegetarian diets. The goal of health professionals must be to help them make the most informed choices possible within their individual philosophic frameworks. In order to achieve this, individual dietary practices must be ascertained. A nonjudgmental, supportive environment will facilitate this goal and help assure that the vegetarian adolescent is prepared to make appropriate choices that will provide for nutritional adequacy as well as a healthful diet. Obtaining the needed nutrients is not impossible for those choosing vegetarian diets, but it does become more difficult with more restrictive patterns. Adolescents and their families must be made aware of the implications of dietary choices and provided with alternate nutrient sources should they choose to delete certain food items from their diets. Parents need to be assured, however, that well-planned vegetarian diets can meet the nutrient needs of the adolescent.

Table 4.7   Food Groups and Serving Sizes for Vegetarian Diets

Food Group	Daily Servings	Serving Size
Breads, grains & cereals	6–11	slice of bread ½ cup of cooked cereal, rice, or pasta 1 6-in. tortilla 1 small roll or muffin ½ bagel or English muffin
Legumes	1–2	½ cup of cooked dry beans, lentils, peas, or limas ½ cup of tofu, soy products, or meat analogs
Vegetables, dark green and green leafy vegetables*	3–5	½ cup of cooked vegetable 1 cup of raw leafy vegetables or salad ¾ cup of vegetable juice
Fruits	2–4	1 medium apple, banana, or orange ½ cup of chopped, cooked, or canned fruit ¼ cup of dried fruit ¾ cup of fruit juice
Nuts and seeds	1–2	1 oz of almonds, walnuts, seeds, etc. (¼–⅓ cup) 2 tbsp of peanut butter, almond butter, or tahini
Milk, yogurt, and cheese	2–3	1 cup of low-fat (or nonfat) milk or yogurt and/or 1½ ounces of lowfat cheese ½ cup part skim ricotta
Milk alternatives (soymilk) & tofu*		1 cup calcium vitamins D & B-12 fortified milk alternative: 1 cup of tofu
Eggs	½	Limit egg yolks to 3/wk (may be deleted)
Fats and oils		1 tsp of oil, margarine, or mayonnaise 2 tsp of salad dressing ⅛ avocado 5 olives
Sugar		1 tsp of sugar, jam, jelly, honey, syrup, etc.

*The total vegetarian meal plan must include at least two servings of calcium-rich food items daily such as 1 cup of milk alternative fortified with calcium, vitamin D, and vitamin-B-12; 1 cup of firm tofu, 1 cup of cooked broccoli, 1 cup of cooked greens (collards, dandelion, kale, mustard, etc.).

E. H. Haddad, *Am J. Clin. Nutr.*, **59**, 1248S (1994). Reprinted with permission.

Table 4.8   Sample Lacto-ovovegetarian Menu

Female	Male

BREAKFAST

Female	Male
1 cup of dry cereal sprinkled with 2 tbsp of seedless raisins and, 2 tbsp almonds	1 cup of dry cereal sprinkled with 2 tbsp of seedless raisins and, 2 tbsp almonds
1 cup of 2% milk	1 toasted English muffin with 2 tsp of soft margarine
½ cup of orange juice	1 cup of 2% milk
1 banana	1 cup of orange juice
	1 banana

LUNCH

Female	Male
1 peanut butter and jelly sandwich	2 peanut butter and jelly sandwiches
2 slices of whole wheat bread	4 slices of whole wheat bread
2 tbsp of peanut butter	4 tbsp of peanut butter
1 tbsp of jelly	2 tbsp of jelly
1 cup of carrot sticks	1 cup of carrot sticks
1 cup of low-fat fruit yogurt	1 cup of low-fat fruit yogurt
1 apple	1 apple

SNACK

Female	Male
1 cup of popcorn	2 cups of popcorn

DINNER

Female	Male
1 cup of spaghetti with ½ cup of tomato-mushroom sauce and, 1 tbsp of Parmesan cheese	2 cups of spaghetti with 1 cup tomato-mushroom sauce and, 2 tbsp Parmesan cheese
Salad made with 1 cup of chopped lettuce, ½ cup kidney beans, ½ cup of green beans, and 2 tsp of Italian dressing	Salad made with 1 cup of chopped lettuce, ½ cup kidney beans ½ cup of green beans, and 1 tsp of Italian dressing
1 cup of 2% milk	1 cup of 2% milk
1 pear	1 pear
1 chocolate chip cookie	3 chocolate chip cookies
Energy: 1900 kcal	Energy: 3000 kcal
Protein: 70 g	Protein: 96 g
Fat: 25% of calories	Fat: 25% of calories

Adapted from P. K. Johnston, E. Haddad, and J. Sabate, in *Adol. Med.: State Art Rev.*, **3**, 417 (1992). Reprinted with permission.

Table 4.9 Food Products in Some Vegetarian Diets

Meat analogues	These are foods designed to look and taste like meat. They are made from vegetable protein sources such as soy, wheat gluten, and nuts. Some are textured and flavored to resemble beef, poultry, or franks, and some contain egg albumin or dried milk solids. The nutrient content of these products varies, and one must read the labels to determine their nutritional contribution.
Milk substitutes	These are commercially prepared products that are intended to substitute for milk. Most use soy protein as a base. Must be fortified with vitamins A, B–12, and D, as well as calcium, in order to adequately replace milk in the vegan diet.
Tofu	Tofu is curd or cheese made from the fluid extracted from ground and pressed soybean, which is precipitated with calcium sulfate, sea water, and other substances. It is a good source of calcium if a calcium salt is used in its preparation.
Miso	Miso is a salty paste made of fermented soybeans, wheat, or barley, with salt and water. It is added to vegetable dishes, soup, or rice.
Tempeh	Tempeh is a fermented soy product made by the action of bacteria and mold on cooked soybeans. It is usually sliced and fried and eaten with soy sauce.
Tahini	Tahini is a spread made from sesame seds in the way that peanut butter is made from peanuts. It is mixed with lemon juice (and garlic) to flavor legumes and vegetables.
Textured vegetable protein	Textured vegetable protein is a dried product made from soybeans. It may be used as a meat extender or may substitute for hamburger in composite dishes.
Nutritional or food yeast	Nutritional yeast is grown on a B-12-enriched medium and, as such, may serve as a source of vitamin B-12 in vegan diets. Brewer's yeast does not contain B-12, but is an excellent source of other B vitamins and chromium.

P. K. Johnston, E. Haddad, and J. Sabate, in *Adol. Med.: State Art Rev.*, 3, 417 (1992). Reprinted with permission.

Table 4.10 Dietary Intake of Vegan Male

Morning		Noon		Evening	
Day 1					
Oats uncooked	2 tbsp	Bagel, whole wheat	1	Beans, black, cooked	½ cup
Soy milk	4 oz	Apple	1	Tortilla, corn	1
Banana	1	Banana	1	Spinach, raw	1 cup
Orange	1	Spinach, raw	½ cup	Carrot, raw, shredded	1 cup
Pears	1	Tomato	½ cup	Potato, baked	2
Nuts, pistachio	1 oz	Mushrooms, raw	⅛ cup		
Herb tea	2 cups	Celery	¼ cup		
		Grapefruit	1		
Day 2					
Orange	1	Pear	1	Potato, boiled	3
Pear	1	Bread, whole wheat	1 slice	Endive	2 cups
Banana	1	Banana	1	Carrot	1
Water	2 cups	Lettuce	1 cup	Lemon	½
Tomato	½ cup	Nuts, pistachio	¼ cup	Olive oil	1 tbsp
Day 3					
Oats, uncooked	3 tbsp	Potato	4	Banana	2
Apple juice	½ cup	Tomato paste	½ cup	Bread, whole wheat	3 slices
Nuts, almonds	¼ cup	Spinach	2 cups	Apple, boiled	3 tbsp
Apple	2	Carrot	1	Orange	2
Banana	1	Bread, whole wheat	2 slices		
Orange	1				
Day 4					
Orange	1	Banana	1	Endive	3 cups
Banana	1	Bread, whole wheat	2 slice	Herb tea	1 cup
Oats, uncooked	3 tbsp	Raisins	1 tbsp	Lemon½	
Soy milk	1.5 oz	Dates	3	Olive oil	2 tsp
Nuts, pistachio	1 tbsp	Strawberries	1 cup	Sauerkraut	1 tbsp
Apple	1			Potato, boiled	3
Orange	1			Leeks, boiled	1
				Dates	6
				Coconut	2 tbsp

CASE ILLUSTRATION

The dietary information in Table 4.10 was collected in a 4-d food record by a 23-year-old male participating in a study of total vegetarians. Steve had been a total vegetarian since he was 17 yr of age and had used no animal products since that time. Prior to that, he had never eaten any meat, fish or poultry. The foods listed were typical of his usual food intake. This case illustrates the type of diet followed by some total vegetarians and raises issues of nutritional adequacy.

As is apparent from the nutritional analysis in Table 4.11, Steve's caloric intake was very low, especially for a 23-year-old male. Since he used no animal products, he consumed no cholesterol and his consumption of fat was also very low, contributing to the low energy intake. Total fat intake contributed only 14% of total calories and saturated fat was less than 3% of total calories (Table 4.12).

Steve's heavy reliance on fruits with some vegetables is reflected in the low protein intake. He ate only ½ cup of dried beans or peas in the 4 d. In spite of the low protein intake, he consumed more than 100% of all essential amino acids; however, because of the low energy intake, it might be questioned whether that level of protein is adequate. When protein is low, amino acids are metabolized to supply needed energy, thus decreasing their availability for tissue synthesis and repair.

Table 4.11 Nutrient Analysis of Diet of Vegan Male

	Subject	RDA
kcal	1701	2900
Protein, (g)	40	58
Fat, (g)	29	
Sat. fat, (g)	4.6	
Mono. fat, (g)	14	
Poly. fat, (g)	5.4	
Oleic fat, (g)	13.7	
Linoleic fat, (g)	4.9	
Cholesterol	0	
Fiber, dietary, (g)	48	
Vitamin A, (RE)	3425	1000
Thiamin, (mg)	1.8	1.5
Riboflavin, (mg)	1.2	1.7
Niacin, (mg)	16	19
Vitamin B–6, (mg)	3.8	2.0
Folate, (mg)	500	200
Vitamin B–12	0	2.0
Vitamin C, (mg)	321	60
Calcium, (mg)	447	1200
Phosphorus, (mg)	906	1200
Magnesium, (mg)	490	350
Iron, (mg)	13.8	10
Zinc, (mg)	6.2	15

Table 4.12 Macronutrients as Percent Calories in Diet of Vegan Male

Protein	9%
Carbohydrate	77%
Fat	14%
Sat. fat	2.5%
Mono. fat	7%
Poly. fat	3%

Table 4.13 Selected Nutritional Indices of Vegan Male

	Subject	Normal Values
Hemoglobin	159 g/L	136–172 g/L
Hematocrit	0.46 L	0.39–0.49 L
Serum B–12	122 pmol/L	150–750 pmol/L
Serum MMA	2182 mg/d	<271 mg/d
Serum homocysteine	30.1 mmol/L	<16.2 mmol/L
Cholesterol	3.03 mmol/L	<5.20 mmol/L
HDL	1.19 mmol/L	0.80–1.80 mmol/L
LDL	1.66 mmol/L	1.30–4.90 mmol/L
Triglycerides	0.77 mmol/L	<1.80 mmol/L

Steve used very little soy milk and what was used was not fortified. The lack of such a beverage or other rich source resulted in a calcium intake of less than 40% of the RDA. Similar findings have been reported in other total vegetarians. His phosphorus intake was nearly twice that of calcium. The long-term implications of low calcium intake when protein intake is also low are under investigation.

Low zinc intake combined with a high-fiber intake merit further study. No indices of zinc status were available. The adequacy of iron intake was indicated in his hemoblobin and hematocrit values as found in Table 4.13; however, serum feritin was not available to indicate iron stores.

Steve consumed no vitamin B-12 in the diet and indicated that he took a B-12 supplement on an irregular basis. This is evidenced by his low serum B-12 levels and more dramatically in the very elevated levels of methylmalonic acid and homocysteine in the serum. The latter two are biochemical indices of a functional B-12 deficiency.

The diet reported here would be improved with a greater inclusion of legumes, more whole and enriched cereals and grains, and additional sources of fat, such as nuts and nut butters, olives, avacodos, and added oil. An appropriately fortified soy beverage would contribute calcium and B-12. It is important that a reliable source of vitamin B-12 be identified and used consistently. If the fortified soy beverage is not used, a vitamin supplement is advised.

If suggestions for improving dietary intake are expected to be followed they must fit within an individual's personal convictions and philosophy. Thus, it is esential to determine just what those convictions are and why they are important.

REFERENCES

1. M. J. Maloney, J. M. Guire, S. R. Daniels, and B. Specker, *Pediatrics*, **84**, 482 (1989).

2. R. J. Freedman, *Wom. Health*, **9**, 29 (1984).

3. W. Feldman, E. Feldman, and J. T. Goodman, *Pediatrics*, **81**, 190, (1988).

4. E. Gellert, J. S. Girgus, and J. Cohen, *Genet. Psychol. Monogr.*, **84**, 109 (1971).

5. B. Edelman, *J. Am. Diet. Assoc.*, **80**, 122 (1982).

6. M. B. Harris and S.D. Smith, *Inter. J. Obes.*, **7**, 361 (1983).

7. K. D. Brownell, *J. Am Diet. Assoc.*, **84**, 406 (1984).

8. J. D. Killen, C. Hayward, I. Litt, L. D. Hammer, D. M. Wilson, B. Miner, C. B. Taylor, A. Varady, and C. Shisslak, *AJDC*, **146**, 323 (1992).

9. R. C. Casper and D. Offer, *Pediatrics*, **86**, 384 (1990).

10. R. T. Gross and P. M. Duke, *Ped. Clin. North Am. Adol. Med.*, **27**, 71 (1983).

11. E. D. Rothblum, *J. Psychol.*, **124**, 5 (1990).

12. E. B. Peck and H. D. Ullrich, *Children and Weight: A Changing Perspective*, Nutrition Communications Associates, Berkeley, CA, p.10–11 (1988).

13. H. Bruch, *Can. Psych.*, **26**, 212 (1981).

14. R. H. Striegel-Moore, L. R. Silberstein, and J. Rodin, *Am. Psychol.*, **41**, 246 (1986).

15. A. Yates, *J. Am. Acad. Child Adol. Psych.*, **28**, 813 (1989).

16. S. L. Gortmaker, A. Must, J. M. Perrin, A. M. Sobol, and W. H. Dietz, *N. Engl. J. Med.*, **329**, 1008 (1993).

17. M. T. Pugliese, F. Lifshitz, G. Grad, P. Fort, and M. Marks-Katz, *N. Engl. J. Med.*, **309**, 513 (1983).

18. F. Lifshitz and N. Moses, *J. Am. College Nutr.*, **7**, 367 (1988).

19. N. Moses, M. M. Banilivy, and F. Lifshitz, *Pediatrics*, **83**, 393 (1989).

20. J. T. Dwyer, J. J. Feldman, and J. Mayer, *Am. J. Clin. Nutr.*, **20**, 1045 (1967).

21. S. M. Desmond, J. M. Price, N. Gray, J. K. O'Connell, *J. Youth Adol.*, **15**, 461 (1986).

22. C. J. Key, *Clin. Nutr.*, **6**, 163 (1987).

23. R. L. Huenemann, L. R. Shapiro, M. C. Hampton, and B. W. Mitchell, *Am. J. Clin. Nutr.*, **18**, 325 (1966).

24. D. C. Moore, *J. Am. College Nutr.*, **12**, 505 (1993).

25. L. Emmons, *J. Am. Diet. Assoc.*, **94**, 725 (1994).

26. T. B. Miller, J. G. Coffman, and R. A. Linke, *J. Am. Diet. Assoc.*, **77**, 561 (1980).

27. J. C. Rosen and J. Gross, *Health Psychol.*, **6**,131 (1987).

28. K. M. Allen, D. L. Thombs, C. A. Mahoney, and E. L. Daniel, *J. Sch. Health*, **63**, 176 (1993).

29. P. A. Conner-Greene, *Wom. Health*, **14**, 648 (1988).

30. M. Story, K. Rosenwinkel, J. H. Himes, M. Resnick, L. J. Harris, and R. W. Blum, *AJDC*, **145**, 994 (1991).

31. National Institutes of Health, *Technology Assessment Conference Statement. Methods for Voluntary Weight Loss and Control*, March 30–April 1, (1992).

32. L. M. Mellin, L. A. Slinkard, C. E. Irwin, Jr, *J. Am. Diet. Asso.*, **87**, 333 (1987).

33. G. R. Arrignton, J. Bonner, and K. R. Stitt, *J. Am. Diet. Assoc.*, **85**, 483 (1985).

34. C. L. Rock and A. M. Coulston, *J. Am. Diet. Assoc.*, **88,** 44 (1988).

35. C. W. Callaway and C. Whitney, *The Callaway Diet*, Bantam, NY (1990).

36. M. H. Mallick, *Am. J. Pub. Health*, **73**, 78 (1983).

37. D. M. Paige, *Postgrad. Med.*, **79**, 2233 (1986).

38. J. T. Dwyer, *Ann. Rev. Nutr.*, **11**, 61 (1991).

39. C. Jacobs and J. T. Dwyer, *Am. J. Clin. Nutr.*, **48**, 811 (1988).

40. P. K. Johnston, E. Haddad, and J. Sabate, *Adol. Med.: State Art Rev.*, **3**, 417, (1992).

41. J. Robbins, *Diet for a New America*, Stillpoint Publishing, Walpole, NH, (1987).

42. J. Gussow, *Am. J. Clin. Nutr.*, **59**, 1110S (1994).

43. Nutrition Committee, Canadian Paediatric Society, *Can. Med. Assoc. J.*, **129**, 692 (1983).

44. P. K. Johnston, *Am. J. Clin. Nutr.*, **48**, 901 (1988).

45. R. Kadambari, S. Gowers, and A. H. Crisp, *Am. J. Eat. Dis.*, **5,** 539 (1986).

46. D. M. Huse and A. R. Lucas, *Am. J. Clin. Nutr.*, **40**, 251 (1984).

47. E. Shur, R. Alloway, R. Obrecht, and G.F.M. Russell, *Br. J. Psych.* **153**, 72 (1988).

48. M. A. O'Conner, S.W.W. Touyz, S. M. Dunn, and P.J.V. Beumont, *Med. J. Aust.*, **147**, 540 (1987).

49. D. G. Kissinger and A. Sanchez, *Nutr. Res.*, **7**, 471 (1987).

50. J. Sabate, K. Lindsted, R. Harris, and P. Johnston, *AJDC*, **144**, 1159 (1990).

51. M. Tayter and K. L. Stanek, *J. Am. Diet. Assoc.*, **89**, 1661 (1989).

52. J. Sabate, K. Lindsted, R. Harris, A. Sanchez, *Eur. J. Clin. Nutr.*, **45**, 51 (1991).

53. J. Sabate, M. C. Llorca, A. Sanchez, *J. Am. Diet. Assoc.*, **10**, 1263 (1992).

54. F. De Waard and D. Trichopoulos, *Int. J. Cancer*, **41**, 666 (1988).

55. E. Kemmann, S. A. Pasquale, and R. Skaf, *JAMA*, **249**, 926 (1983).

56. M. A. Pops and A. D. Schwabe, *JAMA*, **205**, 533 (1968) .

57. W. W. Page, *N. Z. Aust J. Obstet. Gynecol.*, **11**, 32 (1971).

58. A. B. Pederson, M. J. Bartholomew, L. A. Dolence, L. P. Aljadir, K. L. Netteburg, and T. Lloyd, *Am. J. Clin. Nutr.*, **53**, 879 (1991).

59. S. M. Brooks, C. F. Sanborn, B. H. Albrecht, and W. W. Wagner, Jr, *Lancet*, **1**, 559 (1984).

60. J. Slavin and J. Lutter, *Lancet*, **1**,1474 (1984).

61. N. Hanne, R. Dlin, and A. Rotstein, *J. Sports Med.*, **26**, 180 (1986).

62. D. C. Nieman, *Am. J. Clin. Nutr.*, **48**, 754 (1988).

63. M. G. Hardinge and F. J. Stare, *Am. J. Clin. Nutr.*, **2**, 73 (1954).

64. R. D. Harris, R. L. Phillips, P. M. Williams, J. W. Kuzma, and G. E. Fraser, *Am. J. Pub. Health*, **71**, 1342 (1981).

65. W. L. Beeson, P. K. Mills, R. L. Phillips, and M. Andress, G. E. Fraser, *Cancer*, **64**, 57 (1989).

66. H. S. Wright, H. A. Guthrie, M. Q. Wang, and V. Bernardo, *Nutr. Today*, **26**, 21 (1991).

67. W. J. Craig, *Am. J. Clin. Nutr.*, **59**, 1233S (1994).

68. A. Locong, *Can. Diet. Assoc. J.*, **47**, 101 (1986).

69. L. S. McKendree, C. V. Kies, H. M. Fox, *Nutr. Rep. Intern.*, **27**, 199 (1983).

70. J. H. Freeland-Graves, *Am. J. Clin. Nutr.*, **48,** 859 (1988).

71. J. H. Freeland-Graves, M. L. Ebangit, and P. S. W. Bodzy, *J. Am. Diet. Assoc.*, **77**, 648 (1980).

72. J. Treuherz, *J. Plant Foods*, **4**, 89 (1982).

73. C. Kies, E. Young, and L. McEnree, in *Nutritional Bioavailabiltiy of Zinc*, (G. E. Inglett, ed.), ACS series No 210, American Chemical Society, Washington, DC, p.115–126 (1983).

74. R. S. Gibson, *Am. J. Clin. Nutr.*, **59**, 1223S, (1994).

75. P. C. Dagnalie and W. A. Van Staveren, *Am. J. Clin. Nutr.*, **59**, 1187S (1994).

76. R. S. Gibson, P. D. Smit-Vanderkooy,and L. Thompson, *Biol. Trace Elem. Res.*, **30**, 87 (1991).

77. V. R. Young and P. L. Pellett, *Am. J. Clin. Nutr.*, **59**, 1203S (1994).

78. S. Havala and J. Dwyer, *J. Am. Diet. Assoc.*, **88**, 352 (1988).

79. A. Sanchez, I. Hernando, G. W. Shavlik, U. D. Register, R. W. Hubbard, and K. I. Burke, *Nutr. Res.*, **7**, 629 (1987).

80. V. Matkovic, D. Fontana, P. Goel, and C. H. Chestnut, *Am. J. Clin. Nutr.*, **52**, 878 (1990).

81. V. Matkovic and R. P. Heaney, *Am. J. Clin. Nutr.*, **55**, 992 (1992).

82. P. M. Guenter, *J. Am. Diet. Assoc.* , **86**, 493 (1986).

83. M. B. Zemel, *Am J. Clin. Nutr.*, **48**, 880 (1988).

84. E. H. Haddad, *Am. J. Clin. Nutr.*, **59**, 1248S (1994).

85.   R. P. Heaney and C.M. Weaver, *Am. J. Clin. Nutr.*, **51**, 656 (1990).

86.   C. M. Weaver, *Am. J. Clin. Nutr.*, **59**, 1238S (1994).

87.   M. Hellebostad, T. Markestad, and K. Seeger-Halvorsen, *Acta Paediatr. Scand.*, **74**, 191 (1985).

88.   J. B. Henderson, M. G. Dunnigan, W. B. McIntosh, A. A. Abdul-Motal, G. Gettinby, and B. M. Glekin, *Quar. J. Med.*, **63**, 413 (1987).

89.   P. Millet, J. C. Guilland, F. Fuchs, and J. Klepping, *Am. J. Clin. Nutr.*, **50**, 718 (1989).

90.   J. T. Salonen, K. Nyyssonen, H. Korpela, et al., *Circulation*, **86**, 803 (1992).

91.   W. E. Willett, M. J. Stampfer, G. A. Colditz, et al., *N. Engl. J. Med.*, **326**, 201 (1992).

92.   S. Ashkenazi, R. Weitz, I. Varsano, and M. Mimouni, *Clin. Ped.*, **12**, 662 (1987).

93.   M. C. Wighton, J. I. Manson, I. Speed, E. Robertson, and E. Chapman, *Med. J. Aust.*, **2**, 1 (1979).

94.   J. J. Doyle, A. N. Langevin, and A. Zipursky, *Ped. Hematol. Oncol.*, **6**, 161 (1989).

95.   S. M. Graham, O. M. Arvela, and G. A. Wise, *J. Peds.*, **121**, 710 (1992).

96.   J. I. Manson, personal communication, (July 2, 1991).

97.   V. Herbert, *Am. J. Clin. Nutr.*, **48**, 852 (1988).

98.   V. Herbert, *Am. J. Clin. Nutr.*, **59**, 1213S (1994).

99.   J. T. Dwyer, *Am. J. Clin. Nutr.*, **48**, 712 (1988).

100.   P. K. Johnston, ed., Proceedings Second International Congress on Vegetarian Nutrition, *Am. J. Clin. Nutr.*, **59**, 1099S (1994).

101.   M. G. Hardinge, H. Crooks, and F. J. Stare, *Am. J. Clin. Nutr.*, **10**, 516 (1962).

102.   J. Ruys and J. B. Hickie, *Br. Med. J.*, **2**, 87 (1976).

103.   J. M. Rees, in *Nutrition In Infancy and Childhood,* (P. L. Pipes and C. M. Trahms, eds.), Mosby, St. Louis, MO, (1993).

104.   Michigan Department of Health, *Toward Safe Weight Loss*, Lansing, MI (1990).

105.   C. M. Trahms, in *Nutrition in Infancy and Childhood*, (P. Pipes and C. M. Trahms, eds.), Mosby, St. Louis, MO, p. 265–287 (1993).

Disease Prevention Among Youth: Atherosclerosis and Hyperlipidemia

CHAPTER

5

Martha R. Arden, M.D., and
Janet E. Schebendach, M.A., R.D.

INTRODUCTION

Hyperlipidemia, elevated blood cholesterol and/or triglyceride levels, is an important risk factor for atherosclerotic heart disease (Table 5.1). Other risk factors include family history, hypertension, smoking, obesity, glucose intolerance, and physical inactivity. It is now clear that reduction of risk-factor levels can lead to a measurable decrease in the incidence of heart disease,[1] and a major public health initiative addressing these risks, the National Cholesterol Education Program, is currently underway in the United States.[2]

The relationship between diet, hyperlipidemia, and subsequent heart disease has received an increasing amount of attention among adolescents over the past several years. Information about nutrition and disease risk is provided by the media, the educational system, public information campaigns, family, and peers. The health care provider sometimes serves as an expert source to a well-informed patient who wants more detailed information.[3] More often, though, the health care provider must correct nutritional misconceptions and myths. This is especially true for nutritionists, nurses, and physicians serving adolescents.

Table 5.1   Mean and 95th Percentile Plasma Lipid Concentrations (mg/dL) Among Adolescents

Age	Cholesterol		Triglycerides		LDL-Cholesterol		HDL-Cholesterol		
	Mean	95%	Mean	95%	Mean	95%	5%	Mean	95%
10–14-YEAR-OLD									
Female	160	201	75	131	97	136	37	52	70
Male	158	202	66	125	97	133	37	55	74
15–19-YEAR-OLD									
Female	158	203	75	132	96	137	35	52	74
Male	150	197	78	148	94	130	30	46	63

Adapted from National Heart, Lung, and Blood Institute, *Lipid Research Clinics Population Data Book, Vol. 1*, NIH Publication Pub. no. 80-1527, Bethesda, MD, (1980).

Importance to Adolescent Health

The clinical manifestations of atherosclerosis, including angina, myocardial infarction and stroke, rarely occur during adolescence or young adulthood. The process of atherosclerosis, i.e., the gradual reduction of arterial diameter, begins in childhood and progresses throughout life.[4] Thus, the presence of hyperlipidemia and other risk factors increases the risk to future health, but the adolescent is essentially unaffected by his or her cholesterol level. The lack of immediate effects of hyperlipidemia makes the job of the clinician even more difficult. With an "occult" process, only evident when laboratory results are obtained, the adolescent feels little motivation to follow recommendations, and there is no pain or illness or other obvious evidence that alerts parents the patient is noncompliant. Thus, professional intervention in adolescent hyperlipidemia hinges on the development of a relationship with the adolescent in which the importance of future health is successfully conveyed.

Associated Morbidities

Hyperlipidemia is most often seen among adolescents with a family history of hyperlipidemia or evidence of atherosclerotic heart disease, and the American Academy of Pediatrics Committee on Nutrition recommends that blood lipid screening be performed only in children with a positive (or unobtainable) family history.[5] Nonetheless, a significant number of adolescents with no known family history have hypercholesterolemia, and some authors advocate measuring blood cholesterol testing on all children and adolescents.[6]

The causes of hyperlipidemia are listed in Table 5.2. Among adolescents with a genetic form of hypercholesterolemia, there are often no associated findings. However, other adolescents have hypercholesterolemia that is more environmental in origin. These teens are often overweight and in poor physical condition.

Hyperlipidemia is occasionally secondary to other conditions, and lipid levels often normalize when the primary condition is treated. Hypothyroidism and drug-induced hyperlipidemia can easily be overlooked if a complete history, physical examination, and laboratory examination are not completed before beginning nutritional treatment.

Although hyperlipidemia is generally asymptomatic in adolescents, physical manifestations are sometimes seen. Cutaneous signs of hypercholesterolemia, including xanthomas (cholesterol deposits overlying tendons and other areas), xanthalasmas (deposits on the eyelids), and corneal arcus (deposits in the iris, resulting in a halo appearance), may be found in adolescents with familial hypercholesterolemia with total cholesterol levels exceeding 300–400 mg/dL. Acute pancreatitis, presenting as an acute abdomen, may occur in adolescents with triglyceride levels exceeding 500 mg/dL.

Table 5.2   Causes of Hyperlipidemia

Primary hyperlipidemia
Hypercholesterolemia (with or without hypertriglyceridemia)
    Familial Hypercholesterolemia
    Familial combined hyperlipidemia
    Mixed genetic-environmental hypercholesterolemia, or "polygenic hypercholesterolemia"
Hypertriglyceridemia
    Familial hypertriglyceridemia
    Familial combined hyperlipidemia
    Familial lipoprotein lipase deficiency
    Familial apoprotein C-II deficiency

Secondary Hyperlipidemia
Endocrine: Diabetes mellitus, hypothyroidism, pregnancy, lactation, exogenous estrogen, exogenous corticosteroids
Renal: Nephrotic syndrome, dialysis, transplant
Hepatic: Biliary cirrhosis or biliary atresia, pancreatitis, alpha–1 antitrypsin deficiency
Connective tissue disease: Systemic lupus erythematosus, Juvenile rheumatoid arthritis, mixed connective tissue disease, dermatomyositis
Drug-induced: Alcohol, thiazides, beta blockers, isotretinoin, estrogens, progesterone, corticosteroids

---

ASSESSMENT

Regardless of the cause or degree, primary hyperlipidemia in adolescents is treated initially by nutritional intervention to decrease the intake of cholesterol, total fat, and saturated fat. In general, the diet of American youth greatly exceeds the current recommendations for intake of cholesterol, total fat, and saturated fat.[7] However, individual intake varies widely, so the diet must be carefully assessed before recommendations are made. Indiscriminate modifications of the diet to decrease cholesterol and fat may also decrease the intake of other essential nutrients.

Public cholesterol-reduction information campaigns are geared to reduce the lipid levels of all Americans, whereas individual treatment is geared toward adolescents with specific risk from hyperlipidemia. The extent of the individual assessment and treatment effort is determined by the specific risk of the individual patient. Overtreatment of an adolescent who is not at particular risk for early atherosclerosis is not cost-effective or warranted, while the broad, public health approach is not adequate for the adolescent at high risk for premature coronary artery disease. A number of variables must be evaluated in the clinical assessment, including physical and psychosocial development, gender, and culture, as well as lipid levels and other determinants of cardiovascular risk (see Table 5.3).

Growth and Development

The physical and psychosocial developmental stages of the adolescent are crucial in the dietary assessment. As is the case with other nutrients, physical growth is the most important factor in determining appropriate intake. In addition to height and weight, the degree of sexual maturation must be considered when assessing intake. The adolescent growth spurt, which occurs early in sexual maturation in females and later in males, is accompanied by significant increases in food intake.

The adolescent's level of psychosocial development is an equally important consideration. During adolescence, children grow into independent adults with individual identities. This growth occurs in three stages, usually referred to as early, middle, and late adolescence. During early adolescence (11–13 yr of age), the separation from parents begins, but the young teen often looks to other adults for guidance. In middle adolescence (14–16 yr), high school students classically reject parents and other adults while deriving their identity and values from peers. By late adolescence (17–21), parental rejection is decreased as self-identity and independence become established.

The clinician must assess an adolescent's level of psychosocial development while assessing the diet in order to determine how much independence the teen has in making dietary choices. This assessment is also critical in order to select

Table 5.3   Completing the Clinical Assessment

Determination of risk
History
  Family cardiovascular history
  Exercise/activity level
  Smoking
  Medications and concurrent illnesses that affect lipid levels and/or cardiovascular risk
Physical examination
  Blood Pressure
  Weight
  Evidence of peripheral lipid deposition
  Signs of other illnesses
Laboratory examination
  Lipid profile
  Others, if indicated, including serum glucose, liver function tests, urine protein, human chorionic gonadotropin

Assessment of Diet
Physical and psychosocial development
Gender, cultural, and ethnic Issues
Appetite, allergies, food preferences, and other factors affecting intake
Assessment of current intake: 24-h recall, food frequency questionnaire, 3-d food record

the appropriate treatment approach. An older adolescent should be assessed and treated independently, whereas a younger teen should be assessed with the family. However, in order to gain an alliance with the early adolescent, the clinician should allow him or her to make independent dietary choices among offered acceptable alternatives. The adolescent from 14–16 yr of age should be interviewed alone after the family assessment is completed. This gives the adolescent a chance to discuss away-from-home eating habits independent from his or her parents, while continuing the family's involvement in meals at home.

Gender, Culture, and Ethnicity

Eating patterns, dietary restrictions, types and methods of preparation of foods, and the extent of interest in food, weight, and healthy eating are influenced by gender, culture, and ethnicity. These factors must be assessed by an individual patient interview including food frequency checklists, dietary recall, and questioning about patterns, restrictions, and nutritional beliefs. For young teens who may have little knowledge of the family's food beliefs, these issues should be carefully explored with the family. The frequency and character of special occasions, school lunches, and other variations from the usual diet should be explored. For teens over the age of 14 yr, an assessment of the extent and type of eating away from the family in social situations is necessary as well. The intake of alcohol and foods that the parents may forbid must be discussed confidentially.

Lipid Levels

Nutritional intervention is recommended for all adolescents with an LDL-cholesterol level exceeding the 95th percentile for age (Table 5.1). The degree of intervention should be based on the extent of lipid elevation and assessment of other cardiovascular risk factors. Adolescents with increased risk require more strict dietary treatment, whereas those without other risk factors may be treated less aggressively.

As the interest in lipid levels has increased over the past several years, an increasing number of primary care physicians have installed cholesterol-testing equipment in their offices.[8] In addition, cholesterol testing frequently occurs at community health fairs and other nontraditional sites. Unfortunately, the transport of testing machines and use of relatively untrained operators may significantly affect the accuracy of values obtained in these settings.[9]

Before nutritional treatment is begun, an accurate fasting lipid profile, including cholesterol, triglyceride, and HDL levels, should be obtained from a clinical laboratory that adheres to the rigorous standardization protocol as recommended by the Heart, Lung and Blood Institute.[10] Needless treatment may be avoided and more accurate data are obtained using a standardized laboratory. In addition, it is preferable to obtain two measurements, at least 1 mo apart, before committing an adolescent to treatment.

Other Cardiovascular Risk Factors

The assessment of cardiovascular risk is made by evaluating the presence of elevated lipid levels and other risk factors including family history, smoking, exercise, obesity, blood pressure, diabetes, and other illnesses. After the presence of increased risk is established and the diet has been assessed, an individualized treatment plan is formulated.

MANAGEMENT

The lipid-lowering diet prescribed for adolescents should be based on the National Cholesterol Education Program (NCEP), which is outlined in Table 5.4.[2] Step 1 guidelines are appropriate for all healthy adolescents and those with increased risk factor levels, such as moderately elevated lipids, hypertension, family history of cardiovascular disease, or obesity. Other risk-factor intervention is provided

Table 5.4 National Cholesterol Education Program Dietary Reccommendations

---

Step 1:
Total fat: ≤ 30% of total calories
  Saturated fat: < 10% of total calories
  Polyunsaturated fat: Up to 10% of total calories
  Monounsaturated fat: Remaining fat calories
Cholesterol: Less than 300 mg/d
Carbohydrates: Approximately 55% of total calories
Protein: 15–20% of total calories
Calories: Sufficient to reach or maintain desirable body weight, growth, and development

Step 2:
Same as step 1, but with saturated fat less than 7% of total calories and cholesterol less than 200 mg/d.

Expert Panel on Blood Cholesterol Levels in Children and Adolescents, *Pediatrics*, **89**(suppl.), 525 (1992). Reproduced by Permission of Pediatrics.

as needed. Adolescents with significant hypercholesterolemia (i.e., exceeding the 95th percentile) on this diet should be advanced to step 2. Because fat intake recommendations are percentages of the total daily caloric intake, age-, development- and gender-specific dietary prescriptions are not required.

Although requirements for essential fatty acids have been defined, Recommended Dietary Allowances have not been formally established for fat or cholesterol.[11] However, deficiencies of essential fatty acids have been reported only in patients on formulas or intravenous feeding lacking these fats or patients with severe malabsorption.[11]

Concern that the unsupervised institution of a fat-restricted diet could lead to failure to thrive and deficiencies of other nutrients continues to proliferate.[12] However, a study of patients in our atherosclerosis prevention center has demonstrated that a medically/nutritionally supervised low-fat diet is adequate in vitamins, minerals, and macronutrients.[13]

Formulating the Treatment Plan

It is inappropriate, and fruitless, to give an adolescent a copy of the NCEP dietary recommendations without individualized counseling. We also do not recommend having adolescents count grams of fat and milligrams of cholesterol in all their food: this is impractical at best and essentially impossible for an adolescent with a normal social life. Table 5.5 outlines the educational model of our nutrition counseling approach, which we believe empowers the adolescent to make appropriate food choices without making lifestyle changes.[14] After teaching the basics, the teen is given specific recommendations for substitutions of

Table 5.5   The Educational Model of Nutritional Counseling

1. Teach how to reduce cholesterol intake.
2. Teach how to reduce total fat intake.
3. Teach how to improve fatty acid balance.
4. Teach how to read and understand food labels.
5. Teach how to make appropriate substitutions.
6. Teach how to dine out.

more acceptable foods based on his or her usual diet as determined by the nutritional assessment. By giving the adolescent concrete suggestions and goals that reflect actual eating patterns, we allow him or her to reduce saturated fat and cholesterol intake with a minimum of disruption and an increased chance of success. Rather than presenting the required dietary changes as a whole, we teach six specific topics sequentially, enabling the teen to gradu ally develop the skills needed to achieve and maintain the NCEP dietary recommendations.

Cholesterol reduction.   The adolescent is first taught the sources of dietary cholesterol. Most patients are surprised to learn that cholesterol is found only in animal sources, and this simple piece of information allows them to lower their intake of cholesterol. In the average American diet, 45% of cholesterol intake is from egg yolks, with another 35% from meat, fish, and poultry and 20% from dairy products.[15] An adequate reduction of cholesterol intake can be achieved by eliminating the intake of "visible" egg yolks (i.e., those in whole eggs and home-prepared recipes); limiting meat, poultry, and fish to 5–7 cooked oz daily (may go up to 9 ounces for adolescent males in growth spurt); and switching to low-fat dairy products, which are also cholesterol-reduced.

Total fat reduction.   Added fats are targeted first: Patients are taught to identify the fats that are added to prepared foods, such as butter, margarine, salad dressing, mayonnaise, cream, and gravy. After becoming aware of these sources of fat, the patient is urged to cut portion size and, when possible, substitute lower-fat products. For example, a teen who typically eats a bagel with a thick layer of cream cheese would be urged to have his or her bagel with a thinner layer of low-fat cream cheese. A number of these substitutions are provided in Table 5.6.

"Invisible" fats are more problematic because they are harder to identify and vary more in the individual diet. Valuable information on hidden fat is uncovered during the evaluation from the food frequency questionnaire and diet records, and specific foods are identified as having excessive invisible fat. In general, we urge patients to limit the intake of fried foods, processed meats, peanut butter and nuts, baked goods, snack chips and crackers, and whole milk and other

Table 5.6 Substitution List

Food	Suggested Substitution
Dairy	
Milk: whole or 2%	Skim milk or 1% low-fat milk.
Whole milk yogurt	Non-fat or low-fat yogurt.
Cream	Evaporated skim milk.
Sour cream	Light or non-fat sour cream.
Whipped cream	Whipped evaporated skim milk.
Cheese	Limited amounts of part-skim cheese with less than 3g of fat/ oz, or nonfat cheese as desired.
Cream cheese	Light or nonfat cream cheese.
Nondairy whipped topping	Whipped evaporated skim milk or nondairy product free of coconut oil, palm and palm kernel oil.
Nondairy milk substitute	Nondairy milk substitute free of coconut oil, palm and palm kernel oil.
Butter	Tub margarine or squeeze margarine, regular or light.
Meats and other entrées	
Bacon	Lean ham.
Salt pork	Lean ham.
Fried foods	Baked, broiled or grilled foods.
Sausage, salami, pepperoni	Lean meats, skinless poultry, fish.
Luncheon meats	Lean sliced meats such as turkey, turkey cold cuts, roast beef, ham.
Frankfurters	Lowfat chicken, turkey, or beef franks.
Pasta with cheese	Pasta with marinara sauce and nonfat cheese.
Pizza	Blot oil, limit portion size and frequency, or homemade with nonfat mozzarella.
Eggs	Eliminate egg yolks, use egg whites and egg substitute as desired.
Peanut butter	Use "all natural" types made from whole peanuts without added vegetable shortening or tropical oils.
Poultry	Skinless poultry.
Snacks	
Chocolate candy	Jelly beans, gum drops, gummy bears, hard candy.
Pie, pastry	Fresh fruit or home-prepared pie or pastry from appropriate ingredients.
Cake	Commercial angel food cake or home-prepared cake and frosting from appropriate ingredients.

continued on next page

Table 5.6 *Continued*

Food	Suggested Substitution
Cookies, crackers	Read labels carefully: Select those without tropical oils, lard, butter, and vegetable shortening from undisclosed oils. Use nonfat products when available. Commercial or homemade cookies from appropriate ingredients (limit portion).
Snack chips	Pretzels or fat-free popcorn.
Ice cream	Nonfat or low-fat ice milk and low-fat frozen yogurt, fruit ice, sherbert (without cream).
Pancakes and French toast	Prepare with egg whites or egg substitute, limit added fat.
Fast food	
Fried fish or chicken sandwich, chicken nuggets, specialty burger, or cheeseburger	Plain burger or grilled chicken sandwich.
French fries, Onion rings	Salad.
Milk shake	Soda or juice.

Adapted from J. Schebendach and L. Beseler, in *Atherosclerosis Prevention: Identification and Treatment of the Child with High Cholesterol*, (M. S. Jacobson, ed.), Harwood Academic Publishers, Chur, Switzerland, pp. 105–134, (1991).

dairy products. Substitutions from Table 5.6 are used to replace these items. In addition, patients are advised to choose lower-fat cuts of meat, skinless poultry, and fish and to trim away all visible fat.

Fatty acid balance.   After reducing fat intake, we concentrate on improving the balance of the different types of fat in the diet, increasing the monounsaturates while decreasing the saturated fats. Many teens are surprised to learn that saturated fats come from both animal and vegetable sources. Patients are taught to avoid products containing tropical oils (coconut, palm kernel, and palm oils), which are the most highly saturated dietary fats, and to select products with higher percentages of monounsaturated and polyunsaturated fats (canola, olive, safflower, sunflower, and corn oils). Consumption of animal fats, which are more saturated than the nontropical vegetable fats, is decreased by portion control of animal products. Because red meats are higher in saturated fat, increasing consumption of skinless poultry and seafood (while continuing to limit portion size), and decreasing the number of red meat meals, is also recommended.

Food labels.   Instruction on the interpretation of food labels is an especially important tool for high school students who have in creased independence and freedom to choose less familiar foods outside the home. The 1990 National

Labeling and Education Act mandated labels that have appeared since mid 1994. Food labels include the list of ingredients in order of content and a panel listing the serving size and calories, fat, saturated fat, cholesterol, sodium, carbohydrate, and protein per serving. Patients are taught to compare fat type and content by checking ingredient lists for tropical oils (often disguised as "vegetable shortening") and checking the number of grams of fat and saturated fat per serving, in order to select healthier choices among comparable products. It is important, of course, to compare serving size when comparing fat and cholesterol content per serving, but the new regulations should result in more realistic servicing sizes.

Substitutions. Armed with the knowledge of the sources of cholesterol, fat, and saturated fat in the diet and with the ability to interpret food labels, the adolescent is encouraged to make acceptable substitutions for foods in his or her usual diet. This should be done in a way that allows variety and flexibility in order to maximize the teen's chance of continuing the dietary changes for a prolonged period of time. Examples of substitutions recommended in our Center for Atherosclerosis Prevention are listed in Table 5.6. Making these substitutions will generally reduce intake to within the step 1 guidelines and, with portion control and more strict avoidance of high-fat foods, will reduce intake to step 2 or 3.

Dining out. Because eating outside the home is a very important part of teen social life, it is crucial to teach the hyperlipidemic adolescent the skills needed for dining out. Most of the information needed to successfully choose appropriate foods will have been presented to the adolescent before this issue is addressed, and in the nutritionist's office, the adolescent often can properly decide between two options presented. However, it is much more difficult for the adolescent to make selections differing from those of friends if he or she is unprepared for this choice. For this reason, our nutritional counseling focuses on choices in specific settings based on the adolescent's usual habits. We typically discuss the proper selections at a fast-food hamburger outlet, pizza parlor, delicatessen, and diner with our adolescent patients, with the offerings of other types of restaurants reviewed as needed. Teens who frequent a particular establishment discuss their options with the nutritionist, and they may choose to bring in a menu for review. Adolescents are urged to choose the lowest-fat items available, limit the portions of high-fat items, and balance higher-fat meals with very low-fat selections the rest of the day.

Evaluating the Treatment Plan

In general, a repeat lipid profile and dietary assessment 2–3 mo after the initial dietary instruction will serve to demonstrate whether the diet has been adequately modified by the adolescent. A decrease of 10–15% in LDL-cholesterol level can be achieved with dietary modification. If a significant decrease in not seen, or the level remains above the 95th percentile, the teen's adherence to the diet should be evaluated by individual interview and 3-d diet records. Further substitutions and, possibly, elimination of a few specific foods may be required in order to meet dietary goals. Because a lower-fat diet is usually lower in calories, it is important at follow-up to check the patient's weight and determine if a conscious effort to increase the caloric intake is required. Conversely, if a patient needs to lose weight, the diet may have to be made more strict than the lipid values would suggest.

Adherence

Deteminants of adherence.   The variables that influence adherence to diet include disease/treatment variables, patient/family variables, and health care provider variables.[16] Disease/treatment variables include the severity of the disease, complexity and frequency of the treatment, and discomfort associated with nonadherence. Since hyperlipidemia is an asymptomatic condition associated with the increased risk of disease in the distant future and is treated with fairly complex decision-making at every meal, the disease/treatment variables against adherence to the therapeutic diet are quite strong.

Patient/family variables include the individual differences in personal and family functioning that can affect one's ability to adhere to a treatment regimen.[16] In addition to the adolescent's level of psychosocial development, which will affect his or her ability to consume a noticeably different diet from peers, the general level of emotional adjustment and self-esteem will also affect the ability to adhere. Family conflict, especially when it is focused on the imposed diet, can further impair adherence, although the availability of social support is an important factor in maximizing adherence.[16] Attitudes and beliefs about the importance of health, seriousness of hypercholesterolemia, and benefits of the therapeutic diet are major factors that the adolescent and his or her family will consider when the food choices are made.

The relationship between the health care provider and patient is critical in the establishment of and continued adherence to a therapeutic regimen, especially when the patient is an adolescent with an asymptomatic condition. The adolescent's perception of the provider's interest and concern, coupled with the provider's efforts to involve the adolescent in the development of the diet, can significantly improve adherence.

Methods to maximize adherence.

EDUCATION.   The physician, nutritionist, or nurse can provide a number of interventions to increase the adolescent's adherence to a cholesterol-lowering diet. Education is foremost, and it should not be limited to dietary guidelines.

In addition to nutritional counseling, the provider must teach the adolescent about the importance of cardiovascular disease and the relationship between diet and health. Specific skills necessary for implementing the diet, including social skills to select foods different from those chosen by peers or to specifically request alternative foods, must be taught and rehearsed. Role-playing, in which the teen practices specific social eating situations, can be useful in helping the adolescent convert theoretical nutritional information into practical eating habits. It is desirable to provide written materials, reinforcing the most important points, after each verbal discussion.

BEHAVIORAL METHODS.   In addition to the educational approach, other strategies may be used to further improve compliance with the therapeutic diet. Positive reinforcement of appropriate food choices by parents or another significant adult is often useful for young teens, but older adolescents may not respond to this approach. However, improved cholesterol values can be an important source of positive reinforcement for patients of all ages. Having parents and other older relatives set a good example, consuming heart-healthy meals and snacks at home and at social occasions, aids the early adolescent adhere to his or her diet. Maintenance of a food diary can be useful for adolescents of all ages who have a tendency to snack frequently, because the act of writing down all intake forces them to be more aware of their foods, allowing them to consider the appropriateness of each item before eating it.

COGNITIVE APPROACH.   Cognitive approaches can be used concurrently with educational and behavioral approaches to help maintain dietary changes once active interventions have ended.[16] The health care provider can help the adolescent develop a positive attitude toward his or her treatment plan by emphasizing the flexibility, rather than the restrictions, of the diet. The health care provider also can contribute to the development of a positive attitude during all patient encounters by conveying realistic expectations, acknowl edging that problems and lapses may occur, but they are not a sign of failure or misbehavior. Problems should be discussed at visits in a positive way, using them as a springboard for further nutritional and skill-building education. The use of phrases with negative connotations, such as "cheating on the diet" or "being bad," must be avoided in order to maintain a positive relationship between the patient and provider, and this attitude should be conveyed to parents as well.

Conclusions

Multiple strategies to promote change in our adolescents' eating habits, which are outlined in Table 5.7, have been endorsed by the NCEP.[2] By promoting a population-based strategy of changing the foods available and spreading awareness of healthier eating habits throughout the adolescent community, individual

Table 5.7   National Cholesterol Education Program Population Strategies

Schools
  School lunchrooms should provide low fat and low cholesterol meals.
  Health education including recommended eating patterns and heart disease
    prevention.
  Physical education to encourage physical activity as a lifelong habit.
  Family involvement to educate parents on healthful eating.
Health professionals
  Health maintenance visits as source of dietary education.
  Community education by health professionals.
Government
  Food labeling regulations to enable consumers to understand contents.
  Food assistance programs that preferentially include healthier selections.
  Public education through federal, state, and local agencies.
Food industry
  Food labeling understandable by adolescents.
  Restaurants and other sources of food outside the home should offer and promote
    more healthful foods.
Mass media should provide accurate, understandable information.

Expert Panel on Blood Cholesterol Levels in Children and Adolescents, *Pediatrics*, **89**(suppl.), 525 (1992). Reproduced by Permission of Pediatrics.

adolescents who have a specific need for dietary intervention will be able to follow a step 1 diet without as much effort as is currently required. In addition, these adolescents will be able to avoid standing out among their peers when these dietary strategies are universal.

In addition to changes in the foods and information provided to adolescents, the future holds scientific advances, such as genetic screening, which will better delineate cardiovascular risk. Improved treatment of the various risk factors is also expected.

Hyperlipidemia is a widespread problem among American adolescents. This problem is being addressed on a population level by the NCEP, but adolescents who are at increased risk for cardiovascular disease because of elevated cholesterol levels require individual intervention as well. Health care providers should address this by recommending individualized dietary changes in the context of the adolescent's developmental, cultural, and dietary history. The dietary recommendations of the NCEP are not particularly difficult for most adolescents to adopt for a brief period of time. Studies have shown, however, that changes are difficult to maintain over the long-term, unless continued reinforcement of the necessary changes and strategies to achieve them is provided. Providers of adolescent health care are in the unique position of being able to help adolescents develop these dietary strategies as they progress from childhood to adulthood, gaining independence over their nutritional and health care choices.

CASE ILLUSTRATION

Robert is a healthy, normal-weight, 16-year-old American male who presented to us after his primary physician found a total cholesterol level of 235 mg/dL on routine screening. After a fasting lipid profile confirmed hyperlipidemia, Robert was referred for evaluation and treatment. He exercises regularly and does not smoke, but his paternal grandfather had a myocardial infarction at age 55 and his 42-year-old father has high cholesterol. The nutritional assessment revealed that Robert's diet was that of a typical, always hungry adolescent male, with breakfast "on-the-run," daily lunches in the school cafeteria, frequent after-school snacks with friends, and dinner at home.

The following menus illustrate the use of the dietary principles discussed, with modifications made to Robert's original eating habits:

ORIGINAL MENU	NUTRITIONAL ANALYSIS*	
Breakfast (on way to school)	Calories:	3659
bagel with 2 tsp of butter	Carbohydrate:	35%
8 oz of whole milk	Protein:	15%
	Fat:	50%
Lunch (school cafeteria)	Mono.:	5%
6 chicken nuggets	Poly.:	18%
1 cup of French fries	Sat.:	23%
8 oz of whole milk	Cholesterol:	516 mg
Chocolate-covered ice cream bar		

Snack (Burger King)
Whopper with cheese
Large order of French fries
Small chocolate shake

Dinner (home)
4 oz of beef brisket
Medium baked potato
½ cup of carrots
1 tsp of butter
8 oz of whole milk

---

* Nutritional analysis was performed on an IBM personal computer using the Nutrition Data System Version 2.3/5A/20 software from the University of Minnesota School of Public Health Nutrition Coordinating Center.

Snack (home)

½ cup of ice cream

The modified menu represents the results of making appropriate substitutions according to recommended dietary guidelines. Notably, the fast food outing and beef dinner are retained.

MODIFIED MENU	NUTRITIONAL ANALYSIS	
Breakfast (on way to school)	Calories:	2699
bagel with 2 tsp of margarine	Carbohydrates:	50%
8 oz of skim milk	Protein:	20%
	Fat:	29%
Lunch (school cafeteria)	Mono.:	13%
3 oz of turkey on large hard roll	Poly.:	3%
2 tsp of mustard	Sat.:	11%
1 cup of French fries	Cholesterol:	264 mg
1 cup of skim milk		
Popsicle		

Snack (Burger King)

2 regular hamburgers

Regular-size order of French fries

Large cola

Dinner (home)

4 oz of flank steak

Medium baked potato

½ cup of carrots

1 tsp of margarine

8 oz of skim milk

Dessert (home)

½ cup of ice milk

It is critical to note that the calorie value of the modified menu is 26% less than the original menu. Although this would be highly desirable for an overweight teen, a normal adolescent such as Robert would have to add a considerable number of extra foods to replace the calories lost when the fat intake was decreased. The following menu, with added foods in addition to the substitutions made above, provides the same number of calories as the original menu, while keeping the fat intake well within the NCEP guidelines. Interestingly, because the total number of calories is increased, the total amount of fat on the menu can also be increased without exceeding 30% of the total calories. This allows even more flexibility.

ISOCALORIC MODIFIED MENU	NUTRITIONAL ANALYSIS	
Breakfast (before school)	Calories:	3612
1 ½ cups of Kix cereal	Carbohydrates:	56%
1 ½ cups of skim milk	Protein:	18%
½ medium banana	Fat:	26%
	Mono.:	11%
Morning snack (at school)	Poly.:	3%
bagel with 2 tsp of margarine	Sat.:	9%
1 cup of orange juice	Cholesterol:	290 mg

Lunch (school cafeteria)
3 oz of turkey on large hard roll
2 tsp of mayonnaise
1 cup of French fries
2 cups of pretzels
1 cup of skim milk
1 popsicle

Snack (Burger King)
2 regular hamburgers
Regular-size order of French fries
Large cola

Dinner (home)
4 oz of flank steak
Medium baked potato
½ cup of carrots
1 tsp of margarine
1 oz of wheat crackers
8 oz of skim milk
½ cup of ice milk

Dessert (home)
8 oz of fruit yogurt (1–2% milkfat)

It is obvious from the differences in the two modified menus that it can be difficult to maintain adequate caloric intake when modifying a very-high-fat original diet. For this reason, weight and growth must be carefully monitored when such extensive changes are made. With on-going individual nutritional counseling, Robert was able to maintain these dietary changes and his weight without excessive difficulty.

Acknowledgements.   The authors thank Nancy Copperman, R.D., for her assistance with the computerized nutritional analysis of the sample menus. The Center for Atherosclerosis Prevention is supported by a generous grant from Irving Schneider.

REFERENCES

1.   D. H. Blankenhorn and H. N. Hodis, *Arterioscler. Thromb.*, **14**, 177 (1994).

2.   Expert Panel on Blood Cholesterol Levels in Children and Adolescents, *Pediatrics*, **89** (suppl.), 525 (1992).

3.   National Heart, Lung, and Blood Institute, *Lipid Research Clinics Population Data Book,* Vol. 1, NIH Publication Pub. no. 80–1527, Bethesda, MD, (1980.)

4.   Pathobiological Determinants of Atherosclerosis in Youth (PDAY) Research Group, *Arterioscler. Thromb.*, **13**, 1291 (1993).

5.   American Academy of Pediatrics, Committee on Nutrition, *Pediatrics*, **90**, 469 (1992).

6.   R. E. Garcia and D. S. Moodie, *Pediatrics*, **84**, 751 (1989).

7.   S. Abraham and M. D. Carroll, *NCHS Advance Data*, **54**, 1 (Feb. 27, 1981).

8.   M. S. Jacobson and D. E. Lillienfeld, *J. Peds.*, **112**, 836 (1988).

9.   B. Schucker and R. H. Bradford, *Clin. Lab. Med.*, **9**, 29, (1989).

10.   H. K. Naito, *Clin. Lab. Med.*, **9**, 37 (1989).

11.   National Research Council, *Recommended Dietary Allowances*, National Academy Press, Washington, DC, (1989).

12.   R. Lifshitz and N. Moses, *AJDC*, **143**, 537 (1989).

13.   N. Copperman, J. Schebendach, M. R. Arden, E. Eisenberg, M. S. Jacobson, *Ped. Res.*, **29**, 89A (1992).

14.   J. Schebendach and L. Beseler, in *Atherosclerosis Prevention: Identification and Treatment of the Child with High Cholesterol*, (M. S. Jacobson, ed.), Harwood Academic Publishers, Chur, Switzerland, pp. 105–134 (1991).

15.   W. E. Connor and S. L. Connor, in *In Coronary Heart Disease: Prevention, Complications, and Treatment*, (W. E. Connor and J. D. Bristow, eds.), J.B. Lippincott, Philadelphia, PA, p. 53 (1985).

16.   L. Altshuler and A. Adesman, in *Atherosclerosis Prevention: Identification and Treatment of the Child with High Cholesterol*, (M. S. Jacobson, ed.), Harwood Academic Publishers, Chur, Switzerland, pp. 135–153 (1991).

PSYCHOSOCIAL ISSUES AND NUTRITION

PART
II

Psychosocial Development

*Rose M. Mays, Ph.D., R.N. and
Donald P. Orr, M.D.*

INTRODUCTION

The second decade of life, the years of 11–20, has been termed the adolescent years. Individuals negotiating this period are confronted with many new and unique challenges. They must adjust to structural and functional changes in their bodies, learn to think in a different manner, and establish new ways of relating to individuals in their environments. By the end of adolescence, most individuals have developed a coherent sense of themselves and taken on responsible adult roles in society.

Adolescence is a complex and exciting time of developmental transition during which one enters as a child and emerges as an adult. It is a critical time for developing health behavior patterns independent from family. The health habits and practices that may have begun in childhood or initiated in adolescence have the potential for not only influencing well-being during this period, but also affecting health later in adulthood.

The needs and behaviors of adolescents presenting for clinical services are at times inadequately understood by providers because of the acceptance of myths, or a tendency to overgeneralize or use one particular phase of adolescence as the standard by which all youth encountered in practice are evaluated. However, in order to make accurate assessments, the clinician must recognize and appreciate the large variability in adolescent development. Those individuals who are *beginning* adolescence are coping with largely different issues when contrasted with those individuals who are in the *final phases* of this developmental transition. As an example, for the young adolescent, adjusting to the physical changes of puberty is typically a primary focus. However, for individuals late in the period, accommodation to the physical changes has usually occurred successfully and the task of becoming independent assuming a career and moving out of the family home becomes the most pressing developmental challenge. An understanding of and respect for the timing and individual variability of developmental changes that occur during the time between childhood and adulthood is a prerequisite for providing individualized health care to youth.

Since the psychosocial challenges that confront adolescents are related to the intellectual and biological changes that take place during this period in the context of specific social environments, this chapter will present an overview of these changes as a background for discussing the chief psychosocial tasks of adolescence and the important social contexts of adolescent developmental change. It is clear that adolescence is part of a continuum from childhood to adulthood. Teenagers do not develop in a vacuum. Neither are the processes and areas we discuss separable. We do so only in an attempt to achieve clarity. In reality, they are carefully interwoven networks of developmental changes often proceeding out of synchrony.

Developmental Changes

Physical.   Adapting to quantitative and qualitative body transformations is one of the first major challenges of the period. During adolescence, individuals continue their physical growth, as they did in childhood, but this growth does not occur at the uniform pace experienced previously. With adolescence, there is an increase in the rate of growth during which the height of an individual may increase by 3–4 in. in a single year.[1] Both the rate of growth during this period and the timing of the onset of this growth are quite variable. Gender differences account for a portion of the variability. Although puberty begins at nearly the same age for boys (mean, 11.5 yr; range, 9.5–13.5 yr) and girls (mean, 11 yr; range, 9–13 yr), on average boys experience their growth spurt at age 14, which is 2 yr later than girls who reach peak height velocity at an average of 12. Aside from gender differences in timing, there remain large individual differences in tempo and quantity of growth so that a group of adolescents of the same age and gender will vary markedly in height. Increases in weight and modifications in the distribution of body fat accompany gains in height; these changes are also variable. Young adolescents must adjust to this rapid yet variable growth.

Adolescents must also adapt to sexual development that produces additional conspicuous alterations in their bodies. Primary and secondary sex characteristics mature due to hormonal changes.[1] For boys there is rapid growth of the penis and testis, growth of genital and facial hair, deepening of voice, and production of semen. Girls experience breast development and growth of axillary and pubic hair, and menarche. Although there is a general predictable developmental sequence for these physical transformations, their onset and rate vary from individual to individual, and from the perspective of the adolescent, these changes are like none previously experienced.

The physical changes of adolescence have indirect psychological and social effects. Adolescents are cognizant of changes in their bodies and the degree to which these changes render them similar to or different from peers. The awareness of physical changes by the adolescent necessitates adjustment of self-perception. As individuals in the social environment (parents, peers, siblings, and teachers) discern growth and sexual changes, they alter their expectations of the adolescent. In turn, the adolescent generally accommodates behaviorally to these expectations. Adolescents' views of themselves are also probably influenced by the broader social environment via such mechanisms as the media.[2]

The hormonal changes that occur with puberty have been found to be associated with changes in emotion and behavior. Although adolescents do experience more negative emotions and more sexual activity than younger children,[3] the effect of hormones on mood and behavior is a complex phenomenon and appears to be moderated by a host of factors including gender, age, pubertal status and timing, temperament, reactivity, genetic differences, and social factors in the environment.[4] Since most studies of hormones and adolescent socioemotional behavior are correlational, at present there are little data to support the thesis that adolescent behavior is singularly determined by biology.

The time of the onset of puberty, in relation to that of peers, appears to have a mixed relationship to psychosocial functioning. Generally, early-maturing boys fare better than their same-age peers in terms of self-image and popularity.[5] Late-maturing boys are seen by their peers as more childish and less likely to be leaders. For girls, early maturation relative to peers seems to be a disadvantage. Early-maturing girls have lower self-esteem and a poorer self-image than late-maturing girls, but are more popular than their peers.[6,7]

The presumed effects of the timing of physical maturation are thought to be due in part to societal response to the adolescent's development. The early-maturing boy is often a more competent athlete, which supports his self-esteem and popularity. The early-maturing girl no longer has the thin body silhouette of a child, which is valued by society, and this is thought to contribute to her dissatisfaction with her self-image.[2] However, both early-maturing females and males are at risk for engaging in more health-compromising behaviors. They are more likely to be sexually active and use a variety of potentially harmful substances.[8,9] Some data suggest that these timing-related differences in health behaviors are no longer present in young adulthood.[9]

Cognitive. The cognitive processes used by adolescents differ from those used in childhood as new cognitive competencies emerge. Compared to younger children, adolescents are no longer bound by concrete referents and begin to be able to think abstractly and in a more complex manner using propositional logic. Adolescents become able to generate hypotheses, consider alternatives and consequences, and take the perspectives of others. According to Piaget,[10] the changes in cognitive function that occur in adolescence are characteristic of the fourth stage of cognitive development termed formal operational thought.

Thinking in this new mode may begin around 11 yr of age but, like most skills, *develops* over time and does not suddenly appear. Inconsistent use of these higher-order thinking skills by adolescents is commonly noted. In fact, inconsistence is common among adults. In addition, because cognition is influenced by the broader psychosocial context, adolescent thinking may have a less mature quality in social environments that are highly stressful or situations in which decisions must be made quickly. It must also be remembered that a significant proportion of the adult population does not attain formal operational thought.

Schroeder and Hunt's[11] notion of conceptual levels is a useful framework for describing cognitive development in adolescence. According to their view, the conceptual level encompasses both cognitive complexity and interpersonal maturity. Individuals at higher conceptual levels process information in a more complex manner, have increased understanding of themselves and others, and are more capable of acting responsibly than individuals at lower levels. As individuals become more cognitively complex, they are described as less immature, unsocialized, dependent, egocentric, and conforming. Positive correlations between age and levels of cognitive complexity have been found, with the majority of adolescents demonstrating more mature cognitions around the age 17 yr.[12] Higher cognitive complexity appears to be protective for adolescents because it is associated with greater resistance to peer pressure, self-management of health behaviors such as independently complying with diabetic regimes, and less engagement in health-risk behaviors.[13,14]

Psychosocial Tasks

Identity. The physical and cognitive changes of adolescence are associated with one of the most important psychosocial tasks of the period, which is consolidating identity. According to Erickson's model of development, consolidation of identity is the fifth of eight psychosocial crises to be resolved during the life span.[15] From an Ericksonian point of view, the successful resolution of the crisis of identity vs. identity diffusion is influenced by the degree of success the individual has had resolving the previous four crises of development. If the individual has established healthy trust, autonomy, initiative, and industry, the complex task of identity development proceeds on a strong foundation. However, if there are major unresolved issues in any of these areas, there may be difficulties with developing a coherent sense of self.

Identity formation is a lengthy and multifaceted process that encompasses not only an individual's ability to define self in a more differentiated and better organized manner, but also decide on and plan for the societal roles he or she will adopt as an adult.[16] Adolescents' more advanced cognitive skills allow them to describe themselves using abstract generalizations, hypothesize about themselves, and recognize that their self-descriptions are dependent on social roles and contexts. The internalization of a sense of one's self that is integrated, realistic, and positive contributes to identity consolidation, is usually completed late in the period for most adolescents.

Autonomy.   Concomitant with changes in physical appearance, cognitive abilities, and self-conceptions, there is a move toward increasing autonomy. Adolescents spend progressively more time away from parents and make more independent decisions as they increase in age. Steinberg[2] classifies adolescent change in autonomy into three different types: emotional autonomy, behavioral autonomy, and value autonomy. Growth in emotional autonomy entails a transformation or modification in the parent-child relationship in which the adolescent becomes more independent and responsible, but also remains emotionally close to parents. Behaviorally, adolescents become increasingly more autonomous as the result of societal expectations, their own improved decision-making skills, and increased susceptibility to social influences outside the family. Development of value autonomy is reflected in adolescents' adopting more mature political, moral, and religious ideas and beliefs.

In past years, the prevailing view of adolescence depicted the typical teen in immense psychological turmoil and extreme conflict with parents. Such turmoil and conflict were thought to be necessary precursors to independence and autonomy. This traditional conception of adolescence was advanced by psychoanalysts whose theories were based on clinical work with disturbed adolescents. Several studies of large numbers of adolescents of varying ages have revealed that, although a minority of individuals in the adolescent years have psychosocial difficulties, the vast majority traverse the period with minimal distress.[2] Adolescent criticism of parents and family conflicts are generally related to routine daily living issues and regarded as the norm for most families.[17] Extreme psychological distress and disturbed family relationships are not normative during any developmental period and, if encountered by the dietitian, should not be dismissed as inevitable consequences of adolescent development.

Social Contexts

The interacting influences of individual developmental growth and the adolescent's environment further contribute to the diversity of developmental outcomes seen in adolescence. Development occurs in an ecological context that both affects and is affected by developmental change in the individual. As a consequence of this reciprocal interaction and the diversity of ecological contexts, individuals probably experience developmental change differently. Families, the institution where the majority of socialization occurs, vary widely in the values they hold and their structure and functioning. Peer groups, which likewise are important socializers of adolescents, also vary in their form and values. Other important sociocultural contexts for adolescents are schools and work settings. Since these contexts may support or inhibit healthy development and health behaviors, an understanding of their nature and influence is important in clinical work with adolescents.

Family.   Optimally, the developmental changes of adolescence prompt a renegotiation or transformation of the parent-child relationship into one in which there is more mutuality or shared decisionmaking. Such family processes allow adolescents to express their opinions and individuality, yet stay connected to parents. Family researchers have found that adolescents develop most competently in family environments that simultaneously promote autonomy and relatedness to family.[18]

Baumrind's work on the relationship of parenting style and adolescent development has highlighted the importance of parenting approaches that are highly responsive to and supportive of individual needs, but demanding and firm.[19] This type of parenting style, which has been termed authoritative, has been associated with more competent adolescents, as reflected by a number of indices such as higher academic achievement, better psychological health, less delinquency, and less problem drug use. Parents classified as authoritative are democratic in their interactions with adolescents, clearly set and consistently monitor standards for behavior, and sensitively time relinquishing control to correspond with adolescents' ability to assume it. However, an authoritative style of parenting may be difficult to consistently execute if parents are stressed by economic hardships, lack of social support, negative life events, or psychological distress.[20,21]

Peers.   As adolescents become more independent, they spend more time with same-age peers or friends. Peer relationships provide important arenas for developing identity, autonomy, and intimacy. Peers may serve as models, provide feedback, and provide an environment for experimentation. The nature of the peer group changes as the adolescent ages. Peers of young individuals consist of small groups of the same sex. Peer groups of those midway in the period are of both genders and by late adolescence the peer group narrows to a dyadic or couple configuration.[22] In addition to being members of peer groups, adolescents are also affiliated with crowds that are much larger reputation-based groups of individuals. Individuals do not necessarily spend much time with a crowd but are categorized by peers based on certain characteristics. Some examples of crowd designations are "jocks," "brains," "nerds," "preppies," and "hard-rockers."

In combination with parents, peer groups serve important developmental functions, but peers also can be a source of negative influence if they practice and model behaviors that endorse health-compromising activities. Younger adolescents are influenced more strongly by peers than older individuals perhaps due to their being less cognitively complex and a stronger need to conform. Adolescents who have nonconformist peers are more likely to participate in a number of problem or health-risk behaviors[23]; however, the causal nature of this relationship has not been clearly established. Individuals may seek out friends who support their deviant behavior rather than be influenced by their peer group to engage in unhealthful activities.

Schools. It is difficult to widely generalize about the influence of schools on the psychosocial development of adolescents because of the variability in school environments and paucity of empirical data. Individuals in this developmental period spend a significant portion of their lives in school. In today's society, a high school education is believed to be a necessary prerequisite for success in most adult roles. In addition to job-related knowledge and skills, schools provide adolescents with opportunities to develop identity, exercise autonomy, and participate in and practice social relationships. However, a large number of adolescents are dissatisfied with school, some to the point of dropping out. Students who leave school are more likely to come from disadvantaged backgrounds, be members of minority ethnic groups, and have histories of poor school achievement and participation.[23]

One characteristic of the school experience that has been documented to affect the psychosocial development of adolescents is school transition or changing schools. Declines in self-esteem, decreases in participation in extracurricular activities, declines in academic achievement, and increases in feelings of anonymity have been observed when adolescents move from elementary to middle schools and from middle to high schools.[24] These effects are most dramatic for younger adolescents and girls. Such transitions are especially challenging to adolescents when school moves coincide with pubertal changes, involve large contrasts in environments (such as going from small, intimate elementary schools to large, impersonal middle schools), or disrupt peer relationships.

Work. Taking on a part-time job is quite common for older adolescents. Thus, the work setting is another influential context for the development of many youth. Most studies examining the developmental consequences of youth employment have researched career- or school-related outcomes and have documented both positive and negative effects. One critical variable affecting the relationship between youth employment and development is the degree of investment in work. When this aspect of work is examined, adolescents who are heavily invested in work (more than 15–20 h/wk) have significantly more negative outcomes than those less invested or who do not work at all.[25]

Overinvestment in work is linked to negative adolescent outcomes in not only achievement-related areas but also activities related to health such as alcohol, smoking, and marijuana use. Previously, data on this phenomenon came from cross-sectional studies; hence, the causal direction of these relationships was unknown. However, recent longitudinal research with a large heterogeneous sample of Wisconsin and California students suggests that the negative consequences that accrue when adolescents work excessive hours are not the result of preexisting behaviors or attitudes, but directly due to adolescent's amount of time at work.[26]

Alienated Youth.   Although most adolescents reside in families and participate actively in school and/or work, a growing number youth do not have the luxury of such supportive developmental settings.[27, 28] Adolescent developmental needs and behaviors may create conflict and tension that challenge family integrity to the point of the adolescent becoming separated or disconnected from family. The environments of youth who are estranged from their families can create threats to healthy development.

There is no typical profile of a homeless adolescent, yet a common characteristic is his or her inability to maintain a supportive living situation at home. An adolescent may be estranged from family because of running away or being asked or forced to leave by parents. Preceding events and circumstances to adolescent homelessness may include verbal and/or physical abuse by parents, parental substance abuse, adolescent substance abuse, school failure, school suspension, adolescent pregnancy, conduct disorder, criminal or delinquent activity, and a generally chaotic homelife. Families' intolerance of gay and lesbian youth's sexual preferences may precipitate homelessness for some adolescents. The family status of these children may be unknown to the major institutions, such as schools, the juvenile justice system, and health care system, whose mission it is to serve them.

To meet survival needs, homeless adolescents without adequate education may engage in activities that may further compromise their healthy development. Some adolescents who are disconnected from their families may drop out of school, use and/or sell drugs, engage in prostitution, steal or become pregnant. Many feel socially isolated and become depressed about their living conditions. Some may gravitate to gangs that have been associated with interpersonal youth violence. In an effort to satisfy basic needs for food, shelter, and clothing, health and developmental growth may be compromised for young persons who are without a stable home environment.

ASSESSMENT

Clinically adolescents present with problems that may have complex biopsychosocial causes. Examining problems within a framework of normative development is helpful for differentiating normal, commonplace behaviors from pathological, aberrant ones. To this end, it is useful to obtain an accurate picture of the adolescent's total lifestyle in addition to data regarding presenting symptoms or concerns. Information about the amount and quality of time spent with parents and peers, school achievement, participation in extracurricular activities, cultural background, general life circumstances, and self-perceptions enables the clinical dietitian to more precisely evaluate nutrition behaviors. Disturbances in eating behavior (excessive or decreased) may be not be the core problem, but a *symptom* of negative social circumstances such as sexual abuse or parental divorce. Eating problems may also be a sign of psychopathology such as depression or the result of deviant behavior such as drug abuse. A through exploration of psychosocial domains enables the dietitian to more accurately frame nutrition problems.

In collecting psychosocial data, it is necessary to directly interview the adolescent regardless of his or her age. Generally, some portions of this interview should be done separately from parents. Adolescents are usually competent, capable historians and rich data obtained can be supplemented or clarified with parental interviews when necessary. However, clinical interviews with adolescents must be carefully *guided* to explicitly explore the various areas of psychosocial functioning. Such guidance is needed because adolescents most always do not comprehend the interrelatedness of different domains or relate psychosocial issues to health problems. For example, during an interview a late adolescent female may not readily disclose information about her college plans if she does not fathom how her decreased appetite may be related to her sadness and disappointment about not being accepted to a prestigious college.

Most adolescents, especially younger teens, benefit from structure when presenting a medical history and during a clinical interview. They often have little or no experience in providing information to a health provider and thus will welcome an initial overview about the array of information that will be discussed and the rationale. This is especially useful in helping them understand when an adult wants to know about sensitive areas such as sexuality, emotions, and substance use. This overview or interview map will reduce anxiety, focus the adolescent and provider on important areas, and increase the adolescent's ability and willingness to provide accurate information.

Adolescents who are alienated or whose primary reference group is the peer group or gang may be particularly lacking in requisite communication skills when being interviewed by the dietitian. Such youth may also be hostile and distrustful of professionals. Open, respectful communication that focuses on the adolescent's strengths and interests is especially helpful in establishing rapport.

MANAGEMENT

Nutritional interventions should be tailored to the adolescent's developmental stage and unique social situation. For example, the management strategy for an obese, prepubescent, 12-year-old whose meals are prepared by her mother should have a decidedly family focus until she achieves greater cognitive complexity and more independence from family relative to food choice and preparation.

From a health education perspective, adolescents are one of the more receptive age groups because of their heightened concerns about physical appearance and cognitive ability to conceptually understand the relationship between nutritional intake and health. Eliciting the adolescents' concerns prior to exploring negative or maladaptive behaviors is key to both understanding the meanings of the behaviors and developing more appropriate and realistic interventions for change. It will also increase the likelihood of obtaining accurate information. Adolescents often make unhealthy nutritional decisions due to inadequate or inaccurate information or being swayed by the media or peers who are poor role models. Adopting a new or different diet may be an appropriate adolescent behavior when it meets developmental needs for trying on new roles or asserting autonomy from parents. However, if that diet is nutritionally unsound, there may be adverse outcomes. Therefore, a major challenge for dietitians who educate adolescents about nutrition is to impart accurate nutritional messages that are psychosocially relevant to the developmental level of that teen.

Youth whose nutritional problems are secondary to alienation from family, parental maltreatment, or mental health difficulties present unique management opportunities. Adolescents disengaged from families are frequently transient and may be encountered by the dietitian in nontraditional facilities such as drop-in centers, emergency overnight shelters, or transitional living programs. These youth may have other health problems or be engaging in health-compromising behaviors that require referrals for care to additional health and social service providers. Adolescents with eating disorders who are being maltreated by their caretakers likewise often require a broad range of services and may also benefit from having a case manager to coordinate needed care. If mental health problems are affecting dietary intake, arrangements should be made for a formal mental health assessment and treatment. Thus, nutritional management will be most effective when developmental and social circumstances are taken into consideration.

CASE ILLUSTRATION

Kelly is a 12-year-old African American female referred because her mother is worried that her daughter has "anorexia." Although her daughter was always a "picky" eater, Kelly's mother became concerned that she was "too skinny" and "not eating enough" approximately 12 mo prior to the present visit. At that time, her tonsils were "enlarged" and a tonsillectomy was recommended. Kelly's mother initially refused onsent for the procedure for unclear reasons but it was performed without complications 6 mo prior to this visit. At that time Kelly weighed 29.5 kg, but her height was not available. Her appetite did not change following surgery.

Kelly's mother reports that her daughter "plays with her food, just pushing it around on her plate" and frequently complains that she is "too full to eat more." Meal times have become confrontational between Kelly, her mother, and grandparents, with whom the family lives. There is continual encouraging, bribing, and at times threats to Kelly to eat "more." Despite repeated family efforts, she refuses to increase her food intake.

Kelly's mother believes her daughter is "just skin and bones" because she is "so small and her ribs stick out. She is just too weak to even open the door. Sometimes she cannot go to school because of it." Kelly has told her mother that she is worried about "getting too fat" and at times thinks her stomach is "too fat." She is also "afraid of getting her period" and would prefer that it not start.

The family history is positive for obesity, hypertension, and type II diabetes. The maternal grandfather was recently found to have prostatic cancer; the extent of disease is unknown. Younger siblings have chronic asthma, "milk intolerance during infancy," and learning disabilities. There is no family history of eating disorders, substance abuse, or depression.

Kelly attends a suburban middle school and is in the sixth grade. She is unhappy at this school because her friends attend the school across the street from her house. The school boundaries were recently changed and she was assigned to a different school than her neighborhood friends. She is currently bused approximately 3 miles. She dislikes school and reports, "kids are mean, they pick on me and tease me." Because of frequent "sore throats, headaches and colds," she has missed an excessive amount of school. Her grades do not seem to have suffered, as she reports receiving A's and B's.

During the interview, Kelly is a very verbal, articulate young adolescent. She readily acknowledges that she "did not want to get fat like the rest of her family" and at times wondered if her abdomen wasn't already "fat." She denies vomiting, laxative use, or regular exercise outside of physical education at school. Kelly reports frequent "nightmares" about "someone hurting me—just like in the scary movies I watch." She also readily admits being scared of things, such as riding the bus, kids at school, and her grandfather's health. She does not want to begin menarche—"it's nasty." She denies sadness, insomnia (other than "bad dreams"), or sexual abuse.

A physical examination of Kelly reveals that her weight is 31.8 kg (10th percentile for her age), height 142 centimeters (15th percentile for her age), body mass index (BMI) 15.8 k/m² (15th percentile for her age), and blood pressure 95/70. She is a petite and pleasant young adolescent. Sexual maturity rating is the following: breasts 3, pubic hair 3. The physical examination is within normal limits.

On initial presentation, it appears that this young adolescent may have anorexia nervosa. She is thin, has eccentric eating patterns with a refusal to alter them, has expressed repeated concerns about becoming obese and pubertal development, and may have some distortion of body image. Her family is overly focused on eating and weight with open conflict between family members about Kelly's nutrition. However, examination of her growth curve indicates that she has continued to grow at the 10–15th percentile. On physical examination, she is both short and thin. Further exploration of her life situation indicates that there is some basis for her concern about obesity in that all family members including her siblings are obese. She, in fact, is the only member of appropriate weight for height. Given this family background (genetic and environmental), she is realistically at risk for obesity. Her anxiety, however, is somewhat exaggerated. In talking with her, it is clear that this level of anxiety related to body weight and pubertal development exists in proportion to her generally heightened state of anxiety and fearfulness. Indeed, she is equally frightened about many things in addition to weight (school, social encounters, intruders, death). The relationships between her and her family are developmentally inappropriate with their attempting to control aspects of her life (eating and bathing) that should no longer be in the forefront. The nutritional evaluation found that she probably consumed approximately 2100 cal/d, sufficient for her weight and height. Her eating patterns were clearly eccentric and used in an attempt to control her family. Nutrition, in the context of growth during early adolescence, was discussed.

Kelly was referred for a more complete psychological evaluation and subsequent psychotherapy. The psychologist agreed that the primary problem related to generalized anxiety and a distorted maternal view of development. This became the focus of treatment in the context of family therapy directed at developing more appropriate patterns of interpersonal relationships and family communications. She continued to grow at the 10–15th percentile.

REFERENCES

1. J. M. Tanner, in *Adolescent Behavior and Society*, (R. E. Muuss, ed.), McGraw-Hill, New York, pp. 39–50 (1990).

2. L. Steinberg, *Adolescence*, 3rd ed., McGraw-Hill, New York, (1993).

3. J. Brooks-Gunn and E. O. Reiter, in *At the Threshold: The Developing Adolescent*, (S. S. Feldman and G. R. Elliott, eds.), Harvard University Press, Cambridge, MA, pp. 16–53 (1990).

4. C. M. Buchanan, J. S. Eccles, and J. B. Becker, *Develop. Psychol.*, **111**, 62 (1992).

5. A. Petersen, *Gen., Soc., and Gen. Psychol. Mon.*, **111**, 205 (1985).

6. D. Blyth, R. Simmons, and D. Zakin, *J. Youth Adol.*, **14**, 227 (1985).

7. R. Simmons, D. Blyth, and K. McKinney, in *Girls at Puberty*, (J. Brooks-Gunn and A. Petersen, eds.), Plenum Press, New York, pp. 229–272 (1983).

8. D. Orr, M. Beiter, J. Ryser, and G. Ingersoll, *Ped. Res.*, **29**, 5A (1991).

9. D. Magnusson, H. Stattin, and V. Allen, *J. Youth Adol.*, **14**, 167 (1985).

10. B. Inhelder and J. Piaget, *The Growth of Logical Thinking from Childhood to Adolescence*, Basic Books, New York, (1958).

11. D. E. Hunt, *Rev. Ed. Res.*, **45**, 209 (1975).

12. D. Orr, C. Brack, and G. Ingersoll, *J. Adol. Health*, **9**, 273 (1988).

13. G. Ingersoll, D. Orr, A. Herrold, and M. Golden, *J. Peds.*, **108**, 620 (1986).

14. G. Ingersoll, D. Orr, M. Vance, and M. Golden, in *Emotion, Cognition, Health, and Development in Children and Adolescents*, (E. Susman, L. Fagans, W. Ray, eds.), Lawrence Earlbaum Associates, Hillsdale, NJ, pp. 121–132 (1992).

15. E. Erickson, *Childhood and Society*, Norton, New York, (1950).

16. S. Harter, in *At the Threshold: The Developing Adolescent*, (S. S. Feldman and G. R. Elliott, eds.), Harvard University Press, Cambridge, MA, pp. 352–387 (1990).

17. R. Montemayor, *J. Early Adoles.*, **3**, 83 (1983).

18. H. Grotevant and C. Cooper, *Hum. Develop.*, **29**, 82 (1986).

19. D. Baumrind, *J. Early Adoles.*, **11**, 56 (1991).

20. J. D. Lempers, D. Clark-Lempers, and R. L. Simons, *Child Develop.*, **60**, 25 (1989).

21. V. C. McLoyd, *Child Develop.*, **61**, 311, (1990).

22. B. B. Brown, in *At the Threshold: The Developing Adolescent*, (S. S. Feldman and G. R. Elliott, eds.), Harvard University Press, Cambridge, MA, pp. 171–198 (1990).

23. J. G. Dryfoos, *Adolescents at Risk*, Oxford University Press, New York, (1990).

24. R. G. Simmons and D. A. Blyth, in *Moving into Adolescence: The Impact of Pubertal Change and School Context*, Aldine de Gruyter, New York, (1987).

25. E. Greenberger and L. Steinberg, in *When Teenagers Work: The Psychological and Social Costs of Adolescent Employment,* Basic Books, New York, (1986).

26. L. Steinberg, S. Fegley, and S. Dornbusch, *Develop. Psychol., **29**,* 171 (1993).

27. J. A. Farrow, *AJDC,* **147**, 509 (1993).

28. U. S. Congress, Office of Technology Assessment, *Adolescent Health Vol. II: Background and the Effectiveness of Selected Prevention and Treatment Services,* U. S. Government Printing Office, Washington, DC, (1991).

Behavior Change and Compliance: The Dietitian as Counselor

CHAPTER

7

Vaughn I. Rickert, Psy..D., F.S.A.M. and
M. Susan Jay, M.D., F.S.A.M.

INTRODUCTION

Population-based surveys suggest that the diets of many adolescents are inadequate.[1-3] For example, many adolescents report skipping meals,[1,2] consuming a large proportion of their total energy requirement from snack foods,[1-3] and engage in preventive dieting.[4] A study comparing skinfold thickness data from 1963–1980 found a 39% increase in obesity among adolescents.[5] Moreover, adolescent females are bombarded with mixed media messages on nutritional intake, dieting, and fitness.[6] The dieting industry has revenues in excess of $30 million dollars and adolescents are key marketing targets.[4] Unfortunately, the dietary behaviors of adolescents do not appear to be related to their nutritional knowledge or developmental needs.[6] It has been suggested that nutritional behaviors are multifactorial and impacted by a variety of sources such as the media, modeling, and social expectations.[6] Thus, the dietary practices of youth require special attention in order to establish sound nuritional patterns that last a lifetime. The dietitian is pivotal to this process in not only providing needed information and education surrounding nutrition, but also as a facilitator of positive health behavior.

123

ASSESSMENT

General Considerations

When approaching the adolescent who may or may not have requested the nutritional consultation, it is important for the dietitian when conducting the nutritional interview to maintain an upbeat and positive approach. Experienced clinicians are well aware that it is difficult to accurately predict the degree of compliance or resistance that an individual teen will demonstrate even with the use of an extensive battery of psychological tests. However, any condition, physical or mental, that interferes with the teen's ability to remember, respond to cues, or carry out complex behaviors will jeopardize the treatment regimen offered by the dietitian. Obviously, youth with underlying psychiatric conditions, cognitive or developmental delays, or learning problems may have difficulties adhering to a detailed proscriptive regimen. Another subset of teens who can present challenges to the nutritional consultant are those who seek nutritional counseling, but have a "hidden agenda." This subset of adolescents is frustrating to the provider because they appear to have the necessary skills and behaviors to comply with preventative and ongoing nutritional regimens, but because of unexpressed pressures, they do not adhere to the dietitian's recommendations. It is imperative that the dietitian assesses who is the "customer" and what the "goals of treatment" are at the onset of the clinical assessment.[7,8]

All too often, the dietitian's customer is the physician who refers the adolescent or parent who accompanies the patient and this places the nutritional consultant in the awkward position of trying to provide treatment to a "resistant" teen. The customer is that individual who is complaining, wanting the behavior to change, or perceives the problem.[7] In the initial interview with the teen, it is important to ask what he or she desires and what the real "problem" is. It is most helpful to conduct a portion of the dietary interview with the teen alone because it provides the opportunity to establish a confidential relationship and allows the dietitian to better differentiate the customer from the patient. The dietitian must be prepared to address the fact with the parents or physician that their goals for behavior change may be unrealistic at the present time. However, changes in the parents' nutrition-related behavior can impact their teen's dietary habits. For example, reducing intakes of sweets may not be important to the teen, but terribly important to the health care provider and parents. The parent influences the adolescent's behavior indirectly by not purchasing these items.

The language that the dietitian employs during the initial assessment can and does affect the perceptions and experiences of the teen's nutritional problem.[7,8] What the dietitian chooses to focus on and how questions are phrased shape the assessment. Avoiding language heavily laden with medical jargon is most helpful.[7] When the teen discloses the problem, it is helpful to restate the problem as a challenge. For example, " When you begin to reduce using table salt, you will experience a lowering of your blood pressure." Finally, the use of the words "will" or "so far" suggest that sometime is the future, things will be improved and this is not viewed by the teen as a major undertakening that must be accomplished immediately. In general, the manner in which questions regarding dietary practices, behaviors, and patterns are asked should be phrased in a nonjudgemental fashion to elicit information about the resources, strengths, and abilities of the teen.

Another basic rule of thumb when asking about behaviors or dietary practices is to phrase questions in an open-ended manner and avoid the use of "yes" or "no" questions.[7] For example, instead of asking, "Were there good things that happened when you increased your exercise program?" ask, "What good things happened when you increased your exercise program?" This allows the dietitian to discover previously used strategies that were effective and accentuate positive health behaviors.

Finally, the dietitian throughout the course of the interview needs to be attentive to determine whether the teen's self-esteem is linked to his or her nutritional problem. For example, consider the teen who repeatedly states that he is "a dieting failure" or she is "anorexic." It is crucial to for the dietitian to separate the disorder from the teen's "persona" and support the teen with this challenge. For example, the dietitian could say to the teen who ackowledges past difficulties adhering to diets, "You have not been successful with dieting in the past" or to the anorexic, "When you weren't overly concerned with weight, what were you like?" The purpose of these statements is to attempt to separate the problem from their persona, so they two are not one in and the same. Other comments such as "welcome to the club," or "that sounds familiar," are all phrases that normalize commonly experienced difficulties. Adolescents as a group are often sensitive and genuinely concerned about being like their peers. Statements that reaffirm their problem as one that is encountered by many adolescents are constructive and reduce their personal fears of being "crazy," different, or a failure.

Interview

During the initial interview with the teen, it is important for the dietitian to spend a few minutes talking with the teen about his or her overall life. This initial conversation can be accomplished by using the HEADS[9] assessment, rather than immediately addressing the reason for the medical or nutritional visit.[7] Conversation about the teen's current school schedule, or movies or music he or she enjoys is helpful to make the teen feel more comfortable. The amount of time spent "talking" depends on how quickly the teen relaxes. If the dietitian feels rushed to complete the assessment, the teen is likely to also experience this feeling and the therapeutic relationship can be significantly jeopardized.

The next phase of the interview is to generate the teen's perception of why a nutritional consultation or assessment was requested.[7] If the teen has requested nutritional assistance, a brief description of the problem is easily generated. On the other hand, when another customer (doctor or parent) has requested the consultation, the role of the dietitian is to extract the adolescent's perception of the problem and whether this is a "true" concern. When there is some agreement between the teen and customer, the clinical dietitian must gain a consensus between both parties. However, the teen's expressed concerns should be given priority. The most difficult situations are those in which the teen has no identifiable concern and fails to see the need for nutrional counseling. For example, an adolescent with an eating disorder is likely to deny that a problem exists and will be resistant to changing daily eating patterns and habits. Obviously, the interview and dietary assessment must continue, but obtaining and developing workable nutritional therapeutic goals are more difficult. However, even in these uncomfortable situations, the teen can be asked to comment about the concerns expressed by others; this may allow the dietitian the opportunity to gain greater insight into working with the adolescent.

Through out the remainder of the assessment, the clinical dietitian needs to listen with a good "ear" in order to detect any nutritional concerns that might serve as short-term target goals that the teen may be interested in solving. In this way, the teen becomes the customer and is a willing participant in the "change" process. Using statements such as "humor me," or "I know you don't think this is a problem, but I need to get a better understanding of why others may see this as a concern," often will allow the clinician to obtain needed dietary information.

The most extreme situation occurs when the teen refuses to talk with the dietitian. In this scenario, it is advisable for the dietitian to invite the parent, who is the likely customer, to join the interview process. Normally, the dietitian will interview the teen privately, but in these situations, the parent is the only remaining and available information source. It is appropriate to tell the teen that you are going to invite the parent to join in order to understand his or her nutritional concerns. During the remainder of the interview, the dietitian should attempt to gain confirmation from the teen about what the parent has disclosed. Often, the teen will begin to respond to what the parent has said, allowing the dietitian to seek clarification of the teen's dietary history, family concerns, and related mental health issues. It may be necessary to defer dietary intervention until family conflicts and related mental health problems can be addressed by another health care provider, i.e., psychologist, social worker, or psychiatrist. Although the dietitian may not want to spend an excessive amount of time in this phase of the interview, this inquiry often helps the dietitian to formulate hypotheses about workable nutritional therapeutic goals.

Most of the interview is devoted to finding when "exceptions" to the nutritional problem occur.[7,8] Regardless of the magnitude or chronicity of the dietary patterns and behaviors, there are or have been times or situations during which the behavior does or did not occur.[7] For example, even the most severe anorectic eats something she felt was forbidden or the teen with diabetes does not eat a real candy bar. The dietitian needs to amplify and expand on these situations because they offer tremendous information about what is needed in order to solve the presenting problem. Strategies can be discovered by examining the differences between times when the problem occurs and times when it has not. The "exception" question can catch the teen off-guard because he or she does not expect to disclose positive happenings. The focus of this phase is to demonstrate to the teen what has worked in the past and to orient the possibility for change in the future. The following series of questions illustrate how to elicit information about these exceptional situations:[7]

1. What is different about the times when _____ (you are able to reduce snacking between meals, you are able to eat more than half a cheese sandwich, etc.)?
2. How did you get that to happen?
3. How does it make your day go differently when _____ (the exception happened)?
4. Who else noticed that _____ (you lost 10 lb, you had energy, were in a better mood)? In what way could you tell that they noticed; what did they say or do?

These series of questions provide the opportunity for the dietitian to discover differences between problematic and nonproblematic situations.[7,8] Some teens may be unable to immediately recall exceptions, but if the dietitian persists, most can describe one or more situations in which their nutritional behaviors were either healthy or appropriate. Moreover, these questions and responses are the beginnings of identifying workable goals.[7] The dietitian might ask, " When you were eating three meals per day" vs. "When you were just eating once per day." Once the slightest exception is expressed, the dietitian needs to congratulate the teen for overcoming the problem on this occasion. The next question allows the teen to recall other events and feelings that were associated with this change. The purpose of the third question is to demonstrate how nutritionally related behaviors may affect other areas of the teen's life. If during the course of the assessment, there are other family members present, each individual, in turn, should be asked to comment on this question.

These series of questions are particularly useful for the teen who has been referred for nutritional noncompliance. Traditionally, there are three general reasons for noncompliant behavior. These include lack of skill or knowledge, thoughts or beliefs that interfere with adherence, and environmental factors that support noncompliance. The use of these exception questions allows the dietitian to focus on positive behaviors and enumerates the resources and strengths of the teen. In addition, the responses provide valuable information about how the teen overcame environmental barriers to solve his or her problem. The dietitian can asked two additional questions if the teen expresses a pattern or cycle of nutritional behaviors.[7] The first question is phrased, "How did you _____ (follow your diet that day, allow yourself to eat more than you had planned)? In other words, how did the teen make a change from a noncompliant behavior pattern to a pattern of adherence. Compliance should be viewed as a continuum where adherence varies daily. Thus, the identification of clear times when the teen has voluntary ended noncompliance demonstrates the connection between something the teen did with something he or she could do, and the cessation of unpleasant consequences. For the noncompliant teen, he or she may have "found" something new or different that day which helped the teen adhere to a dietary regimen. For example, the teen may state that he was feeling guilty about not following his diet or that he was tired of people nagging him. Another useful follow-up inquiry might be, "How is the guilt you felt or people nagging you on that day different from what you had experienced one month (or any time period) that made you able to handle your diet?" Thus, these questions amplify the resources and strengths of the teen, as well as foster responsibility and his or her ability to effect a personal behavioral change.

Finally, during the final moments of the interview, the dietitian should attempt to compliment the teen.[7] Often, the teen is viewed as a passive partner in a therapeutic relationship. Although the teen holds the information, it is the clinician who is viewed as the expert. This attitude does not foster behavior change or compliance. It is important for the dietitian to remember that the teen is the "expert" when it comes to his or her nutrition behaviors and practices. The dietitian must articulate to the teen instances where significant changes in behavior were made and how difficult this must have been. This feedback is designed to reflect back to the teen what changes have already occurred, possible solutions, and offer the view that continued change can be a reality.

MANAGEMENT

The purpose of the initial assessment aside from gaining specific dietary information is to focus on the teen's attention on the exceptions, solutions, and strengths as much as possible.[7,8] The dietitian's role is to take an active role in assessing that the desired goals are possible and concrete, so when they are achieved, both the dietitian and teen will know.[7] Goal setting or more traditionally phrased as the therapeutic contract are those statements that direct and guide the therapy process. The process of goal definition and selection is a negotiation between the teen and dietitian. Goals must be mutually agreed on, descriptive, and concrete.[7,8] One of the cardinal rules is to start small.[7] Selecting the initial goal can be done by asking the teen to indicate the very first sign that things are moving in the right direction.[7,8] Abstract descriptions such as eating a balanced diet or reducing overall sodium intake are poor goal statements. Rather, well-developed goals consist of actions that the teen can take, or conditions that can be brought around by his or her own behavior. These statements may include time elements of frequency, duration, or perhaps a deadline. For example, "by May 1, I will not use added salt at dinner, or I will exercise 20 minutes per day, 5 out of 7 days," are preferred goal-oriented statements. It is the dietitian's role to guide these goals so that they are realistic, reasonable, and achievable. It is appropriate to tell the teen that you have difficulty coming up with a nutritional goal when you are unclear or confused about the nutritional goal, i.e., "I am having trouble figuring out when we will know that we have been successful and can stop meeting because I want to make sure we are working on your goals, not mine or your parents." Remember, goals are selected by the teen and need not be inclusive of the entire dietary regimen, but should relate to overall nutritional health. Dietary counseling should be viewed as a therapeutic process and several booster sessions across time may be required.

To facilitate and maintain behavior change, it is important that the dietitian be consistent, compliment small changes and progress, and not become discouraged when a problem emerges or reappears. It is not uncommon that once the "new" solution is generated and it works, the adolescent relaxes and returns to older, more established patterns of behavior.[7] The dietitian should avoid becoming angry with the teen and minimize the teen's helplessness. During these transitional times, the dietitian needs to point out that success has been experienced and return to the series of exception questions. Other factors to consider include breaking the goal into smaller components, selecting a different goal, or using adjunctive behavioral strategies.

At the end of the initial workup, it is useful to have the teen engage in some small, but mutually agreed on behavior change. The homework assignment to the teen involves him or her observing or noticing what happens over the next week or two that helps to foster this change.[7,8] The purpose of the homework assignment is to generate a small change in behavior that in turn, will generate larger, more lasting changes. For the diabetic teen, it may be having a diet soda with friends instead of candy, and correspondingly, the homework for the teen would be identifying how others responded to this change, how hard it was to perform this new behavior, or other related events that were experienced. More generic assignments at subsequent sessions include having the teen observe and report what good things happened since the last visit, how the diet goes, or times when he or she was able to eat "forbidden" foods and not binge or purge. At the return visit, the dietitian always wants to first discuss the positive changes before addressing any problems that the teen may have experienced during the previous week.[7] Thus, the focus is always on facilitating and maintaining behavior change. At times, the teen may want to first discuss the problems of the past week. It is desirable for the clinician to interrupt the teen and state that he or she first wants to hear about the good things that happened. Redirecting the session is valuable because it allows the teen to express the positive behaviors that occurred and the problems experienced to be placed in the proper context.[7] Relatedly, it is important for the teen to understand that the most direct way to solve the nutritional problem is to examine and discuss what works.

Another useful management strategy is to have the teen outline any foreseeable challenge that may occur between now and the next nutritional session. If the teen discloses there is a situation that may present difficulties, the dietitian needs to inquire as to how he or she plans to address this difficulty.[7] After obtaining behavioral descriptors of the potential problem and allowing the teen to offer possible solutions, the dietitian can offer guidance. It may be helpful to role-play these situations in the office and try a number of different solutions to see which one is best suited to that specific teen patient and the situation.

Adjunctive Techniques

The use of other behavioral strategies such as self-monitoring, graduated goal setting, and self-management programs may be of benefit. However, these strategies will not be successful when the adolescent chooses to use dietary management as a weapon to threaten parents. Thus, the professional management team needs to avoid this common trap. For example, there is increasing evidence that the management of the adolescent with diabetes is very different from that of the young child.[10] For the adolescent with a chronic illness who is being referred for dietary noncompliance, it is better to assume that poor compliance is a result of inadequate knowledge, rather than placing the teen in a defensive posture. Recognizing that the adolescent will likely "cheat," the dietitian should provide instruction on how to minimize the impact of cheating on his or her health.[11]

Self-monitoring.   This strategy involves the teen observing, recording, and evaluating his or her own behavior.[12,13] Depending on the age and cognitive status of the teen, many different forms may be employed. For the developmentally delayed teen, a daily "thermometer," in which degrees correspond to calories ingested or minutes exercised, can be colored in by the teen at the conclusion of each meal or exercise period. For the more sophisticated youth, food diaries represent another useful variant of this technique.[14] For adolescents with gastrointestinal disorders, having them monitor associated symptoms of pain or diarrhea after eating may be helpful to determine if certain foods are associated with symptom induction.[14] The accuracy of these reports is dependent on a number of factors, but failure to record accurate information usually is due to parental punishment or nagging, i.e., not meeting stated daily goals or forgetting to record.[15] Punishment and nagging should be discouraged as they lead to lying and poor parent-teen relations and usually places the dietitian in the middle of a family disagreement that jeopardizes his or her effectiveness as a therapist. These techniques can be used sparingly, i.e., every other day for 1 wk or one time/wk, and should be between the dietitian and teen.

Graduate goal setting. This strategy is most useful when oral intake or another related behavior such as exercise needs to be increased systematically.[14] The desired caloric intake is first established and the amount of calories currently ingested by the teen determined. Increases in dietary calories then occur in small steps to ensure success and allow for positive feedback or concrete rewards. As each weekly or monthly goal is reached, another increase in the goal occurs, until the desired caloric intake is reached. For example, if an eating-disordered adolescent needs to ingest 3200 cal and currently is eating 1100 cal, the initial increase may be 300 cal. After the teen is eating this amount consistently, another increase to 1700 cal follows. In this way, each increase is small and the increased amount of food on the plate is not dramatic. Conversely, if reductions in total caloric amount are needed, this strategy can be employed, but is tedious for teen and parent.

Self-management programs. These programs rely on a combination of self-monitoring, self-reinforcement, and some problem-solving skills.[12,16] Thus, this strategy is best suited for the older teen in whom initial dietary compliance already has been established. For example, a teen with Crohn's disease would be instructed to monitor caloric intake from foods that were prepared, provide him- or herself with tangible reinforcers (video game or movie rentals) for meeting established goals, and adjusting oral intake dependent on other factors such as going out to eat or weight maintenance. These types of treatment programs are usually best preceded by small group instruction sessions that provide nutritional information and education, simple elements of behavior modification, and problem-solving skills.[12,16] Self-management programs should be time-limited (8–12 wk) and monitored by a dietitian or another member of the medical team who is knowledgeable about nutrition.

Behavioral contract. The behavior contract between teen and dietitian is a useful technique that may be overlooked.[14] A behavioral contact is a written agreement between the clinician and teen that states a desired goal, and stipulates consequences, and rewards.[12,13,16] These contracts may be unilateral or bilateral. A unilateral contact is one in which the teen obligates him- or herself to complete the desired compliance regimen and is rewarded for completion. The bilateral contract specifies the obligations of both the dietitian and youth, as well as stipulates clear and detailed descriptions of what behaviors are expected of each party. Another, but related option for the more sophisticated adolescent is the use of verbal statements of intent to be compliant that are accompanied by a handshake; this can be effective.[14]

Pitfalls

Education is usually considered the first line of defense and is an important ingredient to facilitate and enhance behavior change.[17] However, a common element in most educational programs is a high fear-arousal message.[18] It is important for the dietitian to avoid using these fear tactics with adolescents as they may inadvertently challenge the teen to continue to practice poor dietary practices or use harmful substances in excess.[19] Another intervention that should be avoided by the clinician is "nagging."[18] Using the same educational message or repeating the same intervention on each visit has been shown to lead to a decline in motivation and interest. It becomes incumbent on the dietitian to vary adjunctive techniques across time and modify specific features.[19]

Nutritional adequacy is not determined by what a diet is called, but the nutrients contained in the eaten foods.[20] Health professionals must put aside their personal preferences in counseling adolescents who see dietary practices that may be different from the norm or dominant culture.[20] With regard to counseling adolescents from different ethnic groups, dietitians must be sensitive to the diversity in language, culture, education, and socioeconomic levels between and within each culture.[21] Data suggest that the most effective approach to improving the diet of youth from diverse ethnic groups is to improve the quality of meals eaten away from the home, when they share the adverse dietary practices characteristic of U.S. culture. When prescribing changes in the eating habits of youth from different cultures, the dietitian must be sensitive to that culture's beliefs, attitudes, and concepts regarding health and nutrition.[21]

Not having a clear goal can be a major impediment in nutritional therapy.[7] Vague or ambiguous goal statements or pursuing the dietitian's own goals will lead to significant problems in management. If the dietitian cannot immediately answer the question, "What are the teen's goals?", then it is likely that problems will emerge. If confusion between the nutritional therapist and teen exist, the dietitian needs and should ask for clarification. Another potential problem occurs when the dietitian suggests an intervention that the teen has tried in the past without success. To avoid this pitfall, the clinical dietitian who is aware that another nutritional intervention has taken place needs to inquire about that experience and what it was that the teen found helpful and not helpful. A related issue is repeating advice and suggestions that have been offered to the teen by parents or friends. Generally, prior to a therapeutic experience, significant others have offered a great deal of advice and curbside guidance. In all likelihood, the teen will be as receptive to hearing the same suggestion from the dietitian as he or she was to hearing it from friends and noncompliance with these suggestions should be expected. Finally, failing to attend to the teen's problem-solving behaviors, statements, and attitudes often leads the nutritional therapist down the wrong track.[7] If during the session, the teen begins to discuss his or her situation as hopeless and more time is spent on the "problem," the dietitian needs to interrupt this process. Similar to an attorney objecting to a line of questioning, the dietitian needs to therapeutically redirect the conversation toward solutions and strategies to solve the problem.

Thus, the purpose of clinical nutrition counseling sessions is to focus on finding solutions. Regardless of the solution size or how distant that goal may be to the teen, the clinical dietitian's role is to assess the resources and strengths of the adolescent in mapping out the road to follow. The number and timing of individual sessions are dependent on both parties, and therapy should be focused on clear, achievable goals.

CASE ILLUSTRATION

Diana is almost a 14-year-old female with type 1 diabetes who was initially diagnosed at age six. During the last year at diabetic clinic visits, increased tension was observed between the patient and parents regarding her diabetic management and recent weight gain. Her mother states, "I feel we've worked too hard all this time for the weight to get out of control." Diana moved from the 50% at age 11 yr to >95% on the NCHS growth curve for weight, with height following the 95%. In the past, the patient had voiced concern about her weight, but on a scale of 1–5 she now described her worry about weight as a "3." Her parents, on the other hand, say that on a scale of 1–5 for concern, they are "5+," regarding Diana's weight.

A request was made that the dietitian see Diana alone. The parents vehemently objected and stated that they believed they would be "left out of Diana's care" if she was seen alone. On subsequent visits, either the mother or father accompanied her to clinic and continued to remain in the room for the entire visit. With a case such as this, the dietitian would ideally like to see Diana individually so that she becomes the "customer" and her concerns regarding care could be individually addressed. This one-on-one encounter with the adolescent also reinforces the idea that her health care is now her responsibility. Developmentally, adolescents seek independence during early adolescence (11–14 yr), and allowing them to be partners in their management is of importance as well as offering them a sense of autonomy regarding the health care system that will remain throughout adulthood. In addition, an individual meeting with Diana would allow for confidential discussion about issues such as dietary indiscretions that Diana may discuss more freely without her parents in attendance. If the family is unwilling to initially allow this individual meeting with their teen, other strategies may need to be utilized.

Obviously, with the family presented in the above case, their goals for Diana's care and weight control were of a higher priority than those reported by Diana herself. The family's dogged insistence on being present at all times during a visit often resulted in their concerns being addressed rather than those of their daughter. To change the focus of this interaction, the dietitian acknowledged the parents' concerns, but gave Diana the task of being the "chief" goal setter for her care. When phrased in this manner, Diana shared in ensuring her dietary content and eating patterns were appropriate. Moreover, she chose the goal of exercising 20 min three times a week in addition to her participation in a softball and bowling league.

In follow-up sessions, the dietitian asked Dianna and her parents to negotiate specific responsibilities that they would assume regarding Diana's on-going care so that everyone, including the dietitian, had clear expectations. Confusion regarding specific care issues can result in conflict between an adolescent and his or her parents when the responsibilities of each member are assumed, but never specifically discussed or detailed. In a counseling session, the dietitian, patient, and parents list their concerns, with everyone formulating what they believe to the highest priority issues or "hot buttons" that need to be addressed. In our case, Diana complained that her father frequently commented about her weight in a derogatory manner and her mother would then begin nagging. The dietitian suggested that a goal for the parents would be to avoid all weight-related comments. Instead, the entire family, including Diana, would focus on positive health behaviors. Specifically, the family could take a walk with Diana to encourage her 20 min of aerobic activity or attend her softball games to offer support. In this manner, the family could still be involved in promoting healthy behavior, but would not get bogged down in a verbal assault of past behaviors. Moreover, the dietitian explained that Diana's positive progress may be obscured if the only focus is weight gain or a single blood sugar result.

Adolescence is a time of transition and can be difficult for both the adolescent and his or her family. Often, as in this case, the parents have been the chief and sole coordinator of their child's care and feel a sense of loss as this responsibility is transferred to their teen. Moreover, the adolescent him- or herself, often lacks basic nutrition knowledge, since from an early age all decisions about the type and amounts of foods consumed at meals and snacks are made by parents, nutritionists, or other health care providers. Additional stressors that supervene during adolescence include less regimented schedules, more meals eaten in a hurried fashion or away from home, and greater limit testing. A family such as Diana's would ideally benefit from psychological counseling, but often due to family resistance or economic constraints such care is not sought or follow-up is lacking. The dietitian in this case serves a dual function as both educator and counselor.

Acknowlegments.   The authors wish to acknowlege the helpful contributions of Patty Morris, R. D. In addition, V. I. Rickert wishes to thank William Hudson

O'Hanlon, M.A., for his teachings, books, and related contributions to the field of psychotherapy.

REFERENCES

1. R. K. Johnson, D. G. Johnson, M. Q. Wang, H. Smiciklas-Wright, and H. A Guthrie, *J. Adol. Health*, **15**, 149 (1994).

2. S. A. French, C. L. Perry, G. R. Leon, and J. A. Fulkerson, *J. Adol. Health*, **15**, 286 (1994).

3. M. C. Farthing, *Nutr. Today*, **26**, 35 (1991).

4. K. D. Brownell and J. Rodin, *Am. Psychol.*, **49**, 781 (1994).

5. C. K. Haddock, W. R. Shadish, R. C. Klesges, and R. J. Stein, *Ann. Behav. Med.*, **16**, 235 (1994).

6. E. O. Guillen and S. I. Barr, *J. Adol. Health*, **15**, 464 (1994).

7. W. H. O'Hanlon and M. Weiner-Davis, *Search of Solutions*, W. W. Norton, New York, pp. 60–74 (1989).

8. B. O'Hanlon and S. Beadle, *A Field Guide to PossibilityLand: Possibility Therapy Methods*, Possibility Press, Omaha, NE, pp.17–78 (1994).

9. R. G. MacKenzie and J. L. Peel, *Adol. Med.: State Art Rev.*, **2**, 291 (1991).

10. S. B. Johnson, in *Handbook of Pediatric Psychology*, (D. K. Routh, ed.), Guilford Press, New York, pp. 9–31 (1988).

11. N. P. Spack, *Adol. Med.: State Art Rev.*, **2**, 523 (1991).

12. A. M. LaGreca, in *Handbook of Pediatric Psychology*, (D. K. Routh, ed.), Guilford Press, New York, pp. 299–320 (1988).

13. J. Dunbar and L. Waszak, in *Handbook of Clinical Behavioral Pediatrics*, (A. M. Gross and R. S. Drabman, eds.), Plenum Press, New York, pp. 365–384 (1990).

14. V. I. Rickert, C. J. Graham, and S. C. Fiedorek, *Clin. Appl. Nutr.*, **2**, 51 (1992).

15. A. M. Gross, in *Handbook of Clinical Behavioral Pediatrics*, (A. M. Gross and R. S. Drabman, eds.), Plenum Press, New York, pp. 147–164 (1990).

16. L. J. Stark, A. Spirito, and S. A. Hobbs, in *Handbook of Clinical Behavioral Pediatrics*, (A. M. Gross and R. S. Drabman, eds.), Plenum Press, New York, pp. 253–266 (1990).

17. K. I. Klepp, A. Halper, and C. L. Perry, *J. School Health*, **56**, 407 (1986).

18. R. I. Evans, in *Handbook of Pediatric Psychology*, (D. K. Routh, ed.), Guilford Press, New York, pp. 321–331 (1988).

19. V. I. Rickert, M. S. Jay, and A. A. Gottlieb, *Med. Clin. N. Am.*, **74**, 1135 (1990).

20. P. K. Johnston, E. Haddad, and J. Sabate, *Adol. Med.: State Art Rev.*, **3**, 417 (1992).

21. E. Luder, *Adol. Med.: State Art Rev.*, **3**, 405 (1992).

CHAPTER

8

Body Image

Leslie J. Heinberg, Ph.D.
Katherine C. Wood, M.A., and
J. Kevin Thompson, Ph.D.

INTRODUCTION

Definition and Relevance to Nutrition

Historically, body image has been discussed in a variety of contexts, within an assortment of disciplines, ranging from neurology to psychoanalysis.[1] However, it is the physical appearance-related aspect of body image that has become almost synonymous with the term "body image."[1,2] Since Slade and Russell's[3] seminal investigation examining physical appearance-related body image was completed approximately 20 yr ago, the published literature has increased dramatically. The component of body image that addresses one's physical appearance and weight will simply be referred to as body image throughout the rest of this chapter.

Currently, researchers tend to identify three separate components that comprise body image: perception of body size (accuracy of perceptions regarding one's size, e.g., the belief that one is larger than one's actual body size), a subjective component (satisfaction with one's body size, anxiety, and concern regarding one's body size and/or specific body parts), and a behavioral aspect (avoidance of situations that may cause body-image anxiety or dissatisfaction).[4-6] Therefore, one's body image refers to the feelings, images and behaviors an individual associates with his or her body.[7] Thus, an identified disturbance of body image can be perceptual, subjective, and/or behavioral.[5]

In order to understand the complex nature of body-image disturbance in adolescents, its relation to eating disorders, unhealthy eating patterns, psychological distress, and the ever-increasing evidence that many individuals have a "normative discontent" about their appearance,[8] it is essential to differentiate the various forms, precursors, and correlates of body-image disturbance.[5,9] Further, a better understanding of the construct of body image may be beneficial in the development of effective screening, treatment, and prevention of dysfunctional eating patterns and eating disorders, areas of particular importance for the dietitian.

Recently, researchers have added information to the body-image literature in a variety of populations, such as adults, athletes, ballet dancers, models, obese individuals, and individuals with eating disorders.[6] In addition, body-image disturbance has been investigated in relation to a variety of factors, including depression,[10] teasing history,[11,12] and self-esteem.[13]

Prevalence

Concern with body weight, shape, and appearance are extremely common among females in Western cultures.[14] The extent of subjective body-image disturbance in "normal" populations has led Rodin and Striegel-Moore[15] to coin the term "normative discontent" to describe the degree of disturbance in asymptomatic females. It is becoming increasingly clear that body-image dysfunction exists in noneating-disordered populations. For instance, Silberstein et al.[16] report that the concern over weight and dissatisfaction with one's body has become so prevalent that "it can be considered to be a normal part of the female experience." As additional evidence, Cash et al.[17] in a national survey, found high levels of body dissatisfaction among both genders. Only 7% of women surveyed and 18% of men stated that they had little concern with their appearance. Comparing these data to a previous survey in 1972, the researchers found an increase in dissatisfaction for both genders.[17] It has been suggested by Rodin et al.[15] that this "normative discontent" occurs on a continuum with individuals at the upper extremes, most at risk for developing eating disorders.

Dissatisfaction and distress regarding one's body size are clearly not limited to adults. Research beginning in the early 1980s has generally found that adolescent girls are more dissatisfied with their bodies than adolescent boys.[6] Davies and Furnham[7] concluded in a study of British adolescent females, that although less than 4% of the sample were overweight, over 40% considered themselves to be overweight. A study examining an American sample found that 33% of

10th grade females judged themselves to be overweight or very overweight, whereas all subjects' weight was within 75% of the ideal age-adjusted body mass index.[18] A study by Wardle and Marsland[20] found that 50% of adolescent girls felt too fat and wished to lose weight and levels of weight concern were almost as high among 11-year-olds as 18-year-olds. Finally, researchers found that 30% of 9-year-olds reported concern that they were too fat or feared becoming fat as they got older.[19] Thus, by the time of adolescence, many normal-weight children, particularly girls, are dissatisfied with their body shape and weight and desire to be thinner.

Although certain subgroups of male adolescents may be concerned about their body size (and often wish to be larger, rather than to lose weight), girls differ greatly from boys with regard to their bodies.[20] For example, Rosen and Gross[21] reported that adolescent girls were four times more likely than boys to be attempting to lose weight, whereas boys were about three times more likely than girls to be trying to gain weight. Based on these conclusions, it appears that weight concern may indeed be a "normative discontent" for many adolescent girls.

Associated Features and Adolescent Populations at Risk

Eating disorders.   Since the relationship between body-image disturbance and anorexia nervosa was first empirically shown in 1973,[22] an abundance of research has demonstrated that a body-image disturbance often accompanies eating disorders.[3,5,22,23] This evidence appears to indicate that the tendency among individuals diagnosed with anorexia nervosa and/or bulimia nervosa to have a body-image disturbance is a cardinal feature of the disorders. This evidence was fundamental in the decision to include body-image disturbance in the *Diagnostic and Statistical Manual of Mental Disorders-4th ed.* (DSM-IV).[24] The American Psychiatric Association lists as disturbances of body image anorexia nervosa and bulimia nervosa. The required criteria for each of the two eating disorders are as follows: Anorexia nervosas, "disturbance in the way in which one's body weight or shape is experienced; undo influence of body weight or shape on self-evaluation, or denial of the seriousness of the current low body weight." Bulimia nervosa, "self-evaluation is unduly influenced by body shape and weight."

Slade and Russell[3] reported a relationship between eating disorders and body image when they found that the degree of body size overestimation constituted a negative prognostic indicator for patients with anorexia nervosa. For instance, greater size overestimation in anorectics is related to poorer weight gain while in treatment[23,25,26] and has been shown to be a strong predictor of relapse.[3,27,28] Therefore, greater body-image disturbances may be indicative of poorer prognosis for eating disorders and more severe psychopathology.[4]

Associated bulimic symptomatology, such as vomiting and related nonpurging behaviors, have also been associated with body-image disturbance.[29] Strober et al.[29] investigated anorexic patients and found that those who engaged in purging by vomiting manifested greater body size overestimation than nonpurging anorexics. A number of studies have concluded that bulimic subjects are more likely to overestimate than asymptomatic controls or other eating-disordered populations.[30–32]

Obesity.   Studies examining obesity and body-image disturbance among adolescents have generally been of two types. One set of studies has examined how the experience of being an obese adolescent affects body image. Other research has examined the role of childhood or adolescent obesity vs. adult-onset obesity on later body-image satisfaction.

Historically, researchers have described the experience of being an obese teen, especially for females, as bleak. For example, Wadden et al.[33] described that obese girls are preoccupied with their weight, isolated, and subject to mental health difficulties. These prior studies had largely relied on clinical samples in dietary settings. As such, Wadden et al.'s[33] examination of a large sample of obese and nonobese adolescent girls led to slightly differing conclusions. They reported that obese girls acknowledged significantly greater dissatisfaction with their weight and figures than nonobese girls. However, nonobese girls also expressed dissatisfaction with their weight and nearly 70% of the total sample had made attempts to lose weight in the preceding year. They concluded that obese girls in the general population are dissatisfied with their weight, but are not significantly more depressed or anxious than their nonobese contemporaries as had previously been suggested. Fowler[34] found evidence to support greater dissatisfaction among overweight adolescent females, particularly for those who had a recent change in their weight status.

Several authors have demonstrated that adults who had been obese since childhood are more likely to express body image dissatisfaction and overestimation than individuals with adult-onset obesity.[35,36] However, more recent research seems to indicate that time of onset differences may dissipate following weight loss,[37] i.e., body image between groups may be equivalent after weight normalization. However, it is important to note that being overweight during adolescence may place individuals at greater risk for developing a body-image disturbance at some point in their lifetime.

Dieting behavior.   Weight concerns and dissatisfaction with body shape or appearance are often associated with attempts to alter appearance by limiting food intake and other dieting techniques.[20] As evidence, weight-loss behaviors for both males and females have been shown to be primarily related to a desire for a thinner body shape, and the greater the discrepancy between ideal and current body size, the more frequent the dieting behavior.[38] However, it is important to recognize that dieting is not harmless and may pose a threat to a healthy nutritional state, and may develop into precursors of a later eating disturbance.[20]

Dieting is big business in Western society and occurs so frequently that it can be considered the norm rather than the exception. Hill et al.[39] assert that the prevailing societal opinion is dieting is available, inexpensive, fairly risk-free, and socially acceptable. Several studies confirm that dieting is a popular activity among teens. Studies examining the numbers of adolescents dieting find surprisingly high numbers of teens engaging in this behavior. For example, one report indicated that 60% of adolescent females and over 16% of adolescent males were currently on a weight-loss regimen.[21] These numbers demonstrate a significant increase over the reported one-third of female teens dieting 20 yr ago.[21] It is generally hypothesized that the increase in dieting behavior is due to increasing cultural pressure for thinness and an angular body shape.[1,6] Indeed, a large majority of both males and females, gainers and reducers, are of normal weight.[21]

Research suggests that dieting behavior increases as adolescents age.[40] However, some authors have found evidence of dieting behaviors at disturbingly young ages. Maloney et al.[41] reported that 37% of children in grades 3–6 had already tried to lose weight.

Although dieting has long been considered a risk factor for eating disorders,[42] the rate of dieting among adolescents is far higher than the reported incidence of eating disorders, approximately 5% within this age group.[24] Nevertheless, at best, young children may be beginning a career of body-image distress and dieting. At worst, large proportions of young people are at risk for developing dysfunctional eating and clinical disorders.[39]

Psychological functioning.   Body-image disturbance has been found to relate to a variety of psychological variables, including eating disturbance, self-esteem, anxiety, depression, and global psychological functioning.[1] However, the majority of these studies have focused on adult populations. The few studies examining psychological correlates of body-image disturbance in adolescents have primarily focused on eating disturbance (as discussed earlier), self-esteem, and depression.

Fabian and Thompson[11] found that body-image dissatisfaction was highly correlated with overall self-esteem for both pre- and postmenarcheal adolescent girls. This study fits with evidence for a relationship between self-esteem and body image and eating disturbance found within adult female populations.[43,44] Cattarin and Thompson[45] have begun the important role of demonstrating causal relationships between body image and psychological functioning. In a 3 yr longitudinal study, teasing (about weight/shape) predicted increases in body dissatisfaction and body dissatisfaction predicted increases in restrictive eating and dieting behavior.[45] Further, bulimic symptomatology predicted increases in general psychological disturbance (self-esteem, anxiety, and depression).[45]

Positive relationships have also been demonstrated between depression and size overestimation for weight-related body sites and body esteem.[11] Like self-esteem, the relationship between depression and lower levels of body dissatisfaction among adolescent girls is consistent with the adult literature, but a direct causal link between depression and body-image disturbance has not been consistently demonstrated.[10]

Athletes.   Researchers have begun to examine body-image and eating disturbance among athletes. Although these studies have focused almost exclusively on college-aged young adults, it is important to note their results, as many individuals begin to become active in sports during adolescence.

Body image and weight may be important to athletes for a variety of reasons. For some sports (wrestling, gymnastics, weightlifting), a certain body weight or shape may be desirable for optimal performance.[6] Alternatively, many individuals engage in athletics as a means of losing weight or achieving an idealized physique.[6] Generally, the results indicate that some athletes, especially individuals who engage in extreme work-outs or exercise while being injured, may have body-image disturbance that is greater than normal controls.[46,47]

It is also important to recognize that adolescent athletes, particularly males, are at risk for steroid use. Although some individuals may be solely motivated by increasing their strength, many adolescent athletes may be using these illegal and dangerous drugs as a means of changing their physique to a more idealized size. Just as adolescent females may engage in disturbed eating patterns in order to lose weight, male athletes may abuse steroids in order to achieve their idealized physique.

Body dysmorphic disorder.   For some individuals, body-image disturbance is characterized by extreme levels of disparagement focused on one particular aspect of the body. This extreme dissatisfaction is coupled with high levels of preoccupation with the disliked body part. Recognition that body-image disturbance can occur to such an extreme has led to the diagnostic entity of body dysmorphic disorder.[24] Diagnostic criteria for this disorder include preoccupation with an imagined defect in appearance (e.g., an adolescent girl imagining that her thighs are unnaturally large when normal in appearance), or if a slight physical anomaly is present, the person's concern is markedly excessive (e.g., a teen with a larger than average nose interprets it as being grossly huge).[24] Although any aspect of the body may be the focus of the disorder, common concerns include the nose, hair, mouth, waist, thighs, and genitals. Individuals with this disorder may have plastic surgery in order to correct the defect and develop concomitant obsessive-compulsive behavior or depression.[6,48] The age of onset for this disorder usually ranges from adolescence through young adulthood.[24] Adolescents presenting with body-image complaints should be carefully assessed in order to rule out body dysmorphic disorder.

Theories of Body-Image Disturbance

Several theories have been offered to explain the development and maintenance of body image disturbance.[1] The following theories will be briefly reviewed: developmental factors, the influence of negative verbal commentary (teasing), perceptual disturbance theories, and sociocultural theory, perhaps the most widely accepted and well-documented explanation.

Developmental theories.   Much of the work in the area of body-image development focuses on the importance of puberty and maturational timing, an area of particular importance for those interested in adolescent populations.[6] For example, Fabian and Thompson[11] compared subjective and perceptual measures of body image for premenarcheal and postmenarcheal girls and found that post-menarcheal girls were more likely to overestimate their thighs. Additionally, for postmenarcheal girls, size overestimation was positively correlated with a history of being teased about their body size.[11]

Several studies have also indicated the importance of maturational timing and body-image dissatisfaction. In general, girls who mature later than their peers (experience menarche after the age of 14 yr) have a more positive body image than those who reach menarche early (before the age of 11 yr) or on time (between the ages of 11 and 14 yr).[6] However, more recent research indicates that it is not the timing of puberty alone that predicts body image dissatisfaction. Instead, it is the cumulative effect of puberty and other synchronous stressful events such as the onset of dating or academic stress.[49]

Negative verbal commentary.   An additional developmental factor that has recently gained more attention is the important role that teasing, or negative verbal commentary, plays on later body-image satisfaction. This may be of particular interest to individuals working with adolescent populations, as this may be the time when body-related teasing is at its apex. Cash et al.[17] reported that adult women who had been teased about their appearance during childhood were more dissatisfied with their appearance than women who had been rarely teased. More recently, the possible effects of teasing were investigated in a sample of 10–15-year-old females.[11] Teasing frequency was significantly related to both body satisfaction and eating disturbance. Similarly, Thompson and Psaltis[12] found strong relationships between teasing frequency/effect and depression, eating psychopathology, and global body satisfaction. In addition, Thompson et al.,[50] using exploratory causal modeling procedures, found that teasing history had a direct influence on body image, eating disturbances, and overall psychological functioning.

Perceptual disturbance theories.   Several theories have also been offered to explain perceptual body-image disturbance. For example, Thompson and Spana[51] developed a theory of cortical disturbance to explain perceptual disturbance. They found that size overestimation was positively related to more general visuospatial abilities.[51] Another explanation of body size overestimation, perceptual artifact theory, proposes that a tendency to overestimate one's body size is related to one's actual body size.[1] That is, individuals who are of a smaller size overestimate to a larger extent than individuals of average or larger size.[52–54] Thus, individuals with anorexia nervosa would be likely to overestimate, but this may not be due to psychopathology. Finally, adaptive failure theory proposes that subjects' perception of their size may not change at that same rate as actual size changes (weight loss or gain).[6,28]

Sociocultural theory.   Most researchers appear to agree that the strongest influence on the development of body image and body-image disturbance in Western societies is the sociocultural factor.[1,55] This explanation of body-image disturbance is best supported by available data. A sociocultural model emphasizes that the current societal standard for thinness for women is pervasive and, unfortunately, often unachievable for the average female. These standards are difficult to achieve, and thus especially distressing, for an adolescent female whose body is in a state of change. In a society in which "what is beautiful is good,"[56] thinness has become almost synonymous with beauty.[6,57] Conversely, researchers have found that just as thinness is valued by a society, its opposite, obesity, is seriously denigrated.[8,58,59]

Throughout history, ideals of feminine beauty have varied and changed in accordance with the aesthetic standards of the particular period of time.[55,60–62] Recent research suggests that there has been movement away from a preference for an hourglass figure to a less curvaceous and more angular body shape.[63]

For example, Garner et al.[61] examined the archival data of reported height and weight measurements of Miss America pageant winners from 1960 until 1978 and the reported bust, waist, and hip measurements of 240 *Playboy* centerfolds over a span of 20 yr and concluded that the weights had decreased significantly. These data also indicated that bust, waist, and hip measurements have evolved from a curvaceous standard to a more tubular one.[61] A recent update of this study[64] found that Miss America contestants from 1979–1988 indicated body weights 13–19% below expected weights for women their height. Interestingly, Garner et al.[61] also discovered that while the prevailing female role models have been getting thinner, average women of similar age in the United States have become heavier. Wiseman et al.[64] conclude that the majority of "ideals" in our society, based on their low body weight, could be classified as having one of the major symptoms of anorexia nervosa.

Although the ideal figure has become thinner while the average woman's figure has become larger,[61] it appears that females continue to accept the thinner societal ideal as a goal. A recent study by Collins[65] indicates that expectations of thinness among females may be evident as early as 6 and 7 yr of age. As females enter adolescence, they become more concerned with their appearance and the associated bodily changes and weight gain, continuing to adhere to the idealized societal standard.[66-67] This adherence to a thin ideal continues into adulthood.[68]

Based in part on the importance of socioculturally endorsed ideal weights and appearances, Thompson[6] proposed a self-ideal discrepancy hypothesis to explain the development and maintenance of body-image disturbance. This theory focuses on individuals' tendency to compare their perceived appearance with an imagined ideal or an other ideal.[1] The result of such a comparison process may be a discrepancy between the perceived and ideal self and thus comparison may lead to dissatisfaction.[1,6] Recent research supports the hypothesis that a self-ideal discrepancy exists and a greater discrepancy may be related to higher levels of eating disturbance and body-image dissatisfaction.[12,68-70] Further evidence maintains that a tendency to compare one's physical appearance to others appears to be strongly related to body dissatisfaction.[1,57,70-71] Again, adolescents may be at higher risk for developing body-image disturbance given the importance of "fitting in," teens' need to conform to sociocultural norms, and insecurity related to being different from others.

ASSESSMENT

Adolescents are far more likely to initially report disordered eating, body-image dissatisfaction and distress, regarding appearance to a health care provider than a mental health professional. These providers can have a powerful influence on the education, assessment, and treatment of adolescents regarding body image.

Although adolescents may be aware of some of the changes that occur at puberty, dietitians and other health care providers can be especially helpful in educating individuals about bodily changes that affect appearance. Rosen and Gross[21] assert that adolescents are confused regarding what constitutes over-weight, normal weight, and underweight. What is especially needed is more accurate information about normal weight, normal changes in body constitution, and the importance of maintaining a healthy weight for optimal physical health.[21] For example, it is important for premenarcheal girls to understand the important and necessary role that weight gain and body fat contribute to puberty. Weight gain and increasing hip and thigh circumferences are normal changes that occur during female adolescence. Young girls can be educated that these are not necessarily a cause for concern or dieting. Further, adolescents can be helped to recognize the strong influence of personal and sociocultural pressures that make body size and shape such a focus of attention.[21] Professionals can help adolescents assess realistically the need for weight loss and, if unnecessary, help them resist these pressures.

To adolescents who are overweight or voice concerns about their body size or shape, dietitians need to furnish information about safe weight management and discourage the use of extreme diets, purging, excessive exercise, or steroid abuse. Dietitians may be especially helpful in teaching adolescents healthy ways of maintaining or losing weight, rather than having them rely upon the plethora of erroneous diet information available to youth. Adolescents interested in weight-loss should be encouraged to develop lifestyle changes and educated on the dangers inherent in drastic weight loss plans.

Dietitians can also play an important role in identifying those teens who may be at greater risk for developing body-image disturbance or eating-disordered behavior. The following behaviors, developmental events, and factors may be recognized as "warning signs" that an adolescent is at higher risk for developing a body-image disturbance: (1) constant complaining about weight, size, or body site, (2) frequent weighing, measuring, or checking of overall size or a specific body site, (3) frequent comparing of oneself to an idealized other, (4) puberty, (5) frequent teasing by others, and/or (6) frequent dieting. Once identified, interventions may be immediately provided or the level of severity may indicate a referral to a mental health care professional.

Measures

Although a vast number of measures have been developed to assess body-image dissatisfaction and overestimation, very few have been evaluated on adolescents or children. Table 8.1 organizes measures that have been selected because they possess good psychometric features and/or have been utilized in younger populations. Each measure is followed by the author's name and address, and readers are encouraged to write for more information on measures of interest.[14,50, 67, 72–79]

The Schematic Figure for Children[67], (see Figure 8.1), is a simple measure for determining the discrepancy between the ideal self and how the individual currently views him- or herself. Subjects are simply asked to rate their "ideal" figure and "current" size. The degree of discrepancy is an index of body-image dissatisfaction. The Eating Disorders Inventory[80] has also been widely used with children and has a subscale specifically measuring body image dissatisfaction.

MANAGEMENT

Although a wealth of research has examined the extent of body-image disturbance and how to assess body image, far fewer studies have examined treatment. Even in intervention protocols designed for the treatment of anorexia nervosa and bulimia nervosa, body-image dysfunction is often overlooked.[6] However, re-

Table 8.1 Measures Commonly Used for Body-Image Assessment

Instrument	Author(s)	Description	Reliability	Standardization	Address
Adjustable light beam apparatus (ALBA)	Thompson et al. (1993)[50]	Adjust width of 4 light beams projected on wall to match perceived size of cheeks waist, hips, and thighs	IC*: 0.75	63 female adolescents, (10–15 years)	J. Kevin Thompson, Ph.D. Department of Psychology University of South Florida 4202 Fowler Ave. Tampa, FL 33620–8200
None given	(1) Collins (1991)[65] and (2) Wood et al. (1993)[72]	7 boy and 7 girl figures that vary in size	(1) IC*: Not applicable. TR$^+$: (self=0.71; ideal self=0.59; ideal other child=0.38; ideal adult=0.55; ideal other adult=0.49). (2) TR$^+$: 2 weeks (self=0.70; ideal self=0.63).	(1) 1118 preadolescents., (2) 109 males and 95 females, (aged 8–10 years).	M.E. Collins, H.S.D., M.P.H. Dept. of Health Science Education FLG–5 University of Florida Gainesville, FL 32611–2034

	References	Description	Reliability	Sample	Source
Eating Disorders Inventory/Body Dissatisfaction Scale	(1) Shore & Porter (1990),[73] (2) Wood et al. (1993),[72] and (3) Steiger et al. (1991)[79]	Subjects indicate degree of agreement with statements about body parts being too large	(1) IC*: Female adolescent (11–18 years)=0.91., (2) IC*: Female children (8–10 years)=0.84., (3) IC*: High school females= 0.91 (English) and 0.89 (French).	(1) 196 boys and 414 girls., (2) 109 males and 95 females., (3) 529 English and 395 French .	David M. Garner, Ph.D. c/o Psychological Assessments Resources, Inc. P.O. Box 998 Odessa, FL 33556
Body Esteem Scale	(1) Mendelsohn & White (1985),[74] (2) White (personal communication, 1990), and (3) Hill et al. (1992).[39]	Subjects report their degree of agreement with various statements about their bodies	(1) IC*: split-half reliability (0.85)., (2) TR**: 2 years (0.66), and (3) IC*: None given. TR: None given.	(1) 97 boys/girls (ages 8.5–17.4 years), 48 overweight and 49 normal weight., (2) 105 boys/girls (ages 8–13 years)., (3) 170 girls (ages 8–10 years).	Donna Romano White, Ph.D. Dept of Psychology Concordia University 1455 de Maisonneuve West, Montreal, Quebec Canada H3G–1M8

continued on next page

Table 8.1 *Continued*

Instrument	Author(s)	Description	Reliability	Standardization	Address
Body Shape Questionnaire (BSQ)	Bunell et al. (1992)[14]	34 items that determine concern with body shape	IC*: None given. TR⁺:None given.	81 eating disordered patients (<19 years) and 88 female controls (13–17 years)	Peter Cooper, Ph.D. University of Cambridge Addenbrooke's Hospital, Hills Road Cambridge, CB22QQ Great Britain
Self-Image Questionnaire for Young Adolescents/body image subscale	Peterson et al. (1984)[75]	Designed for 10–15-year-olds. 11-Item body-image subscale assesses positive feelings toward the body.	IC*: Boys=0.81 , Girls=0.77, IR**: 1 year (0.60); 2 years (0.44).	335 sixth grade students who were followed through the eighth grade	Anne C. Peterson, Ph.D. Deputy Director National Science Foundation 4201 Wilson Blvd. Arlington, VA 22230
Goldfarb Fear of Fat Scale	Goldfarb et al. (1985)[76]	10 statements (very untrue to very true) that reflect overconcern with fatness and body size	IC*: 0.85, TR*: 1 week (0.88).	98 high school females	Meg Gerrard Dept. of Psychology Iowa State University Ames, Iowa 50011
Body-Image and Eating Questionnaire for Children/overweight subscale	Thelen et al. (1992)[77]	Subjects respond to 14 items addressing weight concerns, dieting, and restraint	IC*: 0.83, TR⁺: None given.	191 second, fourth, and sixth grade boys and girls	Mark H. Thelen Psychology Dept. University of Missouri-Columbia 210 McAlester Hall Columbia, MO 65211

| None given | Steinhausen and Vollrath (1992)[78] | Subjects describe their body in terms of 16 bipolar adjectives (semantic differential scale) | IC*: "attractiveness" scale =0.93, "body-mass" scale=0.81., TR+: None given. | 46 adolescent anorexic inpatients and 109 secondary school pupils | H. C. Steinhausen, M.D., Ph.D. Dept. of Child and Adolescent Psychiatry University of Zurich Freiestrasse 15 Postfach, CH–8025 Zurich, Switzerland |
| None given | Steiger et al. (1991)[79] | Subjects respond to 6 items addressing concerns about body areas | IC*: English girls=0.83, French girls:0.82. TR**: None given. | 295 English and 456 French girls (ages 11–18 years) | Howard Steiger, Ph.D., Eating Disorders Program Douglas Hospital Centre 6875 La Salle Blvd. Verdun, Quebec HRH IR3 |

*IC = Internal Consistency, +TR = Test-= retest reliability

Note: Internal consistency estimates are not applicable for measures that yield a single index or conceptually distinct indices, e.g., some whole-body adjustment and figural rating scales.

Adapted from J. K. Thompson, in *Body Image Disturbance: Assessment and Treatment*, Pergamon Press, New York, pp. 58–67 (1990).

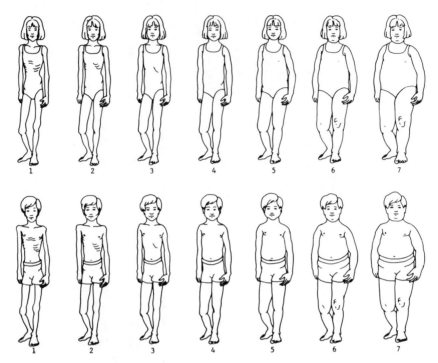

Figure 8-1.   The Schematic Figure for Children.

M. E. Collins, *Int. J. Eat. Dis.,***10,** 199 (1991). Reprinted with permission.

searchers have begun to examine the treatment of body image in a few controlled studies.

Treatment focusing on perceptual body-image disturbance has largely utilized image confrontation procedures. These studies involve exposure to one's image, via a mirror, video feedback, or other specific information. Over time, it is hypothesized that the individual cannot continue to maintain a perceptual distur- bance in contrast to conflicting objective feedback. Although several studies were able to demonstrate increased accuracy over time, they have been criticized for poor maintenance of gains at follow-up, poor subject selection, and only addressing a unitary aspect of body-image disturbance.[1,81]

Recent treatment studies have utilized multimodal interventions designed to focus on the multiple aspects of body-image disturbance. Butters and Cash[82] developed a cognitive-behavioral treatment program focusing on body dissatisfac- tion among noneating-disordered populations. Their program consisted of the following components: education regarding body image, relaxation training, desensitization using imagery for body sites and the whole body, mirror desensitization, addressing irrational cognitions, behavioral assignments designed to ensure a sense of mastery, stress management, and relapse prevention. This treatment produced significant improvement on measures of body image and general psychological functioning and treatment gains were maintained after follow-up.[82] More recent treatment studies have added additional perceptual interventions and addressed behavioral avoidance of body-image-related situations.[83] Thus, cognitive-behavioral treatment programs may be the most effective in producing both statistically and clinically significant improvements in body image.

A recent prevention intervention[84] was designed specifically for adolescent girls. This treatment study had three basic components: education regarding the harmful effects of unhealthful weight regulation, fostering of healthful weight management through the use of nutrition and dietary principles coupled with regular physical activity, and the development of coping skills for resisting sociocultural pressures for thinness and dieting. Although the results demonstrated a significant increase in knowledge and a significant increase in the body mass index among high-risk girls (those engaging in disordered eating behavior), the intervention did not have as great an impact as initially hoped. The authors conclude that such a broad-based intervention is not necessary for all adolescents.[84] Instead, the authors argue for using the curriculum with adolescents who are at high risk for developing eating-disordered behavior.[84]

In several of the above studies, education is an important component of body-image treatment, as is the promotion of healthy methods of weight loss and weight maintenance. Health care providers, especially dietitians, should be vital conduits of this information, perhaps even before a body-image disturbance develops. Additionally, for dietitians especially interested in the treatment of body-image disturbance, Cash[85] has developed a series of audio cassettes that provide a self-directed treatment as well as a patient workbook.

For adolescents who appear to have a severe level of body-image dissatisfaction, body dysmorphic disorder or disturbed eating, the dietitian should clearly communicate concerns and refer the adolescent to a mental health professional.

CASE ILLUSTRATION

Kim, an 18-year-old, Caucasian college freshman, was seen as part of a time-limited, cognitive-behavioral, group treatment for women with binging and purging behavior. As treatment progressed, the case conceptualization of Kim began focusing on a body-image disturbance as the driving force behind her disturbed eating patterns.

Although only about 10 lb overweight, Kim reported extreme distress with her body size and perceived herself to be grossly obese. Her dissatisfaction with her body size began when she was 9-years-old and an active participant in ballet classes. She reported being a talented ballerina and often performed parts more advanced than those assigned to older girls. She indicated that she became increasingly aware of the importance of being small and petite, and noticed that the older girls were often derided by the teachers for weight gain. Kim continued to excel in ballet, until the age of 11 yr, when she began to grow taller. Although she had grown 2 in. in the past year, her teachers punished her for gaining weight by assigning her less important parts. Compounding this message, her pediatrician had teased her that she was getting "thunder thighs" at her yearly physical. She reported that during this time, she tried laboriously to lose weight, but her growing body would not cooperate. During this struggle, older ballerinas taught her to purge on the days prior to weigh-ins, and soon Kim was purging on a regular basis.

At the time of treatment, Kim had internalized the extreme weight demands of ballet, although she had stopped performing 3 yr previously. She continued to struggle to lose weight by exercising several hours a day and attempting to maintain less than a 400-cal daily intake. She would begin each day with an hour of exercise and an apple for breakfast. At lunch, she would eat plain lettuce and exercise for an additional 1–2 h in the afternoon. Inevitably, by the time she would come home she would eat a large meal. She identified this as a binge, but it appeared more likely she was eating a large meal due to hunger than a "true" clinical binge. Feeling guilty and believing that she would never attain her idealized size, Kim would purge by vomiting.

Treatment for Kim followed a multimodal approach. The patient was instructed to keep an eating diary that documented food intake, purges, and thoughts and feelings associated with food intake. A mirror confrontation procedure was utilized and the patient also confronted with information regarding normal weights for women her height. She reported surprise during the confrontation procedures that she was not as "obese" as first imagined. Based on information from her food diary, Kim was educated regarding healthy caloric levels, eating a variety of foods, and spacing eating throughout the day. Behavioral techniques were utilized to reduce triggers for purging, increasing impulse control and relapse prevention. Cognitive techniques were used to help Kim decrease negative thoughts and evaluate her body size more realistically. During the 12 wk of treatment, her purging episodes decreased from a daily occurrence to weekly episodes and she reported less distress with her appearance and less need to exercise excessively. At the time the group treatment ended, Kim was referred for individual therapy in order to maintain her treatment gains.

REFERENCES

1.   J. K. Thompson, in *Progress in Behavior Modification*, (M. Hersen, R. M. Eisler, and P. M. Miller, eds.), Sycamore Publishing, Inc., Sycamore, IL, pp. 3–54 (1992).

2. T. F. Cash and T. Pruzinsky, eds., *Body Images: Development, Deviance, and Change*, Guilford Press, New York, (1990).

3. P. D. Slade and G.F.M. Russell, *Psychol. Med.*, **3**, 188 (1973).

4. T. F. Cash and T. A. Brown, *Behav. Mod.*, **11**, 487 (1987).

5. D. M. Garner and P. E. Garfinkel, *Int. J. Psych. Med.*, **11**, 263 (1981).

6. J. K. Thompson, *Body Image Disturbance: Assessment and Treatment*, Pergamon, New York, (1990).

7. E. Davies and A. Furnham, *Brit. J. Med. Psychol.*, **47**, 349 (1986).

8. J. Rodin, L. R. Silberstein, and R. H. Striegel-Moore, in *Psychology and Gender, Nebraska Symposium on Motivation*, (T. B. Sonderegger, ed.), University of Nebraska Press, Lincoln, NE, pp.267–307 (1984).

9. P. D. Slade, *J. Psych. Res.*, **19**, 255 (1985).

10. S. W. Noles, T. F. Cash, and B. A. Winstead, *J. Consult. Clin. Psychol.*, **53**, 88 (1985).

11. L. J. Fabian and J. K. Thompson, *Int. J. Eat. Dis.*, **8**, 63 (1989).

12. J. K. Thompson and K. Psaltis, *Int. J. Eat. Dis.*, **7**, 813 (1988).

13. A. A. Gleghorn, *The Functional Relationship Between Self-Esteem and Body Image*, unpublished Ph.D. dissertation, University of South Florida, Tampa, FL, (1988).

14. D. W. Bunnell, P. J. Cooper, S. Hertz, and I. R. Shenker, *Int. J. Eat. Dis.*, **11**, 79 (1992).

15. J. Rodin and R. H. Striegel-Moore, *Predicting Attitudes Towards Body Weight and Food Intake in Women*, paper presented at 14th Congress of the European Association of Behavior Therapy (1984).

16. L. R. Silberstein, R. H. Striegel-Moore, and J. Rodin, in *The Role of Shame in Symptom Formation*, (H. B. Lewis, ed.), Lawrence Erlbaum Associates, Hillsdale, NJ, pp. 89, 267 (1987).

17. T. F. Cash, B. A. Winstead, and L. H. Janda, *Psychol. Tod.*, **20**, 30 (1986).

18. J. D. Killen, C. B. Taylor, M. J. Telch, K. E. Saylor, D. J. Maron, and T. N. Robinson, *Am. J. Pub. Health*, **77**, 1539 (1987).

19. L. M. Mellin, C. E. Irwin, Jr., and S. Scully, *J. Am. Diet. Assoc.*, **92**, 851 (1992).

20. J. Wardle and L. Marsland, *J. Psychosom. Res.*, **34**, 377 (1990).

21. J. C. Rosen and J. Gross, *Health Psychol.*, **6**, 131 (1987).

22. H. Bruch, *Eating Disorders: Obesity, Anorexia Nervosa, and the Person Within*, Basic Books, New York, (1973).

23. P. E. Garfinkel, H. Moldofsky, and D. M. Garner, *Psychol. Med.*, **9**, 703 (1979).

24. American Psychiatric Association, *Diagnostic and Statistical Manual of Mental Disorders*, 4th ed., Washington, DC, pp. 545, 550 (1994).

25. R. C. Casper, K. A. Halmi, S. C. Goldenberg, E. D. Eckert, and J. M. Davis, *Brit. J. Psych.*, **134**, 60 (1979).

26. D. L. Norris, *Psychol. Med.*, **14**, 835 (1984).

27. E. Button, F. Franscella, and P. Slade, *Psychol. Med.*, **7**, 235 (1977).

28. A. H. Crisp and R. S. Kalucy, *Brit. J. Med. Psychol.*, **47**, 349 (1974).

29. M. Strober, I. Goldenberg, J. Green, and J. Saxon, *Psychol. Med.*, **9**, 695 (1979).

30. J. K. Thompson, W. W. Berland, P. H. Linton, and R. Weinsier, *Int. J. Eat. Dis.*, **5**, 113 (1986).

31. M. E. Willmuth, H. Leitenberg, J. C. Rosen, and S. S. Cado, *Int. J. Eat. Dis.*, **7**, 825 (1988).

32. M. E. Willmuth, H. Leitenberg, J. C. Rosen, K. M. Fondacaro, and J. Gross, *Int. J. Eat. Dis.*, **4**, 71 (1985).

33. T. A. Wadden, G. D. Foster, A. J. Stunkard, and J. R. Linowitz, *Int. J. Obes.*, 13, **89** (1989).

34. B. A. Fowler, *Adolescence*, **95**, 557 (1989).

35. J. Grinker, *J. Am. Diet. Assoc.*, **62**, 30 (1973).

36. A. Stunkard and V. Burt, *Am. J. Psych.*, **123**, 1443 (1967).

37. S. Fisher, *Development and Structure of the Body Image*, Lawrence Erlbaum Associates, Hillsdale, NJ, (1986).

38. E. H. Wertheim, S. J. Paxton, D. Maude, G. I. Szmukler, K. Gibbons, and L. Hiller, *Int. J. Eat. Dis.*, **12**, 151 (1992).

39. A. J. Hill, S. Oliver, and P. J. Rogers, *Brit. J. Clin. Psychol.*, **31**, 95 (1992).

40. S. J. Gralen, M. P. Levine, L. Smolak, and S. K. Murnen, *Int. J. Eat. Dis.*, **9**, 501 (1990).

41. M. J. Maloney, J. McGuire, S. R. Daniels, and B. Specker, *Pediatrics*, **84**, 482 (1989).

42. R. L. Pyle, J. E. Mitchell, and E. D. Eckert, *J. Clin. Psych.*, **42**, 60 (1981).

43. S. Hesse-Biber, A. Clayton-Matthew, and J. A. Downey, *Psychol. Mon.*, **114**, 511 (1988).

44. J. K. Thompson and C. Thompson, *Int. J. Eat. Dis.*,**5**, 1061 (1986).

45. J. Cattarin and J. K. Thompson, *Eat. Dis.: J. Treat. Prev.*, **2** 114 (1994).

46. K. D. Brownell, J. Rodin, and J. H. Wilmore, *Runn. World*, **XIII**, 28 (1988).

47. S. Nudelman, J. C. Rosen, and H. Leitenberg, *Int. J. Eat. Dis.*, **7**, 625 (1988).

48. T. Pruzinsky, in *Body Images: Development,Deviance, and Change*, (T. F. Cash and T. Pruzinsky, eds.), Guilford Press, New York, pp. 170–189, (1990).

49. M. P. Levine, L. Smolak, A. F. Moodey, M. D. Shuman, and L. D. Hessen, *Int. J. Eat. Dis.*, **15**, 11 (1994).

50. J. K. Thompson, M. Coovert, K. Richards, S. Johnson, and J. Cattarin, *Development of Body Image and Eating Disturbance: Covariance and Longitudinal Analyses*, University of South Florida, Tampa, FL, (1993). (unpublished manuscript).

51. J. K. Thompson, and R. E. Spana, *Int. J. Eat. Dis.*, **7**, 521 (1988).

52. D. L. Coovert, J. K. Thompson, and B. N. Kinder, *Int. J. Eat. Dis.*, **7**, 495 (1988).

53. L. A. Penner, J. K. Thompson, and D. L. Coovert, *J. Abnorm. Psychol.*, **100**, 90 (1991).

54. J. K. Thompson, *Int. J. Eat. Dis.*, **6**, 379 (1987).

55. A. E. Fallon, in *Body images: Development, Deviance, and Change*, (T. F. Cash and T. Pruzinsky, eds.), Guilford Press, New York, pp. 80–110 (1990).

56. S. L. Franzoi and M. E. Herzog, *Person. Soc. Psychol. Bull.*, **13**, 19 (1987).

57. R. Striegel—Moore, G. McAvay, and J. Rodin, *Int. J. Eat. Dis.*, **5**, 935 (1986).

58. C.S.W. Rand and J. M. Kuldau, *Int. J. Eat. Dis.*, **9**, 329 (1990).

59. D. M. Spillman and C. Everington, *Psychol. Rep.*, **64**, 887 (1989).

60. B. Ehrenreich and D. English, *For Her Own Good: 150 Years of the Experts' Advice to Women*, Anchor Press/Doubleday, New York, (1978).

61. D. M. Garner, P. E. Garfinkel, D. Schwartz, and M. Thompson, *Psychol. Rep.*, **47**, 483 (1980).

62. A. Mazur, *J. Sex Res.*, **22**, 281 (1986).

63. A. Morris, T. Cooper, and P. J. Cooper, *Int. J. Eat. Dis.*, **8**, 593 (1989).

64. C. V. Wiseman, J. J. Gray, J. E. Mosimann, and A. H. Ahren, *Int. J. Eat. Dis.*, **11**, 85 (1992).

65. M. E. Collins, *Int. J. Eat. Dis.*, **10**, 199 (1991).

66. R. Freedman, *Beauty Bound*, D. C. Heath, Lexington, MA, (1986).

67. T. R. Kelson, A. Kearney-Cooke, and L. M. Lanksy, *Perc. Mot. Skills*, **71**, 281 (1990).

68. A. E. Fallon and P. Rozin, *J. Abnorm. Psychol.*, **94**, 102 (1985).

69. J. K. Thompson and M. N. Altabe, *Int. J. Eat. Dis.*, **10**, 615 (1991).

70. L. J. Heinberg and J. K. Thompson, *J. Soc. Behav. Pers.*, **7**, 335 (1992).

71. J. K. Thompson, L. J. Heinberg, S. Tantleff, *Behav. Ther.*, **14**, 174 (1991).

72. K. C. Wood, J. A. Becker, and J. K. Thompson, *Reliability of Body Image Assessment for Young Children (ages 8–10)*, University of South Florida, Tampa, FL, (1993). (unpublished manuscript).

73. R. A. Shore and J. E. Porter, *Int. J. Eat. Dis.*, **9**, 201 (1990).

74. B. K. Mendelson and D. R. White, *Perc. Mot. Skills*, **54**, 899 (1985).

75. A. C. Petersen, J. E. Schulenberg, R. H. Abramowitz, D. Offer, and H. D. Jarcho, *J. Youth Adol.*, **13**, 93 (1984).

76. L. A. Goldfarb, E. M. Dykens, and M. Gerrard, *J. Pers. Assess.*, **49**, 329 (1985).

77. M. H. Thelan, A. L. Powell, C. Lawrence, and M. E. Kuhnert, *J. Clin. Child. Psych.*, **21**, 41 (1993).

78. H. C. Steinhausen and M. Vollrath, *Int. J. Eat. Dis.*, **12**, 83 (1992).

79. H. Steiger, F. Leung, G. Puentes-Neuman, and N. Gottheil, *Int. J. Eat. Dis.*, **11**, 121–131 (1992).

80. D. M. Garner, M. A. Olmstead, and J. Polivy, *Int. J. Eat. Dis.*, **2**, 15, (1983).

81. D. Goldsmith and J. K. Thompson, *Int. J. Eat. Dis.*, **8**, 437 (1989).

82. J. W. Butters and T. F. Cash, *J. Consult. Clin. Psychol.*, **55**, 889 (1987).

83. J. C. Rosen, E. Saltzberg, and D. Srebnik, *Behav. Ther.*, **20**, 393 (1989).

84. J. D. Killen, C. B. Taylor, L. D. Hammer, I. Litt, D. M. Wilson, T. Rich, C. Hayward, B. Simmonds, H. Kraemer, and A. Varady, *Int. J. Eat. Dis.*, **13**, 369 (1993).

85. T. F. Cash, *Body Image Therapy: A Program for Self-Directed Change,* (audio cassette series including client workbook and clinician's manual), Guilford Press, New York, (1991).

EATING DISORDERS
AND ADOLESCENTS

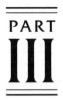

Anorexia Nervosa

Richard E. Kreipe, M.D.
Lori A. Higgins, R.D.

INTRODUCTION

Anorexia nervosa is associated with significant health problems due to nutritional and weight-reduction practices. Therefore, nutritional consultation is of particular importance in the management of this condition.[1,2] Moreover, affected individuals are typically intellectually bright and strong-willed, making them simultaneously receptive and challenging to professional input. However, helping an adolescent recover from anorexia nervosa can be rewarding for the nutritionist. The nutrition consultant requires (1) key facts about the disorder and the individual affected by the disorder, (2) practical information to share about the management of common problems related to food, nutrition, and weight-control, and (3) patience to accept small gains and frequent setbacks in food-related behaviors as the patient moves through the various stages of anorexia nervosa. The professional undertaking nutritional assessment and management may not be the "identified" therapist, but can have an extremely therapeutic impact.

Clinical Features

Weight and food-related characteristics. Anorexia nervosa is an eating disorder characterized by an insufficient and voluntarily restricted caloric intake resulting in weight loss (or failure to gain weight during puberty) that is accompanied by an obsession to be thinner and a delusion of being fat. Weight loss can be extreme, but there is no specific amount of weight loss required to fulfill diagnostic criteria. *The Diagnostic and Statistical Manual of Mental Disorders, IV* (DSM-IV) suggests, as an example, 85% of ideal body weight.[3] However, patients with a significant eating pathology may not experience this degree of emaciation for various reasons, but still require nutritional intervention. Although a desire to be thin is commonly expressed by contemporary females, the obsession to be *thinner* is a key feature that differentiates an eating disorder from mere dieting. That is, a goal weight of 110 lb is abandoned for a lower weight when the initial mark is attained, but that new goal is likewise abandoned once it is attained (in the hope of achieving satisfaction, fulfillment, or a sense of accomplishment) for a still lower target. This obsessive and relentless pursuit of thinness are characteristic of anorexia nervosa. Likewise, the delusion of being fat means that affected individuals believe they are fat, even when emaciated. Although the dieter may verbalize feeling fat, she does not define herself in terms of her body image, as does the youth with anorexia nervosa.

Over 75% of persons with anorexia nervosa exercise compulsively and ritualistically to accelerate weight loss.[4] In addition, a small proportion (less than 20%) may attempt to rid themselves of calories by vomiting or taking laxatives; such purging is more commonly associated with bulimia nervosa (see Chapter 10). Since food restriction reflects willpower, the use of diet pills or other aids suggests a lack of willpower and is uncommon in anorexia nervosa. On the other hand, food preparation for others, while the patient herself partakes of nothing, is common.

Meals. Meals are typically restricted to eating small amounts of a few, monotonous low-calorie, low-fat foods and drinking low-calorie beverages.[5] Breakfast is generally avoided altogether. Patients report not having enough time for breakfast, being too busy in preparing for school, or feeling nauseated when they eat in the morning. Lunch, if eaten at all, often consists of a salad or low-fat yogurt. Teens with anorexia nervosa often report to friends at school that they ate a large breakfast and are too full to eat lunch, then report to their parents that they ate a "huge" lunch and are too full to eat dinner, resulting in the disorder often being "hidden" until significant amounts of weight have been lost. Although dinner tends to be the most nutritious meal of the day, it is customarily eaten under duress as the parents monitor their daughter's inadequate intake with alarm and an overwhelming sense of powerlessness. If not entirely vegetarian, the intake of meat is typically severely restricted, eaten primarily at dinner, and confined to small amounts of skinless poultry or broiled fish. After-dinner desserts, between-meal snacks, and "forbidden foods" (such as candy, cakes, pies, and ice cream) are assiduously avoided.

Personality profile.   The underlying conflicts in anorexia nervosa usually relate to a fear of growing up, difficulty in achieving independence or autonomy, or confusion regarding an emerging identity. These issues are central to the dynamics of adolescence. It is not surprising, then, that anorexia nervosa most commonly emerges during adolescence. Affected individuals may have significant mental health problems, depression, or obsessive-compulsive traits. Also, the label of "dysfunctional" is often attached to the family because of enmeshment, poorly defined interpersonal boundaries, rigidity, and ineffective conflict resolution. However, such labels often divert attention away from the considerable strengths that these individuals and their families exhibit.

Etiology

In the context of nutritional management, it tends to be more useful to consider anorexia nervosa as a final common pathway that allows the affected individual to cope with unresolved adolescent developmental conflicts in a face-saving and empowering way, rather than to search for a specific cause such as an emotional flaw, set of family traits, or precipitating event. At one level, the conflict is metaphorical and has nothing to do with food, eating, or weight. The struggle for control over these concrete and measurable realities is symbolic of the intangible, confusing, and often illusory internal struggles that accompany adolescent development. At another level, however, the conflict has very real consequences for health and nutrition that can perpetuate the vicious cycle of dieting and weight loss. It is essential that both levels be addressed in treatment.

It is possible to provide information and behavioral modification strategies without fully knowing or understanding the unresolved conflicts and tensions underlying the disorder. Nutritional, medical, and psychological interventions can and should occur simultaneously.

Epidemiology

Anorexia nervosa most commonly affects Caucasian, adolescent females, and most adults with anorexia nervosa experience the onset of illness during their adolescence. Prevalence is estimated at between 0.5 and 4% of adolescent females.[6] Certain groups, such as athletes or dancers, may have a substantially higher risk for developing anorexia nervosa. Less than 5% of patients are male or from minority groups in the United States. However, the prevalence of unrecognized, atypical, or subclinical anorexia nervosa is undoubtedly several-fold greater. These individuals may be at greater risk of health consequences since they are less likely to come to clinical attention and more likely to persist in unhealthy nutritional and weight-control habits.

Prognosis

Recent data from our institution and other programs based in adolescent medicine indicate that with early recognition and treatment, anorexia nervosa can have a very good prognosis. Long-term outcome studies from these programs report a recovery rate in excess of 70%.[4] Psychiatric-based programs tend to treat patients who have a longer course of illness prior to treatment and are more likely to have significant psychiatric comorbidities; results from these settings are less favorable, with approximately half of the patients experiencing long-term recovery. The prognosis seems to be best if the adolescent patient is treated with a biopsychosocial approach that is adapted to meet the individual needs of the patient and family by a developmentally oriented interdisciplinary team that is experienced in the treatment of anorexia nervosa.

ASSESSMENT

General Issues

The initial assessment of the adolescent with suspected anorexia nervosa should focus on weight loss and health, per se, and not attempt to determine underlying psychological or emotional factors.[7] The denial that patients so frequently project when threatened with direct confrontation about an eating disorder tends not to be exhibited when they are questioned about their nutritional habits, physical symptoms, and health. The first step in the assessment is to determine if weight loss is intentional and/or desired and ensure that the symptoms are not related to a medical disease, such as inflammatory bowel disease, endocrinopathy, cancer, or an occult infection. However, some patients recover from a medical condition, such as infectious mononucleosis, only to continue to lose weight because they subsequently diet intentionally. This occurs because of the positive reinforcement that they received due to the weight loss that accompanied the initial illness. Pubertal adolescents, on the other hand, may fail to increase caloric intake during their growth spurt, or may increase their caloric expenditure playing sports and lose weight unintentionally. Finally, many adolescents lose weight while attempting to "get in shape" or "look better," without having anorexia nervosa.

The second step in the assessment of a person with suspected anorexia nervosa is to determine if weight-control habits are excessive or unhealthy. Many individuals who do not meet diagnostic criteria for anorexia nervosa may have significant health problems associated with weight control. Questionnaires assessing symptoms related to malnutrition, such as those in Appendix B, can be used to identify individuals who may be experiencing health problems commonly found in anorexia nervosa.

The third step in conducting the nutritional assessment is to determine the degree to which the pursuit of thinness is an overriding concern and a driving force in the individual's daily activities. Typically the adolescent with anorexia nervosa restricts intake to less than 1000 cal/d, is unwilling to accept a body weight of greater than 85% of the average weight for her height, and has a self-concept that is directly linked to her weight or how she feels about her weight. It is useful to have the patient identify a desired goal weight, especially if she is still within a normal-weight range. Adolescents with anorexia nervosa either have an unrealistically low goal weight, or cannot identify a specific weight with which they would be satisfied. Although a distorted body image is included in diagnostic criteria for anorexia nervosa, many adolescent females without eating disorders are also dissatisfied with their bodies, especially their hips, buttocks, and thighs, limiting the specificity of this finding. Instruments such as the Eating Disorder Inventory (EDI) can also be used to measure features including body dissatisfaction or drive for thinness (see Chapter 8).

If the evidence indicates that the adolescent has anorexia nervosa, the fourth step is to determine an immediate plan of action. We advocate the biopsychosocial model in treatment, which recognizes that patients require attention to their biological, psychological, and social needs. For patients who have lost a significant amount of weight and are exhibiting signs of starvation and hypometabolism, immediate hospitalization must be considered. However, with early recognition, hospitalization can usually be avoided, as long as appropriate outpatient treatment is available.

Health

No organ system is spared the effects of the malnutrition that occurs in anorexia nervosa.[8] The medical complications of anorexia nervosa is a topic beyond the scope of this chapter. Most physiologic changes are adaptations to inadequate nutritional intake. Among these, the most concerning are persistent amenorrhea, hypothermia, bradycardia, and orthostatic cardiovascular instability. Low weight, amenorrhea and poor nutrition predispose women with anorexia nervosa to osteoporosis.[9-13] Hypothermia can be extremely uncomfortable, especially in cold climates, and can predispose to cardiac rhythm disturbances. Cardiovascular instability can lead to weakness, fatigue, dizziness, loss of energy, fainting, and death.[14,15]

The laboratory evaluation of patients with anorexia nervosa is primarily directed at detecting unsuspected underlying medical conditions. Nutrition-related tests include levels of hepatic secretory proteins, measures of immune function, and measurement of vitamin or mineral levels.[16,17] Serum albumin and prealbumin, with half-lives of 20 and 2 d, respectively, can be used to assess energy balance and protein synthesis in the liver. Levels of these proteins are typically normal, due to adequate protein intake in the context of extreme restriction of carbohydrates and fat, or to dehydration. Transferrin, a beta-globulin with a half-life of 8 d, tends to be nonspecifically increased in anorexia nervosa. Visceral protein levels can be assessed with the calculation of creatinine height index (CHI) and then compared to reference standards. A 20–40% reduction of CHI is evidence of moderate visceral protein depletion, whereas severe depletion is indicated by a reduction of more than 40%. Measurement of the immune function by various methods has not produced consistent results in the literature, but can sometimes be useful in assessing the physiologic response to nutritional status. Vitamin and mineral levels in circulating compartments, such as the serum, may not be related to actual deficiencies at the tissue level. In vitro assay of dependent enzymes with and without the vitamin cofactor may be a more useful measure, but is not routinely available.

Routine laboratory tests obtained during medical evaluation usually include a complete blood count and erythrocyte sedimentation rate, SMA_6 and SMA_{12}, and urinalysis. These are usually normal, a reflection of the remarkable ability of the body to maintain homeostatic balance. An electrocardiogram may be indicated if there is significant bradycardia or rhythm disturbance. Thyroid screening is often obtained, but rarely useful, since the clinical picture in anorexia nervosa combines symptoms of hyper- and hypo-thyroidism. An unusual finding is elevated serum cholesterol, with both elevated and normal LDL fractions being reported, despite extremely low fat and cholesterol intake.[19–22]

Anthropometry

The most important anthropometric measurements in the assessment of an adolescent with anorexia nervosa are height and weight. The latter should be determined with the patient in a gown, immediately after voiding but before being examined by a health care provider.

The body mass index, BMI, is a calculated anthropometric variable that standardizes weight for height. BMI = weight (kg) ÷ height (m)^2. Values for patients with anorexia nervosa generally fall below 18. Levels below 16 tend to be associated with significant symptoms, especially if weight loss is rapid.

Skinfold thickness, either as triceps or multiple-site determination, can be used to assess subcutaneous fat, but the standards apply only for older adolescents and the measurements must be obtained by skilled personnel using research-quality instruments (see Chapter 18). Thus, plastic calipers are unreliable and should not be used. The four-site (triceps, biceps, subscapular, iliac) method of body fat determination is probably the most accurate. Also, the measurement may not be accurate in states of dehydration and there have been few studies in which skinfold thickness in adolescents with anorexia nervosa has been compared to reference methods of body composition determination. The primary use of this tool is in following the progress of a patient during treatment, rather than to define a level of body fat at any one time.

Diet and Activity Records

The recording of actual food and drink intake by an adolescent is helpful in both assessment and treatment. It aids the professional to identify dietary patterns, deficiencies, excesses, and strengths as well as helps the teen become more aware of her nutritional habits.[23,24] We recommend a 7-d food diaries rather than 24-h recall. Although some adolescents seek a high degree of monotony and sameness in their diet, there can also be a large degree of day-to-day variability, often based on mood, events, thoughts, or feelings. It is worthwhile to assess intake in the context of these variables and a food journal can assist in this process (see Table 9.1). However, since adolescents with anorexia nervosa frequently overestimate their serving size, it is important to verify their reports. A helpful tool in this respect are food models that simultaneously inform the professional about the patient's intake and teach the patient how to estimate serving size.

Table 9.1   Assessment of Eating Attitudes, Behaviors, and Habits

Eating attitudes
Fat content
Food aversions
"Safe" foods
Magical thinking
Binge trigger foods

Eating behaviors
Small bites of food
Ritualistic behavior
Unusual food combinations
Atypical seasoning of food
Atypical use of eating utensils

Eating habits
Intake pattern
   Number of meals and snacks
   Time of day consumed
   Duration of feedings
   Eating environment: where and with whom
   How consumed: sitting or standing
   Monotonous food choices

Adapted from E. Luder and J. Schedenbach, *Top. Clin. Nutr.*, **8**, 48 (1993).
Reprinted with permission.

To fully understand the balance between energy intake and output, it is important to record the type, intensity, frequency, and duration of exercise. In addition, one should determine if there are other ways in which energy is expended without qualifying as formal exercise. For example, walking to and from school while carrying a heavy bookbag, bounding repeatedly up and down stairs at home to "get some things," or "stretching" twice a day all add to the daily expenditure of calories, but generally go unmeasured.

The journals to evaluate nutrition can also be used by other professionals on the team to determine dysfunctional habits (such as the teen eating a rice cake for breakfast), associated mood disturbances (such as not eating dinner because of an argument with her mother), and episodes whereby the patient makes a breakthrough toward recovery (such as eating a "forbidden food" like chocolate). Therefore, we encourage adolescents to bring their journals with them to outpatient visits, regardless of whether or not they are seeing the nutritionist.

Body Composition

If body composition is measured, we believe that it is more clinically useful to focus on lean mass rather than fat mass. Fat tissue is that which the adolescent is most interested in eliminating. However, clinicians sometimes emphasize the importance of reaching a critical amount of body fat to regain normal physiology, including menstrual function, in treatment. The Frisch hypothesis, which postulated that the initiation or maintenance of menstrual cycles requires the persistence of a minimal level of body fat, has numerous empirical and methodological shortcomings. Some women do not menstruate on regaining normal body fat and others continue to menstruate despite being far below the predicted threshold. In addition, the symptoms that the patient experiences are primarily due to a reduction of lean body mass, and the return to normal physical functioning is primarily effected through increases in the lean compartment. Therefore, focusing on the health benefits of gaining lean body mass is both physiologically more appropriate and clinically more therapeutic.

Early in recovery, over two-thirds of the weight gained is lean.[25] As the body approaches more normal distribution of lean and fat, an increasing amount of tissue laid down is fat. The composition does not appear to be influenced by diet, but can be influenced by activity.[26–31] That is, if patients increase their energy intake in a well-balanced diet and also engage in a combination of aerobic exercise and resistance training, then the majority of tissue that is added will be lean.

Energy Intake and Needs

The measurement of metabolic rate by indirect calorimetry can be very helpful in determining the metabolic needs of the patient. Schebendach and Nussbaum recommend prescribing 130% of resting energy expenditure (REE).[32] This also allows the expected increase in REE that occurs with refeeding to be monitored over time.

Vitamins and Minerals

Elevated plasma levels of retinol (the primary form of vitamin A in plasma) and retinyl esters (a transient form of vitamin A associated with chylomicrons) have been reported by some investigators.[33-35] These changes are not typical of protein-energy malnutrition and may be due to altered metabolism (closely related to low T_3 levels[36]) or the delayed clearance of chylomicrons. It is not clear why adolescents with anorexia nervosa have a tendency to become hypercarotenemic. The intake of beta-carotene can be quite high in patients whose diet consists largely of yellow vegetables. However, Rock and Swendseid[37] reported that elevated plasma carotenoids in anorexia nervosa may also indicate a diminished ability to clear or metabolize these compounds. However, there is little evidence for these increased levels posing a risk of hypervitaminosis A.

Investigators have reported increased, decreased, and normal plasma concentrations of tocopherol.[17,18,34,38] Because vitamin E is known to be associated with lipoproteins, levels may reflect the effects of binding to blood lipids rather than tissue concentrations. Vitamin E deficiency has been related to cognitive and neuropsychological problems and is therefore of clinical interest, even though there is no consistent recognized pattern of deficiency. Further investigation is required to elucidate the circumstances in which an alteration of vitamin E status might be expected. Thiamin, riboflavin, and vitamin B-6 may also contribute to cognitive problems and physiological features associated with semistarvation in many anorectic patients. The dietary requirements for these vitamins are determined by substrate utilization, the severity of malnutrition, the refeeding process, and the stage of recovery. Measurement of blood levels is of little clinical use unless the history and physical exam suggest the presence of a specific deficiency.

The primary minerals that are of concern in anorexia nervosa are calcium and zinc. Although calcium intake is typically much less than the RDA, serum levels are usually normal and urinary excretion is often increased. This may be due to the resorption of bone that commonly occurs in association with the low estrogen and high cortisol levels typically found in anorexia nervosa. There is little evidence that variation in calcium intake has measurable effects on bone density, possibly because the high resorptive state makes skeletal calcium available, even if dietary calcium is reduced.[13] Zinc is known to be lost in catabolic states such as occurs in anorexia nervosa, but serum levels are difficult to measure and interpret; balance studies are probably more useful clinically than serum levels. There is also theoretical evidence to consider zinc deficiency as possibly related to some of the symptoms of anorexia nervosa,[17] but little evidence to suggest that it is clinically relevant. A double-blind, placebo-controlled clinical trial of zinc supplementation demonstrated improvement in some psychological functioning, but no effect on weight gain.[39] Furthermore, it is important to note that excessive zinc supplementation can cause copper deficiency.[1,40-42]

MANAGEMENT

Psychosocial

Just as with the medical consequences, the psychological and emotional conflicts that underlie the eating behaviors of many adolescents with anorexia nervosa are beyond the scope of this chapter. However, there are specific issues that should be addressed with respect to psychological factors in relation to nutritional management of anorexia nervosa.

Therapeutic approach.   A primary treatment goal should be the attainment and maintenance of health, not merely weight gain. In this context, weight gain becomes a means to an end, the higher goal of wellness, replacing weight loss as a means to the end of attaining a sense of control.[7] The professional providing nutritional consultation can foster the development of confidence and trust in this goal by recognizing certain psychological features of the adolescent with anorexia nervosa. First is the need for flexibility rather than rigidity in meal planning. Since rigidity characterizes the patient's approach to eating, it is countertherapeutic to propose a rigid nutrition prescription. Instead, the exchange system of meal planning is most productive. This provides sufficient structure to ensure adequate nutrition if followed, but sufficient flexibility to give the patient a sense of control over her eating. Second is the need for compromise rather than protocol in treatment. A patient's sense of efficacy is enhanced when she perceives that she is being listened to and can influence professionals caring for her. Protocols tend to force the patient into a treatment regimen and are best left to experimental interventions. True compromise, in which both parties move toward a common ground, however, reinforce the therapeutic relationship.

Third is the need to recognize the patient as an individual, not as a disease. Although patients with anorexia nervosa share many features in common, often with disconcerting similarities, each person with the diagnosis is a unique individual who deserves a nutritional treatment plan adapted to her special needs. Fourth it is worthwhile to recognize and explicitly acknowledge a patient's desire for sameness and the difficulty that she has adapting to change. By acknowledging how frightening change may be and conceding that making the necessary changes in meal planning and eating can be extremely difficult, the professional demonstrates empathy that can build trust and confidence. A professional who makes a nutritional plan appear as if it is easy to accomplish may alienate the patient, even though the content of the plan is scientifically accurate and well conceived.

It is important to give encouragement for small gains. The change from drinking skim milk to 1% milk may not appear to be a major accomplishment to members of the family of a patient with anorexia nervosa, but it is important for the clinician to recognize this as a major step forward in recovery. One should avoid being overly solicitous in this regard, however, since adolescents are often ambivalent about such changes and may feel guilty about being so recognized. Finally, it is helpful to reframe negative, pejorative concepts that are frequently applied to patients with anorexia nervosa, such as "manipulative," in more positive terms. Patients often consider themselves to be powerless and may believe that the only way they can get their way is to be manipulative. Therefore, the challenge is to help the patient gain a sense of empowerment, so that manipulation of others is not necessary. Open communication among all team members, listening to patients, expecting honesty and trusting are all means of minimizing negative behaviors.

Communication.   The professional management of nutritional issues in anorexia nervosa should focus on facts rather than opinions, health rather than fashion, the objective rather than the subjective. These are the manifestations of authority and the primary sources of credibility with a patient. Compare, for example, the statements "You look too thin to me" and "Your loss of menstrual periods, low body temperature, cold hands and feet, low pulse and blood pressure all indicate that your weight is too low." The latter is much more clinically useful. However, the professional must also be aware of how powerful opinions, fashion, and subjective perceptions can be for individuals with anorexia nervosa, and assist the patient in developing alternative strategies to counteract these messages. In addition, the nutritionist must remain scrupulously honest. Parents may ask a professional to try to influence their daughter to eat by telling her "all the terrible things that she's doing to her body." It is appropriate to respond to such a request with "All I can do is give Susie the facts. They may scare you and me, but they may not scare her. I won't try to control or coerce her. She needs to trust me, and I won't do anything to jeopardize that, even if it might get her to eat for a little while. In the long run, my professional advice will not be of any value if she doesn't believe me." This is best said in the presence of the patient, to emphasize the value that the professional places on honesty and trust in the therapeutic relationship.

When an adolescent realizes that the clinician is not interested in punishing or judging her and there are no expectations other than being honest with herself and everyone else (even if that means disclosing fears and phobias about eating and weight gain), she is often able to avoid the significant problems, such as denial and resistance, that may preclude effective therapeutic interactions. These defensive mechanisms become unnecessary when the clinician has the confidence and trust of the patient.

General Treatment

The methods used to lose weight, possible symptoms or signs associated with excessive weight loss, and the target goal weight must be determined. The functions that the nutritional consultant brings to the therapeutic team include (1) evaluating the diet and identifying specific deficiencies or excesses; (2) educating the patient and family regarding nutritional needs during adolescence; (3) dispelling dietary myths or misconceptions held by the patient; (4) developing a balanced meal plan within a target caloric range to achieve either weight gain or maintenance; (5) applying a food exchange system to allow variety and flexibility in food selection; (6) assessing diet journals to identify dysfunctional eating habits or patterns; and (7) providing feedback to the patient to encourage continued progress toward health.

An adolescent with a distorted body image feels fat despite having lost weight. She may have fallen below her goal weight, but continues to perceive a need to lose more weight. Or, she may desire to fit into the next smaller size of clothes. The clinician should not challenge her perceptions. To the contrary, it is helpful to acknowledge her desire to lose weight, because she believes that she is fat. However, this reality must be balanced against the reality that she is also too thin, manifested by the symptoms and signs of excessive weight loss. The therapeutic potential of this maneuver can be tremendous. Her *feeling* fat cannot be challenged (because only she can know her feelings) and the fact of her *being* too thin cannot be challenged (because of objective data); the clinician must acknowledge to the patient an awareness of the dilemma that the patient faces. This understanding furthers the development of trust in the professional and is much more therapeutic than "How can you possibly feel fat, when you are so thin?" or "Why don't you just eat?", which are often heard from insensitive or uninformed family members or friends.

Daily structure.   Should include eating three meals a day. Eating an adequate breakfast (not merely a rice cake) maximizes the likelihood of adequate daily caloric intake and deserves repeated emphasis. We suggest that half of the daily energy requirement be consumed by the end of lunch; otherwise, patients tend to put off eating until late in the day and find themselves unable to take in adequate nutrition without binge eating. The consequence of eating an insufficient amount of food at meals will be failure to gain weight, which will elicit responses by the treatment team. Thus, parents should be encouraged to ensure that healthy food is available and mealtimes are planned into the patient's day, but not to assume responsibility for her eating. If parents feel it is their duty to make their child eat, eating becomes a battle that cannot be won. If the adolescent acquiesces and eats merely to please her parents, the likelihood is great that she will develop purging as a means of avoiding weight gain after she is "forced" to eat.

Nutrition prescription. The initial caloric prescription is generally between 1000 and 1400 kcal/d, although the use of 130% of REE as determined by indirect calorimetry or adjusted an Harris-Benedict equation are more precise methods of determining actual resting energy requirements. These values need to be adjusted for estimated energy expenditure in daily activity especially for adolescents involved in sports or vigorous physical exercise.[43-45] The nutrition prescription should work toward gradually increasing weight at the rate of about ½–1 lb/wk, by increasing energy intake at 100–200 kcal increments every few days. In addition, the gradual inclusion of "forbidden foods" should be part of the nutrition prescription once the adolescent has shown evidence of being able to eat adequately to gain weight. A standard nutritional balance of 15–20% protein, 55–60% carbohydrate, and 20–25% fat is appropriate. However, the fat content may need to be lowered to 15–20% early in treatment because of continued fat phobia.

Rock and Curran-Celentano[1] note that if refeeding is accomplished with an increased energy diet consisting of a variety of regular foods, sufficient amounts of vitamins and minerals will be provided, so that a correction of deficiencies without supplementation is anticipated. Treating the nutritional problems with nutrient-dense foods will also help to correct the multitude of metabolic and physiological abnormalities associated with semistarvation, in addition to reversing specific micronutrient deficiencies. Low-dose multiple vitamins with minerals at RDA levels may be appropriate for chronically ill adolescents who are unable to maintain adequate nutrition. On the other hand, the use of high-dose supplements can have unfavorable effects through either excessive levels of the micronutrient itself or adverse interactions with other elements (such as occurs between zinc and copper).

Nutritional concerns. It is useful to return to the physical evidence that nutrition is inadequate when discussing meal-planning with an adolescent with an eating disorder. Emphasizing food as fuel for the body, the source of energy in our daily lives, grounds the goal of increasing a patient's energy level, endurance, and strength in the need for food. Likewise, cold, blue hands and feet can be interpreted as evidence that the body is conserving heat, because the patient is not supplying her body with the major source of heat, food. To highlight the relationship between energy, heat, and calories, we point out that a calorie is the amount of energy required to raise the temperature of 1 g of water by 1°C.

It is also important to recognize cognitive distortions of adolescents with anorexia nervosa. Examples include dichotomous, all-or-none thinking; overgeneralization; jumping to conclusions; catastrophizing; emotional reasoning; personalization; and the use of "should" statements. These generate behaviors such as breaking foods down into "good" or "bad" categories, having a day "ruined" because of one unexpected event, or choosing foods based on rigid restrictions rather than personal desires or wishes. In combination with the perfectionism that characterizes adolescents with anorexia nervosa, cognitive patterns can lead to extreme levels of fat restriction (<5 g/d) or strict vegetarianism.

Finally, delayed gastric emptying occurs with malnutrition, leading to early satiety and fullness with small meals. Although this generally abates within a few weeks of healthy eating, it can preclude adequate nutrition, especially if low-calorie foods and drinks continue to be ingested. Therefore, we recommend frequent, small meals that are relatively nutrient-dense and high in carbohydrates, starting early in the day. Some patients find liquid nutritional supplements especially helpful, since they occupy a small volume and have more rapid transit time than solid food. Prokinetic agents, such as cisapride or metoclopramide, can be used if these symptoms are debilitating.

Parental involvement.   We urge the parents to recognize their role in making healthy food available, and the patient's role in taking responsibility for maintaining her health. Then, the parents can avoid being monitors, or assuming a policing function. This is not always possible and frequently needs to be a focus of family therapy, as the members of the family determine their roles and responsibilities as they develop together.

Hospital admission.   Some clinicians include falling below a predetermined minimum weight as an indication for hospitalization for an adolescent with moderate anorexia nervosa. Low weight is only one index of malnutrition. Weight should not be used as the sole criterion for admission to the hospital. Most adolescents with moderate anorexia nervosa realize the wisdom in the adage "a pint is a pound the world around." They may drink fluids, or hide heavy objects in their underwear, prior to "weigh-in" if weight alone determines hospital admission. This may result in acute hyponatremia or dangerous degrees of unrecognized weight loss. A focus on health that includes a physical examination and consideration of body temperature, pulse, blood pressure, and orthostatic cardiovascular changes generally is more physiologically defensible than an arbitrary minimum. However, some patients need to know a concrete minimum threshold to avoid hospitalization.

Hospitalization

Energy needs and dietary prescription.   Most adolescents with severe anorexia nervosa who are hospitalized require at least 1500 cal/d to maintain weight. Their reduced basal metabolic rate (BMR) may be as low as 800–1000 cal/d, and maintenance requirements are 130–150% of BMR. Approximately 1 g of weight is gained for every 5 cal of intake in excess of output; to accrue 100 additional g of weight requires an excess of 500 cal. At low weight, few calories are expended in exercise than at higher weights; even with 1 h of vigorous exercise the patient expends ≤400 cal. If an adolescent appears to eat >3000 cal daily and still does not gain weight, it is likely that food is being vomited or discarded, or unrecognized exercise is occurring. Younger patients require slightly more energy to gain weight than older patients, since some of their intake is allocated to growth.

In prescribing the initial caloric intake, the clinician must recognize that few concepts are as frightening to an adolescent with anorexia nervosa as that of gaining weight and patients who demonstrate decreased metabolic rate (hypothermia, bradycardia, hypotension, lethargy) may gain weight more readily than physiologically stable individuals. Initial weight gain can be rapid for three reasons. First, many malnourished adolescents are hypovolemic and gain weight in the form of extracellular fluid. Second, their basal metabolic rate can be half of what is normal. This reduction in energy expenditure enables calories ingested to exceed calories expended even at low levels of intake, resulting in weight gain in the form of body tissues. Third, these newly formed tissues are two-thirds lean, not entirely fat as presumed by most patients, regardless of the protein content of the diet. It requires much less energy to produce protein-rich lean tissues than fat-rich storage tissues (that are formed in quantity only after restoration of the lean body mass). Thus, more weight is gained initially for each excess calorie over expenditure than will be gained later as the patient approaches normal weight (see Table 9.2) and body composition.[25,46]

Therefore, although her daily requirement may eventually exceed 2500 cal, one should not attempt to prescribe an initial increase of more than 50% over her present average daily intake of energy. Not only is she unlikely to respond favorably to a "normal" diet, but also it is unnecessary and can be physically and psychologically dangerous if the patient gains weight too quickly. Parents, especially, need to recognize that "more" is not necessarily "better" with respect to eating and weight gain. By focusing on a gradual, monitored increased in intake, the nutritionist can often lessen the adolescent's resistance to changing her eating habits.

The minimal daily caloric intake generally begins at about 1000–1200 cal, but may need to be lower if the patient was ingesting only a few hundred calories/day prior to admission. Intake is increased, as necessary, at 200–400 calorie increments every 2 or 3 d. In the severely malnourished patient, fluid retention, congestive heart failure, hypophosphatemia, and other manifestations of the "refeeding syndrome"[47] can occur with too rapid replacement. Rarely is it advisable to decrease the daily caloric minimum, once it is established at a higher level. Only if the patient has demonstrated consistent weight gain not attributable to fluid should lowering energy intake be considered.[48]

Food choices. An adolescent with anorexia nervosa typically agonizes obsessively over decisions relating to choosing and consuming food because eating

Table 9.2   Factors Affecting Rate of Weight Gain in Anorexia Nervosa

Fluid balance
Urine output increased in semistarvation and may "load" with fluids to
    falsify weight gain
Edema
  Famine
  Refeeding
Hydration ratios
  Glycogen
  Protein

Changes in the metabolic rate
Resting energy expenditure (REE)
Termic effect of food
Activity (measured and unmeasured)

Energy cost of the tissue gained
Lean body mass (majority of tissue formed in early stages of refeeding)
Adipose

Adapted from E. Luder and J. Schedenbach, *Top. Clin. Nutr.*, 8, 48 (1993). Reprinted
with permission.

means she will disappoint herself by "giving in," but not eating means she will
disappoint those whom she would like to please. Therefore, she should be allowed
≤10 min to make menu selections and ≤45 min to complete a meal. She may
argue that under such conditions she will be unable to gain weight and it will
be the fault of the doctors and nurses. But these are reasonable and necessary
limits if the patient is to make changes to recover. If she has not chosen sufficient
food within the 10-min allotment, additional foods are chosen for her by the
nutritionist. If she does not clear her food tray within the 45 min allotment, the
tray is removed, and the uneaten portions can be returned at the next meal time
or replaced with fresh food. Alternatively, the balance of her caloric needs for
the meal can be taken as a liquid supplement. In extremely resistant cases in
which the medical stability of the patient is tenuous, that nutrition may need to
be supplied via nasogastric tube (NG) as described below. This prevents food
and meals from occupying all of her time and attention. As successful treatment
progresses, such restrictions usually do not need to be enforced, because she
has incorporated healthy behaviors into her previously dysfunctional repertoire.

Rigid adherence to calorie counting should be avoided; an approach that
considers the nutritional value of food is preferable. Many patients are acutely
aware of the calorie content of food and select foods solely on this criterion.
Other patients can become obsessed with calories if the hospital team focuses
on this aspect of nutrition. The hospital staff must recognize that the caloric

values of foods listed in various reference sources are rough approximations and not worthy of the debate that patients frequently initiate.

Nasogastric tube feedings. Feeding by NG tube is indicated when the patient demonstrates that she is unable to consume sufficient calories by mouth to maintain health. This technique should never be considered a punishment, as "forced feeding," or a means to "teach the patient a lesson." The NG tube may be inserted for each feeding and then removed, or it may be left in place, but its location in the stomach must be ensured prior to use. With an indwelling tube, feeding can be intermittent or continuous. Continuous feeding is especially advantageous in the early stages of nutritional rehabilitation, since slow rates of administration are possible.

The potential advantages of NG tube feeding are numerous. Control over nutritional rehabilitation can be attained, but may require a closed feeding system that allows the patient no means of discarding liquid from an open container, such as can occur with a Kangaroo^R bag. In addition, the patient often feels less guilty about weight gain, since she is not eating when she is being fed by NG tube. Also, many patients express relief (days to weeks later) at not needing to make decisions about eating, while knowing that their health is being secured. Finally, by eliminating habitual conflicts about food and eating, treatment can often focus on more important psychosocial issues underlying the eating disorder. Obviously, NG tube feeds should only be considered as a temporary measure that will eventually be replaced with healthy eating, once nutritional balance has been restored.

Although concerns that a patient may become "dependent" on tube feedings, lose her desire to eat, "forget" how to eat, or "give up" are sometimes raised, these consequences are more feared than real. These fears reflect ambivalence about tube feedings more than realistic complications. Despite the superiority of the enteral over the parenteral route with respect to both the adequacy of nutrition and safety of administration, intravenous feeding is sometimes chosen over NG tube feeding. Intravenous feeding has a place in the emergency management of acute fluid and electrolyte imbalance, but the use of intravenous or total peripheral nutrition is rarely indicated. Concerns that tube feeding is too invasive or punitive seem overstated, but the requirement for prolonged tube feedings indicates a serious underlying pathology that needs to be addressed in treatment. The goal, when using any alternative methods of nourishing, is always to return the patient to normal levels and methods of food consumption. Certainly, prior to discharge a patient must demonstrate the ability to plan, choose, and ingest an adequate diet of normal food and liquids, including "forbidden foods."

Expected weight gain. Regardless of the treatment model used, after stabilization of weight, a healthy average daily weight gain is determined for the patient, usually between 100 and 300 g/d. Her diet is planned with the nutritionist and based on the principles of food exchange. The responsibility for weight gain is explicitly made the patient's. Otherwise, the staff may be blamed for not giving the patient enough food when she does not gain weight or she has her activities restricted. However, weight gain should not be the total focus of the program. The attainment of physical health is merely the foundation for long-term treatment focused on the various developmental conflicts confronting the patient. A behavioral program is a means to the end of physical health. Expectations for weight gain should also include the eventual acceptance by the patient of responsibility to ensure that she is feeding herself adequately to maintain her health after discharge. To that end, patients should gradually work toward eating in the hospital cafeteria, at a restaurant, and at home prior to discharge. Otherwise, the patient often reverts to her preadmission habits of eating and reverts to losing weight immediately after discharge. We find that working with the patient to deal with these realities of life while she is still hospitalized helps her and her family have the confidence that the gains made during hospitalization will continue at home. Then, it is important to continue to follow the adolescent as an outpatient, to minimize the likelihood her of returning to dysfunctional eating habits and weight-control methods. The need for follow-up may continue for months to years, but we have found that the majority of patients benefit from hospitalization and do not require readmission. With proper guidance, most patients recover.

CASE ILLUSTRATION

Amy was a 14½-year-old female who experienced a 17 lb weight loss over the previous 4 mo by limiting her intake of food and increasing her exercise. At the onset of her intentional weight loss, she was 64 in. and weighed 119 lb. She began to diet because she felt that she was "out of shape" for soccer and thought that her thighs looked "too fat" in her soccer uniform.

She acknowledged feeling cold and tired over the last few weeks, which she attributed to not getting enough sleep because of studying for midterm examinations. Although she had been menstruating regularly since age 13 yr, she had not had a period in 3 mo. Amy attributed her amenorrhea to exercising 1 h daily. Her parents noted that she had become increasingly withdrawn and irritable, especially at meals. In fact, they reported that she preferred to go to her room to study while the rest of the family ate dinner. Recently, Amy's parents reported having more arguments about her eating habits and weight loss. In addition, her father had tried to "make her eat," but this only led to increased resentment between the two. Amy's mother indicates that nothing is working despite trying to fix "foods that Amy liked to eat."

Amy reports that she does not eat breakfast at home or school because of time constraints, i.e., 7:20 A.M. music class. She typically has a salad with fat-free dressing for lunch because "all my friends are on diets." When she comes home after school, she reports eating two rice cakes and a diet soda. Dinner, if eaten at all, usually consists of 1–2 oz of chicken breast, a few ounces of plain pasta or potatoes, and a few bites of a vegetable. She never eats dessert with the rest of the family, but does eat 3 oz of frozen fat-free yogurt two to three evenings per week. On weekends or school holidays, she reports eating a small bowl of puffed wheat with skimmed milk for breakfast and fat-free yogurt for lunch. She denies any binge eating, noting that eating large amounts of food is a "sign of weakness and would make me even fatter than I already am." She also denies vomiting or using laxatives or diuretics to lose weight, because they are "not healthy."

Amy's exercise routine consists or 45 min on a stair-stepper machine and 15 min on a stationary bicycle at least five times per week. She reports planning to join a health club in order to have easy access to resistance training equipment, noting that she wants to not only lose fat, but also have stronger leg muscles for soccer.

Amy would like a healthy diet that would help her lose weight to about 100 lb. Amy's mother is worried that she has anorexia nervosa and is going to die (having just seen a television show on this topic). The father is frustrated and withdrawn, believing that Amy is "just doing this for attention" and "all she needs to do is to start eating again."

Physical examinations reveals a thin, Caucasian female who appears apprehensive. Her vital signs reveal hypometabolism (temperature 35.9° C, pulse 52 sitting and 78 standing, blood pressure 78 over 40). Her skin was cool and her hands and feet were blue with poor capillary refill. Her hair was thin and lackluster. The remainder of the findings from her physical exam was consistent with excessive weight loss, but without evidence of an underlying organic etiology. Laboratory studies revealed a low white count ($3200/cm^3$) and blood glucose (59 mg/dL), with no evidence of thyroid dysfunction.

Amy was counseled on the unhealthy effects of her weight-control practices, as demonstrated by her symptoms, physical exam, and laboratory findings. A 1200-cal/d exchange meal plan was provided, with the expectation to advance her intake by 400 cal every week until she reached approximately 2400 cal/d. She was advised to limit her exercise to only 15 min every other day in order to conserve her energy and was requested to return to the clinic in 1 wk.

On follow-up, Amy had lost another 1½ lb. She had tried to increase her intake, but became afraid that she would "blow up like a balloon." Although she reported eating breakfast regularly, she was only able to do so by also increasing her exercise the night before. In addition, she stated that she had felt dizzy and almost fainted during gym class. Her temperature and pulse had fallen to 35.4°C and 48 beats/min, respectively. Because of her physical state and inadequate intake, she was advised to eliminate exercise altogether at both home and school. Amy was referred for mental health services, since she was becoming increasingly more withdrawn and hopeless and her parents felt that family life was becoming "unbearable."

The following week, Amy's weight was down again to 100 lb. She thought that she would stop the weight loss when she got below 100 lb. Although she reported eating "huge amounts of food," parents reported that her intake had, if anything, decreased. The psychologist who saw Amy and the family several days before thought that Amy feared growing up, was depressed, and did not believe Amy would discontinue her weight-loss practices. Amy reported that "everything would be fine if everyone would leave me alone."

Intensive outpatient treatment focused on her biological, psychological, and social status, eventually resulting in significant improvement. When she reached 98 lb, she was put on the waiting list for admission to the hospital. After visiting the unit where she was to be admitted, she realized that hospitalization was imminent and agreed to gain weight and work with the treatment team. After 8 mo of treatment, her weight was up to 109 lb, but menstruation has not returned. However, she is physically stable and making good improvement. Acting as a "coach's assistant" on the soccer team, she will be able to play when her weight reaches 110 lb.

REFERENCES

1. C. L. Rock and J. Curran-Celentano, *Int. J. Eat. Dis.*, **15**, 187 (1994).

2. D. M. Huse and A. R. Lucas, *J. Am. Diet. Assoc.*, **83**, 687 (1983).

3. American Psychiatric Association, *Diagnostic and Statistical Manual of Mental Disorders, IV ed.*, American Psychiatric Association, Washington, DC, pp. 544 (1994).

4. R. E. Kreipe, B. H. Churchill, and J. Strauss, *AJDC*, **113**, 1322 (1989).

5. H. E. Gwirtsman, W. H. Kaye, S. R. Curtis, and L. M. Lyter, *J. Am. Diet. Assoc.*, **89**, 54 (1989).

6. A. S. Whitaker, *Ped. Ann.*, **21**, 752 (1992).

7. R. E. Kreipe and M. Uphoff, *Adol. Med.: State Art Rev.*, **3**, 519 (1992).

8. A. S. Kaplan, and P. E. Garfinkel, in *Medical Issues and the Eating Disorders*, (A. S. Kaplan and P. E. Garfinkel, eds.), Brunner/Mazel, New York, pp. 1–256, (1993).

9. B. K. Biller, V. Saxe, D. B. Herzog, D. I. Rosenthal, S. Holzman, and A. Klibanski, *J. Clin. Endo. Met.*, **68**, 548 (1989).

10. M. M. Newman and K. A. Halmi, *Psychol. Res.*, **29**, 105 (1989).

11. N. A. Rigotti, S. R. Nussbaum, D. B. Herzog, and R. M. Neer, *N. Engl. J. Med.*, **311**, 1601 (1984).

12. C. L. Rock, I. F. Hunt, M. E. Swendseid, and J. Yager, *Am. J. Clin. Nutr.*, **46**(suppl.), 527 (1987).

13. J. J. Salisbury and J. E. Mitchell, *Am. J. Psych.*, **148**, 768 (1991).

14. D. D. Schocken, J. D. Holloway, and P. S. Powers, *Arch. Int. Med.*, **149**, 877 (1989).

15. J. M. Isner, W. C. Roberts, and S. B. Heymsfield, J. Yager, *Ann. Int. Med.*, **102**, 49 (1985).

16. C.J.M. van Binsbergen, J. Odink, H. van Den Berg, H. Koppeschaar, and H. J. T. Colelingh Bennink, *Eur. J. Clin. Nutr.*, **42**, 929 (1988).

17. R. C. Casper, B. Kirschner, H. H. Sandstead, R. A. Jacob, and J. M. Davis, *Am. J. Clin. Nutr.*, **33**, 1801 (1980).

18. M. Mira, P. M. Stewart, and S. F. Abraham, *Am. J. Clin. Nutr.*, **50**, 940 (1989).

19. P. J. Nestel, *J. Clin. Endo. Met.*, **38**, 325 (1974).

20. R. Mordasini, G. Klose, and H. Greten, *Metabolism*, **27**, 71 (1978).

21. M. R. Arden, E. C. Weiselberg, M. P. Nussbaum, R. Shenker, and M. S. Jacobson, *J. Adol Health Care*, **11**, 199 (1990).

22. K. Halmi and M. Fry, *Biol. Psych.*, **8**, 159 (1974).

23. C. L. Rock and J. Yager, *Int. J. Eat. Dis.*, **6**, 167 (1987).

24. P.J.V. Beaumont, T. L. Chambers, L. Rouse, and S. F. Abraham, *J. Hum. Nutr.*, **35**, 265 (1981).

25. G. L. Forbes, R. E. Kreipe, B. A. Lipinski, and C. H. Hodgman, *Am. J. Clin. Nutr.*, **40**, 1137 (1984).

26. W. H. Kaye, H. E. Gwirtsman, E. Obarzanek, T. George, D. C. Jimerson, and M. Ebert, *Am. J. Clin. Nutr.*, **44**, 435 (1986).

27. W. H. Kaye, H. E. Gwirtsman, E. Obarzanek, and D. T. George, *Am. J. Clin. Nutr.*, **47**, 989 (1988).

28. D. D. Krahn, C. L. Rock, R. E. Dechert, K. K. Nairn, and S. A. Hasse, *J. Am. Diet. Assoc.*, **93**, 434 (1993).

29. A. Luke and D. A. Schoeller, *Metabolism*, **41**, 450 (1992).

30. N. Vaisman, M. Corey, M. F. Rossi, E. Goldberg, and P. Pencharz, *J. Peds.*, **113**, 925 (1988).

31. N. Vaisman, M. R. Rossi, E. Goldberg, L. J. Dibden, L. J. Wykes, and P. B. Pencharz, *J. Peds.*, **113**, 919 (1988).

32. E. Luder and J. Schedendach, *Top. Clin. Nutr.*, **8**, 48 (1992).

33. C. L. Rock, *Eating Disorders Review*, **5**, 1 (1994).

34. S. M. Langan and P. M. Farrell, *Am. J. Clin. Nutr.*, **41**, 1054 (1985).

35. N. Vaisman, D. Wolfhart, and D. Sklan, *Eur. J. Clin. Nutr.*, **46**, 873 (1992).

36. J. Curran-Celentano, J. W. Erdman, R. A. Nelson, and S. J. E. Grater, *Am. J. Clin. Nutr.*, **42**, 1183 (1985).

37. C. L. Rock and M. E. Swendseid, *Meth. Enzymol.*, **214**, 116 (1993).

38. E. Phillipp, K. M. Pirke, M. Seidl, R. J. Tuschl, M. M. Fichter, M. Eckert, and G. Wolfram, *Int. J. Eat. Dis.*, **8**, 109 (1988).

39. R. L. Katz, C. L. Keen, I. F. Litt, L. S. Hurley, K. M. Kellams-Harrison, and L. J. Glader, *J. Adol. Health Care*, **8**, 400 (1987).

40. L. Humphries, B. Vivian, M. Stuart, and C. J. McClain, *J. Clin. Psych.*, **50**, 456 (1989).

41. C. J. McClain, M. A. Stuart, B. Vivian, M. McClain, R. Talwalker, L. Snelling, and L. Humphries, *J. Am. Coll. Nutr.*, **11**, 694 (1992).

42. S. Sufai-Kutti and J. Kutti, *Am. J. Clin. Nutr.*, **44**, 581 (1986).

43. K. M. Pirke, P. Trimborn, P. Platte, and M. Fichter, *Biol. Psych.*, **30**, 711 (1991).

44. R. C. Casper, D. A. Schoeller, R. Kushner, J. Hnilicka, and S. T. Gold, *Am. J. Clin. Nutr.*, **53**, 1143 (1991).

45. J. Walker, S. L. Roberts, K. A. Halmi, S. C. Goldberg, *Am. J. Clin. Nutr.*, **32**, 1396 (1979).

46. D. T. Dempsey, L. O. Crosby, M. J. Pertschuk, I. D. Feurer, G. P. Buzby, and J. L. Mullen, *Am. J. Clin. Nutr.*, **39**, 236 (1984).

47. R. L. Weinsier and C. L. Kurmdieck, *Am. J. Clin. Nutr.*, **34**, 393 (1980).

48. R. E. Weltzin, M. H. Fernstrom, D. Hansen, C. McConaha, and W. H. Kaye, *Am. J. Psych.*, **148**, 1675 (1991).

Bulimia Nervosa

Cheryl L. Rock, Ph.D., R.D.

INTRODUCTION

Bulimia nervosa is the most common eating disorder occurring in the population at large. Nutritional problems in the patient with bulimia nervosa are not as obvious as those of the low-weight patient with anorexia nervosa, yet dietary patterns appear to play an important etiologic role in the susceptible individual. Abnormal eating patterns, as well as their physiologic consequences, serve to perpetuate the disorder and contribute to its often intractable nature.

Clinical Features

As defined in the *Diagnostic and Statistical Manual of Mental Disorders: IV* (DSM-IV) of the American Psychiatric Association (APA), central features of bulimia nervosa are binge eating, compensatory behavior to prevent weight gain, and an overconcern with body shape and weight.[1] These criteria illustrate the refinement that has occurred in the definition of this disorder since it was first proposed as a diagnosable eating disorder by Russell in 1979.[2]

The syndrome was first described simply as bulimia, characterized by the

181

primary features of episodic binge eating and compensatory behavior. In 1987, the DSM III-R criteria were modified to include minimum criteria for how often and how long the binge and purge behavior was present in order to make the diagnosis. Bulimia nervosa is now clearly identifiable as distinct and separate from anorexia nervosa and binge eating in obese patients, although there is some overlap in behaviors among the various eating disorders. For example, DSM-IV criteria[1] recognize that a subgroup of patients with anorexia nervosa also exhibit binge and purge behavior. Criteria for binge eating disorder (considered a subtype of the category, eating disorder not otherwise specified) encompass the obese patient who binges, perceiving a similar loss of control over eating, but who does not practice compensatory behavior that effectively prevents weight gain. The distinguishing feature of bulimia nervosa, compared with these other diagnoses, is maintenance of normal body weight, which has nutritional implications, especially when compared with anorexia nervosa. All patients with bulimia nervosa experience binge eating episodes, and the majority of them also purge (by self-induced vomiting or inappropriate use of laxatives or other medications), whereas others prevent weight gain with excessive exercise or fasting. Much of what is known about this disorder is based on research with older adolescent and young adult patients. However, some differences in the etiologic factors, pattern of onset, and the expected course of illness and therapy may be present in the young adolescent with bulimia nervosa.

The nature of the binge eating behavior of patients with bulimia nervosa has been the focus of numerous studies.[3] Rosen et al.[4] evaluated food records over a minimum of 2 wk in a group of 20 patients, who averaged 22 yr of age and had a mean duration of bulimia nervosa of 5 yr. The typical binge was determined to provide 6104 kJ (1459 kcal), but the range was wide [188–21,497 kJ (45–5138 kcal)]. The usefulness of defining a binge is illustrated by these data, due to the variability of definitions among patients and subjectivity involved in using such terminology. As specified in the current diagnostic criteria, a binge episode by clinical definition involves eating significantly more than what most people would eat in those circumstances.

Laboratory studies, which are conducted in situations designed to mimic the environment of spontaneous behavior (including the availability of bathrooms for private patient use), have provided more information about the actual binge behavior of patients with bulimia nervosa, as well as details about other characteristics of their eating patterns. For example, Walsh and others[5,6] examined the behavior of patients with bulimia nervosa compared with controls by presenting an array of food choices and instructing them to purposely binge or eat normally. With this approach, patients were observed to eat faster than control subjects when both groups were instructed to binge. Also, under these circumstances, patients ate larger amounts of desserts and snacks and ate them earlier in the binge meal, when compared with controls. Of equal importance, patients with bulimia nervosa consumed foods and amounts providing significantly less energy than controls during the nonbinge meals.

By evaluating the content of food choices from monitored vending machines, the predominance of desserts and snacks in patients' binges was also observed by Weltzin et al.[7] The patients, who ranged in age from 17–42 yr, were stratified based on evident over- and undereating during the period of observation. Undereating bulimics, who were presumed to be exhibiting the restrictive component of the syndrome, ate fewer meals and consumed a significantly smaller proportion of energy from fat, as well as less energy overall. In a more recent laboratory study by this group,[8] the average binge of a group of 17 women with bulimia nervosa was found to provide 8916 kJ (2131 kcal), and the energy content of the purged (vomited) portion was 4096 kJ (979 kcal). Despite variations in the energy content of the binges, a similar amount of energy [approximately 5021 kJ (1200 kcal)] was retained.

As observed by Mitchell et al.,[9] self-induced vomiting is the most common compensatory behavior used by bulimic patients, reportedly experienced daily or more often by 71.8% of the patients in their series. Binge eating and vomiting are coupled behaviors, because most patients binge eat with full intention of purging afterward. Some patients also use the toxic over-the-counter emetic Ipecac to induce vomiting. Daily use of diet pills was reported by 25.1%, laxative use by 19.7%, and diuretics by 10.2% of the group in this study.[9] Patients who use laxatives as a component of purging typically ingest a dose of 10–40 tablets at a time. In comparative studies, laxative use has been shown to have minimal effect on absorption of energy-producing macronutrients,[10] but instead may be associated with greater dietary restraint in bulimic patients who report this purging tactic.[11]

Prevalence

Although bulimia nervosa is the most prevalent of the defined eating disorders, it does not appear to be nearly as common as estimates several years ago might have suggested. As discussed by Stunkard[12] in a recent review the more rigorous the design and conduct of the study, the lower the prevalence reported. For example, if the problem is identified by loosely defined bulimic behaviors such as binge eating (but without fearing loss of control over eating), prevalence is considerably overestimated. In one study of 1965 university students, 32.0% of college-aged women reported binge eating at least twice per month, yet only 1.3% reported the combination of binge eating, often or usual loss of control associated with the binge, and a perception that the behavior was abnormal.[13] Careful interpretation of reported figures is particularly important in studies of adolescents, because experimental eating patterns, some impulsive behaviors, and occasional conspicuous overeating are often a normal component of this phase of development. The frequency and persistence of the behaviors, in addition to the associated cognitions, are important modifiers.

Using the DSM III-R criteria, Drewnowski et al.[14] assessed the prevalence of bulimia nervosa with a national probability sample of 1007 students from a stratified group of 53 U.S. universities and colleges. They found prevalence rates of 1.0% for the women and 0.2% for the men. In another survey of college freshmen at a single midwestern university,[15] point prevalence was estimated to be 2.9%, with incidence (based on data from a second survey of the same group 6 mo later) estimated at 4.2 cases/100 women/yr. The disorder does occur in both men and women and at any age, but the overwhelming majority of patients described in the literature are female and adolescents or young adults. Increased rates of occurrence are also reported in younger vs. older birth cohorts, when subgroups can be separated and compared.

Etiology

Historically, the onset of bulimia nervosa has been described as typically following a period of dieting to lose weight.[16] A causative link between dietary restraint and bulimia is strengthened by similar observations among obese patients who binge eat[12] and subjects in research studies in which food deprivation has been imposed.[17] Sociocultural factors are also involved in this connection, because chronic dieting is associated with societal pressures to be thin. The compensatory behaviors that patients adopt may thus be regarded as ingenious solutions, enabling them to maintain the approved female appearance despite the ultimate failure of restrictive regimens that are tacitly encouraged and reinforced in the culture. Patients with bulimia nervosa have been described as being failed anorexics; excluding binges, the restrictive diets they often aim to achieve are similar to those of many patients of the restrictive subtype of anorexia nervosa.

In studies of clinic populations, other factors implicated in the etiology of bulimia nervosa include family history of an eating disorder, affective disorder, or alcohol or substance abuse.[18] A link between bulimia nervosa and affective disorders has been hypothesized to be attributable to a basic neuroendocrine dysfunction that may determine biologic vulnerability to both disorders. Identifying cause and effect in this link is difficult to establish, however, because mood disturbances as well as altered neuroendocrine functions occur as a result of malnutrition and the chaotic eating patterns of the eating disorder itself.[19] At many points during adolescent development, susceptibility to bulimia nervosa may exist, due to heightened self-awareness, social anxiety, and poor self-esteem.[20] Several familial patterns and individual personality characteristics, such as impulsivity, have also been proposed to be among the etiologic factors that increase the risk for the disorder to develop in association with dieting. Overall, the importance of these various factors is unknown, due to inadequate or inconsistent data.[18] Similar to anorexia nervosa, the development of bulimia nervosa in the individual patient is usually multifactorial, with several causative and sustaining factors.

Prognosis

Compared with anorexia nervosa, little is known about the long-term outcome of bulimia nervosa. The disorder has been recognized and diagnosable as a distinct clinical entity relatively recently, so long-term follow-up studies are lacking. Recent evidence from a short-term (6-mo) longitudinal study indicates that spontaneous (although usually only partial) remission may occur as one possible natural course of the illness.[15]

Patients provided psychosocial or pharmacologic treatments are likely to experience a 50–90% short-term reduction in binge eating and purging.[21] Although some symptoms may persist, those treated as outpatients are reported to maintain improvement for up to 6 yr, with the severity of illness an important influence on outcome. Also, relapses appear to be a normal occurrence during the recovery process. In one study,[22] more than 80% of a group of recovered patients reported that they had relapsed, in episodes lasting for an average of 5.4 mo, when they thought they were over their disorder.

ASSESSMENT

Most patients with bulimia nervosa experience a great deal of symptom distress, presenting with their own treatment goals such as stopping the binges and assistance with weight control. For the initial diagnosis of the degree and severity of the eating disorder, assessment tools include self-report questionnaires, e.g., the Eating Disorder Inventory,[23] and clinical interviews. The purpose of the questionnaire instrument or clinical interview is to identify the nature of the eating disorder, if present, and the risk of serious complications or need for hospitalization.

Initial assessment of the patient focuses on historical information, such as weight and dieting history, and cognitions and feelings about food, meals, and body weight. Anthropometric data typically reveal a patient who is within the range of desirable or expected body weight and not overtly malnourished. However, reports of frequent and significant weight fluctuations are typical in these patients, as well as a desire for a body weight that is unrealistically low. Physically, "chipmunk cheeks" may be evident, due to purging behavior (which is discussed below), and symptoms of mild to moderate dehydration are often present. Dietary assessment and discussions of food choices typically uncover a pattern of extreme efforts to lose weight or prevent weight gain through excessive dieting. Until a rapport has been established, patients are unlikely to feel comfortable discussing the details of binges and purging behavior with the nutrition professional. The most important attitude with which to approach the patient with bulimia nervosa is nonjudgmental.

As described in the APA Practice Guidelines for Eating Disorders,[21] a multidimensional, comprehensive approach to assessment is recommended.

Medical Complications

Medical complications associated with bulimia nervosa occur due to semistarvation or as a result of the purging behavior, as listed in Table 10.1. Fatigue, lethargy, weakness, and impaired concentration are common complaints that may be related to inadequate retention of energy and other nutrients.[17,24] Similar to patients with anorexia nervosa, malnutrition itself can cause preoccupation with thoughts of food and various endocrine changes, including menstrual dysfunction. As a result of dietary restriction, signs of hypothyroidism, such as hypothermia, hypercholesterolemia, and constipation, may also be present.

Serious medical complications can result from self-induced vomiting, which can occur 20 or more times daily.[25] Signs of this behavior include hypertrophy

Table 10.1   Medical Complications of Bulimia Nervosa

Problems related to malnutrition
Weakness, lethargy, and fatigue
Inability to concentrate
Menstrual dysfunction
Constipation

Problems related to purging
Dehydration and volume depletion
Electrolyte abnormalities
  Hypokalemia
  Hypochloremia
  Alkalosis
Elevated serum amylase
Erosion of tooth enamel
Esophageal reflux and esophagitis
Ecchymoses
Arrhythmia
Hypertrophy of the salivary glands
Renal damage
Gastric dilatation and rupture
Cathartic colon

of the salivary glands and lesions on the skin over the dorsum of the hand (resulting from the use of the hand to induce vomiting). It has been postulated that increased serum amylase, which is observed in approximately one-third of patients with bulimia nervosa, may relate to parotid gland inflammation,[24] but data to support this are inconsistent. If used by patients to induce vomiting, Ipecac causes severe and life-threatening cardiovascular and neuromuscular damage over time.

Dehydration and electrolyte abnormalities, primarily hypokalemia and hypochloremic alkalosis, are commonly seen in patients with bulimia nervosa.[24,25] Secondary problems, such as arrhythmia and renal tubular damage, can result. Gastrointestinal complications caused by frequent vomiting include esophagitis, esophageal reflux, gastritis, and (in rare case reports) gastric dilatation and rupture. Prolonged overuse of laxatives causes laxative dependency and a cathartic colon.

Clinical laboratory work-up that is appropriate for patients with bulimia nervosa includes complete blood count, electrolytes, blood urea nitrogen, creatinine, and basic urinalysis tests. Severely symptomatic patients should also have their serum calcium, magnesium, phosphorus, and amylase quantified, in addition to liver function tests and an electrocardiogram.[21]

Psychological Concerns

A substantial number of patients with bulimia nervosa have depressive symptoms, which Russell noted in his early report of this syndrome.[2] However, depression may be state-related, i.e., a secondary problem resulting from the eating disorder. Addictive disorders are also seen in many bulimic patients. Compared with nonpsychiatric controls, patients with bulimia nervosa (including both high school- and college-aged students) have higher rates of problems with alcohol and substance abuse, although the reported figures for lifetime comorbidity vary widely (ranging from 9–55%).[24] One interesting explanation for this link is that dietary restraint and deprivation lead to both binge eating and substance abuse, with psychoactive substances serving as alternative consummatory reinforcers.[26] Whatever the cause, the alcohol or substance abuse problem must be addressed and treated either prior to therapy for the eating disorder or concurrently, if treatment strategies for managing the bulimic behaviors are to be effective.

An increased comorbidity of personality disorders and anxiety disorders has also been reported to occur in eating disorder patients, although the majority of the research findings are based on adult populations.[24] Such problems may be less likely to occur in the adolescent patient, but evaluation by a mental health professional is essential in this component of the assessment and therapy. Shoplifting is among the behavioral problems that have been reported to be more common in patients with either anorexia or bulimia nervosa.

Nutritional Issues

Patients with bulimia nervosa often enter treatment with the goal of losing weight despite being at or slightly below average weight for height. Results from several studies conducted during the past few years suggest that when they are prevented from practicing binge and purge behaviors, patients with bulimia nervosa appear to have low baseline energy requirements for weight maintenance. Estimates of energy requirements are derived from observations of the energy intake needed to maintain weight, measurements of resting energy expenditure using indirect calorimetry, and newer techniques, such as the doubly labeled water method.

Obarzanek et al.[27] measured resting energy expenditure (REE) in 15 women (who averaged 26 yr of age) with bulimia nervosa following 2–3 wk of hospitalization, when body weight was believed to have stabilized. They found REE to be significantly reduced (an average of 11% lower) than that of normal controls when adjusted for differences in lean body mass. Oxygen consumption with exercise was also found to be blunted in the bulimic patients, when the effect of exercise was examined in these patients. Plasma triiodothyronine and norepinephrine levels were also significantly lower in bulimics than controls. Although the goal during the study was weight maintenance, analysis of the patients' weights revealed a negative linear trend.

In observational studies of dietary intake in a controlled setting, patients with bulimia nervosa have also been observed to require less energy for weight maintenance than normal controls [averaging 92.5 vs. 124.3 kJ/kg/d (22.1 versus 29.7 kcal/kg/d)], in a group that averaged 24 yr of age.[28] In a study comparing the energy intake of various groups of patients with eating disorders, 20 weight-stable hospitalized patients with bulimia nervosa were found to be consuming 108.4 kJ/kg/d (25.9 kcal/kg/d), which was significantly lower than the anorexia nervosa patients who had recently regained weight due to refeeding regimens.[29]

Pirke et al.[30] used the doubly labeled water method to measure total energy expenditure in a group of eight women with bulimia nervosa, with an average age of 24 yr, who were permitted to practice usual binging and purging behavior during the study period. Exercise and sports activities were also permitted and monitored. Low triiodothyronine levels were observed in the patients with bulimia nervosa, but total energy expenditure was not different from that of controls. Bulimic patients were observed to be more active than the controls, but the difference between the groups was not significant when hours of sports activities were quantified.

Observations of low REE could be interpreted as being an indicator of genetic susceptibility to weight gain, which might stimulate the dieting behavior and preoccupation with weight that precede the eating disorder. An alternate hypothesis is that this phenomenon results from chronically restricted energy intake in an effort to maintain a lower body weight than is physiologically appropriate.

When patients are free-living, total daily energy expenditure can apparently be maintained at a normal level due to exercising, binging, and purging, despite reduced REE.

Patients with bulimia nervosa typically describe a pattern of restrained eating and rigorous dietary restriction, with episodic binges that may occur several times a day or week. Assessment of the specific food patterns is of interest in diagnosis and treatment. Foods are typically categorized dichotomously, as either safe or forbidden. In a group of 21 patients with bulimia nervosa and an average age of 23 yr, Kales[31] compared the cognitive attributions of patients and dietary records. The frequency order of the most "forbidden" foods named (from most to least) was cake, cookies, fried foods/bread/ice cream, butter, snacks, pizza, candy, and chocolate. A similar ranking of the "safest" foods (from most to least) was vegetables, fruit, chicken/fish/lean meat, yogurt, whole grains, popcorn/rice cakes, soup/cottage cheese, jello, and tofu. An evaluation of differences in macronutrient content between these two groupings revealed the most significant difference to be in the fat content. As anticipated, the forbidden foods were highly likely to be among the binge foods, and the safe foods were eaten at nonbinge meals and snacks, when food records were examined.

A few case reports of micronutrient deficiencies have been reported,[32–34] and in a few studies, the micronutrient status of patients with bulimia nervosa has been evaluated. Using enzyme activity indices, Philipp et al.[35] reported evidence of biochemical deficiencies of riboflavin and vitamin B-6 in one of 24 bulimic patients who ranged in age from 18–37 yr. Three were found to have elevated plasma retinol concentrations. Mira et al.[36] reported biochemical measures of vitamins A, B-6, and E in two groups of several types of adult eating disorder patients (aged 23–38 yr). The groups consisted of patients with either anorexia or bulimia nervosa or atypical eating disorder. A higher mean plasma concentration of retinol was observed in the patients when compared with a control group, and higher tocopherol levels were found among the patients who reported vitamin supplement use.

In circumstances of inadequate overall dietary intake, it is likely that micronutrient deficiencies may occur in these patients, contributing to the physiologic and psychologic alterations associated with malnutrition. As is true in anorexia nervosa, elevated plasma concentrations of the fat-soluble vitamins may reflect the delayed clearance of lipids, in association with semistarvation.[37] If treatment results in a normalized eating pattern consisting of a variety of foods, these deficiencies are likely to be corrected without the need for supplements.

MANAGEMENT

The first goal of treatment is nutritional rehabilitation and restoration of normal eating patterns, as described in the APA Practice Guidelines.[21] Longer-term treatment can then more effectively address the psychological, familial, and behavioral problems to reduce the likelihood of relapse.

The majority of patients with bulimia nervosa can be managed on an outpatient basis or in day treatment programs. Cases complicated by life-threatening medical problems, severe concurrent substance abuse, or evident risk for suicide require hospitalization. In patients whose chaotic eating patterns cannot be improved during a trial of outpatient therapy, hospitalization for 2–3 wk may also be necessary.[21]

Psychosocial

Cognitive-behavioral therapy, provided individually or in groups, has been shown to reduce binge eating and purging by nearly 80%, with 40–60% of patients becoming completely abstinent from these behaviors.[38] In comparative studies, the cognitive-behavioral approach has been shown to be superior to nondirective therapy and is now considered to be the first-line treatment of choice for bulimia nervosa.[39] Based on a cognitive-behavioral model of bulimia nervosa, the primary theory behind this approach is that societal pressures to be thin lead to dietary restraint, which ultimately leads to binge eating and purging.[39] This type of treatment intervention usually lasts approximately 20 wk and is conducted as a semistructured, problem-oriented program. In comparison with interpersonal or general psychotherapy, the focus in cognitive-behavioral therapy is on the factors and processes that are maintaining the eating disorder, rather than other issues or the past. The cognitive component involves challenging the rigid food rules and overconcern with body shape and weight. Elements of behavioral therapy include attention to environmental factors that promote dieting and bingeing, and self-monitoring is an important component of the approach. Detailed manuals for conducting a cognitive-behavioral treatment program are available.[40]

Once symptoms are under control, psychodynamically oriented or interpersonal therapy appears to be a useful treatment approach.[21,39] The theory underlying interpersonal therapy is that an unsatisfactory interpersonal situation set the stage for the eating disorder, with interpersonal stress, low self-esteem, and dysphoria causing food to be used as a way of coping with negative feelings.

Medical

Several pharmacological approaches have been employed in the treatment of bulimia nervosa. As discussed in the APA Practice Guidelines,[21] antidepressants that have been shown to be efficacious in reducing bulimic symptoms include imipramine, desipramine, trazodone, and fluoxetine. Monoamine oxidase inhibitors (phenelzine and isocarboxazid) also may be useful, although the ability of the patient to avoid tyramine-containing foods must be assessed prior to the use of these agents. Current evidence suggests that carbamezapine and lithium are less effective pharmacologic treatments.

In a controlled trial of imipramine vs. placebo with or without psychosocial therapy, Mitchell et al.[41] found that the antidepressant was superior to placebo, but psychosocial therapy was more effective at reducing symptoms and increasing the likelihood of complete abstinence. There was no additive effect of the two treatments on bingeing and purging, although patients who received the drug had fewer depressive symptoms.

Nutrition

Nutrition is actually an integral component of the cognitive-behavioral therapy milieu. Planning meals and a pattern of regular eating, and avoiding dieting, are all part of the first stage of this intervention, in addition to providing information about body weight regulation, adverse effects of dieting, and physical consequences of bulimic behavior.[39,40] Establishing a pattern of regular eating is believed to be the most essential element in the program[40] and is usually interpreted as being three planned meals plus two or three planned snacks per day. Other strategies traditionally used in nutrition therapy, such as food records and establishing a routine of weekly weighing, are involved in this type of psychosocial treatment as well.

As mentioned above, stimulus control is also a component of cognitive-behavioral therapy, and this is translated into directions for the meal plan. Some examples are limiting the quantity of binge food in the house, not doing other activities while eating, and shopping for food when not hungry. Patients are strongly encouraged not to eat too little [a minimum of 6276 kJ/day (1500 kcal/d) is typically suggested], and to plan for incorporating forbidden foods into the diet. By using the approach common to all behavioral programs, suggested changes are implemented in steps, starting with the easiest and moving on to the most difficult.

Specific dietary counseling and management may be helpful as a component of treatment of bulimia nervosa.[21] One of the most important benefits of providing nutrition intervention sessions in the overall treatment program is that they can function as the arena for discussions about food and food content, so therapy sessions may be devoted to behavioral challenges and psychological exploration.[42] The emphasis in a cognitive-behavioral therapy program is on the regularity of eating, rather than the composition of the meals and snacks, and many patients benefit from more detailed assistance in meal planning. Also, the dietetic or nutrition professional can provide reassurance with planning and estimating portion sizes and reinforcement in modifying abnormal food and weight cognitions and beliefs. Patients have intense concern with the energy content of foods and the meal plan, weight and body composition, and other issues that have become, to them, of critical importance as a characteristic of the eating disorder. These intense concerns must be addressed and not dismissed as unimportant. Empathetic and knowledgeable guidance is the basis of effective nutrition counseling in bulimia nervosa.

Dietary counseling is available in most facilities that provide treatment programs for patients with bulimia nervosa, and the strategies used have been described in a few reports. As described by Story,[43] components of the nutrition approach may include education, weight issues, the food diary, and a dietary plan. The educational component involves providing basic information about the physiological and psychological effects of starvation, energy balance and nutritional requirements, and misconceptions about dieting and weight control. A critical aspect of dealing with weight issues is clarifying that weight loss and achieving a reduction in bulimic symptoms are incompatible goals. Any desired weight loss cannot be addressed until symptoms are under control and a regular eating pattern has been established. Patients are typically instructed to avoid weighing themselves and keep records of dietary intake, purging, and exercise behavior. The dietary plan, as described above, consists of regular planned meals and snacks, and these are typically structured using exchange lists for meal planning. Specific tools that adapt the food group exchange system for use with eating disorder patients are available.[44]

In addition to the general guidelines, strategies to help patients maximize meal satiety have been suggested.[45] Well-balanced meals with adequate amounts of fat and fiber, eaten while sitting down, are examples of these strategies. Patients who are being weaned off laxatives need adequate dietary fiber to encourage normal gastrointestinal function. Fluid retention and dramatic weight fluctuations should be anticipated following a reduction in vomiting, laxative and diuretic abuse, and should be discussed with the patient. Secondary hyperaldosteronism and reflex peripheral edema are the result of volume depletion and dehydration[24]; this problem resolves with the discontinuation of purging behavior. Working with individual food attributions and beliefs is the basis of expanding the diet to include formerly forbidden foods and eliminating food avoidance. As another example of specific strategies, food that is preportioned and labeled with caloric and nutrient content can provide some reassurance to patients who are expanding their allowed food choices. Adding foods to formerly restricted meals can be approached in a stepwise manner, beginning with one meal and then moving on to the next.

The pace of nutrition intervention will vary depending on the treatment setting. For the hospitalized patient, a daily energy level must be prescribed and fed to the patient, but in the outpatient setting, normalized eating patterns may require months of counseling to achieve. An approach that is gaining in popularity is to provide intensive therapy in the controlled setting of a day hospital treatment program.[46] All treatments, including nutrition education, typically occur in groups in these programs. Although a daily energy intake may be prescribed, only one or two supervised meals per day take place in the facility. Other nutrition-related activities for patients in day treatment programs may include supervised meals taken out of the hospital (i.e., in a restaurant), group shopping and cooking experiences.

Reports of studies of the efficacy of the specific nutrition and dietary strategies in the management of bulimia nervosa are extremely limited. These elements of intervention are usually part of an overall program or therapy protocol in which other modalities of treatment are involved. In one study,[47] subjective evaluation of several aspects of treatment, including the nutritional strategies, was obtained from 75 patients with bulimia nervosa using telephone follow-up at 12–15 mo. Components rated as quite helpful included encouragement to eat a balanced diet, eating regular meals, and avoiding binge foods. Regarded less positively were making meal plans, recording food intake, and recording bingeing and vomiting episodes.

A few nutrition approaches to the management of bulimia nervosa are considered more controversial. There has been some consideration of regarding eating disorders as addictive behavior,[48] although the concept is not strongly supported, so the self-help abstinence approach originally applied to alcoholism has also been applied to binge eating.[49] Among obese binge eaters, involvement in Overeaters Anonymous (OA) has been a community-based self-help option for weight control since the organization was founded in 1960. The use of similar 12-step programs for eating disorders are now sponsored by some medical facilities. A primary feature of this intervention strategy is the complete avoidance of all foods believed to be binge-triggering, which sometimes extends to common ingredients such as refined flour. For the binge eating individual involved in such a program, abstinence means eating three meals per day plus the food avoidances described. In a descriptive study[49] of 40 nonrandomized selected adult bulimic patients (aged 20–40 yr) who had been involved with OA, meetings were reportedly attended an average of five times a week, with 52.5% reporting that they become abstinent within the first month of joining the group. Nearly half were also involved with some form of psychotherapy in addition to being in OA. The major problem with the 12-step approach as it is usually applied to eating disorders patients, particularly from a nutritional perspective, is that it reinforces (as a central theme) the need for food avoidances. Also, these avoidances can encompass a wide range of food choices that are likely to be encountered in usual lifestyles. Continued food restrictions do not seem likely to be conducive to long-term normalization of eating patterns.

Another issue is the use of fat- or calorie-reduced food products, which are now a significant portion of the food supply.[50] The patient with bulimia nervosa may rely excessively on these products in the restrictive dieting phase (and if associated with low meal satiety, probably will increase susceptibility to binges).

In some eating disorder treatment programs, these modified food products are not permitted for patient use. However, educating patients in their use in occasional or appropriate circumstances may be more compatible with normalized eating patterns. Similarly, caffeine-containing beverages are often overused by patients with bulimia nervosa[51] so that in the initial phases of therapy, specific limitations may be indicated. Table 10.2 summarizes the basic principles and goals of nutritional care for patients with bulimia nervosa.

Practical Problems

Working with the patient with bulimia nervosa poses some distinct challenges for the dietetic or nutrition professional. Multidisciplinary teams that manage eating disorder patients must be mutually supportive, with shared treatment goals. These patients are often chronically ill, unstable, and are themselves involved in an intensive treatment program that challenges their deeply held beliefs and behavioral patterns. Because he or she is usually involved in enforcing food rules and meal planning, which are the focus of the patients' distress and disordered cognitive and behavioral patterns, the dietetic professional is particularly vulnerable to stress and burnout in this situation. Concepts of transference and countertransference, and dealing with one's own emotional responses to patients, are not typically taught in dietetic training programs. Understanding these concepts and maintaining close communication with the mental health professionals involved in the patients' treatment can be very helpful.

It has been suggested that dietetic professionals, as well as other groups whose jobs or careers involve food or nutrition, have an increased prevalence of eating disorders. Results of an investigation[52] of the occurrence of eating disorder behaviors in various university populations do not support this theory. Students enrolled in a lower-division introductory nutrition course were found to have a

Table 10.2   Basic Principles and Goals of Nutritional Care

1. Regular pattern of nutritionally balanced, planned meals and snacks.
2. Adequate but not excessive levels of energy intake, with the goal of weight maintenance.
3. Adequate dietary fat and fiber intake, with the goal of promoting meal satiety.
4. Avoidance of dieting behavior, excessive exercise, and associated strategies (such as overuse of caffeine-containing beverages and modified food products).
5. Inclusion of formerly forbidden categories of foods in the diet, with the goal of minimizing food avoidances.
6. Dietary record-keeping and review.
7. Stimulus control strategies, with the goal of controlling exposures and high-risk situations.
8. Weighing at scheduled intervals only.

higher degree of pathology in comparison to other student groups, but the dietetic majors did not have a greater degree of abnormal eating patterns or behaviors resembling eating disorders.

In hospital units and day treatment programs, patient meals must be selected from a limited-choice food-service menu, so it is essential that written guidelines are well known to all staff members. For example, specific patient requests should be accommodated only within certain limits; e.g., each patient may select only a certain number of foods (usually three to five) that may be excluded from the diet. Ovo-lacto-vegetarian preferences can usually be accommodated, but permitting long lists of foods that a patient may refuse to eat will simply reinforce the eating disorder, as does permitting excessive exercising. Similarly, limitations on coffee, soft drinks, and condiments provided in the meal are often necessary. The long-term goal is to ensure adequate dietary intake and minimize restrictions and overconcern with food and weight.

CASE ILLUSTRATION

Carole, an 18-year-old college freshman, presented with primary complaints of depression and bulimia nervosa. She reported that throughout high school, she had been bingeing and vomiting at least twice per week. She described being obsessed with her looks and her weight. When she entered high school at age 14, she weighed 56.8 kg and began dieting that year, after her parents commented on her appearance. Carole eliminated breakfast and lunch and designed a very-low-fat dinner plan, and also joined an informal after-school running group. About 2 mo later, after struggling with the self-imposed diet, she began self-induced vomiting following any dinner that contained fat or sweets, and this remained her only planned meal throughout high school. Once she had deviated from the diet at dinner, she would continue to eat more of everything with the intention of purging later.

At college, increased availability of food at the dormitory cafeteria and living with roommates (rather than parents) facilitated the pattern of bingeing and purging, so it became a daily ritual. Carole injured a knee but continued exercising (now cycling as well as running) for a minimum of 3 h/d. Because she was having difficulty concentrating and was unable to complete assigned reading or homework assignments, her grades suffered. It was recommended by the university Student Health Center personnel that she take a leave of absence, return home to her parents, and seek treatment.

Initial laboratory values included the following: albumin 42 (normal 35–50 g/L); hemoglobin 120 (normal 120–160 g/L); hematocrit 41 (normal 37–48%); serum amylase 127 (normal 4–25 U/mL). Electrolytes were normal. Physical findings revealed a height of 162.5 cm, weight of 58.2 kg, and swollen-appearing face.

Carole's initial therapy was a cognitive-behavioral therapy group, and her binges decreased but she still complained of crying all the time. She was extremely unhappy with the gain of 4.5 kg that followed her attempt to institute a three meal per day food plan and the reduction in vomiting and excessive exercise. Not until she was prescribed imipramine did her mood and attitude about recovery improve.

The focus of nutrition counseling sessions was on increasing Carole's allowed (nonpurged) foods to include adequate fat and calories. For example, her planned dinner at the beginning of treatment consisted of ½ cantaloupe, 1 cup nonfat yogurt, and 2 bagels. This dinner was typically followed by a binge of several packages of reduced-fat cookies and culminated with foods from the family kitchen that would not be missed, such as bread with peanut butter. The goal of counseling was to achieve a weight-maintenance energy intake level with 30% kcal from fat. The first successful nonpurged meals that consisted of formerly forbidden foods occurred in a restaurant meal, when no leftovers were available to tempt a binge. Food records were reviewed with the dietitian weekly, and Carole continued in individual psychotherapy. With continued improvement, her return to college is likely, with referral to eating disorder professionals in that community to provide follow-up and continuing care.

REFERENCES

1. American Psychiatric Association, *Diagnostic and Statistical Manual of Mental Disorders*, IV ed., American Psychiatric Association, Washington, DC, pp. 549 (1994).

2. G.F.M. Russell, *Psych. Med.*, **9**, 429 (1979).

3. B. T. Walsh, in *Binge Eating*, (C. G. Fairburn and G. T. Wilson, eds.), Guilford Press, New York, pp. 37–49 (1993).

4. J. C. Rosen, H. Leitenberg, C. Fisher, and C. Khazam, *Int. J. Eating Dis.*, **5**, 255 (1986).

5. C. M. Hadigan, H. R. Kissileff, and B. T. Walsh, *Am. J. Clin. Nutr.*, **50**, 759 (1989).

6. B. T. Walsh, C. M. Hadigan, H. R. Kissileff, J. L. LaChaussee, in *The Biology of Feast and Famine*, (G. H. Anderson and S. H. Kennedy, eds.), Academic Press, New York, pp. 4–20 (1992).

7. T. E. Weltzin, K. G. Hsu, C. Pollice, and W. H. Kaye, *Biol. Psych.*, **30**, 1093 (1991).

8. W. H. Kaye, T. E. Weltzin, L. K. Hsu, C. W. McConaha, and B. Bolton, *Am. J. Psych.*, **150**, 969 (1993).

9. J. E. Mitchell, D. Hatsukami, E. D. Eckert, and R. L. Pyle, *Am. J. Psych.*, **142**, 482 (1985).

10. G. W. Bo-Linn, C. A. Santa Ana, S. G. Morawski, and J. S. Fordtran, *Ann. Int. Med.*, **99**, 14 (1983).

11. J. H. Lacey and E. Gibson, *Hum. Nutr. Appl. Nutr.*, **39A**, 36 (1985).

12. A. J. Stunkard, in *Binge Eating*, (C. G. Fairburn and G. T. Wilson, eds.), Guilford Press, New York, pp. 15–34 (1993).

13. D. E. Schotte and A. J. Stunkard, *JAMA*, **258**, 1213 (1987).

14. A. Drewnowski, S. A. Hopkins, and R. C. Kessler, *Am. J. Pub. Health*, **78**, 1322 (1988).

15. A. Drewnowski, D. K. Yee, and D. D. Krahn, *Am. J. Psych.*, **145**, 753 (1988).

16. B. G. Kirkley, *J. Am. Diet. Assoc.*, **86**, 468 (1986).

17. A. Keys, J. Brozek, A. Henschel, O. Mickelson, and H. L. Taylor, *The Biology of Human Starvation*, University of Minnesota Press, Minneapolis, MN, (1950).

18. C. G. Fairburn, P. J. Hay, and S. L. Welch, in *Binge Eating*, (C. G. Fairburn and G. T. Wilson, eds.), Guilford Press, New York, pp. 123–143 (1993).

19. W. H. Kaye and T. E. Weltzin, *J. Clin. Psych.*, **52**, 21 (1991).

20. R. H. Striegel-Moore, in *Binge Eating*, (C. G. Fairburn and G. T. Wilson, eds.), Guilford Press, New York, pp. 144–172 (1993).

21. American Psychiatric Association, *Am. J. Psych.*, **150**, 207 (1993).

22. M.P.P. Root, *Psychotherapy*, **27**, 397 (1990).

23. D. M. Garner, *Eating Disorders Inventory–2*, Psychological Assessment Resources, Odessa, FL, (1991).

24. J. E. Mitchell, S. M. Specker, and M. deZwaan, *J. Clin. Psych.*, **52** (suppl.), 13 (1991).

25. R. C. Casper, *Ann. Rev. Nutr.*, **6**, 299 (1986).

26. D. D. Krahn, *J. Sub. Abuse*, **3**, 239 (1991).

27. E. Obarzanek, M. D. Lesem, D. S. Goldstein, and D. C. Jimerson, *Arch. Gen. Psych.*, **48**, 456 (1991).

28. H. E. Gwirtsman, W. H. Kaye, E. Obarzanek, D. T. George, D. C. Jimerson, and M. H. Ebert, *Am. J. Clin. Nutr.*, **49**, 86 (1989).

29. T. E. Weltzin, M. H. Fernstrom, D. Hansen, C. McConaha, and W. H. Kaye, *Am. J. Psych.*, **148**, 12 (1991).

30. K. M. Pirke, P.Trimborn, P. Platte, M. Fichter, *Biol. Psych.*, **30**, 711 (1991).

31. E. F. Kales, *Physiol. Behav.*, **48**, 837 (1990).

32. R. Alloway, E. H. Reynolds, E. Spargo, and G.F.M. Russell, *J. Neurol. Neurosurg. Psych.*, **48**, 1015 (1985).

33. D. J. Eedy, J. G. Curran, and W. J. Andrews, *Postgrad. Med. J.*, **62**, 853 (1986).

34. K. Nijya, T. Kitigawa, M. Fujishita, S. Yoshimoto, M. Kobayashi, J. Kuboniski, H. Taguchi, and J. Miyoshi, *JAMA*, **250**, 792 (1983).

35. E. Philipp, K. M. Pirke, M. Seidl, R. J. Tuschl, M. M. Fichter, M. Eckert, and G. Wolfram, *Int. J. Eating Dis.*, **8**, 209 (1988).

36. M. Mira, P. M. Stewart, and S. F. Abraham, *Am. J. Clin. Nutr.*, **50**, 940 (1989).

37. C. L. Rock and J. Curran-Celentano, *Int. J. Eating Dis.*, **15**, 187 (1994).

38. C. G. Fairburn, W. S. Agras, and G. T. Wilson, in *The Biology of Feast and Famine*, (G. H. Anderson and S. H. Kennedy, eds.), Academic Press, San Diego, CA, pp. 317–340 (1992).

39. W. S. Agras, *J. Clin. Psych.*, **52** (suppl.), 29 (1991).

40. C. G. Fairburn, M. D. Marcus, and G. T. Wilson, in *Binge Eating*, (C. G. Fairburn and G. T. Wilson, eds.), Guilford Press, New York, pp. 361–404 (1993).

41. J. E. Mitchell, R. L. Pyle, E. D. Eckert, D. Hatsukami, C. Pomeroy, and R. Zimmerman, *Arch. Gen. Psych.*, **47**, 149 (1990).

42. American Dietetic Association, *J. Am. Diet. Assoc.*, **88**, 68 (1988).

43. M. Story, *J. Am. Diet. Assoc.*, **86**, 517 (1986).

44. C. M. Patterson, D. P. Whelan, C. L. Rock, and T. J. Lyon, *Nutrition and Eating Disorders: Guidelines for the Patient with Anorexia Nervosa and Bulimia Nervosa*, PM Publications, Los Angeles, CA, (1989).

45. C. L. Rock and J. Yager, *Int. J. Eating Dis.*, **6**, 267 (1987).

46. N. Piran and A. S. Kaplan, *A Day Hospital Group Treatment Program for Anorexia Nervosa and Bulimia Nervosa*, Brunner-Mazel, New York, (1990).

47. M. A. Gannon and J. E. Mitchell, *J. Am. Diet. Assoc.*, **86**, 520 (1986).

48. E. A. Riley, *Nurs. Clin. N. Am.*, **26**, 715 (1991).

49. R. Malenbaum, D. Herzog, S. Eisenthal, and G. Wyshak, *Int. J. Eating Dis.*, **7**, 139 (1988).

50. A. Drewnowski, *Postgrad. Med.*, **87**, 111 (1990).

51. D. D. Krahn, S. Hasse, A. Ray, B. Gosnell, and A. Drewnowski, *Hosp. Comm. Psych.*, **42**, 313 (1991).

52. C. Johnston and F. S. Christopher, *J. Nutr. Ed.*, **23**, 148 (1991).

Obesity

Barbara McCarty, R.D.
Laurel Mellin, M.A., R.D.

INTRODUCTION

Adolescent obesity represents the most prevalent nutritional problem among American adolescents between the ages of 12–17 yr.[1] Currently, at least 27% of children and 21% of adolescents are obese. This represents a 54% increase in child obesity and a 39% increase in adolescent obesity during the last two decades.[2] With this alarming trend of increasing childhood and adolescent obesity, it is estimated that 70% of obese adolescents will become obese adults.[2] And even more unsettling is that these individuals are likely to be even more severely overweight in their adult years.[1] Further, it has been well documented that obesity in adults is strongly associated with increased risk for a variety of disorders such as diabetes, orthopedic problems, and respiratory disease.[3]

Adolescent obesity is diverse in causation including both genetic and environmental factors. The increase in the prevalence of childhood obesity is environmental and appears to be another sign that children are not doing well, and that families and social institutions appear not to have provided children with the nurturing and guidance needed to develop healthful nutritional habits.

The National Cholesterol Education Report on Obesity[3] states that "obese children are at greater risk for a number of health problems including diminished work capacity (orthopedic and pulmonary complications), insulin resistance, and hypertension. They also experience difficulties in social and psychological adjustment. Obesity in children is positively related to increased VLDL cholesterol and LDL cholesterol and inversely related to HDL cholesterol and is also associated with clustering of multiple coronary heart disease risk factors." In addition, obese children enter puberty earlier than their nonobese peers, resulting in a shorter duration of long bone growth and, ultimately, shorter stature. The psychosocial consequences of obesity are varied. Most frequently, obesity for the young is a psychosocial disability. Obese children are often ridiculed by peers and seen as laughable or pathetic. Many obese children or adolescents avoid or dislike school because of the hostile social climate. Obesity often results in social isolation, negative body image, low self-esteem, and delayed psychosocial development for children. By adolescence, the obese are often excluded from sports, dating and peers.

The American Heart Association's[4] clinical recommendations regarding child obesity are also appropriate for adolescents (see Table 11.1). However, obesity is a symptom of an underlying problem(s) and without identifying that problem, behavioral intervention alone will be limited in helping the adolescent with the long-term management of his or her obesity. Teaching adolescents about internal cue responsivity vs. external cue responsivity, how to eat to take care of their hunger, to stop eating when they are satiated, and to trust that no one will take

Table 11.1 Clinical Recommendations Regarding Adolescent Obesity

1. Select a healthy diet in which fat provides no more than 30% of calories.
2. Dietary moderation, not restriction, so that favorite foods are not forbidden.
3. First helpings but not seconds to reduce overall intake of calories, but not to leave the child deprived.
4. Snack foods are acceptable when healthy snacks like fruit and vegetables are favored and snacking is limited.
5. Food should not be used as a reward.
6. Increase levels for physical activity including, walking or riding bikes to school.
7. Add a formal exercise program to the daily schedule.
8. Individualize the exercise program so that children enjoy their activity.
9. Make exercise time a priority rather than something to fit in as time permits.
10. Parents should be healthy role models of appropriate dietary and physical activity habits.
11. Maintain realistic expectations of appearance. Look at relatives to get a realistic idea of the shape and type of body a child will have. Weight gains are normal during growth and only unusual gains should be of concern.

Adapted from W. B. Strong et al., in *Integrated Cardiovascular Health Promotion in Childhood*, American Heart Association, Dallas, TX, (1992). Reprinted with permission.

the food away from them is a necessity. In addition, the teen needs to discover those issues that he or she is trying to avoid and address these through communication and cognitive restructuring. Most important, treatment must be handled in such a way as to decrease the diet/weight conflict that is currently plaguing our society. Many parents of obese teens struggle with these conflicts and/or food-control issues from their past. These parents have their own ideas on how to deal with obesity and when those ideas become actions, they often end up perpetuating the problem. The role of the dietitian is to help the parents identify the current family's attitudes toward obesity and related eating problems and to teach them a positive parenting role for empowering their adolescent to make the needed changes for long-term weight management.

Health professionals need to emphatically stress overall fitness and well-being vs. fatness, while reinforcing the notion that thinness is not the ideal. Also, health professionals will have to evaluate their own attitudes toward weight in order to effectively and empathically treat this population, or refer to an appropriately trained team. If not done skillfully, the health professional can become part of the ever-increasing problem of decreased self-esteem, poor body image, and/or disordered eating.

Although diet, exercise, and behavioral approaches to adolescent obesity have shown no significant long-term effectiveness, the family-based treatment of obesity has demonstrated remarkable long-term maintenance of weight loss. These programs target not only changes in family lifestyle, but also the psychosocial development of the adolescent and functioning of the family. The approach supports disengaged families in becoming more cohesive and supporting enmeshed families to allow their adolescent to separate and individuate. In addition, adolescents develop a broad range of skills that enhance their social interactions, body and self-image and affect. The orientation of these interventions is to use the presenting complaint of obesity to examine a host of its potential correlates that will impede the adolescent's psychosocial and physical health and to address them within the context of weight-management care.

ASSESSMENT

Overview

Many obese teens were not identified as children and were not referred for treatment. We now know that as the obese child grows older with untreated obesity, the problems often become more difficult to treat with the increased risk of both medical and psychological consequences. Therefore, early detection and proper intervention by a trained adolescent obesity specialist team using a biopsychosocial approach are essential for the prevention of morbid obesity and weight normalization for the obese teen. Figure 11.1 outlines the recently established screening guidelines for overweight adolescents.

The physician usually first makes the diagnosis of obesity in the teen. Although adolescent obesity is a sensitive issue with patients, all rapid weight gain and other obesity aspects in patients must be evaluated. Obesity in adolescents is often the only visible sign of psychological or physical distress. If it is ignored, sexual, physical, emotional, and other forms of abuse and neglect that otherwise could be identified and responded to are ignored. Nonetheless, clinicians can address obesity in sensitive ways, including asking if the teen's weight gets in the way of his or her happiness, thus suggesting care for their well-being rather than judgment and rejection of them based on body size. In addition, reviewing growth charts (height/weight percentiles) with the parent(s), discussing the adolescent's activity level and overall health, and asking the parent(s) if they are concerned about their adolescent's weight are ways to sensitively inquire about weight. In addition, obtained information will help to determine the parent(s) level of concern or reactions to a diagnosis of obesity. Once the level of concern of the parent is established, the physician might suggest family involvement in a good-quality educational (nutrition) program in order for the family to adopt a healthy lifestyle as the initial intervention. Thus, the obese teen will feel less likely that he or she is being identified as the "problem." If the obesity persists

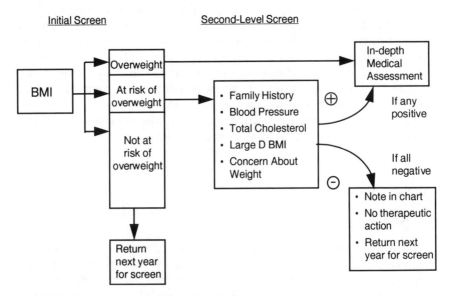

Figure 11-1. Recommended Screening Guidelines for Adolescents.

From J. H. Himes and W. H. Dietz, *Am. J. Clin. Nutr.*, 59, 312 (1994). Reprinted with permission.

or the parent begins talking about a diet for the teen, further evaluation by a dietitian who has had specific training in adolescent obesity and uses a biopsychosocial approach to obesity management should be recommended. Without this kind of guidance from the physician, the family may decide to just go on a diet together or have their adolescent put on a diet that often begins a lifetime of "yo-yo" dieting or preoccupation with weight and/or food for the teen. In this scenario, the teen experiences repeated feelings of failure and negative body-image messages, with decreasing self-esteem often leading to depression.

Nutritional Interview

To complete the assessment, the dietitian should conduct a thorough clinical interview as well as utilize standardized tools of measurement, to assess the biological, psychological, and social areas to determine the patient's present clinical status. The only standardized measure of these factors is the Youth Evaluation Scale (YES).[9] Clinicians could construct their own measures, compiling psychometric testing, family systems measures, behavioral, fitness, and other measures to function in the same way as this computerized tool. Unfortunately, it is more common to address medical problems and lifestyle habits with the genetically predisposed and psychological areas are often neglected. However, if the psychological areas are not assessed, any underlying problem may be hidden only to be uncovered at a later stage of life after causing increased psychological difficulties.

There are six specific areas contributing to adolescent obesity that need to be assessed.[6–10] These are medical problems (diabetes, orthopedic problems, asthma, etc.), lifestyle habits, genetic predisposition, and the psychological aspects of emotional eating, the too comfortable adolescent situation, and the too uncomfortable adolescent situation. As any one of these can occur alone or in any combination, a thorough assessment of each factor involved prior to determining treatment is critical for a long-term positive outcome.

Medical problems.   A thorough evaluation of medical history is necessary to discover if there are any medical problems that complicate the obesity. Particular attention should be paid to diabetes, asthma, medications, or orthopedic complications. In diabetes, the weight gain may be secondary to binge eating that the adolescent has learned to hide with increased insulin usage. The asthmatic adolescent often curbs his or her activity level in an effort to avoid uncomfortable asthma attacks. Orthopedic problems can also encourage an adolescent to be less active. Medications can often stimulate weight gain and may need reevaluation based on the adolescent's history and current symptomatology.

Lifestyle.   Characteristically, the obese adolescent eats a high-fat or calorically dense diet, has irregular meal patterns, often skipping meals and eating large quantities in the late afternoon and evening, and is usually very inactive. These traits are identifiable through the use of a dietary recall, which includes a recall of a typical weekday and weekend, as well as a weekly recall of after-school and family activities. In completing the dietary recall, the dietitian skill-fully helps the adolescent to quantify the foods eaten and completes a computer-ized analysis (when available) to determine the density and nutritional quality of the teen's habitual food intake. It is important to note that obese adolescents are often unaware of how much they eat, are fearful of being judged, and sometimes feel there is something intrinsically wrong with them. Therefore, it is imperative that the health professional has a good rapport with the teen and remains nonjudgmental regardless of the information shared.

Genetics.   Genetic predisposition is determined by identifying if any of the parents and/or grandparents have had child or adolescent obesity, are presently obese, or have struggled with obesity.

Emotional overeating.   Obese teens tend to eat in response to feelings and events rather than hunger and satiety. It is recommended that standardized ques-tionnaires such as the Eating Disorder Inventory (EDI),[10] Eating Disorder Exami-nation (EDE),[11] or YES[5] be used by a trained professional for accurate assessment.

Too comfortable teen.   Characteristically, this is the case that is often referred to as the enmeshed family where the teen has been overindulged with an overpro-tective, permissive parent. Parental expectations are usually low, the teen is often acting as a surrogate spouse, and as a result, the adolescent has too much power. The falseness of the relationship impairs the parent-child intimacy, creat-ing a sense of isolation in the adolescent that excessive food, television, or reading diminish. Interestingly enough, the permissiveness is usually associated with indulgent food and inactivity behaviors. Standardized questionnaires such as the EDI, EDE, and YES can be employed to assess this area.

Too uncomfortable child.   Characteristically, this is the case known as the disengaged family where the child is neglected or deprived in some way. Often, the parents seem removed from the adolescent's life. The adolescent often has a depressed affect or expresses anger at one or both parents. These adolescents often respond to their uncomfortable emotions with compulsive eating or exces-sive inactivity (watching a lot of television or excessive reading). For assessment in this area, standardized methods such as EDI, EDE, or YES may also be helpful.

Anthropometrics

Obesity is body fatness significantly in excess of that consistent with optimal health and can be reliably measured. The most reliable race-specific and population-based measurements for determining adolescent obesity at this time are body mass index (BMI) and triceps skinfolds (TSF).[5] However, height/weight percentiles from the National Center for Health Statistics (NCHS) Growth Curves for Children can be used to show a pattern of increased weight gain for height as an indicator as well. For example, an individual consistently falling in the 95th percentile or above for weight for a period of 2 or 3 yr while their height is in the 50th or 60th percentile should be evaluated for weight-management intervention.

BMI is an index of a person's weight in relation to height, determined by dividing the weight in kilograms by the square of the height in meters[8]:

$$\text{BMI} = \frac{\text{weight (kg)}}{\text{height}^2 \text{ (m)}}$$

However, for simplicity, a nomograph (Figure 11.2) can be used to determine the adolescent's BMI. First, obtain the adolescent's height and weight. Then, plot their height on the left-hand height scale and their weight on the right-hand side of the scale. A straight edge is placed on the marked height and marked weight and a straight line is drawn between these two points. The point where the line crosses the central scale designates the individual's BMI (see Chapters 9 and 10). Once the BMI has been determined, refer to Table 11.2 (on p. 207) in order assess the level of obesity risk.

Height should be measured with the individual in his or her stocking feet and the person's back up against a flat surface that has been marked by height gradations. The individual should stand as straight as possible with the buttocks, shoulders, and head touching the vertical flat surface. The individual's head should be straight with his or her line of vision horizontal. A flat block should be brought down to the crown of the individual's head and the measurement noted.[6] Weight should be measured with a balance beam scale that employs nondetachable weights. The individual should be weighed in his or her stocking feet and light clothing.[6]

TSF is a measure of the thickness of the fatfold site on the tricep that is a vertical fold on the back of the upper arm, midway between the shoulder the tip of the elbow (see Chapter 18). Briefly, to obtain the tricep skinfold measurement, the following steps have been recommended:[9]

1. Be sure to work with the adolescent's bare pendant right arm.
2. Have the adolescent bend his or her arm at the elbow to a 90 degree angle with the palm up.
3. Measure the length between the shoulder and elbow, divide the length by 2 and mark the midpoint with an ink pen or a felt-tipped pen.

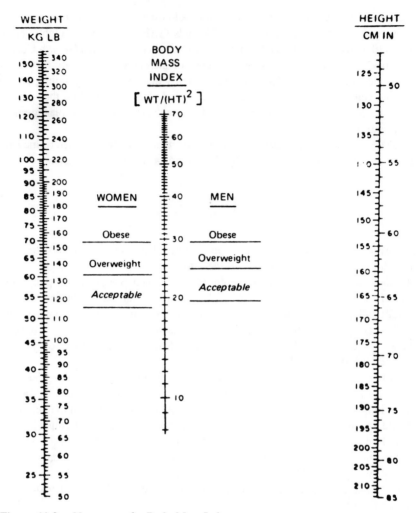

Figure 11-2. Nomogram for Body Mass Index.

From Bray, in *Obesity in America*, National Institute of Health, Pub. no. 79–359, Washington, DC, pp. 6 (1979).

4. Using the thumb and forefinger of your left hand, lift the skinfold parallel to the long axis of the arm and ask the adolescent to lower his or her arm.
5. Apply a pair of calipers to the skinfold so that the point marked is midway between the caliper jaws.
6. Release your thumb from the caliper handle, letting the tips of the caliper have

Table 11.2 Recommened Cutoff Calues for Body Mass Index for Adolescents who are Overweight or At-Risk of Overweight

Age (yr)	At risk of overweight		Overweight	
	Males	Females	Males	Females
10	20	20	23	23
11	20	21	24	25
12	21	22	25	26
13	22	23	26	27
14	23	24	27	28
15	24	24	28	29
16	24	25	29	29
17	25	25	29	30
18	26	26	30	30
19	26	26	30	30
20–24	27	26	30	30

From J. H. Himes and W. H. Dietz, *Am. J. Clin. Nutr.*, 59, 313 (1994). Reprinted with permission.

full exertion of the skinfold (do not release the pinch on the skinfold); read the value immediately after the first rapid fall.

7. Repeat the reading three times and take the average of the three readings as the triceps skinfold measurement.

Once the TSF is determined, compare the measurement to the National Health and Nutrition Survey (NHANESI) Reference Data Table (see Chapters 17 and 18) for the 85th and 95th percentiles for TSF to determine obesity or superobesity, respectively.[5]

The BMI is reasonably constant across all heights for a given body weight and allows more convenient comparisons of weights.[8] The BMI would be the indicator of choice as it requires only the normal height and weight measurement (which the medical practitioner would normally require upon any physical), a nomograph, and the BMI percentile chart. The TSF, on the other hand, requires a set of reliable calipers and a trained, experienced staff person to perform the measurement.

MANAGEMENT

Rather than narrowly focusing on the excess adipose tissue, adolescent obesity should be addressed within the context of the overall development of the teen, the family, and the teen's social system.

Family-Based Approach

The family-based management modalities run by multidisciplinary teams are the programs that usually have the best resources for dealing with adolescent obesity.[12-14] Treatment should be provided by trained child and adolescent specialists so that all issues can be addressed adequately, and appropriate referrals made for dealing with underlying family issues that require psychotherapy, such as substance or psychiatric intervention.

The recommended treatment team may include a dietitian or nutritionist as the primary provider along with a person who has a background in exercise physiology as support. Additionally, a mental health care person and physician or nurse practitioner would serve as consultants to this team. Unfortunately, this structure is not always possible due to the cost constraints. However, the primary provider must have consultants who specialize in adolescent obesity and are familiar with the provider's approach to management to ensure continuity of care.

The ideal management approach is one in which the family would minimally commit to a 10–12 wk program that focuses on the development of a healthy family lifestyle while building good effective communication within the family. The American Heart Association's clinical recommendations for child obesity (see Table 11.1) with the addition of satiety recognition should be used as the guide for behavioral change. This can best be accomplished through nutrition education regarding the frequent use of light foods vs. heavy or junk foods; by not forbidding any food; and by encouraging additional physical activity and less television viewing.[19] Often, this information is received best by the teen if it is presented by an outside educator rather than a parent.

One family-based program is SHAPEDOWN and it is an in-depth format for self-directed change.[16-19] This approach utilizes workbooks for children of various ages, including workbooks for the parents as well. It emphasizes excellent techniques for improving family functioning while concurrently supporting the development of healthy lifestyles. For communication purposes, John Gray's Love Letter[20] is an excellent tool to help individuals identify feelings, begin to process feelings, and then negotiate solutions and problem-solving. Usually, one or more of the following six previously identified areas will need to be addressed.

Medical problems. Upon reviewing the medical history and youth's present medical status, referral to the primary care physician may be necessary. One situation might be that the parents referred the patient to the dietitian on their own without the physician's consent. The dietitian needs to notify the physician that the parents have referred their teen for obesity treatment and request recent physical examination findings, laboratory data, and a listing of any medical constraints that would inhibit treatment. Second, a referral may be necessary after a significant amount of weight loss or gain has been determined. For example, in the case of an obese insulin-dependent diabetic (IDDM), the teen should be referred back to his or her physician for insulin adjustment. The dietitian should request that the adolescent visit his or her physician for additional medical assessment to examine related factors such as hypertension, hyperlipidemia, and the like.

Lifestyle. The goal of treatment is to improve the family's, as well as the adolescent's, health behaviors related to weight. More specifically, to increase physical activity, decrease caloric density of the diet, increase the nutritional adequacy of the diet, decrease excessive quantities, improve regularity of meals, decrease television viewing, and increase after-school activities with structured sports, household chores, walking, and family outings.

Genetics. The treatment goal in this area is to facilitate the adolescent's and parent's acceptance of one's genetic build. Weight loss in the genetically obese may be biologically refractory; therefore, failure to accept one's genetic body build can result in restrictive dieting, binge eating, psychological distress, and weight gain.

Emotional overeating. The treatment goals are to decrease the teen's emotional overeating through identification of feelings and improvement of communication skills (i.e., assertiveness, expressiveness, and substituting adaptive responses to difficult emotions); increase his or her ability to eat in response to hunger and satiety (develop internal cue responsivity); decrease dysphoric moods through increasing physical activity; decreasing social isolation; decreasing negative cognition; and developing an active and enriching lifestyle. Generally, once these goals are reached, the quality and quantity of the diet improve.

Too comfortable adolescent. The treatment goal is to decrease the adolescent's apparent but not actual comfort by altering the functioning of the family. This is done by improving the parental limit-setting skills and practices; identifying and addressing barriers to parental limit-setting, including necessary family system changes; encouraging the teen's and family's recognition and expression of feelings and needs; and supporting the closer parent in separating from the teen while encouraging the other parent to become more involved. Referral for psychotherapy/family counseling may be necessary and is usually determined by the amount of resistance to recommended changes in other areas.

Too uncomfortable adolescent. The treatment goal is to increase the teen's comfort by improving family relations. This is done by improving the parental nurturing skills, identifying and addressing barriers to parental nurturing including necessary family changes, encouraging the family's recognition and expression of feelings and needs. Referral for psychotherapy/family counseling may be necessary and is usually determined by the amount of resistance to recommended changes.

Other Alternatives

Individual family management.   In this style of management, at least one parent, but preferably both parents, and the adolescent are involved in treatment. Often, only one parent will commit to treatment because of divorce, work, or other outside commitments, or mental health difficulties such as substance abuse. As the presenting teen is often the symptom of the family dysfunction, this is an opportunity to engage the family in an initial treatment plan of understanding obesity and its contributing factors while guiding them toward the ultimate treatment plan needed by this family.

The benefits of individually working with a family include more time available for problem-solving; increase comfort experienced by the adolescent allowing discussion of sensitive issues such as alcoholism, verbal abuse, or family violence; private time for youths and parents; and having ample time to discuss issues with the facilitator. The suggested format is 25 min with the adolescent, 10 min with the parent(s), and 10 min for family time. Frequently, more time is spent with the adolescent especially when he or she is struggling with a sensitive issue. Parents should be informed of this possible variation in format at the onset. The main disadvantage of this management alternative is that there is little, if any, peer support.

Group family management.   Adolescents are grouped according to age and management is based through group experiences with other adolescents. Parents are involved in their own support group. The benefits in working with families include the following: teens do not feel alone and may find new accepting friends; parents can share their concerns with other parents and there is parent-specific problem-solving; and both parents and teens find support groups and learn to appreciate the value of a support network. The suggested format is 60 min for the adolescents group, 60 min for the adult group, and 30 min for the combined group of parents and adolescents. The drawbacks to this approach are a possible decreased sharing due to lack of peer approval or disapproval, time limitations, and/or fear of parental retribution; space requirements; and staffing requirements. The ideal method is to have two obesity specialists working with each group simultaneously and coming together in the combined group to discuss issues of concern.

Practical considerations.   The teen years tend to be tumultuous for any family, but obesity usually exacerbates these difficulties. The main issue for adolescents is their struggle for independence by continually testing and stretching parental limits. Parents also struggle with setting appropriate limits while allowing their teen some independence and problem-solving experiences. Nurturing is often difficult during these stressful growing periods. These issues provide the foundation of self-esteem as well as personal growth and are often camouflaged by teen obesity. The following problems contribute to the teen's obesity: the parent's need to place the teen on a diet to fix the problem, the parent's own struggle with "weightism",[6] and the parent's resistance to role modeling. Thus, the initial role of the dietitian is to facilitate the establishment of the appropriate roles in weight management and encourage open lines of communication. Table 11.3 provides specific suggestions regarding these problems. Additional psychological training in family dynamics, communication, and relationship work is very helpful in dealing with these families. Attending eating disorder seminars and other psychological seminars can help to further insight into working with these sorts of cases.

Adolescent obesity must be treated and, much like cancer, needs to be put into remission. Thus, the ideal mode of treatment should be a family-based with services provided by a multidisciplinary team where the team leader is certified as a child and adolescent obesity specialist. Clearly, obesity is multifaceted, and evaluation techniques should include standardized subscales that address biological, psychological, and social factors in order to identify all the overt and covert problems of obesity. Obese adolescents are telling us that something in their lives is not working for them. Providers need to teach families healthy eating habits, the benefits of increased physical activity, improved parental communication skills (assertiveness, emotional expression, and listening), and behavior-management suggestions. It is believed that by providing these educational experiences, adolescents will become empowered and have an improved chance of arresting their condition of obesity. Moreover, the acquisition and practice of these survival skills will impact on the teen's family, friends, and future children.

CASE ILLUSTRATION

Allison, a 15-year-old, presented for care with her mother Linda. Instead of the dietitian seeing the adolescent alone for the first part of the assessment, mother and daughter were seen together because Linda appeared confused and anxious. Allison appeared listless, distracted, and was a poorly groomed, massively obese adolescent. As the assessment began, she plopped into the chair, chewing gum. Linda was thin and looked tired, sat forward on her chair, and inquired anxiously as to the length of assessment because she had to return to work. Linda was told that the assessment would take an hour that day and another hour in a week or two to review test results. Precipitating events were then explored.

Linda responded that Allison's physician had previously recommended the program, but because of other priorities, they were just now able to participate.

Table 11.3   Practical Problems

Problems	Solutions
The need for a diet by parent	
Parents present their obese adolescent and want you to put them on a diet. If you won't, the parents will take the teen to a commercial program to be placed on a diet. The outcome is that the teen experiences one of two possibilities: (1) initial success only to regain weight later ("failure") or (2) learns weight can *only be* controlled when on a diet and therefore begins his or career in weight cycling or "yo-yo" dieting.	Explain to the parents that you will not place the adolescent on a diet, but guidelines will be provided to indicate what a healthy intake would be for that individual adolescent. Stress to the parents that the guidelines are based on the food guide pyramid for healthy individuals and it is just that, a guide. Often, the parent needs to see the guidelines more than the teen so that they will not place unrealistic restrictions on the adolescent. On the other hand nutrition, is not emphasized a great deal in schools and some guidance in this area is helpful for snack and meal planning.
	Help the parents relinquish the responsibility of the adolescent's weight to the adolescent. Explain to the parents what their role is in their adolescent's eating which is, to provide regular wholesome (low-fat, nutritious foods) meals and snacks. The teen's role is to choose the foods he or she wants to eat while learning how to deal with how his or her body feels based on what he or she has chosen. Learning to eat in response to internal cues is critical and outside pressures and constraints will not allow this to occur. Parents must relinquish their role as food cop or eating buddy, whichever the case may be. This is difficult for parents as they will find it hard to watch their teen make their choices that may not always show weight loss. But this is where the work gets done regarding balancing calories over time to reach the goal desired while taking care of oneself. If judgments are not made and problem-solving is done ba sed on how the body feels, personal growth and change can occur.

continued on next page

Table 11.3 *Continued*

Problems	Solutions

*Weightism**

"Weightism" is prejudice or discrimination based on weight; it is racism but against people that are overweight. Therefore, people who don't accept another person's appearance are weightists and our society is full of them. As a result, many of the parents of these adolescents feel that having an obese teen means having a defective teen or that they as parents are inadequate in some way. Many of the parents are weightist based on their own weight issues (experiences of being discriminated against due to their own weight) or other society or familial influences. Either way, these kids know and feel weightism though it has never been explained to them as prejudicial discrimination.

Teach the parents and teen about weightism.

Help the parents accept their teen's body build through fitness testing and anthropometric data.

Help the parents to reframe weight, explaining their teen's genetic body build being rounder or more solid, not necessarily unhealthy and most of all not unworthy of love and acceptance.

Special note: The adolescent will feel the underlying rejection that the weightist parents exhibit even though parents frequently covers up their feelings through distancing or indulging the adolescent inappropriately.

Parent's resistance to role modeling

Parents bring their obese adolescent to the dietitian to fix the problem. They do not understand that their teen learns from what they see modeled at home.

Their beliefs are: It's not my problem. I'm not overweight. Why do I have to change my eating habits or exercise—it's my child I'm concerned about.

Explain thoroughly to the family that health and its benefits are a family affair and everyone can benefit from this healthy lifestyle program.

Explain that teens learn from what they see modeled or experienced. For example: If a wife gives her husband the silent treatment when she is angry at him, the child may give her friend the silent treatment when she is angry with her.

Inform the parents (minimally) and other family members (ideally) that they ideally need to participate in the weight-management program by setting goals regarding lifestyle changes that they are willing to work on each week. When they come in with their goals unmet have them problem-solve how they can reach their goal for

continued on next page

Table 11.3   *Continued*

Problems	Solutions
	the next week. Point out how hard it is to change even if the change seems small. (This will help them to develop an understanding and tolerance of their teen's struggles with change.) If they seem uncomfortable with having to make changes, explore with them what that is about. What are the resisitances, roadblocks, etc.?
Communication barriers Parents often do not know how to support their teen in his or her efforts to make lifestyle changes. The adolescent often does not know how to ask for parental support in making these changes.	Teach the parent and the teen ways to identify their feelings and needs. Using Love Letters[21] can open up communication regarding hidden feelings that families often are unable to verbally express. By using this writing method the myriad of feelings that lead to anger can be explored. This process helps individuals to express their anger, fear, sadness, guilt, and finally their understanding of a situation; can be a very clarifying process. Teach the teen strategies for expressing his or her needs and getting them met. Teach the parents to listen actively to their adolescent and respond in an empathic manner.
Separation from parents During adolescence, the individual begins experimenting with independence. It is important that parents understand their role here is to set limits and the job of the adolescent is to test those limits.	Teach parents limit-setting skills. Teach parents to be clear and firm when setting limits. Teach parents to be firm and consistent in carrying out consequences when limits are broken. Teach parents that this process can be stressful.

As the interview continued, Allison was asked about other family members. Linda began to answer for Allison, but was interrupted by the dietitian. The conversation was redirected to Allison with the question, "If you don't mind, Linda, I need to know what Allison thinks on this. Allison, I know your mom is important to you, but who else is important to you that didn't come today?" Allison replied, "My father." At this point, Linda became agitated and blurted out, "Her father cannot be involved in this. He hasn't seen her in four years and I can't stand the sight of him. What he did to me and the children was horrid and . . ." and she began to cry. Allison stared blankly into space and was asked by the dietitian, "How is that for you to hear your mother say those things?" "I don't know. I can't say," Allison responded.

Linda was extremely agitated and it was felt by the dietitian that a response to her suffering needed to be conveyed. Otherwise, it was likely that Linda would terminate treatment despite Allison's severe obesity. The dietitian provided verbal support as Linda described how she had left her home without a car, with two children because her alcoholic husband had verbally assaulted her again. She had lived with her mother for several months until she secured a job and found an apartment for them. The divorce settlement was reached quickly, and although Allison's father Jack had joined AA, stopped drinking, and taken up running, he did not see them again. Jack still lived nearby and had expressed interest in seeing the children, but had not pursued seeing them because of Linda's behavior. Neither parent had remarried or developed a significant long-term relationship since their divorce. At this time, the dietitian acknowledged, "I know how hard it is for you to let Allison's dad into her life. You have been very hurt. But Allison is half you and half her dad. It's easy for her to get the message that, if her dad is no good, part of her is no good, too." During this interchange, Allison became more attentive. After discussing the assessment process and use of the YES questionnaire, Allison indicated a desire to complete the assessment process. In addition, the dietitian stated, "Linda, it is a very personal matter whether Allison's dad comes to the session. You know best what your daughter needs. My concern is that weight problems in adolescence often have to do with an absent or removed parent. If we don't include that parent, we are not dealing with one of the causes. There is often far less chance that Allison will be successful in losing weight. The YES assessment sessions are often very healing and supportive to the teenagers, particularly so if both parents are involved." Linda responded positively to this interchange by asking her daughter if she would like her father to attend these sessions. Allison nodded in affirmation.

With the first hour of the assessment nearly over, the normal interview process was suspended and both mother and daughter were asked if they would be willing to schedule a longer session at the next visit. Further, it was suggested to Linda that Allison needed some time alone with the dietitian to complete the fitness testing. During the remaining and confidential time with Allison, general psychosocial questions about her school, her interests, and her future plans were addressed. Allison was asked about how weight got in her way. Using the SHAPEDOWN categories, it was hypothesized that she was a "too uncomfortable adolescent." The dietitian was careful to touch her in a gentle and nurturing manner during the anthropometric and fitness testing. Throughout the interview, the dietitian mirrored her behaviors and listened attentively to her feelings and needs.

Linda and her daughter were instructed to complete the standardized YES questionnaires and it was emphasized that their individual responses were confidential. In order to support Allison's autonomy, the dietitian gave Allison the responsibility of mailing back the questionnaires to the office. Linda said she would call Jack and drop off a questionnaire to him.

In reviewing the YES results prior to the second session, the following data were revealed: a weight of 208 lb with a relative weight of 196, high because of her relative shortness. Central obesity with a hip-to-waist ratio of 0.84. Low fitness on all tests. Both lifestyle and emotional overeating problems. All three psychological functioning tests abnormal. Scores on lifestyle and parenting were also somewhat low. Allison reported poor communication with her father. Although her father had not spoken with her in several years, he nonetheless evaluated their communication as good. There was no family history of obesity and the onset of Allison's weight problems had coincided with her parents' marital difficulties, at about the age of 9 yr.

At the next visit, Allison and then her parents were greeted. Linda appeared relaxed and even flirtatious with Jack, her ex-husband. Jack, an office manager, appeared neatly attired in a gray suit with a humble, but concerned attitude. The dietitian explained that initially Allison would be seen first and then the entire family would join them.

Although much information had been obtained via the questionnaire, the following questions also required responses. Had someone touched her? Hurt her? Did she know why her parents were divorced? Who nurtured her, hugged her, and said she was wonderful? Who said "no " to her and made her do things she didn't want to do? What did she do after school? To whom did she talk when she was upset? If she could have three wishes, what would they be? How did she feel when she was around her dad? Her brother? Her mother?

When her parents joined the session, the conversation was directed toward Jack. The dietitian responded, "Thank you for coming. Linda has done much to care for Allison during the last years, but you are her father and adolescence often brings on a heightened need for the parent that has been less involved. Linda supported us all in getting together as a sign of her love for her daughter. However, I am interested in your concerns about Allison's weight." The session continued slowly as the results of her YES questionnaire were disclosed. The dietitian frequently "checked" in with both parents and Allison to obtain their individual opinions.

Allison's obesity was summarized by the dietitian as follows: "The medical risk is high because Allison is very heavy and she carries her weight in the middle. Also there was hypertension and diabetes on both sides of the family. The psychosocial seriousness was also high, as Allison's self-esteem about her weight was low. Contributors to the problem included her depression, her emotional overeating, and her lifestyle. Allison has some hurts from the time of your separation and later that were difficult to heal as Allison is very sensitive to others. What's more, she does not usually discharge these negative feelings by opening up and talking about her feelings and needs." Recommendations to the family were psychotherapy for Allison and family therapy to improve the relationship between Allison and her father. In addition, Allison could participate in the teen obesity group, either now or preferably after therapies had begun. They agreed to begin counseling and Linda agreed to allow Jack to attend the session with her.

Both parents and Allison participated in the teen family-based adolescent obesity group. Several incidents were notable. When Allison and Jack completed an exercise in which they wrote Love Letters,[11] Allison was able to confront her father and express her anger toward him. He, in turn, expressed his sadness and guilt about not being a better parent and his love for her. Previously, Allison had eaten mainly from cans, the freezer, and fast food at school. Linda began keeping vegetables and fruits in the house. Although she was struggling with her own difficulties, she was paying more attention to Allison.

Unfortunately, 6 wk into the group Linda lost her job. Linda who in the past had relied on Allison for emotional support reverted to letting go of her parenting responsibilities and Allison, again, had to fend for herself. Although Linda stopped attending the group, Jack continued to provide support for Allison. He pulled the dietitian aside after one parent meeting and said how grateful he was to be back together with his daughter.

Although Allison was desirous of continuing her care with the advanced support group, at the end of the initial 10-wk program, she completed a YES follow-up that revealed some important findings. Clear improvements in health-related behaviors were reported. Allison indicated exercising almost daily, eating regular meals, and choosing low-fat foods. However, her affect had deteriorated. She demonstrated a common pattern, in that although she made some improvements in her eating habits, removing her behavioral coping mechanism of eating had actually worsened her mental health. The dietitian explored this issue with the family and discovered that Allison had not entered psychotherapy and no family counseling had been initiated.

A family planning session was requested by the dietitian. At this meeting, only Jack and Allison appeared. The dietitian met with them briefly, indicating that this was a critical point in Allison's care and the decision making of both parents was required. The dietitian inquired of Jack as to the reason Linda was not able to make this scheduled meeting. He stated that due to Linda's new job, she was unable to attend and he had failed to emphasize the need for Linda's support of Allison. Allison and Jack left, rescheduling the visit for the following week.

The following week, both parents appeared with Allison and the follow-up results were reviewed. Both parents acknowledged the findings presented, i.e., improved nutritional behaviors and decreased weight, but overall well-being had deteriorated. Although Jack felt his communication with Allison had improved, Allison who was just beginning to express her anger at him saw it worsening. Allison wanted to continue with the advanced teen weight support group. She enjoyed the attention and being with other overweight teens. However, the dietitian questioned Allison about whether or not she would get the results she wanted if she was depressed and anxious. Was it fair to her to target changes in diet and exercise when television and food were important outlets for her difficult feelings? Allison said probably not.

It was difficult for Linda to focus on what her daughter needed as she, herself, was still in turmoil about her employment. However, with careful discussion facilitated by the dietitian, Linda cautiously suggested that family therapy as well as individual sessions for Allison may be helpful. It was agreed that starting and continuing psychotherapy was a precondition to entering the advanced teen weight management program. Within 2 wk, Allison was in both the advanced support group and therapy.

REFERENCES

1. W. H. Dietz, *Ob. Health*, **5**, 41 (1991).

2. S. L. Gortmaker, W. H. Dietz, A. N. Sobol, and C. A. Wehler, *AJDC*, **141**, 535 (1987).

3. National Cholesterol Education Program (NCEP), *Report of the Expert Panel on Blood Cholesterol Levels in Children and Adolescents*, NIH Pub. no. 91–2732, National Institute of Health, Rockville, MD (1986).

4. W. B. Strong et al., in *Integrated Cardiovascular Health Promotion in Childhood*, American Heart Association, Dallas, TX (1992).

5. A. Must, G. E. Dallal, and W. H. Dietz, *Am. J. Clin. Nutr.*, **53**, 839 (1991).

6. J. B. Marcus, in *Sports Nutrition*, (J. B. Marcus, ed.), American Dietitecs Association, Chicago, IL, pp.3 (1986).

7. A. Grant and S. DeHoog, in *Nutritional Assessment and Support*, North Gate Station, Seattle, WA, pp.42 (1991).

8. B. T Burton and W. R. Foster, *J. Amer. Diet. Assoc.*, **85**, 1117 (1985).

9. L. Mellin, *The Youth Evaluation Scale, II ed.*, Balboa Publishing, San Anselmo, CA (1987).

10. D. M. Garner, in *Manual for Eating Disorder Inventory–2*, Psychological Assessment Resources, Inc., Odessa, FL, pp. 1–31 (1991).

11. Z. Cooper, P. J. Cooper, and C. G. Fairburn, *Br. J. Psych.*, 154, 807 (1989).

12. L. H. Epstein, A. Valoski, R. R. Wing, and J. McCurley, *JAMA*, **264**, 2519 (1990).

13. W. H. Dietz, *Child. Adol. Ob.*, **9**, 8 (1993).

14. L. Mellin, L. A. Slinkard, C. Irwin, *J. Amer. Diet. Assoc.*, **87**, 333 (1987).

15. W. H. Dietz and S. L. Gortmaker, *Pediatrics*, **75**, 807 (1985).

16. L. Mellin, in *SHAPEDOWN: Weight Management Program for Children & Adolescents Leader's Guide, IV ed.*, Balboa Publishing, San Anselmo, CA (1991).

17. L. Mellin, in *SHAPEDOWN: Weight Management Program for Teens: Teen Workbook Level 3, V ed.*, Balboa Publishing, San Anselmo, CA (1994).

18. L. Mellin, in *SHAPEDOWN: Weight Management for Teens: Teen Workbook Level 4, V ed.*, Balboa Publishing, San Anselmo, CA (1994).

19. L. Mellin, in *SHAPEDOWN: Weight Management Program for Teens: Parent's Guide, V ed.*, Balboa Publishing, San Anselmo, CA (1994).

20. J. Gray, in *What You Feel You Can Heal: A Guide For Enriching Relationships*, HEART Publishing, Mill Valley, CA, pp. 158–183 (1984).

ADOLESCENTS WITH SPECIAL NEEDS

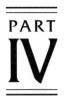

PART
IV

The Competitive Athlete

Suzanne Nelson Steen D.Sc., R.D.

INTRODUCTION

There are a number of factors that contribute to being a successful athlete. Dedication and training techniques are still an athlete's most effective means of developing natural abilities, but nutrition is also an important component of the conditioning process. With regard to nutrition, the most important concept for the adolescent athlete to remember is that *proper sports nutrition is balanced nutrition*. The key to health and performance cannot be found in any one food or supplement, but in a proper combination of foods that provide many different nutrients the body requires.

There are six classes of nutrients: water, carbohydrates, protein, fats, vitamins, and minerals. When balanced correctly, these nutrients will contribute to overall health and physical performance. However, an excess or inadequacy of one or more may be deleterious. One should rely on variety and moderation as the best strategy to achieve balance.

Although appropriate emphasis should be placed on nutrition, an obsession with minor fluctuations in calorie and nutrient intake can lead to unbalanced nutrition. Eating disorders such as anorexia nervosa and bulimia nervosa may be the result.

ASSESSMENT

Dietary Intake

How does the health professional assess whether an athlete is consuming adequate amounts of calories, carbohydrate, protein, vitamins, and minerals? Evaluation of eating patterns and nutrient intake in athletes is a challenge. To obtain dietary information about an individual without influencing typical habits is difficult, as the report of food intake may depend on what the athlete believes the sports dietitian wants to see or hear. To obtain an accurate description of nutrient intake and dietary patterns, objectivity and skill on the part of the nutritionist are required. Several techniques for assessment may be used, depending on the information desired.

24-h recall.   To obtain a brief overview of what an athlete is consuming, a 24-h recall can be used. The athlete is asked to recall foods and beverages consumed within the previous 24 h. Because 1 d is not representative of the season, 24-h recalls are most appropriate to characterize eating patterns for a specific day. For example, a recall may be taken on a group of runners the day of a race to characterize preevent and postevent meal patterns.

Food frequency.   Food frequency questionnaires provide information about the quality of the diet by having the individual indicate the number of times per day, week, or month he or she consumes particular foods and beverages. The food frequency may include questions about all foods or it may be selective for specific foods suspected of being adequate or excessive in the diet. For example, a food frequency given to female athletes may focus on consumption of foods high in calcium and iron (see Table 12.1). These questionnaires are useful for categorizing individuals and groups by food intake characteristics.

Food intake records.   A more complete picture of food intake can be obtained from a food record in which the athlete records all foods and beverages consumed during a specified length of time, usually 4 or 7 d. This allows for an evaluation of the types of foods eaten, nutrient intake, and food patterns. In addition to asking the athlete to write down what he or she eats, the time, location, feelings, and any other information deemed important can also be recorded. Patterns emerge from keeping daily records that provide important information about how often the athlete eats, where food is typically eaten and during what time of day. Based on this information, strategies to promote optimal intake can be

Table 12.1 Selective Food Frequency Form for Calcium and Iron

Food Item	Frequency of Consumption					
	Daily	3–4 times/wk	Once/wk	Every 2wks	1/month	Never
Milk						
Whole						
Lowfat						
Skim						
Buttermilk						
Cheese						
American						
Cheddar						
Swiss						
Cottage						
Yogurt						
Plain						
Fruit						
Frozen						
Ice cream						
Ice milk						
Sherbet						
Sardines						
Dark, leafy green vegetables						
Oysters						
Enriched cereals						
Dried beans						
Beef						
Pork						
Poultry						
Fish						
Eggs						
Supplements						
Calcium						
Iron						
Multimineral						

recommended. For example, the eating patterns of an adolescent figure skater are illustrated in Table 12.2.

Because of early practice, this athlete was only eating an apple until noon because of early morning practice and school immediately afterward (last recorded intake was at 8:00 P.M. the previous day). She consumed the majority of calories

Table 12.2 Eating Patterns of an Adolescent Female Figure Skater (1 d from a 3 d food record)

Time	Food/Beverage	Amount Eaten	Place Eaten	Feelings
6:00–7:30 A.M. (practice)				Tired
8:00 A.M.–12:00 P.M. (school)				Tired
9:30 A.M.	Apple, water	1 medium	School	
12:00 P.M.	Salad with:		School	
	Iceberg lettuce	2 pieces (6 in. × 4 in.)		
	Tomato	2 slices	Brought from home	
	Carrots	1 small		
	Cucumber	4 pieces		
	Non-fat dressing	1 tsp		
	Low fat frozen yogurt	1 cup		
	Diet soda	1 12-oz can		Worried about weight
12:30–2:00 P.M. (school)				
2:00	Diet soda	1 12-oz can		
	Pretzel rods	4		
2:30–4:30 P.M. (practice)				
5:00 P.M.	Water	1 cup	At the skating rink	Very bad practice
6:30 P.M.	Baked chicken	2 oz	Home	
	Bagel	½ plain		
	Corn	¼ cup		
	Sugar-free iced tea	1 cup		
9:00 P.M.	Low-fat frozen yogurt	½ cup	Home	
10:00 P.M. (sleep)				

for dinner. As is evident from her record, the skater complained of being tired, trying to lose weight, and having difficulty practicing.

Food records can also be used to screen for unusual or ritualistic patterns of food consumption that may indicate an eating disorder. For example, in the previous record aside from the overall caloric intake being extremely low, there are no foods listed that contain a significant amount of fat and everything is eaten plain. All the drinks listed are diet. Initiating a discussion about food preferences, recent changes in weight, attitudes about weight loss and dieting, and any unusual dietary practices may provide further insight into a potential problem.

Food records are the best method available for evaluating intake among athletes (aside from direct observation in a metabolic unit that is impractical for this population); however, there are limitations.

For example, some individuals may have difficulty recording or remembering types and amounts of foods eaten or incorrectly estimated portion sizes, leading to an under- or overestimation of nutrient intake. Others may not be motivated to complete the records completely or at all. Certain individuals may resist providing detailed information that would expose the secrecy of an eating disorder. However, despite these limitations, if individuals are given specific instructions on how to keep records by a trained professional and an incentive to do so, valuable information can be obtained.

Evaluating Dietary Intake

In general, two methods can be used to evaluate dietary intake for nutrient adequacy. The first method is a fast, rough estimate that involves estimating the number of servings from the food pyramid (see Figure 18.11) that were consumed during the day recorded and comparing them to what is recommended.

Low intakes of protein, iron, calcium, riboflavin, and vitamins A and C can be detected this way. In addition, the U.S. Dietary Goals can be used for a general evaluation of nutrients consumed in excess, such as fat, cholesterol, sugar, and sodium.

The second method is more precise and involves calculating the nutrients in every food and beverage consumed. This process can be done by hand with the use of USDA food composition books and information from manufacturers and food labels, or with a computerized nutrient data bank or computer software program. (The sources used for nutrient composition vary for computer programs and each should be evaluated carefully before a choice is made for analysis.) In addition, complete information is not available for all foods. For example, not all foods have been analyzed for certain nutrients such as magnesium, B-6, and B-12, limiting the interpretation of results.

After determining the nutrient composition for each food, the nutrient composition of overall daily intake can be calculated. A comparison can be made to a desired standard such as the RDA. From food intake data, conclusions can be made regarding the adequacy of the diet for various nutrients as compared to the RDA. However, one cannot assume that because an individual has a low or inadequate intake of a certain nutrient he or she is deficient in that nutrient. In order to establish whether or not a deficiency exists, blood tests and a clinical exam must be performed.

After the analysis of the food records is completed, the clinical dietitian needs to translate computer output data into specific dietary advice. Based on the interpretation, recommendations can be made that consider the athlete's sport, position, training intensity and frequency, climate, age, and gender.

MANAGEMENT

Energy Requirements

All athletes must adjust their dietary intake to meet the energy demands of the sport. Prior to puberty, nutritional needs are modest compared to the adolescent period of rapid growth and high nutritional demands. To accurately estimate calorie needs, consideration must be given to current dietary intake, rate of growth, age, gender, and weight, as well as the intensity, frequency, and duration of training. The emotional and physical stress of training and competition combined with hectic travel schedules also influence intake.

As a result, adequate calories and essential nutrients must be carefully planned to meet nutritional requirements for training and health. Calorie needs for normal growth and development are presented in Table 12.3. Depending on the specific regimen, additional calories are needed to support training. Caloric equivalents for various activities are presented in Table 12.4.

Table 12.3   Estimate Average Calories and Protien Needs per Kilogram of Body Weight

Age (yr)	Cal/kg	Protein (g/kg)
4–6	90	1.2
7–10	70	1.0
11–14 (m)	55	1.0
11–14 (f)	47	1.0
15–18 (m)	45	0.9
15–18 (f)	40	0.8

Adapted from National Research Council, in
Recommended Dietary Allowances, X ed., National
Academy of Sciences, Washington, DC, (1989).

Table 12.4   Calorie Equivalents in kcal/10 min of Activity

Activity	Body Weight (kg)									
	20	25	30	35	40	45	50	55	60	65
Basketball	34	43	51	60	68	77	85	94	102	110
Calisthenics	13	17	20	23	26	30	33	36	40	43
Cycling										
10 km/h	15	17	20	23	26	29	33	36	39	42
15 km/h	22	27	32	36	41	46	50	55	60	65
Figure skating	40	50	60	70	80	90	100	110	120	130
Ice hockey										
(on-ice time)	52	65	78	91	104	117	130	143	156	168
Running										
8 km/h	37	45	52	60	66	72	78	84	90	95
10 km/h	48	55	64	73	79	85	92	100	107	113
Soccer (game)	36	45	54	63	72	81	90	99	108	117
Swimming										
30 m/min										
Breast	19	24	29	34	38	43	48	53	58	62
Front crawl	25	31	37	43	49	56	62	68	74	80
Back	17	21	25	30	34	38	42	47	51	55
Tennis	22	28	33	39	44	50	55	61	66	72
Walking										
4 km/h	17	19	21	23	26	28	30	32	34	36
6 km/h	24	26	28	30	32	34	37	40	43	48

Adapted from O. Bar-Or, in *Pediatric Sports Medicine for the Practitioner*, Springer Verlag, New York, Appendix IV, (1983).

In general, the adolescent athlete should consume 50–55% of total calories from carbohydrate. The remaining calories should be obtained from protein (10–15%) and fat (20–30%). Planning intake around the food guide pyramid (see Figure 18.11) encourages daily consumption of a variety of foods and serves as a visual guide for planning healthful meals. Each section of the pyramid represents a food category and gives a range for the number of recommended servings to be consumed daily. Depending on the calorie requirements of the adolescent, consuming the appropriate number of servings will supply necessary nutrients and energy.

Carbohydrates

Carbohydrates are the most readily available source of food energy. There are two types of carbohydrates: simple and complex. Simple carbohydrates include glucose, fructose, sucrose (table sugar), and galactose (milk sugar). Examples of simple (refined) carbohydrates are candy, cake, soda, and jelly. Complex carbohydrates are chains of glucose molecules hooked together and include foods such as pasta, bread, grains, corn, and beans. During the digestive process, all carbohydrates are broken down into glucose that then circulates in the blood to be used as the body's principal energy source.

Both simple and complex carbohydrates are important components of the athlete's diet. However, the emphasis should be on consuming more complex carbohydrates because they contain B vitamins, minerals, fiber, and protein, which contribute to a nutritionally balanced diet. Refined carbohydrates are a concentrated energy source, but offer no other nutritional value.

Physical training.   Glucose is stored in the liver and muscle tissue as glycogen. With repeated bouts of training, carbohydrate intake is important on a regular basis to maintain glycogen stores. As shown by Costill and colleagues, only minimal glycogen synthesis will occur for athletes who consume a low-(40%) carbohydrate diet containing 300–350 g of carbohydrate.[1] On such a diet, the athlete is susceptible to fatigue and premature exhaustion because muscle glycogen stores are easily depleted. On the other hand, a high-(70%) carbohydrate diet of 500–600 g carbohydrate/d, provides near maximal repletion of muscle glycogen stores following strenuous training.[1] However, consuming more than 600 g of carbohydrate/d does not result in proportionately greater amounts of muscle glycogen.[1] More importantly, excess carbohydrate will be stored as fat.

Athletes that must meet a certain weight class (scholastic wrestlers), or maintain a low body weight for aesthetic reasons (gymnasts, figure skaters, and ballet dancers), may be at an increased risk for suboptimal nutrient intake.[2,3] Rapid weight-reduction techniques often used by these athletes such as fasting, dieting, or chronically omitting carbohydrate-rich foods will decrease muscle glycogen levels.[4] In addition, athletes who are in negative caloric balance limit their ability to synthesize glycogen.[4] Endurance athletes who train exhaustively on successive days must also consume adequate carbohydrate to minimize the threat of chronic exhaustion associated with the cumulative depletion of muscle glycogen.

If the athlete finds that normal exercise intensity is difficult to maintain, performance gradually deteriorates, or a sudden weight loss occurs, glycogen depletion is a probable cause. Training glycogen depletion can be prevented by a carbohydrate-rich diet and intermittent rest days to permit adequate muscle glycogen synthesis. Examples of high-carbohydrate foods are listed in Table 12.5.

Because of the energy demands of training, some athletes have difficulty consuming sufficient amounts of carbohydrate from food. In this case, a commercial high-carbohydrate beverage may be necessary to boost carbohydrate calories. It is important to emphasize to the teen that the products listed in Table 12.5

Table 12.5   Examples of High-Carbohydrate Foods

Food	Carbohydrate (g)
Apple	21
Applesauce (½ cup)	25
Bagel	31
Baked potato (large)	51
Banana (medium)	27
Beans (refried) (½ cup)	23
Bread (whole wheat) (2 slices)	22
Cereal (corn flakes) (1 oz)	24
Cereal (raisin bran) (1 oz)	21
Corn (½ cup)	21
Cranberry juice (1 cup)	37
Grapes (1 cup)	16
Orange juice (1 cup)	26
Pear	25
Raisins (2/3 cup)	79
Rice (1 cup)	50
Spaghetti (with sauce) (1 cup)	37
Tortilla (flour)	15
Waffle (buttermilk) (2 waffles)	29
Yogurt (low-fat) (1 cup)	42
Commercial high-carbohydrate drinks (12 oz)	
Gatorlode	70
Carboplex	81
Exceed High Carbohydrate Source	89

are designed to provide supplemental carbohydrate and calories and should not be used to replace regular food.

Pre exercise intake.   The preevent meal serves two purposes. First, it keeps the athlete from feeling hungry before and during the event. Second, carbohydrate feedings prior to exercise maintain optimal levels of blood glucose for the exercising muscles during training and competition.[5,6]

Adolescents notoriously skip breakfast. However, it is imperative that the adolescent athlete includes breakfast as an integral part of the eating plan, particularly if the athlete trains early in the morning such as figure skaters and rowers. Aside from the positive impact of breakfast on academic performance, nourishment is important to replenish suboptimal liver glycogen stores that are reduced by 80% overnight. Without breakfast, morning workouts and competition may prove difficult, particularly if the exercise regimen involves endurance training.

Breakfast can be facilitated by providing the adolescent with suggestions for quick and easy meals on the run.

While allowing for personal preferences and psychological factors, the preexercise meal should include familiar foods that are high in carbohydrate, low to moderate in protein, low in fat and fiber.[5,6] For example, fruit juice, fruit, breads, pasta, and yogurt are appropriate choices. High-fat foods such as hot dogs, candy bars, and cheeseburgers should be avoided because fat slows gastric emptying time. Exercising with a full stomach also may cause indigestion and nausea.

Current guidelines indicate that 1–4 g of carbohydrate/kg of body weight should be consumed 1–4 h prior to exercise.[5] To prevent gastrointestinal distress, the carbohydrate content of the meal should be reduced the closer to the event or exercise period that it is consumed. For example, a carbohydrate feeding of 1 g/kg is appropriate an hour before exercise, whereas 4 g/kg can be consumed 4 h before exercise.[5]

Liquid meals can be consumed closer to competition than solid meals because of their shorter gastric emptying time. This may help to avoid precompetition nausea for those athletes who are anxious and have an associated delay in gastric emptying.[6]

When should the preevent meal be eaten? In the past, athletes have been cautioned not to eat large amounts of sugar prior to exercise. This advice was based on data that suggested consuming 50–75 g of glucose 30–45 min prior to exercise reduced endurance by causing a hypoglycemic response.[7] Findings from a recent study showed that 75 g of glucose consumed 45 min prior to bicycling to exhaustion did not negatively affect exercise time.[8] These contradictory results suggest that individuals may differ in their susceptibility to a lowering of blood glucose during exercise.[5]

Preexercise sugar consumption may benefit the endurance athlete by providing glucose to the exercising muscles when glycogen stores have dropped to low levels.[5] However, even though new evidence suggests that sugary foods may be consumed 30–45 min prior to exercise, for some athletes this practice could harm performance if they are sensitive to fluctuations in blood sugar. Athletes should be advised to evaluate whether they are sensitive to a lowering of blood glucose by trying various amounts of carbohydrate before exercise during training.[5]

Carbohydrate loading is a technique that can increase muscle glycogen levels to above normal. For 3–5 d before competition, the athlete consumes a high-carbohydrate (7–10 g/kg) and concurrently tapers training.[6] The final day before the event requires total rest and maintaining the high-carbohydrate intake. This strategy will only help athletes who are enduranced-trained (endurance training increases the activity of glycogen synthetase, the enzyme responsible for glycogen storage) and those who engage in continuous endurance exercise for longer than 90 min.[6] There is no advantage to having greater than usual glycogen stores for athletes involved in shorter duration exercise. To the contrary, the stiffness and heaviness often associated with increased glycogen stores may harm performance.

During exercise. Research has shown that for endurance activities lasting longer than 90 min, carbohydrate feedings may enhance performance.[9] The liver supplies glucose to the bloodstream to maintain levels for optimal functioning of the central nervous system. During exercise, as muscles become glycogen-depleted, they will begin to utilize blood glucose. As a result, liver glycogen stores are drained. When liver glycogen is depleted, the blood glucose declines (remember that muscle glycogen stays in the muscle and cannot contribute to blood glucose levels). Hypoglycemia occurs and exercise intensity is reduced due to muscle fatigue.

Dietary carbohydrate feedings during exercise provide the muscles with a source of glucose when their glycogen stores are diminished. Therefore, blood glucose can be maintained, allowing the individual to exercise longer.

It is recommenced that endurance athletes consume 30–60 g of carbohydrate every hour.[9] Depending on the sport, this can be obtained through carbohydrate-rich foods such as crackers or bananas, as well as sports drinks containing 6–8% carbohydrate.

Post exercise. The time period in which carbohydrate is consumed relative to completion of exercise is important. Research suggests that the rate of muscle glycogen storage is increased during the 2 h postexercise.[10] Practically, this suggests that delaying the carbohydrate intake for too long after exercise will reduce muscle glycogen storage and may impair recovery. Thus, an athlete should consume 1.5 g of carbohydrate/kg within 15–30 min postexercise, to be followed by additional 1.5 g/kg feedings every 2 h thereafter.[10]

Typically, most athletes are not hungry after exercising. Therefore, the most effective strategy may be to encourage the athlete to consume a high-carbohydrate drink or fruit juice immediately after exercise, to be followed later by high-carbohydrate meals. Examples of high-carbohydrate meals are presented in Table 12.6.

Fat

Even though maximal performance is impossible without muscle glycogen, fat also provides energy for exercise. Fat is the most concentrated source of food energy and supplies more than twice as many cal (9 cal) by weight as protein (4 cal) or carbohydrate (4 cal). Fats provide essential fatty acids and are necessary for cell membranes, skin, hormones, and transporting fat-soluble vitamins. The body has total glycogen stores (in muscle and liver) that equal about 2500 cal, whereas each pound of body fat supplies 3500 cal. This means that an athlete weighing 74 kg (163 lb) with 10% body fat has 16.3 lb of fat, which equals 57,000 cal!

Table 12.6   Examples of High-Carbohydrate Meals

BREAKFAST

Orange juice	Cranberry juice
Bluebery pancakes with syrup	Raisin bran or oatmeal
Bagel	Low-fat milk
Low-fat yogurt	Apple bran muffin
Banana	

LUNCH

Chicken sandwich on whole wheat roll	Baked potato with chili
Fruit cup	Cornmeal muffin
	Vanilla milkshake
Frozen low-fat yogurt	

DINNER

Pasta with tomato sauce	Thick-crust cheese, mushroom, and Green pepper pizza
Salad with tomato, carrots, cucumbers, and mushrooms	Low-fat milk
Italian bread	Fresh fruit
Fresh fruit	
Low-fat milk	
Sherbet	

Note: Caloric needs depend on age, gender, and activity level.

Fat is the major, if not most important, fuel for light- to moderate-intensity exercise. Although fat is a valuable metabolic fuel for muscle activity during longer-term aerobic exercise and performs many important functions in the body, no attempt should be made to store fat (as you can store glycogen), because as is evident from the previous example, more fat is stored than is ever needed. In addition, athletes that consume a high-fat diet typically consume fewer calories from carbohydrate. Following a low-fat diet is also important because a high intake of fat has been associated with cardiovascular disease, diabetes and obesity. Adolescent athletes should consume between 25–30% of their daily calories from fat.

Protein

Protein is essential for the growth and development of almost all tissue of the body. Proteins are composed of amino acids and found in both plant and animal sources. The body combines specific amino acids to create a particular protein. Eight (nine in children) of the 20 amino acids are considered essential because they cannot be synthesized by the body, but must be obtained from the diet.

Many athletes erroneously believe that the body requires large amounts of protein for optimum performance. Athletes in sports where strength is a critical factor, such as football and weightlifting, often consume a high-protein diet and/ or take protein supplements to increase strength and muscle mass.[10,11] However, contrary to popular opinion, the consumption of excess protein does not influence muscle size. If daily needs are met, muscle size will be dictated by the specific training regimen and genetic potential.

Protein requirements depend on a number of factors including growth, the type of sport (strength vs. endurance), intensity of training, stage of training, and most important, the energy balance of the diet. For any given protein intake, increasing energy intake will improve nitrogen balance.

Available evidence suggests that some athletes may require 50–150% more protein than the RDA.[12] This means that athletes may need 1.2 g/kg and may benefit from up to 1.5 g/kg during periods of muscle building or prolonged heavy-endurance exercise.[12] Athletes that chronically restrict cal, also require slightly higher intakes of protein (1.2–1.5 g/kg) to allow for the adequate synthesis and repair of muscle tissue.[13]

Athletes can easily obtain protein from foods and do not need protein supplements. Protein supplements in the form of powders, pills, or bars are not necessary and should be discouraged. Taking large amounts of protein or amino acid supplements can lead to dehydration, weight gain, increase calcium loss from the body, and stress the kidneys and liver.[14] Ingestion of single amino acids or in combination, such as arginine and lysine, may interfere with the absorption of certain essential amino acids.[14] An additional concern is that substituting amino acid supplements for food may cause deficiencies of other nutrients found in protein-rich foods such as iron, niacin, and thiamin.[14] Amino acid supplements have not been shown to increase muscle mass or burn body fat. Additionally, no margin of safety is available for ingesting large doses of amino acids and the long-term risks have not been identified. It is important for the health professional to develop effective strategies to approach and discuss supplement use with both athletes and coaches.

Some athletes follow a vegetarian diet. When carefully planned, a diet that derives its protein from vegetable sources can provide adequate protein, carbohydrate, and vitamins and minerals that the young athlete needs to sustain growth and prolonged workouts. Protein intake on a lacto-ovo vegetarian or semivegetarian diet should provide adequate high-quality protein from eggs and dairy products. However, on a strict vegetarian diet, the adolescent may have difficulty obtaining necessary protein and other nutrients such as calcium, vitamins D and B-12. Because growth is paramount for the adolescent, planning intake with a health professional is advised to ensure adequate cal and nutrients (see Chapter 4).

Fluid Requirements

Water.   The most important nutrient for the athlete during any phase of training and competition. As little as a 2 % decrease in body weight from fluid loss can lead to a significant decrease in muscular strength and stamina.[15] This translates into a 2 ½ lb loss for a 125-lb (57-kg) female; or a 3 ½ lb loss for a 175-lb (79.5-kg) male. As an individual becomes dehydrated, heart rate increases, blood flow to the skin decreases, and body temperature can rise steadily to dangerous levels.[16,17] Exercise in a hot environment places a greater demand on the cardiovascular system and requirement for adequate fluid intake.[16] Relative humidity can be a problem as well because athletes can lose large amounts of fluid and become dehydrated even at cooler temperatures when humidity is high. Because a substantial level of dehydration can be reached before the body ever feels "thirsty", athletes must make a conscious effort to consume fluids before, during, and after exercise. Guidelines to help ensure adequate fluid intake are presented in Table 12.7.

Fluid losses can be monitored by weighing the athlete before and after exercise. The athlete should be encouraged to drink 16 oz of water for every pound of weight lost. Serial weighing (ideally after each practice; minimum two or three times per week) can identify the athlete who has a tendency toward dehydration, and strategies to ensure adequate fluid intake during training can follow.

Sports drinks.   Plain water is the most economical source of fluid to hydrate the body. For exercise bouts lasting less than 60 min, water is an appropriate fluid replacement.[6] However, when the workout period exceeds 60 min, sports drinks that contain 6–8 % calories from carbohydrate can be beneficial as they supply energy and electrolytes that are key ingredients for maximum fluid absorption.[6] Both water and sports drinks have the same favorable influence on cardiovascular and thermoregulatory function.[18,19]

Although carbohydrate feedings during exercise can improve exercise performance, with the vast array of sports drinks available, how does the athlete decide

Table 12.7   Guidelines for Fluid Replacement

Drink 1 ½–2 ½ cups of cool fluid 10–20 min before activity.

During exercise, drink an additional ½–1 cup of cool fluid every 15–20 min.

Weigh-in without clothes before and after exercise. Drink 2 cups of cool fluid for
  every pound of body weight lost.

Drink during training and competition.

Drink on schedule rather than relying on thirst.

---

which one to use? First of all, it is important to keep in mind that although some beverages in the marketplace are touted as "sports drinks," not all measure up to sports science standards of an optimal fluid replacer. For example, carbonated beverages are not recommended because they usually have a high-carbohydrate concentration of 10% or more, which slows absorption.[6,19] When choosing a sports beverage, the source of carbohydrate is important to consider. Glucose, glucose polymers (maltodextrins), and sucrose all stimulate fluid absorption in the small intestine.[6,19] The effect of the ingestion of these types of sugars on exercise performance is similar, and all result in similar cardiovascular and thermoregulatory responses.[20] However, research shows that beverages containing fructose as the sole carbohydrate source are absorbed more slowly than other sugars and do not stimulate as much fluid absorption.[21] In addition, gastrointestinal distress and osmotic diarrhea are common side effects of drinking fructose solutions during exercise.[21] Fructose ingestion during exercise has not been associated with performance improvement.[21]

Sports drinks should be between 6–8% carbohydrate, because at this concentration they are absorbed into the bloodstream as quickly as water.[18,21,22] Drinks less than 5% probably do not provide enough energy to enhance performance, whereas those that exceed 10–12% may cause gastric upset and impair performance.[18,21,22] The amount of carbohydrate in 1 cup of sports drink should be between 15 and 18 g. Calories should fall between 50–80 cal/8 oz.

Ultimately, if the sports beverage meets the above guidelines, personal preference becomes the deciding factor. The athlete needs to choose which product tastes the best and works well with a particular exercise regimen. The athlete should be encouraged to evaluate different products during training, not competition.

Vitamins

Athletes are often looking for an edge, something that will give them an advantage, and many turn to supplements in the form of pills, powders, and liquids in an effort to make the body perform at its best. Unfortunately, many self-proclaimed "experts" are eager to convince athletes that their product will improve athletic performance by improving muscle contractions, preventing fat gain, enhancing strength, or supplying energy. These experts may insist that the athletes' fatigue and muscle soreness are due to a vitamin or mineral deficiency. In fact, when there is a nutritional reason for fatigue, it is usually a lack of calories and/or carbohydrate.

Vitamins function as metabolic regulators that influence the processes of growth, maintenance, and repair. They are organic molecules, that the body cannot manufacture, but are required in small amounts. Vitamins are divided into two groups: water-soluble and fat-soluble. A, D, E, and K are soluble in fat, whereas C and the B vitamins are soluble in water. Table 12.8 lists all vitamins, their physiological function, and major food sources.

Fat-soluble vitamins are stored in body fat, principally the liver. Excess accumulation of fat-soluble vitamins, particularly vitamins A and D, can produce serious toxic effects. Although excesses of most water-soluble vitamins are typically excreted, some may pose toxicity problems. Large amounts of niacin, e.g., can cause burning or tingling, skin rash, nausea, and diarrhea. High doses of niacin also interfere with fat mobilization and increase glycogen depletion.

Table 12.8   Vitamins

Vitamin	Main Function	Good Sources
A	Maintenance of skin, bone growth, vision, teeth	Eggs, cheese, margarine, milk, carrots, broccoli, squash, spinach
D	Bone growth and maintenance of bones	Milk, egg yolk, tuna, salmon
E	Prevents oxidation of polyunsaturated fats	Vegetable oils, whole-grain cereal, bread, dried beans, green leafy vegetables
K	Blood clotting	Cabbage, green leafy vegetables, milk
Thiamin B-1	Energy-releasing reactions	Pork, ham, oysters, breads, cereals, pasta, green peas
Riboflavin B-2	Energy-releasing reactions	Milk, meat, cereals pasta, mushrooms, dark green vegetables
Niacin	Energy-releasing reactions	Poultry, meat, tuna, cereal, pasta, bread, nuts, legumes
Pyridoxine B-6	Metabolism of fats and proteins, formation of red blood cells	Cereals, bread, spinach, avocados, green beans, bananas
Cobalamin B-12	Formation of red blood cells, functioning of nervous system	Meat, fish, eggs, cells, milk
Folacin	Assists in forming proteins, formation of red blood cells	Dark green leafy vegetables, wheat germ
Pantothenic acid	Metabolism of proteins, carbohydrates, fats, formation of hormones	Bread, cereals, nuts, eggs, dark green vegetables
Biotin	Formation of fatty acids, energy-releasing reactions	Egg yolk, leafy green vegetables, egg yolk
C	Bones, teeth, blood vessels, collagen	Citrus fruits, tomato, strawberries, melon, green pepper, potato

Athletes need to understand that more is not always better. The National Academy of Sciences has established Recommended Daily Allowances (RDAs) for vitamins and minerals as a guide for determining nutritional needs.[23] The RDA is the daily amount of a nutrient recommended for practically all healthy individuals to promote optimal health. It is not a minimal amount needed to prevent disease symptoms as a large margin of safety is included. For example, the body needs approximately 10 mg of vitamin C to prevent the deficiency disease called scurvy. The RDA for vitamin C is set far above that level at 60 mg. Although it has been shown that a severely inadequate intake of certain vitamins can impair performance, it is unusual for an athlete to have such deficiencies.[24] Even marginal deficiencies do not appear to markedly affect the ability to exercise efficiently.[24]

Minerals

Minerals perform a variety of functions in the body. Although some are used to build tissue, such as calcium and phosphorus for bones and teeth, others are important components of hormones, such as iodine in thyroxine. Iron is critical for the formation of hemoglobin that carries oxygen within red blood cells. Minerals are also important for the regulation of muscle contractions and body fluids, conduction of nerve impulses, and regulation of normal heart rhythm.

Minerals are divided into two groups. The first are referred to as macrominerals and needed in amounts from 100 mg–1 g. These include calcium, phosphorus, magnesium, sodium, potassium, chloride, and sulfur. The others fall under the category of trace minerals and are needed in far smaller amounts. These include iron, manganese, copper, iodine, zinc, cobalt, fluoride, and selenium. Food sources and the physiological functions for each mineral are listed in Table 12.9.

Iron. The iron status of the athlete, particularly the female athlete, is of concern as indices of low-serum iron (ferritin, iron, and hematocrit) have been observed.[25,26] Reasons for these low levels may be due to inadequate dietary intake, low bioavailability of iron, or high rates of iron loss.[25] Adolescent females are at an increased risk for iron deficiency because of not only increased physiological needs, but lower caloric intakes and faulty eating habits. In addition, as mentioned earlier, many female athletes are vegetarians. In one report, 42% of the female distance runners studied were modified vegetarians and consumed less than 200 g of meat/wk.[27]

Although the dietary intake of iron is tied to caloric intake, iron absorption depends on the bioavailability of iron. Meats contain heme-iron that is highly bioavailable and, therefore, a superior source of iron. Heme iron also enhances the absorption of the nonheme iron found in leafy greens, legumes, cereals, whole grains, and enriched breads. Combining these foods with a source of vitamin C can significantly enhance the absorption of iron. For example, orange

Table 12.9   Minerals

Mineral	Main Function	Good Sources
Calcium	Formation of bones, teeth, nerve impulses, blood clotting	Cheese, sardines, dark green vegetables, clams, milk
Phosphorus	Formation of bones, teeth, acid–base balance	Milk, cheese, meat, fish, poultry, nuts, grains
Magnesium	Activation of enzymes, protein synthesis	Nuts, meats, milk, whole-grain cereal, green leafy vegetables
Sodium	Acid-base balance, body water balance, nerve function	Most foods except fruit
Potassium	Acid-base balance reactions, body water balance, nerve function	Meat, milk, many fruits, cereals, vegetables, legumes
Chloride	Gastric juice formation acid-base balance	Table salt, seafood, milk, meat, eggs
Sulfur	Component of tissue, cartilage	Protein foods
Iron	Component of hemoglobin and enzymes	Meats, legumes, eggs, grains, dark green vegetables
Zinc	Component of enzymes digestion	Milk, shellfish, wheat bran
Iodine	Component of thyroid hormone	Fish, dairy products, vegetables, iodized salt
Copper	Component of enzymes, digestion	Shellfish, grains, cherries, legumes, poultry, oysters, nuts
Manganese	Component of enzymes, fat synthesis	Greens, blueberries grains, legumes, fruit
Flouride	Maintenance of bone and teeth	Water, seafood, rice, soybeans, spinach, onions, lettuce
Chromium	Glucose and energy metabolism	Fats, meats, clams, cereals
Selenium	Functions with vitamin E	Fish, poultry, meats, grains, milk, vegetables
Molybdenum	Component of enzymes	Legumes, cereals, dark green leafy vegetables

juice together with an iron-enriched cereal, or pasta in combination with broccoli, tomatoes, and green peppers.

Regular monitoring of iron levels in athletes, including biochemical evaluations and dietary assessments, is recommended to ensure optimal training and performance. For individuals with iron-deficiency anemia, supplements are required since it is difficult to overcome this condition through dietary measures alone. However, supplementation should not be given routinely to athletes without medical supervision. Taking excessive amounts of iron does not improve performance and can be toxic when taken in large doses.

Calcium. The adequate consumption of calcium is also important, because low levels can lead to stress fractures and osteoporosis. These complications are most relevant for females because they have thinner bones and, after reaching maturity, lose bone density at a faster rate. In addition, many female athletes have amenorrhea. Studies have shown that these women have decreased spinal bone mass, compared to both active and sedentary women who are menstruating. The cause of this decrease in bone mineral content is not clear since amenorrhea is associated with a number of variables including low body weight and low body fat, weight loss, low caloric and nutrient intake, physical stress, energy drain, and chronic hormonal alterations.[28,29] There is increasing evidence that disordered eating, menstrual dysfunction, and bone mineral disorders form a triad of disorders in female athletes.[30]

Consumption of foods that are rich in calcium should be encouraged, such as those listed in Table 12.10. If a supplement is necessary, calcium carbonate is preferred because it supplies the amount of elemental calcium and is free from toxins such as those found in dolomite and bone meal. However, calcium supplements can cause nausea and loss of appetite.

Certainly, for the athlete who is chronically dieting, taking a one-a-day multivitamin and multimineral (100% of the RDA) is prudent to ensure the adequate intake of micronutrients. For the athlete with a diagnosed deficiency, supplementation by a health professional is necessary. However, in general, most researchers agree that the indiscriminate use of supplements is ineffective in attaining a high level of performance. Overconsumption can lead to toxicity, and a false sense of security, and may alter the utilization of other micronutrients. The bottom line, megadoses of supplements will not make up for a lack of training or talent, or give one an edge over the competition.

Table 12.10   Increasing Calcium in the Adolescent's Diet

Drink low-fat milk with meals.
Prepare canned soups with low-fat milk instead of water.
Add nonfat dry milk powder to casseroles.
Top salad, cooked vegetables, pasta, or tacos with grated cheese.
Drink orange juice fortified with calcium.
Make desserts calcium-rich: ice cream, low-fat frozen yogurt, puddings.
Have calcium-rich meals: waffles, macaroni and cheese, cheese veggie pizza, lasagna, grilled cheese sandwich.
Include calcium-rich snacks: cheese and crackers, yogurt, low-fat milk, milkshake.

Table 12.11   Warning Signs for Anorexia Nervosa and Bulimia Nervosa

Anorexia Nervosa	Bulimia Nervosa
Weight loss	Weight loss or gain
Preoccupations with weight, calories, and food	Excessive weight concern
Wears layered or baggy clothing	Visits bathroom after meals
Excessive exercise	Sad mood
Mood swings	Dieting followed by binge eating
Avoids social activities involving food	Critical of body image

Note: The presence of one or two of these symptoms does not indicate the presence of an eating disorder.

Adapted from National Collegiate Athletic Association, Kansas City, MO, (1990).

Weight-Loss Practices and Eating Disorders

As children progress in a sport, they may develop compulsive weight-loss behaviors in an effort to reach the "ideal" body weight for competition.[31] Although this is most often a problem for adolescent females, all athletes may experiment with fad diets. Extreme eating patterns can set the stage for an eating disorder such as anorexia nervosa or bulimia nervosa. Compulsive weight-loss behaviors may be triggered by many factors. Crash dieting may be prompted by an unrealistic weight goal set by a parent or coach in an erroneous effort to enhance performance, a desire to succeed coupled with a fear of failure, or a seemingly harmless remark by a parent, coach, or friend about the teen athlete looking "fat."[31] Sports-related expectations can go beyond the physical and emotional challenges already faced by the young athlete.

Athletes believed to have an eating problem should be approached privately by someone they trust. Although it may be difficult to talk to a young adult athlete about the possible presence of an eating disorder, ignoring the issue may jeopardize his or her health. Coaches should be encouraged to provide information in the form of a fact sheet that details where the complications of eating disorders, healthy alternatives, and where the adolescent can find professional help. Warning signs that suggest an eating disorder are listed in Table 12.11.

Identifying who is placing pressure on the adolescent regarding body weight, such as a coach, parent, or teammate, is essential for successful intervention and subsequent recommendations. The unhealthful practices associated with efforts to change body weight can, in part, be prevented by education and establishing appropriate guidelines for weight control.

Making Weight

Scholastic wrestlers must meet a certain weight classification in order to compete. It is a common practice throughout the competitive season for wrestlers to restrict food and fluid intake in order to compete at one to three weight classes below their normal weight.[32] Wrestlers typically believe that this practice, known as "making weight," gives them a competitive edge over smaller opponents. Few wrestlers, coaches, and parents realize the negative physiological impact this practice may have on their bodies.

Studies have shown that making weight lowers blood and plasma volumes, reduces cardiac function during submaximal work (e.g., higher heart rate, smaller stroke volume, and reduced cardiac output), impairs thermoregulation, decreases renal blood flow and renal filtration, and increases electrolyte losses.[33,34] The calorie and micronutrient content of wrestlers' diet during training are typically inadequate.[2]

From a performance standpoint, making weight can lead to liver and muscle glycogen depletion, dehydration, reduced muscular strength, and decreased performance work time.[35] Unfortunately, wrestlers rarely regain all their lost weight after the official weigh-in prior to competition. Thus, they may be wrestling under suboptimal conditions.

In an effort to preclude the use of erratic weight-loss practices commonly observed among adolescent and collegiate wrestlers, it is imperative to establish healthy weight-control guidelines. Through nutrition education, coaches, parents, and the athlete can be apprised about the consequences of rapid and extreme weight reduction by fluid and food restriction and healthy alternatives for achieving a suitable competitive weight.[2]

Sources of Reliable Nutrition Information

Individuals at all levels of the sports community can have an impact on promoting sound nutrition for the teenage and young adult athlete. Athletic directors can play a key role by supporting the efforts of health professionals to provide seminars and workshops on sports nutrition within the high school or university. Better still is having a sports nutritionist as part of the sports medicine team. Doing so will help athletes perform at their best and establish healthy eating habits that can last a lifetime.

Having the support and cooperation of the coaching staff is of the utmost importance when educating a team or player about nutrition. The result can be a enhanced rapport between the nutritionist and athlete. Subsequently, the message conveyed to the athlete may be more readily received and put into practice. Aside from encouraging athletes to seek advice from a sports nutritionist, coaches can also help in the effort to combat misinformation by providing team members with handouts from credible resources. Finally, coaches can serve as role models by making healthy dietary changes themselves. This is particularly important for the young athlete. Parents are also important role models for the adolescent athlete and can have an impact on promoting positive dietary choices by providing nutritious foods at home.

To consult a sports nutritionist in your area, contact Sports and Cardiovascular Nutritionists (SCAN) that is a practice group of the American Dietetic Association (ADA). Members of this group are registered dietitians and have expertise in the area of nutrition and exercise. The address for this group is Sports and Cardiovascular Nutritionists (SCAN), 216 West Jackson Street, Suite 800 Chicago, Illinois 60606 (1-800-877-1600).

CASE ILLUSTRATION

Julia, a talented young figure skater, suffered a disappointing loss in a regional competition. Although her technical marks for execution of jumps and spins were high, her artistic impression marks were low and consequently she lost by a narrow margin. Her parents told her that they overheard the judges say that she was given low marks artistically because "she looked chunky and fat, particularly in her thighs." The coach agreed that losing a few pounds would give her a "more sleek appearance and improve her performance." As a result, this 13-year-old (weight 38.6 kg, height 152.4 cm; 92% IBW) severely restricted intake and within 3 wk had lost 4.0 kg (82% IBW). As she struggled to lose more weight, her performance began to deteriorate; she felt tired all the time and started having frequent respiratory infections.

Physical measures indicated that she was 34.6 kg and 152.4 cm in height (wt/ht: 42.25 kg). She had lost 10% of her body weight (4 kg over 3 wk) by severely resticting food and fluid intake. She was 82% IBW and 97% ht/age (157.5 cm). She was postpubescent (menarche at age 12 ½ yr), but had not menstruated since she initiated dieting.

A 3 d food record revealed that she consumed 900 cal/d (range: 800–1125 cal) that was 50% of caloric needs based on RDA (47 cal/kg). Percent cal from CHO: 54%; PRO: 16%; FAT: 30%. Protein intake was 1.0 g/kg (inadequate due to negative caloric balance). Majority of micronutrients were less than two-thirds of the RDA. Of particular concern were low intakes of calcium, iron, zinc, and vitamin C. On average, she consumed 24 oz of diet soda and 8 oz water). She trained 7 d/wk. Two h were spent on the ice and 2 h/wk were devoted to ballet.

Although Julia was preoccupied with weight and limiting food intake, she did not exhibit a fear of fat or obesity. She recognized that her performance and health were suffering because of dieting. She acknowledged feeling hungry and tired, but wanted to please her coach and parents by winning.

Her parents reported that they were very angry that she had not been awarded first place. They also admitted that another competitor's parent, not the judges, had made a negative remark about their daughter's weight. They reasoned that if she lost a couple of pounds, it couldn't hurt and might, in fact, be helpful to her performance. They thought that telling her the judges had commented on her weight would motivate her to lose the excess pounds. They didn't realize that she would take their advice to lose a few pounds to such an extreme.

The plan consisted of talking with Julia, her parents, and coach about the following:

1. A realistic competitive weight. At present, it was agreed that she would stop losing weight and focus on maintaining current weight by increasing cal by 200 cal/d for 1 wk. Next step was to gradually increase weight to initial goal (negotiated with skater) to 36.0 kg (1.4 kg) over the ne xt 4 wk.
2. Positive body image and how her body will continue to change naturally as part of growth.
3. The importance of nutrition for growth, performance, and health. Explained the relationship of calorie intake and normal menstruation.
4. Nutrition training regimen.

Initially, a 200 cal/d increase for 1 wk was recommended. To achieve this goal, she agreed to drink 8 oz of milk combined with an instant breakfast mix for calories, protein, and micronutrients. Eventual caloric intake would be determined when weight stabilized at desired goal (actual cal to maintain 36 kg were 2100 cal/d; 55% CHO; 30% FAT; 15% PRO).

Fluid needs were reviewed. For the first week Julia agreed to increase her water intake to 4 cups/d. Goal for fluid intake was 6 cups/d plus 16 oz for every pound lost after training sessions. Since she was dehydrated upon assessment (noted darkened color of urine sample), the sports nutritionist reassured her that the initial increase in weight would be due to an increase in fluid (not fat) as she rehydrated. In addition, triceps and subscapular skinfold measures were taken each week as reassurance that weight gain did not represent fat gain.

For the first month, a one-a-day multivitamin/mineral was recommended. Emphasis was placed on increasing calcium-rich foods and foods high in iron eaten in combination with a good source of vitamin C.

As illustrated by this case history, weight loss may lead to decrements in performance and health. Depending on the sport and the particular athlete, there may be many factors that contribute to extreme dieting. These factors must be identified and appropriate steps taken to determine a realistic competitive weight and adequate nutrient intake. For the young athlete, establishing a relationship based on trust and understanding is essential to facilitate recommendations.

REFERENCES

1. D. L. Costill and J. M. Miller, *Int. J. Sports Med.*, **1**, 2 (1980).
2. S. N. Steen and S. M. McKinney, *The Phys. Sportsmed.*, **14**, 100 (1986).

3. L. H. Calabrese and D. T. Kirkendall, *Clin. Sports Med.*, **2**, 539 (1983).

4. D. L. Costill, *Int. J. Sports Med.*, **9**, 1 (1988).

5. W. M. Sherman, *Gatorade Sports Sci. Exchange*, **1** , (1989).

6. E. Coleman, in *Sports Nutrition for the Nineties: The Health Professional's Handbook*, (J. Berning and S. N. Steen, eds.), Aspen Publishers Inc., Gaithersburg, MD, (1991).

7. D. L. Costill, E. F. Coyle, G. Dalsky, W. Evans, W. Fink, and D. Hoopes, *J. Appl. Physiol.*, **43**, 695 (1977).

8. M. Hargreaves, D. L. Costill, W. J. Fink, D. S. King, and R. A. Fielding, *Med. Sci. Sports Exer.*, **19**, 33 (1987).

9. E. F. Coyle and S. J. Montain, *Med. Sci. Sports Exer.*, **24**, 324s (1992).

10. J. L. Ivy, A. L. Katz, C. L. Cutler, W. M. Sherman, and E. F. Coyle, *J. Appl. Physiol.*, **6**, 1480 (1988).

11. S. N. Steen, *Int. J. Sport Nutr.*, **1**, 6 (1991).

12. P. Lemon, *Gatorade Sports Sci. Exchange*, **2** , (1989).

13. G. Butterfield, in *Perspectives in Exercise Science and Sports Medicine, Vol. 4: Ergogenics—Enhancement of Exercise and Sports Performance*, Benchmark Press, Carmel, IN, (1991).

14. J. Slavin, in *Sports Nutrition for the Nineties: The Health Professional's Handbook*, (J. Berning and S. N. Steen, eds.), Aspen Publishers Inc. , Gaithersburg, MD, (1991).

15. E. R. Buskirk, P. F. Iampietro, D. F. Bass, *J. Appl. Physiol.*, **12**, 189 (1958).

16. L. B. Rowell, *Physiol. Rev.*, **54**, 75 (1974).

17. B. Ekblom, C. J. Greenleaf, J. E. Greenleaf, and L. Hermansen, *Acta. Physiol. Scand.*, **79**, 475 (1970).

18. D. R. Lamb and G. R. Brodowicz, *Sports Med.*, **3**, 247 (1986).

19. R. Murray, *Sports. Med.*, **4**, 322 (1987).

20. M. D. Owen, K. C. Kregel, P. T. Wall, and C. V. Gisolfi, *Med. Sci. Sports Exer.*, **18**, 568 (1986).

21. R. Murray, *Med. Sci. Sports Exer.*, **21**, 275 (1989).

22. J. M. Davis, D. R. Lamb, W. A. Burgess, W. P. Bartoli, and R. R. Pate, *Eur. J. Appl. Physiol.*, **57**, 563 (1988).

23. National Research Council, *Recommended Dietary Allowances, X ed.*, National Academy Press, Washington, DC, (1989).

24. D. A. Roe, in *Exercise, Nutrition, and Energy Metabolism*, (E. S. Horton, R. L. Terjung, eds.), Macmillan, New York, pp. 172–179 (1988).

25. R. R. Pate, *The Phys. Sportsmed.*, **11**, 115 (1983).

26. A. C. Synder, L. L. Dvorak, and J. B. Roepke, *Med. Sci. Sports Exer.*, **21**, 7 (1989).

27. S. M. Brooks, C. F. Sanborn, B. H. Albrecht, and W. W. Wagner, *Lancet*, **1**, 559 (1984).

28. B. L. Drinkwater, K. Nilson, C. H. Chesnut, W. J. Bremner, S. Shanholtz, and M. B. Southworth, *N. Engl. J. Med.*, **311**, 277 (1984).

29. R. T. Frizzell, G. H. Lang, D. C. Lowance, and S. R. Lathan, *JAMA*, **255**, 772 (1986).

30. J. H. Wilmore, *J. Appl. Physiol.*, **72**, 15 (1992).

31. S. N. Steen, in *Sports Nutrition for the 90s: The Health Professional's Handbook*, (J. B. Berning and S. N. Steen, eds.), Aspen Publishers, Gaithersburg, MD, pp. 153–174 (1991).

32. S. N. Steen and K. D. Brownell, *Med. Sci. Sports Exer.*, **22**, 762 (1991).

33. American College of Sports Medicine, *Med. Sci. Sports Exer.*, **8**, xi (1976).

34. American Medical Association, Committee on the Medical Aspects of Sports, *JAMA*, **201**, 541 (1967).

35. S. A. Yarrows, *J. Am. Diet. Assoc.*, 88, 491 (1988).

The Pregnant Teen: Pre- and Post-Natal

Catherine Stevens-Simon, M.D., and
Deborah Andrews, R.D.

INTRODUCTION

Each year, over 1 million American teenagers become pregnant and one-half to two-thirds of these young women give birth.[1] After a decade in which the birth rate among adolescents in this country declined, the rate of births to young women under 20 yr of age has begun to rise.[1] This is concerning because current data indicate that pregnancies which are conceived during adolescence are frequently complicated by the numerous maternal and neonatal medical problems listed in Table 13.1.[1]

It has been difficult to determine why the pregnancies of adolescents are high-risk because in most studies age is confounded by other maternal characteristics such as race and poverty. These factors predispose pregnant women of all ages to the adverse pregnancy outcomes listed in Table 13.1.[1] Thus, it is unclear whether the etiology of the risks associated with adolescent childbearing is primarily biologic, due to factors such as incomplete maternal growth, maternal reproductive immaturity, and small maternal size or primarily social, due to factors such as poor health habits, poverty, and stress.[1,2] Current data indicate that adolescents who obtain adequate prenatal care have better pregnancy out-

Table 13.1 Maternal and Neonatal Medical Problems Commonly Associated with Adolescent Children

Maternal	Neonatal
Preterm labor and delivery	Low birth weight and prematurity
Pregnancy-induced hypertension	Minor acute illnesses
Anemia	Failure to thrive
Cephalopelvic disproportion	Sudden infant death syndrome
Obesity	Neonatal and infant mortality

comes than their peers who obtain inadequate or no prenatal care.[1–4] These findings suggest that it may be possible to minimize the risks associated with adolescent childbearing by focusing on the elimination of obstetrical risk factors that can be modified during pregnancy.

Poor maternal nutritional status is a particularly important obstetric risk factor among pregnant adolescents because it is a common medical problem, which, if treated appropriately during gestation, has the potential to decrease the risk of most of the maternal and neonatal complications listed in Table 13.1.[1–5]

Morbidities Associated with Poor Maternal Nutrition

Over the last century, data compiled during periods of acute nutritional deprivation and famine dispelled the traditional view of the fetus.[5–9] Previously, the fetus had been regarded as relatively protected from the nutritional deficiencies of the mother by its ability to parasitize maternal nutritional stores and the capacity of the mother to adapt to an inadequate intake of nutrients.[5–9] However, current data indicate that the human fetus is vulnerable to the adverse effects of inadequate maternal caloric intake, as well as specific maternal vitamin and mineral deficiencies.

Low birth weight and prematurity. These are the two most frequently reported and serious medical complications associated with adolescent childbearing. Even after controlling for potentially confounding high-risk maternal conditions, studies have consistently demonstrated an association between young maternal age and low birth weight and preterm delivery.[1,2] The physiologic mechanisms underlying this association are still not completely understood. Researchers have attempted to partition the individual effects of various maternal characteristics. The results of their studies show that maternal age, maternal prepregnant weight, and maternal weight gain interact, such that as maternal age and maternal prepregnant weight decrease, the effect of maternal weight gain on infant birth weight increases.[5–17] For example, in one study, the investigators reported that maternal weight gain accounted for 5.1% of the variance in the birth weight of infants born to adolescent mothers, but only 1.9% of the variance in the birth weight of infants born to adult mothers.[10] These findings may be due to adolescents' size as they tend to be smaller than adults at conception.[5,10–13] The results of several studies indicate that, regardless of age, maternal weight gain accounts for a greater portion of the variance in the birth weight of infants born to smaller women.[11–14] However, it seems probable that some factor (or factors) other than diminished maternal body size is responsible for the enhanced importance of maternal weight gain for the outcome of adolescent pregnancies.[5,10–13] In one study, the investigators reported that after controlling for prepregnancy weight and other potentially confounding maternal characteristics infant birth weight increased by 38.2 g for each kilogram of weight gained by adolescent mothers who were less than 16 yr of age at conception and by only 5.6 grams for each kilogram of weight gained by older adolescent mothers.[10] Thus, younger gravidas transfer more of the weight they gain during pregnancy to their fetuses than same-sized older gravidas. These findings suggest that as maternal age decreases, the nutritional demands associated with fetal growth take increasing priority over those associated with the deposition of maternal fat and energy stores.

Even though the results of other studies also suggest that maternal age affects the relationship between maternal weight gain and infant birth weight.[5,10–13] it has been difficult to elucidate the physiologic mechanisms underling this interaction. This is because some investigators have reported that adolescent gravidas gain more weight during pregnancy than same-sized adult gravidas to achieve comparable birth-weight outcomes.[5,15–17] For example, in one study, it was reported that regardless of maternal prepregnant weight, infant birth weight increases linearly in relation to maternal weight until maternal weight reached 120% of ideal weight for height among adults and 140% of ideal weight for height among adolescents.[15] These findings appear inconsistent with reports that maternal weight gain accounts for a greater portion of the variance in the birth weight of infants born to adolescent than adult gravidas. They suggest that younger gravidas transfer less (rather than more) of the weight they gain during pregnancy to their fetuses than same-sized older gravidas. This suggests the opposite conclusion. That is, as maternal age decreases, the nutritional demands associated with the deposition of maternal fat and energy stores take increasing priority over those associated with fetal growth. Age-related differences in the pattern and composition of the weight women gain during pregnancy offer one potential explanation for this apparent discrepancy.

During the first half of gestation, when fetal energy needs are minimal, high ambient levels of progesterone direct the flow of nutrients toward the mother, thereby promoting the deposition of maternal fat and energy stores.[6,9,18] Inadequate weight gain during this portion of the gestation has been shown to limit maternal nutrient reserves and compromises the development of the uteroplacental vascular bed.[6,9,18,19] Histomorphometric studies of the human placenta suggest that as maternal prepregnant body size and the size of the placenta decrease, the rate of maternal fat weight gain during the first trimester of pregnancy and the density of fetal capillary tissue within the placenta may become increasingly important determinants of the oxygen diffusion capacity of the placenta.[19]

During the second half of gestation, rising levels of estriol and human placental lactogen induce an increase in the peripheral resistance to insulin, stimulate lipolysis, and redirect the flow of nutrients toward the now rapidly growing fetus.[6,9,18] These metabolic adjustments ensure that the nutritional requirements associated with fetal growth take precedence over those associated with the deposition of maternal fat and energy stores.

Studies of well-nourished, pregnant adults indicate that an inadequate rate of weight gain during the second half of gestation has more serious consequences for infant birth weight than an inadequate rate of maternal weight gain during the first half of gestation.[5,6,8,9,18] By contrast, studies of younger, less well-nourished pregnant women indicate that as maternal age and maternal adiposity decrease, the rate of maternal fat weight gain during the first half of gestation becomes an increasingly important determinant of infant birth weight.[5–9,11,18,20,21] In one study, the investigators reported that the rate of maternal fat weight gain explained 11% of the birth-weight variance among infants born to adolescent mothers who were less than 16 yr of age at conception and less than 1% of the birth-weight variance among infants born to older adolescent mothers.[20] Results of other studies concur with these findings and provide further evidence that the rate of maternal weight gain early in gestation is a particularly important determinant of the birth weight of infants born to young adolescent mothers.[11,21] Studies of the postmenarcheal growth and development of nulliparous adolescent females help to clarify the physiologic mechanisms underlying these age-related differences in the importance of the deposition of maternal fat and energy stores early in gestation.

Although young women grow minimally after menarche, most gain an average of 3–5 kg of fat during the first 3–5 postmenarcheal years.[22,24] Thus, it seems probable that adolescents who conceive soon after menarche have lower body fat stores than same-sized, older, and reproductively more mature adolescent and adult woman.[22–24] To attain body fat stores that are comparable in size to those of same-sized, older, more reproductively mature, females most young women who conceive soon after menarche will therefore need to gain additional weight. The optimal time to gain this additional weight is during the first half of gestation, when the hormonal milieu favors the deposition of maternal fat stores. Since body composition studies indicate that women store both fat and lean weight during gestation,[20,25] it seems probable that in order to gain the requisite amount of fat weight during the first half of gestation, most young women who conceive before they have established a fully mature, adult, body composition must also gain additional lean body weight. As a result of this additional gain in lean body weight, it might be anticipated that these young women will attain a higher percentage of their ideal weight for height at term than older, more physiologically mature gravidas. However, as long as younger gravidas gain the majority of this additional weight early in gestation (during the period of gestation when the intrauterine hormonal milieu naturally favors the deposition of maternal fat over fetal growth), there should be no need for the young mother to compete with her fetus for nutrients. Thus, taken together, the results of these studies suggest that when women of any age fail to store enough fat during the first half of gestation, the development of the placental vascular bed is stunted and the subsequent growth of the fetus limited by the size and oxygen diffusion capacity of the placenta, rather than the preferential flow of blood and nutrients to the mother.[6,7,19–21,25,26] Interventions designed to augment the rate of maternal weight gain early in gestation have the potential to mitigate against the adverse effects that low prepregnant body fat stores have on the size of the placenta and its vascular bed. The additional attention to these dietary and nutritional matters that adolescents receive in comprehensive multidisciplinary maternity programs could be one reason that the incidence of low birth weight and preterm delivery is lower among young women who obtain prenatal care in these special programs than those who are cared for prenatally in traditional adult-oriented settings.[1–4,27,28]

Much less is known about the effect that maternal nutritional status has on the duration of gestation.[29] Although it has been reported that inadequate weight gain during the second half of gestation is associated with an increased incidence of preterm delivery it is unclear if this pattern of weight gain is a cause or symptom of impending preterm labor.[21,29,30] This uncertainty remains because results of dietary supplementation studies indicate that most of the increase in infant birth weight that is associated with the relief of acute and chronic maternal undernutrition reflects an increase in the rate, rather than the duration of intrauterine growth.[29] Further studies are needed as small gains in the duration of gestation have been reported in association with dietary intervention among selected groups of women.[29] Such studies are critical because increasing the duration of adolescent gestations has the potential to change the birth-weight distribution of infants born to adolescent mothers and to significantly decrease the incidence of the other neonatal medical complications listed in Table 13.1. Evidence from a variety of sources suggests that larger gestational weight gains are associated with the birth of larger infants and birth weight is the most important predictor of infant survival during the first 28 d of life.[6–9] Although inadequate gestational weight gain usually causes more concern than excessive gestational weight gain, particularly among pregnant adolescents,[1–5,31,32] caution is critical. In one study, it was found that adolescent mothers who gain more than 0.4 kg/wk during gestation gave birth to larger infants than adolescent mothers who gained weight more slowly during gestation. However, the larger infants were no healthier and did not experience fewer perinatal complications than the smaller infants.[31] Thus, further examination is needed to ensure that interventions designed to increase the amount of weight adolescent mothers gain during gestation do not cause new, unanticipated maternal and neonatal morbidities such as dystocia and postpartum obesity.

Cephalopelvic disproportion. Radiologic studies indicate that the pelvic inlet grows more slowly then the rest of the body during adolescence.[22,24] Since the growth asymptotes of the pelvis and birth canal are usually not reached for several years after menarche, young adolescent mothers tend to have smaller pelvises than same-sized older adolescent and adult mothers.[22,24] The increased risk of cephalopelvic disproportion and its associated morbidities, cesarean delivery, and maternal and infant birth trauma once reported among young adolescent mothers may therefore have been a reflection of attenuated pelvic growth.[28,34] In recent years, the secular trend in pubertal growth and development and better labor preparation has been associated with a decrease in the number of very small, frightened adolescent mothers.[28,35,36] This has virtually eliminated the association between young maternal age and cephalopelvic disproportion.[21,31] However, if current recommendation for augmented adolescent maternal weight gain produce the anticipated enhancement of fetal growth, the relatively small size of the young, early-maturing adolescent's pelvis could again become an obstetric risk factor. The risk of cephalopelvic disproportion may be higher for young African American adolescents because they are more likely to have an android pelvic shape than white and Hispanic adolescents.[22]

Obesity. The importance of gestational weight gain as an etiologic factor in the development of obesity has also been debated.[5,31,32,33,37–39] There is some evidence that the amount of weight women retain after delivery is directly related to the amount of weight they gain during gestation.[31,37–39] It has been demonstrated that for each pregnancy weight-gain category above what could be attributed to physiological changes of pregnancy, there was a progressive increase in postpartum weight retention and obesity.[38] Other investigators found that adolescent mothers who gained more than 0.4 kg/wk during gestation retained more weight and were therefore more often obese after pregnancy then the adolescent mothers who gained weight more slowly during gestation.[31] These findings should prompt caution in the reconsideration of weight-gain recommendations for young adolescent mothers. As we evaluate interventions designed to decrease the incidence of low-birth-weight deliveries by augmenting maternal weight gain, we must balance the long-term potential morbidity of maternal obesity against the benefits of enhanced fetal growth.[30,31,38,39]

Other morbidities. Pregnancy-induced hypertension and its associated morbidities, preeclampsia, eclampsia, placental abruption, renal failure, and maternal cerebral hemorrhage are among the leading causes of fetal and maternal morbidity and mortality in this country.[40] Vital statistic data indicate that the pregnancies of adolescents are more frequently complicated by pregnancy-induced hypertension than the pregnancies of adult women.[1,40,44] This is largely because primiparous women are more likely to develop pregnancy-induced hypertension then multiparous women, and pregnant adolescents are more often primiparous than pregnant adults.[1,40,41] Although the etiology of pregnancy induced hypertension is still uncertain, this complication develops more frequently among pregnant women whose diets are deficient in protein, calcium, and zinc.[40,42–45] These studies suggest that even if pregnancy induced hypertension is no more prevalent among nulliparous adolescents than nulliparous adults, the tendency for adolescent gravidas to consume poorer-quality diets and enter prenatal care later than adult gravidas could increase the risk morbidity associated with the progression of mild pregnancy-induced hypertension to eclampsia.[3,46] Thus, it seems possible that the additional attention to dietary and nutritional matters that adolescents receive in comprehensive multidisciplinary maternity programs could be one reason that the incidence of pregnancy-induced hypertension is lower among adolescents who obtain prenatal care in these special programs than those who obtain prenatal care in traditional adult-oriented settings.[1,3,28,47,48]

Anemia during pregnancy is usually defined as a hemoglobin of less than 11 g.[9,49] Studies indicate that most of the anemia that occurs during pregnancy is normocytic and normochromic.[9,49] The most common causes of anemia during pregnancy are hemodilussion and iron deficiency.[49] The development of anemia during pregnancy is of concern because it reduces the oxygen-carrying capacity of the blood and is associated with an increased incidence of preterm and low-birth-weight delivery, maternal and neonatal infections, and depletion of maternal and infant iron stores during the first year of life.[49–52] Rapid expansion of the red cell mass during adolescence and the typically iron-poor diet that American teenagers consume can deplete their endogenous iron stores and put adolescents at increased risk for iron-deficiency anemia during pregnancy.[46,52] The widespread use of iron supplements among pregnant women in this country may explain why the incidence of anemia is similar among young women who obtain prenatal care in comprehensive, multidisciplinary, adolescent-oriented maternity programs and those who are cared for in traditional adult-oriented prenatal settings.[52]

ASSESSMENT

Prenatal Dietary Requirements

Estimates concerning the nutritional requirements of pregnant women, particularly pregnant adolescent women, have changed numerous times during the last century. Since ethical considerations prohibit the deliberate imposition of nutritional deficiencies during gestation, our understanding of the adverse effects that inadequate and excessive intakes of various nutrients have on pregnant women and their fetuses is based primarily on observational data.[6,8,9] These observations have, at times, resulted in erroneous conclusions and detrimental clinical practices. For example, during the 1950s and 1960s, the observation that excessive weight gain is a prominent feature of preeclampsia led many obstetricians to impose severe caloric restrictions on their patients.[9] This resulted in a significant rise in the incidence of intrauterine growth retardation, but no decrease in the incidence of pregnancy-induced hypertension.[9] If such disasters are to be avoided in the future, it is critical that dietary recommendations for pregnant women be based on a clear understanding of the physiologic mechanisms underlying apparent variation in their nutritional requirements.

Optimal gestational weight, or the total amount and pattern of weight gain, necessary to assure optimal intrauterine fetal growth during pregnancy is disputed, especially for adolescents. Figure 13.1 shows that approximately 9 kg of the weight adolescent and adult women gain during pregnancy can be accounted for by the products of conception (the fetus and placenta), the amniotic fluid, uterine hypertrophy, expansion of maternal blood volume, breast enlargement, and dependent edema. The rest of the weight that is gained during gestation represents

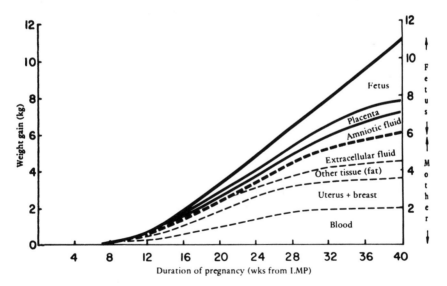

Figure 13-1. Components of weight gain during pregnancy.

R. M. Pitkin, in *Nutritional Support of Medical Practice,* (H. A. Schneider, C. E. Anderson, and D. B. Coursin, eds.), Harper & Row, New York, p.408 (1977). Reprinted with permission.

the growth of maternal fat stores.[9] Studies indicate that the average, healthy, pregnant adult who is eating to appetite gains 12–14 kg of weight during gestation, whereas the average adolescent gravida gains 14–16 kg of weight during gestation.[9,21,53] Most adult women gain weight slowly early in gestation and on average only accumulate 4–5 kg of weight by midgestation.[9] By contrast, adolescent gravidas often gain weight rapidly early in gestation and commonly accumulate 6–8 kg of weight by midgestation.[21,53,54] Thereafter, the rate of weight gain accelerates and most healthy adolescent and adult women gain 0.4–0.5 kg of weight/wk during the rest of gestation.[9,54] Since weight-gain velocities are similar among adolescent and adult gravidas during the second half of gestation, most of the difference in the amount of weight they gain during gestation is the result of increased rates of weight gain among adolescent gravidas during the first half of gestation.[54]

As discussed earlier, the nutritional requirements associated with the increments in maternal fat and energy stores that occur during the first half of gestation may be significantly larger for young women who conceive soon after menarche.[20,23] By contrast, even though many adolescent gravidas have the capacity to grow during pregnancy,[55,56] the nutritional requirements associated with the increments in maternal lean body and bone mass that take place during the 9-mo period of gestation are small compared to those imposed by pregnancy.[5,22,55,57] Figure 13.1 shows that fetal growth predominates during the second half of gestation, when adolescent and adult gravidas gain weight at the same rate. Thus, the tendency for adolescent gravidas to gain more weight than same-sized adult gravidas to achieve comparable birth-weight outcomes should not be misinterpreted as evidence of competition between the young mother and her fetus for nutrients during gestation.

Age-related differences in the requirements for specific minerals and vitamins during pregnancy are more difficult to define than age-related differences in requirements for calories. Currently, there is no evidence that maternal age affects mineral and vitamin requirements during gestation. However, since the premenarcheal growth spurt can deplete endogenous stores of iron and other essential minerals, adolescent gravidas who conceive soon after menarche may need to meet a greater proportion of their pregnancy-related requirements for these minerals from exogenous sources. Iron has received the most attention. It is estimated that during the course of gestation, women transfer approximately 300 mg of iron to the fetus and incorporate approximately 500 mg of iron into their expanded red blood cell mass.[9] To meet these requirements and compensate for daily losses of iron, the average pregnant woman needs to consume approximately 7 mg of iron/d. Supplementation is usually required as most diets do not contain enough iron to meet the demands imposed by pregnancy.[9,58,59] Much less is known about the requirements for other minerals and vitamins during pregnancy.[5] Although current data suggest that supplementation is rarely necessary because most American diets that supply sufficient calories for optimal gestational weight gain also contain a sufficient quality of other vitamins and minerals to prevent deficiencies during gestation, it may be wise to encourage, young, perimenarcheal, adolescent gravidas who have erratic eating habits to take a daily prenatal multivitamin preparation.[5] Similarly, even though pregnant adolescents tend to have lower endogenous calcium stores than pregnant adults, the demand for calcium during pregnancy represents only a small fraction of the total body calcium stores.[58,59] Since calcium absorption is enhanced during pregnancy, supplements are usually unnecessary.[58,59]

Postpartum Weight Loss

Following delivery, most women want to return to their prepregnant body weight. However, it may be physiologically inappropriate for young, still maturing adolescents to return to their pregravid weight.[81] Thus, expectations for postpartum weight loss should be individualized according to the young woman's prepregnant body habitus and her level of physiologic maturity.[81] Although a return to prepregnant weight may not be a reasonable expectation for adolescents who conceive soon after menarche, providers who care for young adolescent mothers must be sensitive to the social pressures to remain thin and physically fit that these young women may face.

Infants and Children

We have focused on the postpartum nutritional needs of adolescent mothers, but the nutritional needs of their children also deserve professional attention. The high incidence of growth, medical, and psychosocial problems noted among the infants and children of adolescent mothers emphasizes the necessity of attending closely to both their physical and psychosocial development.[1] For example, there are several reasons why the infants and children of adolescent mothers are particularly vulnerable to conditions such as the nonorganic failure to thrive. First, lack of knowledge about the changing nutritional needs of their children may foster inappropriate feeding practices and result in a deceleration of growth velocity that causes a physically normal child to fall below the appropriate growth percentile for purely nutritional reasons. This form of nonorganic failure to thrive is easily diagnosed and treated by obtaining a careful dietary history and educating the young mother about her child's nutritional needs.[88] Second, maternal psychologic distress and depression may result in a psychosocial form of nonorganic failure to thrive.[88-90] Although this condition is more difficult to diagnose and treat than the purely nutritional form of nonorganic failure to thrive, a caring, supportive approach that focuses simultaneously on practical solutions to the young mother's real-life problems and mother-infant interactions during feeding times usually proves both diagnostic and therapeutic. Finally, adolescent mothers who are still struggling to resolve their own autonomy and identity issues may have difficulty accepting their toddlers' need and desire for independence. This can lead to conflict at meal time and result in inadequate caloric intake and nonorganic failure to thrive at the time of weaning.

MANAGEMENT

Prenatal

The most recent recommendations for weight gain during pregnancy are based on maternal prepregnant body mass; larger weight gains are recommended for smaller, thinner women.[60] Table 13.2 shows that to optimize fetal growth and minimize the risk of low-birth-weight delivery and intrauterine growth retardation, it is now recommended that average-sized adult women gain 11.5–16 kg of weight during gestation.[60] This represents an increase of 2.5–4.5 kg over earlier recommendations for gestational weight gain. Since epidemiologic studies indicate that younger mothers tend to give birth to smaller babies than older mothers who gain the same amount of weight during gestation, it is recommended that young adolescents strive for weight gains toward the upper end of the range recommended for older women their size.[60]

This recommendation is controversial because the reasons that younger adolescents have smaller babies reflect the complex interaction between several high-risk maternal conditions.[1,5,32] Although augmented maternal weight gain may compensate for small maternal size and an immature maternal body composition, it can do little to ameliorate the adverse effects that factors such as cigarette smoking, substance abuse, and stress have on fetal growth and development.[5] Indeed, data suggest that in such circumstances, interventions designed to decrease the incidence of low-birth-weight delivery by increasing maternal weight gain may compromise fetuses that have adapted to their suboptimal intrauterine environment.[61] Given the striking range in body size and adiposity of perimenarcheal adolescent females and the potential morbidity of maternal obesity

Table 13.2 Recommended Total Weight-Gain Ranges for Pregnant Women by Prepregnancy BMI*

	Recommended Total Gain	
Weight-for-Height Category (BMI)	kg	lb
Low (<19.8)	12.5–18	28–40
Normal (19.8–26.0)	11.5–16	25–35
High (>26.0–29.0)	7–11.5	15–25

* BMI= Body mass index; weight (kg)/height (m^2).

acquired through repeated pregnancies in which adolescents are encouraged to gain more weight than can be attributed to the physiological changes of pregnancy and puberty, it seems unwise to base recommendations for larger gestational weight gains on maternal age. Further studies are urgently needed to ensure that the new recommendations for gestational weight gain do not solve one major public health problem, low-birth-weight delivery, by adding a new one, adolescent obesity.[31,32]

The Food and Nutritional Board's[63] latest recommendations for the dietary allowances of nonpregnant adolescents and pregnant and lactating women are summarized in Table 13.3. Since the recommendations for nonpregnant adolescents are based on chonologic age and therefore do not take into account the state of maturity of the teenager, they may overestimate the needs of young women who are 3 or more yr past their premenarcheal growth spurt.

There is good evidence that only one mineral, iron, provides a demonstrable benefit when given as a supplement to pregnant women.[63] Since iron requirements are small early in gestation the recommendation is that women begin to take 30 mg of iron/d during the second trimester of pernancy.[9] As noted earlier, adolescent gravidas who conceive soon after their premenarcheal growth spurt may benefit from earlier, larger iron supplements. To maximize absorption, patients should be instructed to take their iron supplement with orange juice or other vitamin-C-rich foods and to avoid taking iron with calcium- and magnesium-containing medications such as antiacid. Whereas the need for iron supplementation during gestation is clear, the benefits of augmenting the diets of pregnant women with other nutrients are less certain. Even though protein, folate, calcium, and zinc deficiencies have been implicated in reproductive complications such as intrauterine growth retardation, pregnancy-induced hypertension, and placental abruption, there is no clear evidence that supplementing the diets of pregnant women with these nutrients decreases the risk of any obstetric or neonatal complications.[9,59,63] Indeed, data suggest that the consumption of "high" protein supplements during gestation may increase, rather than decrease, the incidence of low birth weight and preterm delivery.[64] Results of some studies suggest that folate and multivitamin supplementation prior to conception is associated with a decrease in the risk of neurotube defects[58,59] and calcium supplementation during gestation is associated with a decrease in the incidence of pregnancy induced hypertension.[44] However, these data should be regarded as preliminary; the broad implementation of these types of supplementation programs should therefore be discouraged until it is clear that there will not be any unanticipated complications.

The Prenatal Teen

It is generally agreed that patient self-reports concerning food intake and activity are of little help in explaining the wide variation in gestational weight

Table 13.3   Recommended Daily Dietary Allowances for Women 163 cm (64 in.) Tall and Weighing 55 kg (121 lb)

		Increase	
Nutrient	Nonpregnant	Pregnant	Lactating
Kilocalories	2100	300	500
Protein (g)	44[a]	30	20
Vitamin A (RE)[b]	800	200	400
Vitamin D (mg)[c]	7.5	5	5
Vitamin E (mg TE)[d]	10	2	3
Ascorbic acid (mg)	60	20	40
Folacin (mg)[e]	0.4	0.4	0.1
Niacin (mg)[f]	14	2	5
Riboflavin (mg)	1.3	0.3	0.5
Thiamin (mg)	1.1	0.4	0.5
Vitamin B-6 (mg)	2.0	0.6	0.5
Vitamin B-12 (mg)	3.0	1.0	1.0
Calcium (mg)	800	400	400
Phosphorus (mg)	800	400	400
Iodine (mg)	150	25	50
Iron (mg)	18	Supplement[g]	0
Magnesium (mg)	300	150	150
Zinc (mg)	15	5	10

[a] 46 g for under 19 yr of age.

[b] 1 mg retinol = 1 retinol equivalent (RE).

[c] As cholecalciferol; 100 international units = 2.5 mg of cholecalciferol.

[d] TE=tocopherol equivalent.

[e] Refers to dietary sources ascertained by Lactobacillus casei assay; pteroylglutamic acid may be effective in smaller doses.

[f] Includes dietary sources of the vitamin plus 1-mg equivalent for each 60 mg of dietary tryptophan

[g] increased requirement cannot be met by ordinary diets; therefore supplementation recommended (see text).

Adapted from *Recommended Dietary Allowances*, IX ed., National Academy of Sciences, Washington, DC (1979).

gain.[65-69] The poor correlation between reported caloric intake and expenditure and gestational weight gain is a reflection of the difficulties associated with obtaining accurate information on prepregnant body size, diet, and exercise. The large and often variable amount of water that pregnant women retain during gestation and the poorly understood effects of maternal characteristics and behaviors such as cigarette smoking, drug and alcohol abuse, and maternal stress also make it difficult to correlate patients' self-reports concerning energy intake and expenditure with weight gain.[65–67] Nevertheless a 24-h diet recall or 3-d diet record may be helpful in identifying individual dietary deficiencies or excesses and substance use among women who are gaining weight inappropriately during gestation.[69]

The accurate determination of maternal prepregnant weight body size is critical. Maternal prepregnant weight and height are used to individualize recommendations for pregnancy weight gain, predict infant birth weight, and assess the adequacy of the weight women gain during pregnancy. The prepregnant weight and height recorded in the prenatal record are usually obtained retrospectively as part of the prenatal history. Although studies indicate that most pregnant and nonpregnant women report their weight with remarkable accuracy, the tendency for overweight subjects to underestimate their weights and underweight subjects to overestimate their weights may result in unjustified concerns about excessive weight gain among overweight women and weight loss or inadequate weight gain among underweight women.[70] Thus, when concerns about weight gain arise among patients who begin pregnancy below the 90th percentile or above the 120th percentile of ideal weight for height are experienced, it is wise to seek objective validation of the prepregnant weight.[70] If this information is not available, an alternative method of assessing the adequacy of the gestational weight gain should be used. For example, gestational weight gain can be defined as the difference between the woman's weight at delivery and her weight at the first prenatal visit or assessed by determining the percentage of ideal weight for height at term. Although these definitions of gestational gain are attractive because they enable the clinician to avoid concerns about the validity of the stated prepregnant weight, they are less desirable than definitions that incorporate maternal prepregnant weight, because they assume that the amount of weight gained early in gestation is a negligible fraction of the total amount of weight gained during gestation. Furthermore, studies employing these definitions lose two valuable, independent predictors of infant birth weight, i.e., maternal prepregnant body size and the pattern of gestational weight gain. This may be problematic when assessing the adequacy of weight gained by young, perimenarcheal adolescent gravidas, as these young women often gain weight rapidly during the first trimester of pregnancy and enter prenatal care late in gestation.[70]

The usefulness of skinfold determinations for individualizing weight-gain recommendations, predicting infant birth weight, and assessing the adequacy of the weight women gain during pregnancy is also debated.[20,22,26,71] The consensus is that skinfold determinations are a relatively inaccurate method for assessing the total body fat content of individual women, especially late in gestation when the accumulation of subcutaneous edema fluid often jeopardizes the accuracy of these measurements.[20,71] Nevertheless, the results of several studies suggest that the determination of skinfold thicknesses can be helpful in identifying women who might benefit from dietary supplementation because they are underweight at conception and/or have not gained an adequate amount of weight during the first half of gestation.[20,22,26,71]

Several other factors should be considered in assessing the etiology of inappropriately large or small gestational weight gain. These include information about the young person's understanding about how much weight she needs to gain and her attitudes toward weight gain, illicit substance use, psychologic state, eating habits, and the availability of desirable, age-appropriate foods.[65] Attention to these modifiable correlates of inadequate and excessive weight gain may enable dietitians and other health care providers to develop more effective strategies for promoting optimal weight gain among pregnant adolescents. For example, even though maternal compliance with specific weight-gain recommendations is far from perfect, studies indicate that the advice women receive about weight gain has a pronounced effect on the amount of weight they gain during gestation.[72] Professional dietary counseling is particularly important for pregnant adolescents who may otherwise base their expectations for gestational weight gain on the advice of older relatives and attempt to restrict the amount of weight they gain during gestation because they have been told that it will decrease their risk of developing complications such as pregnancy-induced hypertension during pregnancy and obesity following delivery.

One of the major developmental tasks of early adolescence is formulating a satisfactory body image. Health care providers often worry that their young, adolescent prenatal patients may have more negative attitudes toward weight gain and may therefore try to cope with the bodily changes imposed by pregnancy by deliberately attempting to limit the amount of weight they gain during gestation.[73] Although there is some evidence that negative attitudes toward weight gain adversely effect the amount of weight women gain during gestation[72-74] the results of two recently conducted studies help to allay concerns about negative attitudes toward gestational weight gain among younger adolescent gravidas. One study demonstrated that pregnant teenagers actually had a more positive (rather than a more negative) body image than their nonpregnant peers.[75] Another study found that younger pregnant adolescent gravidas reported no more concern about staying slim than older adolescent and adult gravidas.[74] Thus, even though many adolescents verbalize concerns about excessive amounts of weight gain during pregnancy, few appear to allow their concerns to adversely affect their weight gain during gestation or seriously compromise their intake of nutrients. Rather, current data indicate that, regardless of age, women who are overweight at conception and women who are unhappy and depressed during pregnancy judge their bodies more negatively and have more negative attitudes toward weight gain than thinner women and women who are happy and well supported during gestation.[74,76]

Although studies indicate that adult women who smoke cigarettes, abuse substances, and are depressed during pregnancy are more likely to gain an inadequate amount of weight during gestation these characteristics have not been consistently associated with inadequate gestational weight gain among pregnant adolescents.[65,68,77,78] This may be true in part because pregnant teens are less apt to be heavy tobacco and substance abusers than pregnant adults.[1,65,79] Thus, depression may be associated with excessive, rather than inadequate, weight gain among adolescent gravidas.[1,65,79]

Finally, data show that the consumption of less than three snacks/day and delayed (third trimester) enrollment in the Women, Infants, and Children Food Supplement Program are two of the most important predictors of slow, inadequate weight gain during adolescent pregnancies.[65] These data emphasize the importance of reviewing eating habits and the availability of desirable, age-appropriate foods with adolescents who are not gaining an appropriate amount of weight during gestation.[65] Evidence from a variety of sources indicates that the erratic eating habits characteristic of American teenagers increase the importance of snacking and snack foods in their diets; efforts to eliminate snack foods from the diets of pregnant American teenagers can seriously jeopardize their caloric intake and may be associated with an increased incidence of inadequate maternal weight gain in this age group.[80] Although frank starvation is rare in this country, pregnant adolescents often report that the availability of food in their homes limits their nutrient intakes during gestation. Thus, additional emphasis on the importance of early enrollment in food supplementation programs may be one reason that studies have consistently demonstrated that the incidence of inadequate maternal weight gain is lower among adolescents who obtain prenatal care in adolescent-oriented maternity programs than those who are cared for in traditional adult-oriented settings.[3]

The Postpartum Teen

Following delivery, adolescents should be encouraged to avoid starvation diets and diet pills and helped to develop a sound weight-loss program that includes the consumption of regular meals and exercise. An exercise program designed to reestablish abdominal tone may make it easier for some young women to tolerate the necessary retention of an additional 3–5 lb of weight following delivery. The postpartum period is an ideal time to help these new parents develop the sorts of dietary and exercise habits that will enable them to model appropriate, healthy eating behavior for their children.

Many questions remain about the effects of pregnancy on the physical health of the adolescent. For example, growing evidence that adolescent childbearing is associated with an increased risk of obesity and hypertension later in life[31,32,82,83] emphasizes the need for research that separates the effects of early childbearing and early maturation on the adult body habitus of young women who become mothers during adolescence. In addition, studies of the physiologic effects of lactation on adolescents are inconclusive; some investigators have reported increased bone demineralization in lactating adolescent mothers.[84,85] Further research defining the impact of lactation on the health of young adolescents is needed so dietary recommendations can be made that will enable young mothers to breast feed their babies without jeopardizing their own health. Such studies are crucial because it is hypothesized that the depletion of adolescent maternal reserves contributes to the increased risk of adverse neonatal outcome in subsequent adolescent pregnancies.[86,87]

Nevertheless, adolescent mothers should be given the option of breast or bottle feeding their infants. Prenatal health care providers should ensure that each young women has sufficient knowledge to weigh the benefits and disadvantages of breast and bottle feeding her infant. It is critical for providers who care for adolescent mothers during the prenatal and early postpartum period to understand how adolescent development issues may influence their young patients' decisions concerning breast and bottle feeding. For example, younger adolescents who still harbor concerns about the normalcy of their pubertal body habitus may be reluctant to breast feed for fear that it will cause permanent damage or disfigurement to their breasts. By contrast, middle adolescents who are still struggling with emancipation issues may either decide that their school and social lives will not accommodate breast feeding or may elect to breast feed as a means of establishing an independent identity and some autonomy in the care of their infant. A supportive, nonjudgmental attitude is the best way to ensure that the new mother-infant dyad gets off to a good start. It is also important for the contraceptive advice given to young women who choose to breast feed be tempered with the knowledge that the rate of repeat pregnancy ranges from 10–15% during the first 6 postpartum mo in this population. Given the numerous, well-documented medical and psychosocial risks associated with rapid repeat adolescent pregnancies,[86] it may be wiser to help adolescent mothers maintain an adequate supply of breast milk by discouraging supplemental feedings, rather than the use of the most reliable hormonal contraceptive methods. Breast-feeding mothers who are concerned about contraceptive side-effects and therefore leave the postpartum ward with a less effective form of contraception should have ready access to alternative forms of contraceptives during the earlier childbearing period.[81] The additional attention to contraceptive matters that adolescents receive in comprehensive multidisciplinary maternity programs could be one reason that the incidence of recidivism is lower among adolescents who obtain postpartum care in these special programs than those who receive postpartum care in traditional adult-oriented settings.[1]

Infants and children who are not growing appropriately may help the provider identify and treat confused, struggling adolescent mothers, before they become angry, frustrated young women who leave home and school for a life of welfare dependency or delinquency. Teaching adolescent parents how to feed and nurture their children appropriately may be the most effective way to stop the transmission of poor health habits, anger, and poverty from one generation to the next.

Summary

The nutritional status of pregnant women is one of the most important determinants of infant size and well-being at birth. Poor maternal nutrition is a common, easily modifiable problem, which has in recent years become an increasingly important focus in debates over ways to reduce the high incidence of low birth weight and neonatal mortality in this country. We have tried to demonstrate the heterogeneity of factors underlying the interaction among maternal age, nutritional status, and infant outcome. Caution in the reconsideration of age-related dietary recommendation for young gravidas who differ strikingly in body habitus and reproductive maturity is recommended. Until it has been demonstrated that bigger babies are always better, healthier babies, we must carefully evaluate intervention programs designed to decrease the incidence of low birth weight by augmenting maternal weight gain so that we don't inadvertently compromise fetuses that have adapted to their suboptimal intrauterine environment and promote maternal obesity. Finally, we have tried to demonstrate that adolescent pregnancy is a complex problem; simple answers (like inadequate nutrition) and solutions (like augmented gestational weight gain) are unlikely. Rather, rigorous research tactics are needed to ensure that as health care providers, dieticians, social workers, and teachers, we first do no harm.

CASE ILLUSTRATION

Sarah is a 15-year-old white female and presents for her second visit to the adolescent obstetric clinic where you work as a dietician. As you review her medical record, you note that she had her first menstrual period last year and her last menstrual period approximately 5 mo ago. You are surprised to see that this is her second pregnancy; she had a therapeutic abortion last year. She has no chronic or acute medical problems, but she does have a past history of substance abuse. Although she told the nurse that she stopped using drugs over 3 mo ago, when she first learned she was pregnant, you note that her urine drug screen is still positive for THC (the urine metabolite of marijuana). You read on and learn that Sarah lives with her mother and 25-year-old boyfriend. Both are heavy substance abusers, and the boyfriend is currently in jail. It appears that Sarah has known of her pregnancy for more than 3 mo. She had a pregnancy test done secretly at Planned Parenthood and has been trying to hide her condition from her mother since that time so "she wouldn't make me get another abortion." Sarah told the nurse that she has been trying not to eat much so she "wouldn't look pregnant." The nurse's diet history reveals that during the last 24 h, she has had three sodas, two candy bars, a bag of chips, and a taco. It appears that her mother rarely cooks and that she has essentially been on her own at meal time since she was 8 or 9 yr old. Food is in short supply in the home, particularly toward the end of the month. Her mother doesn't go to the grocery store very often because "her boyfriends mostly take her out to eat." Sarah has told the nurse that she can't remember the last time she had a glass of milk, or even saw a carton of milk in her house, and states, "My mother and boyfriend mostly drink beer when they are thirsty and I drink pop." Review of the medical record shows a prepregnancy weight of 105 lb and reported height of 5 ft and 5 in. Her current weight is 105 lb and an initial blood count shows a hemoglobin of 10 g/dL and low mean corpuscular volume. Thus, her apparent failure to gain weight and her ongoing substance use are of immediate concern.

Sarah's apparent failure to gain weight during the first half of gestation is particularly worrisome because she is only 1 yr past menarche. At 5 ft 5 in. and 105 lb you can be certain that her endogenous body fat stores were minimal at conception. Optimally, at this point in her pregnancy, she would have gained 0.5–1 lb/wk. Since studies indicate that underweight women often overestimate their weights and that small women often overestimate their heights, an objective validation of her prepregnant weight and height is required. In this case, the requisite information concerning the prepregnant weight should be available at the local Planned Parenthood office where Sarah had her pregnancy test done at approximately 4 wk of gestation and her height can be measured today.

You obtain Sarah's permission to call the Planned Parenthood office and learn that at the time of her visit she weighed 95 lb. You measure her height and find that she is actually only 5 ft and 2 in. tall. Hence, despite her diet history and efforts to restrict her weight gain, Sarah has gained an appropriate amount of weight. This is consistent with the results of studies showing that even though many adolescents verbalize concerns about excessive amounts of weight gain during pregnancy, their concerns rarely adversely affect their weight gain during gestation. Although Sarah's rate of gain (approximately 0.5 lb/wk) would be more than adequate for a fatter, more mature woman, it is likely to be minimally sufficient to meet the nutritional needs of a thin perimenarcheal woman. Similarly, even though Sarah's diet has not seriously compromised her weight gain, her hemoglobin level is evidence that her diet has not supplied her with a sufficient quantity of micronutrients. Sarah requires intensive nutritional counseling and needs to be monitored closely throughout her pregnancy. In addition she will need vitamin and iron supplements, help enrolling in the Women, Infant's, and Children's (WIC) Food Supplement Program, and help with meal planning. Sarah's needs are probably too pervasive to be handled in the clinic, even if transportation permitted weekly clinic visits. A home visitor or placement in a foster home will probably be necessary to ensure a healthy pregnancy.

Sarah must be told that metabolites of marijuana were found in her urine. However, this can be done in a nonthreatening way by suggesting to her that she may have exposed herself unknowingly by being in a confined space where marijuana was being smoked. She needs to be given a clear, honest explanation about the dangers of drug and alcohol use during pregnancy and warned that you and her other health care providers consider it her responsibility to see to it that she doesn't allow herself to become "passively" exposed to drugs again during the pregnancy. She should be advised that her urine will be tested for illicit substances periodically throughout the pregnancy and informed that this is being done because it is critical that the doctors and nurses who care for her and her baby during labor and delivery be aware of any substance exposure.

Exactly, 3 mo later, Sarah is 34 wk pregnant. As you review her medical record, you are pleased to see that she weighs 119.5 lb, her hemoglobin level has risen to 11.5 g/dL, and her mean corpuscular volume is normal. The results of the last two urine toxicology screens were entirely negative. Although Sarah appears to thriving in her new foster home, the nurse's notes draw your attention to the fact that her boyfriend was released from jail last week and came to visit her. She has already verbalized plans to leave the foster home and move in with him. You glance up from the medical record to see Sarah's foster mother's worried face. She tells you that Sarah has been out past midnight with her boyfriend every night this week, has missed dinner on three nights, and has started sleeping in until noon and doesn't eat breakfast. She goes on to say that she talks of nothing except getting her own place with her boyfriend and seems to have almost forgotten that she is due to deliver the baby next month. "She even forgot to pick up her WIC supplements this week." You note that Sarah's weight has fallen a pound since last week, catch a glimpse of her as she walks into the examination room, and see that she has gone back to wearing too much make-up. During the course of your interview with Sarah, you learn that she has no intention of breast feeding her baby; she finds the thought of it "disgusting." She admits that she doesn't have much for the baby yet, but says that her boyfriend is taking her shopping and to look for an apartment tomorrow. When you point out her weight loss, she replies, "That's OK, my boyfriend says I'm getting too fat. . . . I don't think I'll even be able to lose the weight I've already gained-I just want to have this baby and move into my own place."

Sarah's apparent rapid recovery in the structured environment of a foster home is not uncommon and is illustrative of the necessity of treating nutritional and social problems simultaneously. Sarah's equally rapid relapse into her former lifestyle is also very common. Sarah's story emphasizes the importance of extending comprehensive, multidisciplinary, adolescent-oriented maternity programs beyond the immediate postpartum period and providing intensive medical, nutritional, and social service follow-up for mother, father, and baby through the first 2–3 yr of the infant's life.

Sarah's reaction to the thought of breast feeding as "disgusting" is characteristic of early adolescence; young people at this stage of development are typically very concerned about their bodies and their body image. Hence, the aspect of Sarah's story that is of most immediate concern is her weight loss.

Sarah is in the last trimester of her pregnancy, the period of most rapid growth for the baby. Therefore, the maintenance of adequate weight gain is critical. Like many younger teenagers, Sarah has begun to worry about how much weight she has gained and whether she will ever look like she did before she got pregnant. Sarah must be told that you and her doctors are extremely concerned about her weight loss. You should reassure her that you will help her lose most of the weight she has gained, but not until she delivers. Sarah should also understand that it may not be physiologically appropriate for her to return to 95 lb. The foster mother will need the support of the clinic staff to help Sarah focus on her baby's needs. Early adolescents are concrete thinkers and respond best to immediate rewards and punishments that they feel they have some control over. The clinic staff might therefore help the foster mother set up a reward and punishment system that would make Sarah come home for meals if she wanted to see her boyfriend. Once Sarah's weight-gain pattern has been reestablished, it will be important to begin to help her understand that it is unlikely she will be allowed to live on her own with the baby and her boyfriend.

REFERENCES

1. C. Stevens-Simon and M. M. White, *Ped. Ann.,* **20**, 322 (1991).

2. E. R. McAnarney, *AJDC*, 141, 1053 (1987).

3. C. Stevens-Simon, S. Fullar, and E. R. McAnarney, *J. Adol. Health,* **13**, 298 (1992).

4. T. O. Scholl, L. K. Miller , R. W. Salmon, et al., *Obstet. Gynecol.,* **69**, 312 (1987).

5. C. Stevens-Simon, and E. R. McAnarney, *Am. J. Clin. Nutr.,* 47, 948 (1988).

6. A. Briend, in *Nutritional Needs and Assessment of Normal Growth. Nestle Nutrition Workshop Series,* (M. Gracey and F. Falkner, eds.), Raven Press, New York, pp. 1–21 (1985).

7. M. Lawrence, W. A. Coward, F. Lawrence, T. J. Cole, and R. G. Whitehead, *Am. J. Clin. Nutr.,* **45,** 1442 (1987).

8. M. Susser, *Am. J. Clin. Nutr.,* **34** (suppl. 4), 784 (1981).

9. F. E. Hytten, in *Clinical Physiology in Obstetrics,* (F. Hytten and G. Chamberlain, eds.), Blackwell, Boston, MA, pp. 193–234 (1980).

10. I. L. Horon, D. M. Strobino, and H. M. MacDonald, *Am. J. Obstet. Gynecol.,* **146**, 444 (1983).

11. C. Stevens-Simon, K. J. Roghmann, and E. R. McAnarney, *Pediatrics*, **92**, 805 (1993).

12. M. L. Hediger, T. O. Scholl, I. G. Ances, D. H. Belskey, and R. W. Salmon, *Am. J. Clin. Nutr.*, **52**,793 (1990).

13. R. L. Naeye, *Pediatrics*, 67, 146 (1981).

14. B. Winikoff and C. H. Debrovner, *Obstet. Gynecol.*, **58**, 678 (1981).

15. L. Haiek and S. Lederman, *J. Adol. Health Care* **10**, 16 (1989).

16. S. M. Garn, S. D. Pesick, and A. S. Petzold, in *School-Age Pregnancies and Parenthood: Biosocial Dimensions*, (J. A. Lancaster and B. A. Hamburg, eds.), Aldine DeGruyter, Hawthorne, New York, pp.77–93 (1985).

17. A. R. Frisancho, J. Matos, and P. Flegel, *Am. J. Clin. Nutr.*, **38**, 739 (1983).

18. P. Rosso, *Am. J. Clin. Nutr.*, **34** (suppl. 4), 744 (1981).

19. C. Stevens-Simon, L. Metlay, C. Pruksunanonda, J. Maude, and E. R. McAnarney, *J. Mat. Fetal Med.*, **2**, 294 (1993).

20. C. Stevens-Simon, G. B. Forbes, K. J. Roghmann, and E. R. McAnarney, *J. Adol. Health Care,***11**, 275 (1990).

21. M. L. Hediger, T. O. Scholl, D. H. Belsky, I. G. Ances, and R. W. Salmon, *Obstet. Gynecol.*, **74**, 6 (1989).

22. G. B. Forbes, *Human Body Composition: Growth, Aging, Nutrition, and Activity*, Springer-Verlag, New York, (1987).

23. E. Frish and W. McArthur, *Science*, **185**, 949 (1974).

24. J. M. Tanner, *Growth at Adolescence*, Blackwell, Oxford, England, (1962).

25. J. C. King, D. H. Callaway, and S. Margen, *J. Nutr.*, **103**, 772 (1973).

26. M. J. Maso, E. J. Gong, M. S. Jacobson, D. S. Bross, and F. P. Heald, *J. Adol. Health Care*, **9**, 188 (1988).

27. M. E. Felice, J. L. Granados, I. G. Ances, R. Hebel, L. M. Roeder, and F. P. Heald, *J. Adol. Health Care*, **1**, 193 (1981).

28. J. B. Hardy and L. S. Zabin, *Adolescent Pregnancy in an Urban Environment*, Urban and Schwarzenberg, Baltimore, MD (1991).

29. A. R. Kristal and D. Rush, *Clin. Obstet. Gynecol.*, **27**, 553 (1984).

30. B. Abrams, V. Newman, T. Key, and J. Parker, *Obstet. Gynecol.*, **74**, 577 (1989).

31. C. Stevens-Simon and E. R. McAnarney, *AJDC*, 146, 1359 (1992).

32. E. R. McAnarney and C. Stevens-Simon, *AJDC*, **147**, 983 (1993).

33. M. L. Moerman, *Am. J. Obstet. Gynecol.*, **143**, 528 (1982).

34. F. C. Battaglia, T. M. Frazier, and A. E. Hellegers, *Pediatrics* **32**, 902 (1963).

35. G. Wyshak and R. E. Frisch, *N. Engl. J. Med.*, **306**, 1033 (1982).

36. R. Sosa, J. Kennell, M. Klaus, S. Robertson, and J. Urrutia, *N. Engl. J. Med.*, **303**, 597 (1980).

37. G. W. Greene, H. Smiciklas-Wright, T. O. Scholl, and R. J. Karp, *Obstet. Gynecol.*, **71**, 701 (1988).

38. M. A. Rookus, P. Rokebrand, J. Burema, and P. Deurenberg, *Int. J. Obes.*, 11, 609 (1987).

39. K. Kepple and S. Taffel, *Am. J. Pub. Health,* 83, 110 (1993).

40. F. G. Cunningham and M. D. Lindheimer, *N. Engl. J. Med.*, 326, 927 (1992).

41. D. Graham, *Birth Def.,* 17, 49 (1981).

42. A. F. Saftlas, D. R. Olson, A. L. Franks, H. K. Atrash, and R. Pokras, *Am. J. Obstet. Gynecol.*, 163, 460 (1990).

43. F. F. Cherry, E. A. Bennett, G. S. Bazzano, L. K. Johnson, G. J. Fosmire, and H. K. Batson, *Am. J. Clin. Nutr.*, 34, 2367 (1981).

44. J. Belizan, J. Villar, L. Gonzalez, L. Campodonico, and E. Bergel, *N. Eng. J. of Med.*, 325, 1399 (1991).

45. C. A. Swanson and J. C. King, *Am. J. Clin. Nutr.*, 46, 763 (1987).

46. M. E. Schneck, K. S. Sideras, R. A. Fox, and L. Dupuis, *J. Am. Diet. Assoc.*, 90, 555 (1990).

47. E. R. McAnarney, K. J. Roghmann, B. N. Adams, R. C. Tatelbaum, C. Kash, M. Coulter, M. Plume, and E. Charney, *Pediatrics,* 61, 199 (1978).

48. R. P. Perkins, I. I. Nakashima, M. Mullin, L. S. Dubansky, M. L. Chin, *Obstet. Gynecol.*, 52, 179 (1978).

49. R. C. Goodlin, *J. Reprod. Med.*, 27, 639 (1982).

50. L. B. Bailey, C. S. Mahan, and D. Dimperio, *Am. J. Clin. Nutr.*, 33, 1997 (1980).

51. P. Rosso, *Ped. Ann.*, 10, 21 (1981).

52. T. O. Scoll, M. L. Hediger, R. L. Fischer, and J. W. Shearer, *Am. J. Clin. Nutr.*, 55, 985 (1992).

53. L. P. Meserole, B. S. Worthington-Roberts, J. M. Rees, and L. W. Wright, *J. Adol. Health Care,* 5, 21 (1984)

54. J. M. Rees, K. A. Engelbert-Fenton, E. J. Gong, and C. M. Bach, *Am. J. Clin. Nutr.*, 56, 868 (1992).

55. C. Stevens-Simon and E. R. McAnarney, *J. Adol. Health,* 14, 428 (1993).

56. T. O. Scholl, M. L. Hediger, and I. G. Ances, *Am. J. Clin. Nutr.*, 51, 790 (1990).

57. S. M. Garn, M. LaVelle, S. D. Pesick, and S. A. Ridella, *AJDC,* 138, 32 (1984).

58. D. Rothman, *Am. J. Obstet. Gynecol.*, 108, 149 (1970).

59. A. E. Czeizel and I. Dudas, *N. Engl. J. Med.*, 327, 1832 (1992).

60. Food and Nutrition Board: Institute of Medicine, *Nutrition During Pregnancy,* National Academy of Sciences, National Academy Press, Washington, DC (1990).

61. J. B. Warshaw, *Pediatrics,* 76, 998 (1985).

62. *Recommended Dietary Allowances*, IX ed., National Academy of Sciences, Washington, DC (1979).

63. F. G. Cunningham, P. C. MacDonald, and N. F. Gant, eds., *Williams Obstetrics,* 18th ed., Appleton and Lange, Norwalk, CT, pp.741 (1989).

64. D. Rush, Z. Stein, and M. Susser, *Pediatrics,* 65, 683 (1980).

65. C. Stevens-Simon, E. R. McAnarney, *J. Am. Diet. Assoc.*, 92, 1348 (1992).
66. T. O. Scholl, M. L. Hediger, C. S. Khoo, M. F. Healey, and N. L. Rawson, *J. Clin. Epidemiol.*, **44**, 423 (1991).
67. S. A. Lederman, in *Feeding the Mother and Infant,*(M. Winick, ed.), John Wiley & Sons, New York, pp.13–43 (1985).
68. P. Loris, K. G. Dewey, and K. Poirier-Brode, *J. Am. Diet. Assoc.*, 85, 1296 (1985).
69. C. Stevens-Simon and E. R. McAnarney, *J. Am. Diet. Assoc.*, **93**, 581 (1993).
70. C. Stevens-Simon, K. J. Roghmann, and E. R. McAnarney, *J. Am. Diet. Assoc.*, **92**, 85 (1992).
71. N. R. Taggart, R. M. Holliday, W. Z. Billewicz, F. E. Hytten, and A. M. Thompson, *Br. J. Nutr.* **21**, 439 (1967).
72. S. M. Taffel and K. G. Keppel, *Am. J. Pub. Health*, **76**, 1396 (1986).
73. C. Stevens-Simon, I. I. Nakashima, and D. Andrews, *J. Adol. Health.*, **14**, 369 (1993).
74. J. L. Palmer, G. E. Jennings, and L. Massey, *J. Am. Diet. Assoc.*, 85, 946 (1985).
75. Y. Matsuhashi and M. E. Felice, *J. Adol. Health,* **12**, 313 (1991).
76. O. L. McConnell and P. G. Daston, *J. Proj. Tech.*, **25**, 451 (1961).
77. T. A. Picone, L. H. Allan, M. M. Schramm, and P. N. Olsen, *Am. J. Clin. Nutr.*, 36, 1205 (1982).
78. B. Zuckerman, H. Amaro, H. Bauchner, and H. Cabral, *Am. J. Obstet. Gynecol.*, **160**, 1107 (1989).
79. B. Zuckerman, J. J. Alpert, E. Dooling, et al., *Pediatrics,* **71**, 489 (1983).
80. L. Sands, *Semin. Adol. Med.*, **2**, 191 (1986).
81. C. Stevens-Simon, S. A. Fullar, and E. R. McAnarney, *Clin. Peds.*, **28**, 282 (1989).
82. J. M. Kotchen, H. E. Kotchen, and T. A. Mckean, *Am. J. Epidemiol.*, **115**, 861 (1982).
83. S. M. Garn, M. Lavelle, K. R. Rosenberg, and V. M. Hawthorne, *Am. J. Clin. Nutrit.*, 43, 879 (1986).
84. G. M. Chan, N. Ronald, P. Slater, J. Hollis, and M. R. Thomas, *J. Peds.*, **101**, 767 (1982).
85. F. R. Greer and S. M. Garn, *J. Peds.*, **101**, 718 (1982).
86. C. Stevens-Simon, K. J. Roghmann, and E. R. McAnarney, *J. Adol. Health Care*, **11**, 114 (1990).
87. B. Winikoff, *Stud. Fam. Plann.*, **14**, 231 (1983).
88. M. Colloton, *J. Am. Acad. Phys. Assist.*, 2, 359 (1989).
89. L. A. Hall, C. A. Williams, and R. S. Greenberg, *Am. J. Pub. Health*, **75,** 518 (1985).
90. S. O. Tangerose and S. James, *Am. J. Pub. Health*, **74**, 363 (1984).

Genetic Disorders

Christopher Cunniff, M.D.

INTRODUCTION

With declining morbidity and mortality from infectious diseases in Western society, genetic disorders and birth defects have assumed greater relative importance. It is now estimated that these conditions are the leading cause of infant mortality in the United States,[1] surpassing complications of prematurity and accidents. In addition, a significant percentage of pediatric hospital admissions are for genetic disorders and birth defect complications.[2] Recent survival trends for these conditions indicate better early detection and longer survival for affected individuals,[3] which suggests that dietitians will encounter increasing numbers of adolescent patients with genetic disorders. However, training for dietitians in the recognition and treatment of specific genetic conditions is rare, and when training is available, it often focuses on isolated conditions without providing a clinical overview of the disorder or its relationship to other disorders. The purpose of this chapter is to introduce the reader to a classification of genetic disorders and provide information on special needs and resources that are available for the evaluation and treatment of adolescents with selected genetic conditions. This chapter is not designed to provide a comprehensive list of all disorders the nutritionist may encounter. For these purposes, a number of authoritative texts are recommended.[4-6]

An understanding of the classification of genetic disorders is important for determining the recurrence risk, prognosis, and management of the individual patient. For example, a cleft lip that occurs as one feature of a multiple malformation syndrome such as trisomy 18 syndrome may be managed differently from both a surgical and nutritional standpoint than cleft lip that occurs as an isolated malformation. In all cases, the design of an appropriate nutritional plan will consider growth potential, expected developmental level, associated disabilities and the natural history of the disorder as a basis for treatment.

In the strictest sense, genetic disorders include only those caused by the malfunction of a single gene; however, in common usage genetic disorders can be thought of as all conditions for which a medical geneticist may be consulted. These include disorders caused by an abnormality of the chromosomes such as Down syndrome, single-gene disorders such as cystic fibrosis and sickle cell anemia, contiguous-gene syndromes such as Prader-Willi syndrome, multifactorially determined conditions such as meningomyelocele, and syndromes that are easily recognized but for which a cause is not known, such as Cornelia de Lange syndrome. Selected conditions that are relatively common and therefore likely to be encountered by the clinical nutrition team will be reviewed. For most of these conditions, the affected individual will have at least mild developmental disabilities, so general nutrition issues for the developmentally disabled will apply (see Chapter 16) in addition to the specific recommendations outlined in this chapter.

ASSESSMENT

Assessment of the adolescent and young adult with a genetic disorder must be tailored to the specific needs of the affected individual, for this group of conditions is very diverse and comprises a variety and range of dietary issues that other conditions may not share. Some general assessment and management guidelines will be covered in this and the following section, and specific concerns of individuals with selected conditions will follow. It is expected that the dietitian will evaluate the current feeding practices and level of functioning, specific expectations for the individual and particular disorder, and objective measures of nutritional health.

Evaluation of feeding practices should include information from a variety of domains. The first is the mode of delivery and mealtime practices. This information is usually intimately related to the level of functioning and developmental level of the patient. Although most patients will be receiving oral feedings, many others will require enteral feedings, usually through a gastrostomy tube. Food choices will, of necessity, be limited in the patient with a gastrostomy and particular attention should be given to whether these choices can provide adequate calories and meet vitamin and mineral requirements or whether supplementation will be necesary. The same holds true for the patient receiving oral feedings. Some medications the patient will be taking may also influence appetite or elimination patterns and should be inquired about in the dietary history. A history of strong food preferences or intolerance should be sought and may be helpful in future meal planning.

Specific expectations according to diagnosis are also important for the design of an appropriate diet for the adolescent and young adult. For this, the dietitian will need to consider the natural history and associated features of the primary diagnosis of the patient. For example, for the adolescent who is expected to have regression of motor skills, a balance will need to be struck between the early institution of enteral feedings to maintain weight and continuation of oral feedings to maintain a higher level of independence and competence. For other disorders, the specific diagnosis will allow judgments about diet planning to be made in anticipation of future needs and changes in status. Of particular importance is the use of disorder-specific growth charts. When objective measures of height, weight, and head circumference are made, it is essential that these measures be made in relation to the underlying disorder, which may have very specific and quantifiable differences from measures made in the normal adolescent. In the section on the assessment and management of specific disorders, references to growth charts specific to the underlying condition are cited. Usually, the weight for height from standardized growth charts will be sufficient to assess the appropriateness of weight gain or loss. Objective measurements such as skinfold thickness may be helpful for estimating body fat, as may other measurements the dietitian employs in the normal adolescent population.

MANAGEMENT

Because the disabilities encountered in children, adolescents, and young adults with genetic conditions are so varied, general information about dietary management that applies equally to all members of this population is difficult to formulate. Guidelines developed for the assessment and management of the adolescent with developmental disabilities (Chapter 16) are also useful for management of the patient with a genetic disorder. However, some focused recommendations can be made in regard to patients with specific conditions.

Chromosome Disorders

Chromosomes are the packages of genetic information that direct practically all aspects of growth, differentiation, and development. Humans have 46 chromosomes arranged in 23 pairs: 22 of the pairs are called autosomes, and the 23rd pair contains the sex chromosomes. In the normal situation, males have one X chromosome and one Y chromosome, whereas females have two X's. Chromosomes are derived equally from mother and father. Unlike somatic cells, gametes (sperm cells and oocytes) have only 23 chromosomes, and their union at fertilization produces the normal configuration of 46 chromosomes. Chromosome abnormalities occur with a frequency of approximately 8/1000 liveborns, and these abnormalities are detected by microscopic examination of the chromosomes, most commonly in dividing lymphocytes. In general, autosomal abnormalities result in growth deficiency, mental retardation, and major and minor malformations, and sex chromosome anomalies are associated with growth disturbances (either excessively short or tall), abnormal sexual maturation, and variable developmental disabilities, but rarely with frank mental retardation.

The most common type of autosomal abnormality is trisomy, which is the presence of an extra copy of an entire chromosome, giving a total of 47 chromosomes. Trisomy 21, or Down syndrome, is the most common autosomal trisomy the clinical dietitian or nutritionist will encounter in an adolescent population. For individuals with other autosomal abnormalities, nutritional support is most readily directed toward general recommendations for adolescents with developmental disabilities. Although many of these adolescents will require close supervision, many others can assume all daily living activities. Of those with sex chromosome abnormalities, abnormal growth is the norm. Although girls with Turner syndrome, caused by absence of all or part of one of the X chromosomes, are short, boys and girls with an extra sex chromosome are abnormally tall. Nutritional evaluation will likely be requested for weight gain in these patients since they are relatively underweight for their height.

Down syndrome and other autosomal disorders. Individuals with Down Syndrome have a characteristic group of features, including mild to moderate mental retardation, low muscle tone, congenital heart defects in about 50%, and other minor anomalies. Although low muscle tone may be responsible for poor feeding in infancy, it is rarely a problem in the adolescent. Likewise, congenital gastrointestinal malformations will require careful nutritional management in infancy, but problems rarely persist into adolescence. Treatment of the young adult with Down syndrome and residual heart disease will often require such special dietary measures as low-sodium diets for congestive heart failure. However, for most adolescents with Down syndrome the major nutritional concerns are weight control, food choice, meal planning, and sometimes management of chronic constipation. Additional questions will also arise in regard to vitamin, mineral, and/or hormone treatment, so the dietitian should be familiar with these modalities, their studied effects, and their possible complications.

Both weight and length are decreased in infants with Down syndrome when compared to a normal birth cohort. The decrement in height remains throughout life, with greater differences seen with advancing age. It is of the utmost importance that growth measurements be plotted on a standardized growth chart for the individual with Down syndrome.[7] Since individuals with Down syndrome are shorter than their normal peers at all ages, the use of normal growth curves will falsely identify a linear growth deficiency. Growth data for Down syndrome and many other disorders covered in this chapter are nicely compiled in a recent publication[8] or are available from the medical literature or parent support organization for that particular disorder.

Many individuals with Down syndrome will be overweight and require nutritional treatment to enhance healthy, balanced food choices, weight reduction, and meal planning.[9] It appears that the increased weight in these individuals is from excessive body fat, which has been shown to be increased by about 50% in both males and females. This suggests a genetic predisposition toward obesity for adults with Down syndrome and emphasizes the need to involve parents early on in planning for dietary management so that healthy patterns of eating are instituted early. Previous investigators have indicated a need to control environmental factors such as poor diet and low activity levels to prevent the later development of obesity. Chronic constipation may also be present in the adolescent or adult with Down syndrome. Food choices that are high in fiber are preferable to others and may help to control both weight and constipation. It is important for the dietitian to differentiate functional constipation which is common in this condition, from constipation associated with hypothyroidism, which is also associated with this population.[10]

The dietitian will often be asked for recommendations with regard to vitamin, mineral, or hormone use for improving developmental outcome or immune function. In the past, many controversial therapies have been recommended for individuals with Down syndrome, such as megavitamin therapy for improving cognitive performance. Although some claims have been made in the medical and lay literature for the efficacy of these agents, no discernible improvement has been found in developmental outcome between those taking and those not taking high doses of vitamins in controlled clinical trials.[11] Furthermore, some therapies clearly have risks and should be avoided. For example, serotonin (5-hydroxytryptamine) has been found to be low in the blood of some children with Down syndrome, leading to the use of this compound as a therapeutic agent. Although some investigators report improvement in developmental performance, these findings have not been consistently replicated. Moreover, infantile spasms were seen in 14% of treated children.[12] Because of the abnormal skin findings and impaired immune function in many individuals with Down syndrome, both vitamin A and zinc levels have been measured and found to be low in some studies, although these results have not been reproduced consistently. Each of these compounds, when supplemented, has been found to have beneficial effects in at least one clinical trial, but more study is needed. At this time, it can be said with confidence that no type of dietary or pharmacological therapy has been shown to have a consistently positive and reproducible effect on development or performance in individuals with Down syndrome.

The great majority of adolescents with other autosomal disorders will be found to have at least mild to moderate mental retardation. Their dietary assessment and management issues will be similar to the general dietary issues of patients with developmental disabilities. These measures will include attention to weight gain for those who are growth-deficient, control of gastroesophageal reflux if present, facilitation of oral-motor training and self-help skills, and meal planning. The use of adaptive equipment and a consideration of alternative forms of feeding such as nasogastric or gastrostomy tube feedings may also merit consideration in some patients. Eicher[13] provides another overview of strategies for nutritional assessment and management of individuals with developmental disabilities.

Sex chromosome abnormalities. Turner syndrome is a clinical disorder caused by the absence of all or part of one of the X chromosomes. Girls with this condition have short stature, infertility as a result of ovarian dysgenesis absent secondary sex characteristics, and variable somatic features such as lymphedema, cardiac and renal defects, and characteristic facial features. Although some developmental disabilities such as poor visual memory, deficits in mathematical skills and other nonlinguistic tasks, and immaturity have been identified, the great majority of girls with Turner syndrome are of normal intelligence, have good peer relationships, and are performing well in school.

The growth of girls with Turner syndrome is one of the most extensively studied topics in the growth literature, and standardized growth curves are readily available.[14] In the untreated patient, the final adult stature is between 135–150 cm. It appears that this short stature is more readily apparent in the growth of the extremities rather than the torso. The recent advent of recombinant growth hormone therapy appears to offer the possibility of an increase in final adult stature.[15] A number of other growth-promoting agents have also been tried, including low-dose estrogen and oxandrolone therapy, but none has shown consistent positive results in controlled studies. The estrogen replacement therapy that is recommended to enhance secondary sex characteristics may provide an increase in stature when given prior to epiphyseal fusion. In addition to short stature, many women with Turner syndrome have the visual appearance of a square-shaped torso, which derives primarily from the relative width of the thorax in relation to height. This often makes them appear overweight and may be the source of a poor body image. For this reason, some girls may develop disordered eating behaviors and benefit from social skills interventions to enhance body image (see Chapter 8). For many young women with Turner syndrome, weight for height is increased. Although some investigations have suggested an increase in adiposity, most of this increase appears to be the result of increased muscle mass rather than adipose tissue.[16]

Although linear growth deficiency is almost invariable in Turner syndrome, the dietitian should be aware of secondary conditions that may impact growth in women with Turner syndrome. First, carbohydrate intolerance appears to occur commonly. In one study, abnormal or borderline oral glucose tolerance tests were present in 15% of patients. It should be noted that type 1 diabetes (also called juvenile-onset) does not appear increased over the general population; most investigators consider the carbohydrate intolerance of girls with Turner syndrome to resemble the type 2 disorder. Young women with Turner syndrome are also at increased risk for autoimmune thyroiditis and inflammatory bowel disease, both of which may be responsible for linear growth failure. Therefore, when taking a dietary history in these patients, special attention should be given to signs and symptoms such as constipation that may be a sign of hypothyroidism, abdominal pain and bloody stools that may represent features of inflammatory bowel disease, as well as polyuria, polydipsia, and polyphagia that are common symptoms of diabetes.

The appearance of "osteopenia" on radiographs and findings of decreased bone mineral content or density on specialized testing indicate that women with Turner syndrome have abnormal bone formation and possibly abnormal bony integrity. However, other than an increase in idiopathic scoliosis in affected individuals, clinical manifestations such as increased fractures or bony deformity, at least in patients studied through their 30s, has not been demonstrated. Whether older women with Turner syndrome will manifest clinically significant osteoporosis is yet to be determined. Until more data are reported, it seems reasonable to recommend that girls with this condition follow a regimen designed to enhance normal bone formation. This regimen includes adequate daily calcium intake, frequent weight-bearing exercise, and hormone replacement therapy.[17]

The sex chromosome trisomies, Klinefelter syndrome (47,XXY), 47,XYY, and triple X (47,XXX) have a collective incidence of approximately 1 in 1000. Individuals with sex chromosome trisomy have a variable clinical picture that may range from normal to those with tall stature, abnormal sexual maturation, infertility, mild developmental disabilities and behavioral disturbances. As opposed to most genetic disorders, which will require the nutritionist to assist with healthy food choice and weight reduction, patients with trisomy for one of the sex chromosomes may seek assistance with weight gain because of their thin body habitus. There is no known contraindication to judicious use of calorie supplements in this group of patients. It should be remembered that mild developmental disabilities are present in most patients, so nutrition counseling must consider the developmental level and behavior patterns of the patient. Written dietary plans are very helpful, as are concrete instructions for meal planning.

Single-gene disorders. Genes are the units of heredity and located on the chromosomes. In the normal situation, there are two copies of each gene present, one copy of which comes from the mother and one copy from the father. In contrast to chromosome abnormalities that are diagnosed by the microscopic examination of dividing lymphocytes, either specialized testing, characteristic radiographic findings, or clinical recognition are the methods most commonly used for diagnosis. When the disorder is caused by genes located on one of the autosomes, the disorder can be inherited as either an autosomal dominant or autosomal recessive trait, depending on whether only one or both copies of the gene need be abnormal for the clinical disorder to be expressed. An autosomal recessive disorder is one that occurs only when both copies of the gene are abnormal. Many common disorders such as cystic fibrosis, sickle cell anemia, and Tay-Sachs disease are inherited as autosomal recessive traits. In addition, most metabolic disorders are autosomal recessive disorders (see Chapter 14). Autosomal dominant disorders occur when only one copy of the gene is abnormal. Common conditions inherited in an autosomal dominant fashion include Marfan syndrome, neurofibromatosis, and most skeletal dysplasias. Disorders caused by an abnormality of a gene carried on the X chromosome is known as an X-linked trait, and the great majority of these conditions are X-linked recessive traits, which tend to be carried in females but expressed in males. With very few exceptions, disorders caused by abnormalities of genes found on the Y chromosome are not seen clinically. For a catalog of almost all genetic disorders presently identified, including mode of inheritance and pertinent references, the McKusick book[4] is suggested.

Although weight control is important for all of us, it is particularly important for people with abnormalities of bone structure such as achondroplasia and other skeletal dysplasias. Achondroplasia is the most common skeletal dysplasia, with an incidence of approximately 1 in 10,000–20,000 livebirths. Affected individuals have a characteristic appearance, with a large head size, short stature that primarily involves the proximal portions of the extremities, and distinctive facial features. Final adult stature averages 130 cm for males and 123 cm for females. Children, adolescents, and adults with achondroplasia are also at risk of a number of complications because of their short stature and abnormal bone structure. These complications include upper and lower spinal stenosis with spinal cord compression, obstructive sleep apnea, and recurrent otitis media with hearing loss. Eighty% of patients have achondroplasia because of a spontaneous mutation and therefore have no other affected family members. In addition, many of teens may be isolated and unaware of the potential medical complications of their primary condition, so the dietitian may be able to facilitate referral to a treatment center experienced in the care of youth afflicted with skeletal dysplasias. As with other children with rare conditions that have characteristic growth features, standardized growth curves are available for patients with achondroplasia[18] and should be consulted for measurement of appropriate growth. In addition to monitoring weight gain and linear growth, head growth must also be monitored with achondroplasia-specific curves, as macrocephaly is the norm and may prompt repeated (unnecessary) diagnostic investigations unless it is recognized as normal in this population. Increased weight for height is universal among teens with achondroplasia when standard weight by height curves are used. This has led to the use of other body-mass indices such as weight-to-square of the height ratio (W/H^2) and skinfold measurements to determine obesity. Control of obesity is particularly important in these patients, as it may contribute to lumbar spinal canal stenosis, pain in the weight-bearing joints, exacerbation of sleep apnea, and possibly increased early cardiovascular disease. It has been recommended that weight be monitored closely in all persons with achondroplasia and weight-reduction plans be formulated when the W/H^2 and triceps skinfold measurements are above the 95th percentile for the general population.[19]

Contiguous gene syndromes.   Disorders characterized by microdeletions or microduplications of chromosomal segments associated with clusters of single-gene disorders.[20] These disorders tend to occur sporadically, meaning that first degree relatives of affected individuals have a very low risk of bearing an affected child. A great number of contiguous-gene syndromes are known, but the one that is most likely to require nutrition evaluation and treatment is Prader-Willi syndrome. This disorder is caused by a deletion (missing segment), microscopically visible in 60% of patients, of part of chromosome 15. In infancy, hyptonia dominates the clinical picture and very often prompts nutritional intervention such as nasogastric or orogastric feeding and increased caloric density of formula. Progressive obesity, mild mental retardation, learning disabilities, and behavioral disturbances, particularly in regard to food and eating, predominate the clinical picture in adolescence and adulthood.

Abnormal growth in children with Prader-Willi syndrome is one of the cardinal features of this disorder. Short stature is variable but generally present.[21] Although hypotonia results in a failure to thrive in the newborn and early infant periods, obesity usually begins to become apparent by age 3–5 yr. The obesity in these patients is striking and may assume massive proportions. Consensus diagnostic criteria have been published and should be used as a guide to diagnosis in suspected cases.[22] Excessive daytime sleepiness and sleep apnea have been described often and appear related. In the review of systems for affected individuals, it is important to discuss these items, as complications of sleep apnea are a cause of significant morbidity and mortality, particularly in the obese patient. One of the important benefits of early diagnosis is obesity prevention, which becomes progressively more difficult to control in the older patient. Presumably under the influence of altered hypothalamic control, basal metabolic rate is decreased in affected individuals and they gain weight on a lower calorie intake than normal individuals. For this reason, diets of 1000–1500 cal/d are recommended, as is regular aerobic exercise. In addition to these strategies, the nutritionist should be prepared to discuss some of the more bizarre eating behaviors in these patients. These include relentless food seeking in some, as well as the consumption of nonfood items, which may necessitate strict food-control procedures. Comprehensive recommendations for individuals with Prader-Willi syndrome who live in group homes have recently been published and can serve as a helpful guide.[23]

Multifactorial Conditions

This group of disorders is caused by a combination of genetic and environmental factors and are usually single primary defects in development. Examples include cleft lip and palate, as well as neural tube defects such as spina bifida and anencephaly. Although not considered to be strictly multifactorial, birth defects caused by teratogenic exposures such as alcohol are actually dependent on a number of factors in addition to the exposure itself. In this section, the nutritional management of two particular conditions will be discussed: meningomyelocele and fetal alcohol syndrome. In addition, new recommendations from the Food and Drug Administration in regard to folic acid comsumption in pre-pregnant women to reduce the risk of having a child with spina bifida will be addressed.

Meningomyelocele.   Caused by a failure of caudal neural tube closure and results in an opening in the back, usually in the lower spine, containing neural elements. Children with meningomyelocele usually have paralysis below the level of the lesion, and the associated hydrocephalus that occurs in approximately 85% of patients necessitates placement of a ventriculoperitoneal shunt. The level of the lesion determines functional capacity. For example, lesions below the level of the L-3 dermatome are usually associated with ambulation that requires minimal assistance, whereas lesions above that level will most often require extensive bracing and crutches for independent ambulation. Bladder and bowel incontinence occur in over 90% of affected individuals, since sphincter control for both bladder and bowel is mediated through sacral nerve roots. Because of denervation of the sacral nerves, constipation is also quite common in these patients and may be manifest as abdominal pain, overflow diarrhea, and soiling. Attempts to control bowel function are usually begun sometime between 2–4 yr of age and consist of timed potty-sitting after meals, as well as abdominal straining. For many children and young adults, a nightly suppository or other bowel evacuation treatment will facilitate more effective emptying. Dietary instruction is necessary to ensure that adequate fluids are taken, judicious use of bulking agents is employed, and adequate natural fiber and laxatives are eaten.

Obesity is a common problem in the teen with a meningomyelocele. One of the major reasons for this propensity almost certainly involves their decreased mobility, which results in the utilization of fewer calories than the independently ambulatory patient. It has been estimated that up to two-thirds of patients are overweight and will therefore require weight-reduction treatment, including both calorie reduction and increased activity. Control of obesity is important in helping to prevent decubitus ulcers and removing undue stress from the spine and lower extremities, which are at increased risk of progressive deformity and their attendant physical compromise.

Over the past several years, increasing evidence has been accumulating in regard to the positive effects of folic acid, one of the B vitamins, in the prevention of neural tube defects. Perhaps the most influential of the earlier studies was a controlled clinical trial conducted by Great Britain's Medical Research Council. This study sought to prevent recurrence of a neural tube defect in the offspring of mothers who had already given birth to a child with a meningomyelocele. This study found that high-dose supplementation of 4.0 mg of folic acid daily reduced the risk of having a subsequent meningomyelocele-affected pregnancy by approximately 70%. A subsequent prospective study of pregnancies of women who had *no history* of meningomyelocele showed that lower doses of folic acid appeared to decrease significantly the risk of having an affected child when compared to a group of women who were not supplemented. Because of these findings, recommendations for the use of folic acid to prevent neural tube defects were developed through the efforts of the Centers for Disease Control, the Food and Drug Administration, the Health Resources and Services Administration, and the National Institutes of Health.[24] This recommendation indicates that all women of childbearing age in the United States who are capable of becoming pregnant should consume 0.4 mg of folic acid/d to reduce the risk of having a child with a neural tube defect. These recommendations also caution against higher intakes except under the supervision of a physician, primarily because of the risk of masking B-12 deficiency. The nutritionist will want to recommend foods rich in folic acid for those women who wish to consume the 0.4 mg daily from dietary rather than supplementary sources. For adolescent and young adult women who have already had a neural tube defect pregnancy, it is advised that they consume 0.4 mg/d *unless* they are planning a pregnancy. If they are planning a pregnancy, it would appear prudent that they consult their physician and follow the previous recommendation of consuming 4.0 mg daily of folic acid from at least 1 mo prior conception through the first 2 mo of an established pregnancy.

Fetal alcohol syndrome (FAS).   A specific pattern of abnormal development that is seen in the babies of women who drink throughout pregnancy. It is estimated that FAS occurs in one in 1000–10,000 livebirths, making it one of the leading preventable causes of mental retardation in this country. Concensus criteria for the diagnosis of FAS have been published and include abnormalities of growth, central nervous system structure and/or function, and distinctive facial features.[25] Increasing recognition of FAS has focused attention on all aspects of this condition, including its incidence, prevalence, associated findings, and strategies for prevention.[26] Although much work remains, it is gratifying that public health efforts have been increasingly directed toward public health strategies on warning of the dangers of consuming alcohol during pregnancy.

FAS represents the most severely affected end of the spectrum of children exposed to alcohol prenatally. For every child with full-blown FAS, there are many others who will have lesser effects, but will clearly suffer problems from their exposure, primarily in learning and behavior domains. The primary indication for the nutritional assessment for most children and adolescents with FAS will be poor weight gain and possibly linear growth deficiency. Although no particular difficulty is usually encountered in planning a diet that will promote weight gain, social factors may intervene that will make the nutritionist's job more difficult than the usual referral for weight gain. First, anywhere from 70–80% of children recognized to have FAS are in a nonbiological family setting such as a foster or adoptive home. For those in foster care, there may be multiple caregivers, each of whom will require some type of dietary instruction. Biological living situations may also be chaotic, as maternal alcoholism is a prerequisite for the disorder to be expressed. Whenever possible, maintaining continuity of care through one healthcare professional, providing written diet instructions, and scheduling frequent follow-up visits will ensure that ongoing assessment is available to the patient. Of course, every effort to provide a balanced, high-calorie diet will be helpful, but it should be remembered that, even with the best of diet plans, some children with FAS will never show compensatory growth.

Unknown Genesis Disorders

Despite the tremendous advances in the understanding and, in some cases treatment of genetic conditions, many disorders for which a characteristic clinical picture has been identified have an unknown cause. There are also many individuals with multiple major and minor malformations but no recognizable pattern of malformation. For these conditions, most clinicians should try to concentrate on the individual symptoms which characterize the disorder, recognizing that prognosis and recurrence risk are largely unknown. A comprehensive list of these disorders is beyond the scope of this chapter, but one of the conditions, de Lange syndrome, deserves attention, as feeding and growth problems are two of the more prominent clinical features of this condition.

de Lange syndrome (sometimes called Cornelia de Lange or Brachmann-de Lange syndrome) is a complex multisystem disorder involving multiple major and minor malformations, mental retardation, and growth deficiency. In infancy, feeding problems and failure to thrive dominate the clinical picture. The growth deficiency is striking and involves diminution of linear growth, weight gain and head circumference. As with other disorders discussed in this chapter, normative curves have been developed and should be used in the evaluation of affected individuals.[27] Gastrointestinal findings in these patients have included gastro-esophageal reflux, dysmotility, aspiration, and esophagitis. For the patient with symptoms possibly referrable to the above conditions, referral to a primary care physician or gastrointestinal specialist appears warranted. Full medical management should be attempted, but in those in whom medical management is unsuccessful, consideration should be given to surgical treatments such as Nissen fundal plication and/or gastrostomy tube placement. In some patients, Sandifer complex (torticollis, opisthotonus, and paroxysmal dystonic posturing) has been noted and should prompt the clinical nutrition team to institute aggressive medical therapy, with surgical treatment as a backup for those who do not improve with medical management.

Summary

Nutritional management issues for patients with a wide range of genetically determined or congenitally apparent disorders have been discussed, and recommendations for the treatment of some of these conditions have been made. In all cases, the starting point for the evaluation of growth issues should begin with a careful medical history, consideration of family dynamics and the developmental level of the affected individual, and plotting of growth parameters on growth curves that have been developed specifically for the disorder in question. For cases where the clinical dietitian is evaluating an adolescent with an unknown disorder or one with which he or she has no clinical experience, resources such as the standard genetics references listed in the introduction should be used. Family support groups and clinical geneticists or genetic counselors may be valuable in gaining information about the underlying diagnosis. Appropriate dietary management of patients with genetic disorders will often require the services of many professionals and design of creative approaches in addition to standard nutritional interventions. The provision of a nutritious, varied, and healthful diet is a basic requirement for adequate growth and development and can be made available to all patients without regard to the developmental level or degree of disability.

CASE ILLUSTRATION

Wally, a 14-year-old boy with Cornelia de Lange (CdL) syndrome, was referred for nutritional assessment and management by the chronic care facility in which he was residing. His medical history revealed that his height and weight had always been well below the 5th percentile. As an infant, he had been very orally defensive and a difficult feeder. He eventually required gastrostomy tube placement and fundoplication for severe gastroesophageal reflux and esophagitis. At the time of the consultation, Wally's diet consisted primarily of a total nutritional formula to meet 100% of his calorie requirements. He was allowed to feed himself *ad lib,* but rarely took any food voluntarily. His IQ had been measured at 30, and he required a wheelchair for ambulation. He was found to have recurrent episodes of pneumonia, twice requiring hospitalization and intravenous antibiotic therapy.

At the time of the consultation, Wally's weight was 32 kg (below the 5th percentile on normal curve but at the 50th percentile on CdL growth curve), height 142 cm (also below 5th percentile on normal curve but 75th percentile on CdL curve), and head circumference 49 cm (below 5th percentile on normal curve and 50th percentile on CdL curve). Weight for height was 25th percentile. On observation of feeding, Wally could not feed himself, but he could take food from a spoon. He seemed to prefer foods with a thin consistency and had some episodes of severe coughing when foods with more texture were offered. After a half-hour of attempting oral feedings, he was given his nutritional supplement per gastrostomy tube without difficulty.

In determining a management plan for this boy, it was noted that Wally's growth was appropriate for a boy with CdL. In addition, his weight for height was good, so it was concluded that he was receiving adequate calories. Analysis of the liquid nutritional formula showed that it had more than the recommended daily allowances of all vitamins and minerals. Concern was raised about the coughing episodes noted during oral feedings, and a swallowing study was obtained that showed moderate incoordination of chewing and swallowing, resulting in frequent aspiration of small amounts of food. An occupational therapy evaluation was undertaken, and a regimen of oral-motor training was instituted. During this time, oral feedings were discontinued. After several months of oral-motor training, foods were reintroduced, but limited to those of liquid or near-liquid consistency. In addition, these foods were nonfat, which decreased the risk of a severe reactive pneumonia occurring, should he aspirate. His weight gain remained normal, and Wally had no episodes of pneumonia in the following year. Planning was begun for the graduated introduction of foods with more texture and a corresponding decrease in the calories derived from his formula.

REFERENCES

1. L. Sever, M. D. Lynberg, and L. D. Edmonds, *Teratology,* 48, 547 (1993).

2. J. G. Hall, E. K. Powers, R. T. McIlvaine, and V. H. Ean, *Am. J. Med. Gen.,* 1, 417 (1978).

3. E. Hori, T. Koyanagi, T. Yoshizato, et al., *Fetal Diag.Ther.*, **8**, 388 (1993).

4. V. A. McKusick, *Mendelian Inheritance in Man. Catalogs of Autosomal Dominant, Autosomal Recessive, and X-Linked Phenotypes*, X ed., Johns Hopkins University Press, Baltimore, MD (1992).

5. M. L. Buyse, *Birth Defects Encyclopedia,* Blackwell, Cambridge, MA (1990).

6. C. R. Scriver, A. L. Beaudet, W. S. Sly, and D. Valle, *Metabolic Basis of Inherited Disease*, VI ed., McGraw-Hill, New York (1989).

7. C. Cronk, A. C. Crocker, S. M. Pueschel, A. M. Shea, E. Zackai, G. Pickens, and R. B. Reed, *Pediatrics*, **81**, 102 (1988).

8. R. A. Saul, R. E. Stevenson, C. R. Rogers, S. A. Skinner, L. A. Prouty, and D. B. Flannery, *Proc. Greenwood Gen. Center*, **1** (suppl.), pp. 184–187 (1988).

9. R. Bronks and A. W. Parker, *Am. J. Mental Def.*, **90**, 110 (1985).

10. Z. Sare, R.H.A. Ruvalcaba, and V. C. Kelley, *Clin. Gen.*, **14**, 154 (1978).

11. G. F. Smith, D. Spiker, C. P. Peterson, D. Cichetti, and P. Justice, *J. Peds.*, **105**, 228 (1984).

12. M. Coleman, *J. Peds.*, **21**, 911 (1971).

13. P. M. Eicher, in *Children with Disabilities: A Primer*, (M. L. Batshaw and Y. M. Perret, eds.), Paul H. Brookes, Baltimore, MD, pp. 197–212 (1992).

14. A. J. Lyon, M. A. Preece, and D. B. Grant, *Arch. Dis. Child*, 60, 932 (1985).

15. R. G. Rosenfeld, J. Frane, K. M. Attie, et al., *J. Peds.*, **121**, 49 (1992).

16. T. Ohzeki, K. Hanake, H. Motozumi, H. Ohtahare, H. Urashima, and K. Shirake, *Am. J. Med. Gen.*, **46**, 450 (1993).

17. K. R. Rubin, in *Turner Syndrome*, (R. G. Rosenfeld and M. H. Grumbach eds.), Marcel Dekker, New York, pp. 301–318 (1990).

18. W. A. Horton, J. I. Rotter, D. L. Rimoin, C. I. Scott, and J. G. Hall, *J. Peds.*, **93**, 435 (1978).

19. J. T. Hecht, O. J. Hood, R. J. Schwartz, J. C. Hennessey, B. A. Bernhardt, and W. A. Horton, *Am. J. Med. Gen.*, **31**, 597 (1988).

20. R. D. Schmickel, *J. Peds.*, **109**, 231 (1988).

21. M. G. Butler and J. F. Meaney, *Pediatrics*, **88**, 853 (1991).

22. V. A. Holm, S. B. Cassidy, and M. G. Butler, *Pediatrics*, **91**, 398 (1993).

23. C. J. Hoffman, D. Autlmen, and P. Pipes, *J. Am. Diet. Assoc.*, **92**, 823 (1992).

24. Centers for Disease Control, *MMWR*, **41** (no. RR–14), 1 (1992).

25. R. J. Sokol and S. K. Clarren, *Alcoh. Clin. Exp. Res.*, **13**, 597 (1989).

26. K. L. Jones, *Ped. Rev.*, **8**, 122 (1986).

27. A. D. Kline, M. Barr, and L. G. Jackson, *Am. J. Med. Gen.*, **47**, 1042 (1993).

Metabolic Disturbances

Richard Koch, M.D.

INTRODUCTION

Although the nutritional needs in terms of caloric intake of adolescents with metabolic disorders are similar to those of the nonaffected adolescent, the diet will vary according to the particular diagnoses of each affected individual. The major focus of this chapter is phenylketonuria (PKU) and galactosemia (GA); it is hoped that the principles outlined here will aid the dietitian in treating a variety of amino acid and carbohydrate disorders, as well as the youth with organic acidemia and fatty acid oxidation disorders. However, there are many other metabolic disorders such as propionic aciduria and fatty acid oxidation disorders because not enough is known about these due to the rarity of these conditions and their recent description. The general nutritional needs of normal teenagers and young adults should be followed (see Chapter 1).

We have chosen PKU[1] and GA[2] for in-depth discussion because these two disorders have been known for several decades and are well delineated in terms of diagnosis and treatment. In addition, newborn-screening programs for early diagnosis are present in all states for PKU and 40 states for galactosemia. It is anticipated that newborn-screening programs will significantly expand in the future and thus it is important for health professionals to be familiar with the problems of treatment posed by adolescents, since it is now apparent most of these conditions require life-long nutritional treatment.

ASSESSMENT

Phenylketonuria

The incidence of this disorder is 1/12,000 births and the dietary guidelines for PKU are well described[3] because of the initial efforts at treatment by Bickel et al.[4] Subsequently, they have been modified by many others, based on clinical experience. The defect in the phenylalanine hydroxylase gene on chromosome 12[5] causes an excessive accumulation of phenylalanine in body tissue fluids because of the inability to convert into tyrosine. In some way, as yet unknown, these excess amounts of phenylalanine cause a disturbance in myelin metabolism, which results in severe mental retardation and neurological deterioration. Experience has shown that a well-controlled, restricted phenylalanine diet, when started by 2 wk of age, allows the newborn to develop normally.[6] The Collaborative Study for the Treatment of Children with PKU demonstrated an average intellectual ability at age 6 yr in well-treated children comparable to their normal siblings.[7,8] However, those who started the restricted diet between 2–4 wk of age attained an average IQ of only 85 by 6 yr of age. Thus, it would appear that diagnosis and treatment at less than 2 wk of age are very important.

Although dietary treatment of the young child is well delineated, adolescence and adulthood present unique consideration. During adolescence, peer pressure to participate in normal dietary practices is often overwhelming. While participation in sports is healthy and to be encouraged in adolescents, adequate calories and protein are of critical importance for the athlete. Practices and games can disturb the normal eating routine and after-game visits to the local fast food hang-out bring added peer pressure for dietary indiscretions. These dietary indiscretions are a constant threat to maintaining blood phenylalanine levels between the recommended 120–360 μmol/L range. The adolescent is often on his or her own in regard to eating and may not regularly ingest the recommended amount of the medical food product devoid of phenylalanine. Without an adequate protein and energy intake, growth may be delayed and energy output is decreased. With catabolism, blood phenylalanine levels invariably increase. There will be an increased appetite for foods other than PKU medical foods, so phenylalanine intake may be excessive. Through these periods, regular medical, nutritional and laboratory assessments are critical to maintaining good nutrition and phenylalanine control.

Galactosemia

This enzyme disorder (incidence 1/60,000 births) has presented many more problems to the clinician than PKU because of its rapid onset in the neonatal period, associated with significant mortality and morbidity in survivors. It is transmitted as an autosomal recessive disorder and initially responds to a galactose-restricted diet. The disorder is due to a deficiency of galactose-1-phosphate uridyl transferase (GALT). Galactose is initially converted to galactose-1-phosphate by the galactokinase enzyme and then diphosphouridine galactose by GALT.[9] It is this step that is defective and causes an accumulation of large amounts of galactose-1-phosphate in body fluids and various tissues in affected infants receiving lactose in breast milk or various cow's-milk-based formulae.

The clinical onset in infancy can be acute with vomiting, jaundice, hepatomegaly, sepsis, and early death, or somewhat delayed with intermittent vomiting and failure to thrive. Subsequently, hepatic symptoms of jaundice and hepatomegaly suggest a diagnosis of hepatitis associated with failure to thrive. Unless the diagnosis is made and appropriate dietary treatment instituted, the infant may develop cataracts and becomes mentally retarded and neurologically impaired. As cataracts become more dense, gross tremor develops, interfering with ambulation. Death usually supervenes during childhood, but rare untreated cases have lived to adulthood. Recently, the gene has been located and described by Reichart[10] and Elsas.[11]

The diagnosis can be made clinically by the astute clinician by identifying galactose in the urine. This can be suspected by finding a positive Benedict's test and negative glucose oxidase test on a urine sample from the affected infant. Today, however, a blood sample for the GALT enzyme and erythrocyte galactose-1-phosphate concentration can be readily obtained and are used for confirmatory evidence. Once the infant is placed on a galactose-restricted diet, with either a soy isolate formula with added methionine, such as Isomil®, or Prosobee®, or Nutramigen® (products very low in galactose), the clinical symptoms subside and the infant significantly and rapidly improves.

Maple Syrup Urine Disease

The clinical course of untreated maple syrup urine disease (MSUD) is usually rapidly fatal during the first 1–2 wk of life unless the diagnosis is recognized and treatment instituted. The disorder occurs in about 1/250,000 births; however, there are certain ethnic and cultural groups in which it is much more frequent. In Saudi Arabia and the Amish population in Pennsylvania, it is significantly increased.

The disorder has a rapid onset with lethargy, convulsions, and neurological impairment. Blood leucine, isoleucine, and valine levels are markedly increased due to this enzyme disorder, which is usually fatal unless treatment is instituted.

It is inherited in an autosomal recessive pattern. After diagnosis and institution of treatment, the clinical course and academic performance in school are dependent on the amount of neurologic damage that has occurred prior to diagnosis. There are only 23 states screening for this disorder because of its rarity and generally poor clinical results. In our experience, there has been only one person who has lived long enough to experience a pregnancy. The overall poor prognosis is due to delayed diagnosis neonatally and the difficulty of excluding three different branched-chain amino acids from the diet in sufficient amounts to maintain near normal blood levels of leucine, isoleucine, and valine. Dietary care of the adolescent is complicated and the reader is referred to the work of Snyderman et al.[12]

Homocystinuria

This disorder is also uncommon (1/250,000 births). It is due to a cystathionine synthetase enzyme defect causing an accumulation of cystathionine and methionine, which cause progressive neurologic impairment, lens dislocation, and skeletal changes resulting in a Marfanoid habitus.[13] Although newborn screening is available, few states screen for the disorder because of its rarity and the belief that screening is not efficacious in the first few days of life. Despite this, when the diagnosis is made neonatally, the clinical course is significantly improved when methionine blood levels are normalized. In addition, 25–50% of babies with this disorder are responsive to vitamin B-6 therapy, and strict dietary therapy is unnecessary, although definitive data are not available to substantiate this statement.

MANAGEMENT

Phenylketonuria

Dietary treatment for phenylketonuria traditionally has been based on the restriction of dietary phenylalanine, while maintaining adequate protein and caloric intake.[14] This is defined as the ratio of other essential amino acids to phenylalanine, together with adequate carbohydrate, essential fats, minerals, vitamins, and trace elements. The majority of the amino acids except for phenylalanine are provided by a phenylalanine-free protein product, and the other foods allowed contain the essential amount of phenylalanine. The diet must be calculated for all these nutrients to assure adequacy and bioavailability. The total fat content and sources of essential fatty acids may need to be considered because of the absence of lipids in some products and the specific fatty acids included in others.

Products that are available in North America for adolescents include Mead-

Johnson (Evansville, IN):[15,16] Phenyl-Free, PKU1®, PKU2®, PKU3®; Scientific Hospital Supplies (Gaithersburg, MD): Maxamum XP, Maxamaid XP; Ross Products Division, Abbott Laboratories (Columbus,OH): phenex-2. Nutrient contents are described in the *Final Report of the Task Force of the Dietary Management of Metabolic Disorders Commentary on Nutrition, American Academy of Pediatrics*, June 1985,[17] or the product information from the manufacturers. These products are described as special dietary products and exempt from "Requirements for Infant Formulas" of the Federal Food, Drug & Cosmetic Act. These products are devoid of phenylalanine and are not to be the sole source of nutrition for the adolescent.[17]

Currently, it is recommended that adolescents be treated with a diet restriction of phenylalanine when the blood phenylalanine exceeds 600 μmol/L. The maximum blood phenylalanine is dependent on phenylalanine hydroxylase activity and the intake of phenylalanine. Prescribing phenylalanine 30 mg/kg/d, protein 2–2.5 g/kg/d, and energy 100–105 kcal/kg/d will generally provide satisfactory blood phenylalanine control.[3] If the adolescent is growing rapidly, more may be needed. Initially, careful surveillance is needed for individuals who are active in sports. Medical supervision, serial serum phenylalanine determinations, and calculations of intake of phenylalanine, protein, and calories will prevent phenylalanine deficiency.

A meal plan is designed and serving lists of foods[18,19] guide the parents. The adolescent should be encouraged to take responsibility for his or her own supervision. However, adjustments in the diet prescription are made for blood phenylalanine concentrations, rate of growth, and physical activity. Low-protein baked products and pastas, along with phenylalanine-restricted recipes, are recommended to increase caloric intake, variety, and palatability.[20–22] The absence of fat in several of the low-phenylalanine products requires that linoleic and linolenic fatty acids be prescribed as 5% of the calories. Total fat content of the prescribed diet should contain a minimum of 30% of the ingested calories.

Nutrient needs for minerals and vitamins and trace minerals are usually met by the combination of the phenylalanine-restricted product and additional foods. Although the amino acid-modified products have a vitamin-mineral component, laboratory tests are suggested to measure blood levels to indicate a need for supplementation.

In the past few years, there have been reports of deficiencies in zinc, selenium, copper, and carnitine.[23–27] The need for these nutrients during times of rapid growth is well documented. Monitoring blood values for trace metals is indicated in the management of any PKU subject who is not doing well. We recently observed a severe case of selenium deficiency in an adolescent with persistent vomiting and diarrhea.

Some years ago, objections were raised regarding the beneficial effects of the phenylalanine-restricted diet. However, the evidence is now overwhelming that proper dietary therapy is therapeutic and results in normal development and must be maintained into adulthood.[28,29]

Diet discontinuation. This is, perhaps, one of the most controversial aspects of PKU. Horner et al.[30] was the first to report that perhaps discontinuation of dietary therapy was safe, but in recent years it has become clear that early diet discontinuation is harmful. The pioneering works of Cabalska et al[31] and Smith et al.[32] have now been corroborated by the results of the recent report by Holtzman et al.[28] These reports revealed a detrimental effect on intellectual performance and behavior in children in whom dietary control was lost. These researchers suggested that the children's diets were considered to be out of control when their blood phenylalanine concentration persistently exceeded 900 μmol/L. The age at which control was lost was the best predictor of the child's IQ at the ages of 8, 10, or 12 yr, and of the deficit in the child's IQ as compared with those of his or her unaffected siblings or parents. The age at which control was lost was also the best predictor of deficit achievement scores of children with PKU at the age of 8 yr in comparison with unaffected siblings. The greater deficiencies in all of these outcomes were observed among children who were out of dietary control before the age of 6 yr.

Azen et al[33] evaluated 12-yr IQ and achievement test scores for 95 PKU children, again grouped according to the age at which dietary control was lost. The differences between groups that were apparent at ages 8 and 10 persist through age 12. The group that maintained dietary control at least through 8 yr of age, many of whom were still in good control at age 12, had the highest scores at age 12 years. The single exception was seen in arithmetic achievement where all groups of PKU children showed considerable deficit at age 12, regardless of dietary control.

Thus, recent data indicate that the prudent course is to maintain dietary control through adolescence.[8] This is difficult, but long-term control may be assisted if the physician allows "holidays" every 2 mo, beginning at age 10 yr. A holiday is a day when the child can eat anything he or she wants and does not have to ingest the special formula. At age 12, the number of holidays is increased to one each month. This has allowed the adolescent to eat and taste normal foods at parties and special celebrations. We have found by experience that this approach is helpful and prolongs the period of dietary control.

Life during high school can be hectic and erratic. The pressure of academic achievement and athletics can cause irregular eating habits and peer pressure at parties may result in excessive protein intake. Since liver metabolism is important in maintaining and utilizing protein appropriately, the physician and dietician must provide appropriate advice about avoiding alcohol and drugs, including marijuana. While unrelated to PKU, a discussion of smoking and sexual practices is also important. Regular meals with ingestion of the phenylalanine-restricted medical food product should be encouraged. During this period, blood levels of phenylalanine of 600–720 μmol/L are tolerated.

Maternal PKU. Teenage pregnancy has increased greatly[34] and it is quite clear the PKU teenagers are at risk for pregnancy resulting in microcephalic babies with other congenital defects[35] unless they are treated with the phenylalanine-restricted diet. Ideally, the best results occur with pre-conception dietary control, but this is difficult for teenagers due to the unplanned nature of these pregnancies. Thus, phenylalanine blood level control should be established as early as possible.

The Maternal PKU Collaborative Study has demonstrated that satisfactory fetal development occurs and a normal outcome can be anticipated if blood phenylalanine levels are kept between 120 and 360 μmol/L before the eighth week of pregnancy.[36–38] These results suggest that dietary restriction of blood phenylalanine levels during pregnancy is an effective treatment to reduce the occurrence of congenital anomalies in the offspring of PKU women. The problem is to develop a plan to follow all PKU women so that proper counseling and treatment can be provided prior to conception.

Magnetic resonance imaging. Disturbed myelination in phenylketonuria has now been well documented in several centers.[39,40] The nature and extent of these changes in the cerebral white matter in some persons is remarkable. They consist of bandlike or confluent patchy areas of high signal intensity, predominately in the white matter with extension into the anterior and posterior periventricular regions, and or involvement of the subcortical white matter, according to Bick et al.[39] The curious aspect of these findings is the lack of clinical correlation with intelligence, age of diagnosis, and treatment regimens. In fact, we have observed one 47-year-old severely mentally impaired, nonambulatory woman who does not exhibit these typical magnetic resonance imaging (MRI) findings at all. To date, nearly all classical PKU adolescents who are in the teen years exhibit these changes, but individuals with mild hyperphenylalaninemia with blood phenylalanine levels of 120–360 μmol/L do not. The MRI changes have been reported to resolve in a few cases in individuals who resume strict dietary control, suggesting that permanent brain damage may not be occurring. This presents a problem in counseling an affected adolescent. It would seem prudent to suggest that individuals who are not on a phenylalanine-restricted diet return to dietary therapy, but this is resisted by many who seemingly are mentally unaffected due to the nature of the diet. At this time, the MRI changes are worrisome, but the lack of clinical correlation to date is disconcerting. Our recommendation is to return to dietary therapy until we know what the clinical significance of these changes is as they become further delineated.

Galactosemia

Treatment of galactosemia must begin during the neonatal period for optimal results. Although a surveyhas thrown doubt about the efficacy of the galactose-restricted diet, there is no question about its importance during the early years of life.[41] Traditionally, soy-bean-based formulae are utilized initially. Nutramigen®, a protein hydrolysate formula, also may be acceptable, but the cost is greater.* As the individual grows and matures into adolescence, the elimination of dairy products, such as milk, cheese, whey, etc., a few organ meats and a few vegetables, such as peas, beans, and legumes, are prohibited. However, additional research has shown that galactose is more widely distributed in food-stuffs than was previously realized.[41,42] There is the thought that it is these more obscure sources of galactose that may be the cause of some of the poor results recorded by Buist and his colleagues.

Dietary intake of galactose is usually monitored by nutritional surveillance and serial erythrocyte galactose-1-phosphate measurements every 3 mo. In adolescence, this has not been successful, as shown by the survey of over 300 cases by the Oregon group. Thus, at present, a completely revised dietary approach to galactosemia is occurring as research continues to produce data on the galactose content on various foodstuffs. Gropper et al.'s recent article[44] demonstrates that in the past many foods thought to be free of galactose indeed have clinically significant amounts. There is no question that dairy products and other lactose-containing products are still the primary foods to be avoided by the adolescent. The lack of adequate calcium in the diet of galactosemic persons makes it imperative that a minimum of 1000 mg of calcium be added to the diet to prevent osteopenia. Galactosemic individuals should be carefully followed throughout adolescence. Careful attention to food labeling is important to exclude hidden sources of galactose.

More research is indicated to further delineate foods that may contain galactose to improve dietary therapy. There is controversy regarding the effectiveness of the galactose-restricted diet in terms of overall development throughout the teenage years.[43,44] However, at present a strictly controlled dietary intake of galactose with medical and laboratory monitoring would seem to offer the best chance for long-term good health.

Maple Syrup Urine Disease

The care of adolescents with maple syrup urine disease (MSUD) is complicated because three different amino acids are involved (leucine, isoleucine, and valine). There is no question that dietary treatment with the medical foods presently

---

* Isomil® is produced by Ross Products Division, Abbott Laboratories, Columbus, OH. Prosobee® and Nutramigen® are produced by Mead Johnson Co., Evansville, IN.

available commercially is helpful. The course, however, is stormy. Few affected individuals live beyond the teenage years. The diet should be balanced in the amount of leucine, isoleucine, and valine, but adequate calories and protein must be available in the diet. During acute episodes of ketoacidosis, the adolescent will need to be hospitalized for care since vomiting may make care in the home difficult. Intravenous fluids with adequate carbohydrate, carnitine (100 mg/kg/ d) and careful monitoring of the branched-chain amino acids are usually indicated. With severe acidosis, intravenous bicarbonate may be used, but in our experience is not necessary. The benefits of hemodialysis and intraperitoneal dialysis are preferred by some. Insulin has also been utilized to promote better carbohydrate utilization[44], but frequent blood sugar monitoring is necessary. Adequate caloric intake can be maintained with nasogastric tube feedings of commercially prepared MSUD formulae deficient in the branched-chain amino acids. As blood levels of the latter stabilize, it is mandatory to provide adequate amounts of leucine, valine, and isoleucine since they are essential amino acids.

Prenatal diagnosis is available, and prospective parents are provided information upon which to make rational decisions.[44] There is no question that excellent dietary treatment is beneficial. However, whether it prevents long-term problems remains unanswered.

Homocystonuria

The diet for unresponsive subjects is sufficiently complicated that the reader is referred to a chapter by Mudd and Levy.[12] However, careful attention must be paid to overall mutation and particularly blood methionine levels. The diagnosis is difficult to make clinically in the absence of newborn screening until neurologic or ocular changes occur. Lens dislocation may cause the opthamologist to suspect the disorder. Blood and urine amino acid screening confirm the diagnosis. A trial of vitamin B-6 is indicated in cases of homocystinuria to rule out the vitamin B-6 responsive form and 2–3 g of betaine three times a day may be efficacious as well.

CASE ILLUSTRATION

Michael was diagnosed at age 2 yr with classical phenylketonuria. His initial developmental quotient was 48 on the Gesell scales and the blood phenylalanine level over 20 mg%. He was started on a phenylalanine-restricted diet and made excellent mental progress. By age 17, his intelligence quotient on a standardized measure was in the low-average range (86) and dietary therapy was discontinued. While on the restricted diet his blood phenylalanine levels had been between 3– 12 mg%, whereas when the diet was discontinued, they immediately rose to levels greater than 20 mg%. He was able to graduate from high school, but thereafter his behavior deteriorated. He was unable to work and became involved in child molestation charges. His parents were greatly concerned about the course of events since his phenylalanine-restricted diet was discontinued at age 17 yr. Accordingly, the diet was reinstituted with some difficulty with good control by age 18 yr. Subsequently, he has found steady employment and stabilized his behavior.

Acknowledgment.   Supported in part by the National Institute of Child Health and Human Development, contract NO1-HD–2–3148, Bethesda, MD 20892.

REFERENCES

1.   R. Koch, K.N.F. Shaw, P. B. Acosta, K. Fishler, G. Schaeffler, E. Wenz, and A. Wohlers, *J.Peds.*, **76**, 815 (1970).

2.   G. N. Donnell, R. Koch, and W. R. Bergren, in *Galactosemia*, (D. Y. Hsia and C. C. Thomas, eds.), Springfield, IL, pp. 247–268 (1969).

3.   R. Koch and E. Wenz, *Ann. Rev. Nutr.*, **7**, 117 (1987).

4.   H. Bickel, J. W. Gerrard, and E. M. Hickmans, *Lancet*, **2**, 812 (1953).

5.   S.L.C. Woo, A. S. Lidsky, F. Güttler, T. Chandra, and K.J.H. Robson, *Nature*, **306**, 151 (1983).

6.   M. L. Williamson, R. Koch, C. Azen, and C. Chang, *Pediatrics*, **68**, 161 (1981).

7.   M. L. Williamson, J. C. Dobson, and R. Koch, *Pediatrics*, **60**, 815 (1977).

8.   M. L. Williamson, R. Koch, C. Azen, and E. G. Friedman, in *Inherited Diseases of Amino Acid Metabolism*, (H. Bickel and U. Wachtel, eds.), Georg Theime Verlag, Stuttgart, Austria, pp.151–162 (1985).

9.   L. F. Leloir, *Arch. Biophys. Biochem.*, **33**, 186 (1951).

10.   J.K.V. Reichardt and S.L.C. Woo, *Proc. Natl. Acad. Sci. USA*, **88**, 2633 (1991).

11.   L. J. Elsas, J. L. Fridovich-Keil, and N. D. Leslie, *Int. Ped.*, **8**, 101 (1993).

12.   C. R. Scriver, A. L. Beaudet, W. S. Sly, and D. Valle, in *The Metabolic Basis of Inherited Disease*, (L Sweetman, ed.), McGraw-Hill, NY, pp. 791–819 (1989).

13.   N.A.J. Carson, D. C. Cusworth, E. E. Dent, C.M.B. Field, D. W. Neill, and R. G. Westall, *Arch. Dis. Child.*, **38**, 425 (1963).

14.   P. B. Acosta et al., *Am. J. Clin. Nutr.*, **3**, 694 (1983).

15.   *Milupa Special Products for the Dietary Treatment of Inherited Disorders of Amino Acid Metabolism*, Milupa Corp., Dept. of Scientific Affairs, Darien, CT (1984).

16.   *Pediatric Products Handbook*, Mead-Johnson, Nutritional Division, Evansville, IN, (1993) .

17.   *Final Report of the Task Force of the Dietary Management of Metabolic Disorders of the Committee on Nutrition*, American Academy of Pediatrics, Evanston, IL, (1985).

18. V. E. Schuett et al., *Low Protein Food List*, University of Wisconsin Press, Madison, WI, (1981).

19. P. B. Acosta and P. Fernhoff, *A Parent's Guide to the Child with PKU*, Center for Family Services, Tallahassee, FL, (1983).

20. V. E. Schuett and J. I. Yandow, *Low Protein Breads*, Waisman Center, Madison, WI.

21. E. Read, *The PKU Cookbook*, University of New Mexico Press, Albuquerque, NM, (1976).

22. V. E. Schuett and J. I. Yandow, *Low Protein Cookery for PKU*, II ed. University of Wisconsin Press, Madison, WI (1993).

23. P. B. Acosta et al., *J. Inher. Metab. Dis.*, **5**, 107 (1982).

24. C. J. Taylor, G. Moore, and D. C. Davidson, *J. Inher. Metab. Dis.*, **7**, 160 (1984).

25. J. M. Fraga, *J. Inher. Metab. Dis.*, **6**, 99 (1983).

26. R. S. Gibson, *Food & Nutr. News*, **57**, 21 (1985).

27. P. R. Borum, *Nutr. Rev.*, **39**, 385 (1981).

28. N. A. Holtzman, R. A. Kronmal, W. Van Doorninck, C. Azen, and R. Koch, *N. Engl. J. Med.*, **314**, 593 (1986).

29. F. J. Menolascino and J. A. Stark, in *Preventive and Curative Intervention in Mental Retardation*, Paul Brookes Publishing Co., Baltimore, MD, pp.61–90 (1988).

30. F. A. Horner, C. W. Streamer, L. L. Alejandro, L. H. Read, and F. Ibbot, *N. Engl. J. Med.*, **226**, 79 (1962).

31. B. Cabalska, N. Duszynska, J. Borzymowska, K. Zorska, H. Foslacz-Folga, and K. Bozkowa, *Eur. J. Ped..*, **126**, 253 (1977).

32. I. Smith, M. Lobascher, J. Stevenson, O. H. Woolf, H. Schmidt, S. Grubel-Kaiser, and H. Bickel, *Br. Med. J.*, **2**, 723 (1978).

33. C. G. Azen, R. Koch, E. G. Friedman, S. Berlow, J. Coldwell, W. Krause, R. Matalon, E. McCabe, M. O'Flynn, R. Peterson, B. Rouse, C. R. Scott, B. Sigman, D. Valle, and R. Warner, *AJDC*, **145**, 35 (1991).

34. W. B. Hanley, J.T.R. Clarke, and W. Schoonheyt, *Clin. Biochem.*, **20**, 149 (1987).

35. R. Lenke, H. L. Levy, *N. Eng. J. Med.*, **303**, 1202 (1980).

36. R. Koch, E. Wenz, C. Bauman, E. G. Friedman, C. Azen, K. Fishler, and W. Heiter, *Acta Paediatr Japan.*, **30**, 1410 (1988).

37. R. Koch and F. de la Cruz, *J. NIH Res.*, **3**, 61, (1991).

38. R. Koch, H. Levy, R. Matalon, B. Rouse, W. Hanley, and C. Azen, *AJDC*, **147**, 1224 (1993).

39. U. Bick, G. Fahrendorf, A. C. Ludolph, P. Vassalo, J. Weglage, and K. Ullrich, *Eur. J. Ped.*, **150**, 185 (1991).

40. A. J. Thompson, S. Tillotson, I. Smith, B. Kendall, S. G. Moore, and D. P. Brenton, *Brain*, **116**, 811 (1993).

41. K. C. Gross and P. B. Acosta, *J. Inher. Metab. Dis.*, **14**, 253 (1991).

42. S. S. Gropper, K. A. Gross, and S. J. Olds, *J. Am. Diet. Assoc.*, **93**, 328 (1993).

43. D. D. Waggoner, N. R. Buist, and G. N. Donnell, *J. Inher. Metab. Dis.*, **13**, 801 (1990).

44. S. Schweitzer, Y. Shin, C. Jacobs, J. Brodehl, *Eur. J. Pediatr.*, **152**, 36 (1993).

Developmental Disabilities

Kathleen Selvaggi-Fadden M.D.,
Heidi Puelzl-Quinn, M.S., R.D., and
Theodore A. Kastner, M.D.

INTRODUCTION

Developmental disability is a term used to describe a constellation of disorders that cause an initial impairment of function in infancy, childhood, and adolescence. Cerebral palsy, autism, mental retardation, and severe hearing or visual impairments in childhood are among the most common conditions considered developmental disabilities. However, there are a wide range of causes for these developmental disorders. For example, autism has been associated with all of the following: fragile X syndrome, tuberous sclerosis, neurofibromatosis, phenylketonuria, congenital infection with rubella or cytomegalovirus, trisomy 21, mucopolysaccharidosis type 3, congenital hypothyroidism, pituitary deficiency with septo-optic dysplasia and Rett syndrome. The difficulty in providing nutritional services to adolescents with developmental disabilities is that evaluation and treatment must separately address the effect of etiology on nutritional status and the functional level of the individual. Given the rarity of many disorders associated with developmental disability, this is often difficult.

A developmental disability in and of itself may impact on an adolescent's nutritional status and so might problems associated with that disability. Conversely, nutritional factors can impact on the disability either directly or indirectly. Many factors must be considered when evaluating the nutritional status of the adolescent with a developmental disability. For example, caloric requirements may need to be altered due to level of activity. Nutrient intake may be affected by dysphagia or other eating and swallowing disorders. Enzyme defects may affect the utilization of nutrients (see Chapter 15). In many cases, a developmental disability has no effect on nutritional status and the adolescent has the same health risks as any other member of the general population. For example, a recent study demonstrated that blood lipid levels, obesity, and smoking in a population of adults with mental retardation carry the same risk for cardiovascular disease as the general population.[1]

Nutritional status in an adolescent with a developmental disability may be difficult to ascertain. Typical growth curves cannot always be used for persons with developmental disabilities. The atypical growth pattern in such conditions as Down Syndrome, Prader-Willi syndrome, fragile X syndrome, Turner syndrome and Noonan syndrome has necessitated the generation of syndrome-specific growth charts (see Chapters 14 and 15). Muscle tone abnormalities, such as hypertonicity seen in cerebral palsy, can impact on normal growth so that careful anthropometric measurements must be used to monitor nutritional status.

ASSESSMENT

A comprehensive nutritional assessment is an essential component of the total care plan for the adolescent with developmental disabilities. The comprehensive nutrition assessment includes a medical and feeding history; growth history and anthropometric measurement; dietary assessment; feeding assessment; clinical assessment; and assessment of biochemical indices.

Medical and Feeding History

A review of past medical history is essential to identify potential risk factors associated with poor nutritional status (i.e., gastrointestinal disorders, recurrent infections, anemia, seizures, poor dental health). Medications that may have an impact on growth and nutritional status, i.e., anticonvulsants or corticosteroids, should also be noted. A feeding history is obtained to provide information on feeding practices, feeding skill development, and feeding problems. A history of food allergies or intolerances should also be obtained.

Growth History and Anthropometric Measurement

A growth history is essential for accurately assessing the adequacy of anthropometric measurements in relation to the usual growth pattern. This is especially important for children and adolescents with developmental disabilities because growth expectations, as well as growth patterns, can vary due to multiple factors including syndrome-specific growth patterns, chronic illness, and/or inadequate intake due to poor oral-motor skills.

A standard anthropometric assessment includes current weight and height (or body length if unable to stand), and weight for height. Skinfold measurements (triceps or subscapular) and midupper arm circumference measurements may also be obtained in order to evaluate body fat stores and muscle mass (see Chapter 18). It is important to note that these anthropometric parameters have their limitations.[2] For optimal results, these measurements should be obtained by an experienced dietitian. Appropriate tools should be used and serial measurements monitored. It should also be noted that the reference data for skinfold thickness measurements are derived from a population of Caucasian children and racial differences in skinfold thickness do exist.[3] Despite their limitations, skinfold thickness and arm muscle circumference can be useful if they have been serially evaluated and when used in conjunction with weight and height/length information. Skinfold grids for evaluating these anthropometric parameters are available (see Chapter 18).[4]

Using anthropometric data from only a single point in time, without a growth history for reference, may yield incomplete and potentially misleading information. In addition, the use of standard growth charts for evaluating growth of children and adolescents with developmental disabilities may be problematic due to differences in growth patterns. Therefore, they are useful only if serial measurements of all growth parameters are collected over time.

One of the reasons that standard growth charts are often inadequate for adolescents with developmental disabilities is that these individuals are generally shorter[5] and often have decreased lean body mass[6] than their age-matched peers. Adolescents with developmental disabilities often fall at or below the lowest percentiles for height for age on standard growth charts. However, these growth parameters may be appropriate given the diagnosis and growth history of the adolescent. Alternately, desirable weight goals may be overestimated if standard growth charts are used without a growth history. Additional weight gain may be excess fat rather than fat-free mass and, as such, is not usually desirable.[7] For example, research has found that the children and adolescents residing in one southern state consumed greater than 67% of Recommended Daily Allowances of nutrients and had greater tricep skinfold thicknesses than able-bodied peers, but lower midarm muscle circumference and decreased weight measurements, indicating increased fat stores and decreased muscle mass.[8] In summary, using only one set of growth parameters for an adolescent with developmental disabilities could result in underestimating the adequacy of length and overestimating appropriate weight.

For some adolescents with developmental disabilities, it may be useful to use the weight-for-height guidelines from the growth chart to determine adequate weight for height. However, it is important to note that these weight-for-height guidelines are based on prepubertal growth and do not take into account the changes in body composition that accompany puberty.[7] It is also important to note that this method should be used in conjunction with clinical observation, as using growth charts alone can be misleading. For example, weight for length/height may be overestimated as a result of error in length/height measurement. The adolescent's actual length/height may be longer than measured. Accurate measurement may be compromised by scoliosis and/or contractures. As a result, the weight for length may appear adequate while the adolescent may, in fact, be underweight for their his or her length.

Some of the difficulties in obtaining accurate measurements in adolescents with developmental disabilities can be overcome. Special scales such as wheelchair or sling scales may be required to obtain accurate results. Alternate methods for obtaining lengths may also be needed, especially in adolescents with contractures and/or scoliosis. Segmented lengths are commonly used as an alternative method of measurement in this group. However, this method can overestimate body length due to the increased number of opportunities for measurement error. It can also underestimate body length when measurements are made along the concave surface of the curve in the adolescent with scoliosis.

The arm—span method is another alternate method of measurement used to estimate body length. However, it too has its limitations. For example, it cannot be used in a child with contractures in the arms or hands as it requires measurement from the fingertips of one outstretched hand to the other.[9]

Another alternate method of assessing length is to use a measurement of sitting height (crown-to-rump length). This method can be used to assess length in adolescents whose legs are poorly developed or shorter than normal. There are percentile charts available for assessing these measurements.[4] Recent research has yielded another alternate method of assessing linear growth using measurements of upper arm and lower leg length. These measurements have been shown to be highly correlated with body length, and growth charts have been developed to plot the growth of arm/leg length over time.[10]

As previously noted, there are several syndrome-specific growth charts available that take into consideration the alterations in growth patterns characteristic of the syndrome. These include Down syndrome, Prader-Willi syndrome, Turner syndrome, myelomeningocele, and sickle cell anemia (see Chapters 14 and 15). Most important, consistency in both the method of measurement and, ideally, the personnel obtaining the measurements improves the reliability of these measurements. The difficulties inherent in obtaining accurate anthropometric measurements in this group reinforces the importance of having a growth history for reference of previous growth patterns.

Dietary Assessment

The dietary assessment includes evaluation of past feeding practices and diet intake, current feeding practices and diet intake, including multivitamin and mineral supplements, and information on food intolerances and allergies. It also includes information on medications that may impact nutritional status, such as antibiotic or anticonvulsant medication, as well as elimination patterns (constipation or diarrhea). Information on activity level is also obtained to help determine calorie requirements. It is additionally important to obtain intake information related to food temperature and texture preferences.

Information on current intake may be obtained from a 24-h recall, typical daily intake, or multiday food record. Information obtained from a multiday food record is generally more useful in determining the nutritional adequacy of overall intake, although it has been found that the act of recording may, in itself, alter intake.[2] When recording intake, specific information regarding quantity of foods/beverages, methods of preparation (boiled, fried, or baked), and additions to foods (butter, gravy, or sauces) should be included to improve the accuracy of diet analysis. Information on mineral and vitamin supplements should also be included on the food record. Of importance to note is that estimating actual intake for an adolescent with developmental disabilities may be complicated by food losses due to poor oral-motor ability. Actual intake may be less than recorded intake due to these losses.

Diet intake is generally evaluated based on the Recommended Dietary Allowances (RDAs), guidelines developed for the general healthy population. Requirements for adolescents with developmental disabilities may differ from these guidelines due to illness, malabsorption, medications, or altered activity levels. Energy requirements, in particular, can be quite different. For example, a healthy 12-year-old boy will have different caloric requirements from a 12-year-old boy with athetoid cerebral palsy and increased motor tone and activity, i.e., continuous involuntary movement, or a 12-year-old boy with spina bifida who is nonambulatory. Also, the RDAs for energy requirements are based upon age, sex, and body weight. As a consequence, some clinicians recommend that the initial evaluation of energy needs be calculated based on estimates of basal metabolic rate, with adjustments for activity level and changes in weight.[11] Other calorie estimates include an assessment of calories per centimeter of body height (see Table 16.1).[5,12] In addition, for some adolescents with severe disabilities due to significant central nervous system impairment, caloric requirements may be as low as 4–5 cal/cm of body length. In these individuals, close monitoring of weight and intake is essential. Supplementation with a multivitamin containing minerals is necessary. Additional supplementation of calcium and phosphorus is generally needed to meet recommended daily allowances.

Table 16.1   Guidelines for Estimating Caloric Requirements in Children with Developmental Disabilities

Condition	Caloric Recommendation
Ambulatory, ages 5–12 yr	13.6 kcal/cm height
Nonambulatory, ages 5–12 yr	11.1 kcal/cm height
Cerebral palsy with decreased levels of activity	10 kcal/cm height
Cerebral palsy with normal or increased levels of activity	15 kcal/cm height
Athetoid cerebral palsy, adolescence	Up to 6000 kcal
Down syndrome, boys ages 5–12 yr	16.1 Kcal/cm height
Down syndrome, girls ages 5–12 yr	14.3 Kcal/cm height
Myelomeningocele	Approximately 50% of RDA for age after infancy, may need as little as 7 kcal/cm height

From *Mayo Clinic Diet Manuel: A Handbook of Dietary Practices,* VII ed., J. K. Nelson, K. Moxness, C. F. Gastineau, and M. D. Jensen, eds., C. V. Mosby, St. Louis, MO (1994). Reprinted with permission.

Although there are alternate guidelines available for estimating energy requirements for children with developmental disabilities, there are none available for the remaining nutrients for which RDAs have been established. Therefore, it is important that the RDAs be used in conjunction with clinical observation and biochemical indices to best determine the adequacy of intake, and possible mineral and vitamin supplementation requirements. Nutrients of specific concern during adolescence are protein, calcium, phosphorus, and iron.[13] Intake of vitamin A and riboflavin is also of concern, as adequacy of intake has been found to be marginal in the general population.[9] Supplementation with minerals and vitamins is especially important for adolescents whose dietary intake is limited due to inadequate intake or calorie restriction for prevention of excess weight gain.

Information on elimination patterns should be included in the dietary assessment. Constipation, in particular, is a frequent concern for individuals with developmental disabilities. It can be caused by a number of factors including inadequate intake of fluids, increased fluid loss due to drooling or poor oral-motor control wiht drinking, inadequate intake of fiber due to food preferences, texture modification or dietary restrictions, alterations in muscle tone that may affect bowel motility, decreased activity levels, or medications. Often, constipation is associated with a combination of these factors. It is not uncommon for constipation to interfere with appetite, causing decreased intake. Diarrhea can also be a problem and is often seen in association with certain medications such as antibiotics, food intolerance (lactose intolerance), or malabsorption. Persistent diarrhea can lead to weight loss, as well as nutrient losses.

Feeding Assessment

Observation of feeding is an essential component of the nutritional assessment for the individual with developmental disability. It allows for the observation of skills, including oral-motor function and self-feeding skills. It also provides an opportunity to observe the individual's overall response to the feeding experience. That is, is mealtime pleasant, playful, and fun or stressful, uncomfortable, and difficult? For severely impaired individuals, it also provides an opportunity to observe the interaction between that individual and the feeder. This interaction is especially significant as the feeder must understand and acknowledge nonverbal cues that are used to communicate feeding-related needs. These include food preferences related to texture and temperature of food, and adequate pacing of feeding, i.e., determining whether the adolescent is full or may just need a rest during the mealtime. The feeding observation also gives information about the length of the mealtime, and how much food the individual can consume within that time frame. Further, these observations also provides important information of oral-motor functioning.

Oral-motor ability has a significant impact on overall intake and hence nutritional status, growth, and development. Oral-motor difficulties include problems with sucking, swallowing, chewing, and gagging. These difficulties are related to problems with lip function, tongue mobility, jaw stability, and bite reflex. Each of these is affected by muscle tone (hypotonia, hypertonia, mixed tone, and fluctuating tone), as well as the level of sensitivity to various foods, flavors, temperatures, or textures.

A complete oral-motor assessment is usually accomplished by a speech pathologist or an occupational therapist with a specialty in oral-motor functioning and swallowing. Oral-motor and feeding therapy to improve oral-motor function can be essential for both feeding development as well as prespeech and language skill development. The dietitian works with other therapists to help determine appropriate texture modifications based on the adolescent's oral-motor abilities in order to maximize safe oral intake and minimize the loss of food and fluids (see Table 16.2).

The safety of oral intake should always be recognized as a priority. For adolescents with severe developmental disabilities, inadequate intake due to poor oral-motor function may be compounded by swallowing difficulties. They may result from problems in the oral, pharyngeal, or esophageal phases of swallowing. In addition to inadequate intake, swallowing difficulties can aggravate respiratory problems due to the aspiration of food or fluid. One way to assess the safety of the swallow is by a video-fluoroscopic swallowing study (sometimes called a modified barium swallow).[15] This procedure consists of positioning the adolescent in his or her usual feeding position and presenting the individual with familiar foods of various textures. These usually include a thin liquid, paste, pureed food,

Table 16.2   Progression of Food Texture

Level of Oral Development	Desired Food Texture
Level 1 Child tolerates only commercially prepared strained foods.	Puréed table foods
Level 2 Child tolerates puréed food.	Thickened pureed foods
Level 3 Child begins to show vertical (up and down) chewing motions.	Ground foods
Level 4 Child begins to move food from side to side by using tongue.	Chopped foods
Level 5 Child displays mature rotary chew.	Coarsely chopped foods

From T. E. Shaddix, in *Nutr. Focus*, **6**, 1 (1991). Reprinted with permission.

and food that requires some chewing. Oral-motor manipulation, preparation of the bolus for swallowing, bolus transit time, swallowing mechanism, and aspiration risk with each texture are assessed during the study. The modified barium swallow is usually performed by a radiologist and speech pathologist with expertise in oral-motor function and swallowing. If the swallow is determined to be unsafe, various strategies with regard to positioning and food texture modification may be recommended. If the swallow continues to be unsafe despite these strategies, a supplemental feeding via a feeding tube may be warranted.

Stamina plays an important role in the feeding experience of the adolescent with developmental disabilities. It is often affected by the overall health of the individual and is especially impaired by poor cardiopulmonary function and seizure activity. Optimum positioning is important to gain maximum support during feeding in order to enhance stamina and oral-motor ability. Poor head and trunk control and abnormal reflex patterns that affect feeding are some of the problems that can be improved through appropriate positioning. With improved positioning, decreased effort is required to maintain stability and increased effort can be directed toward oral-motor control (see Table 16.3).[16] Sedatives such as diazepam and felbamate can adversely affect stamina.

Behavioral and environmental issues may also impact feeding. Children with developmental disabilities often use the feeding situation as a time to exert their control or independence or to obtain attention from the feeder.[14] Environmental

Table 16.3 Components of Good Sitting Posture

Neutral head and neck alignment, with head in midline
Stable and relaxed shoulders
Symmetrical upper and lower trunk, extended and aligned
Neutral and stable pelvis
90-deg flexion for hips, knees, and ankles, with hips slightly abducted
Supported and aligned feet

From T. E. Shaddix, in *Nutr. Focus*, **6**, 1 (1991). Reprinted with permission.

considerations include when and where the child is fed, the mealtime schedule, with whom the child eats, and what types of distractions interfere with intake, i.e., excessive noise, light, unfamiliar places or people.[14] Appropriate steps should be taken to modify the environment if it interferes with feeding.

Clinical Assessment

A physical examination to address the general nutritional state should include the observation of skin, hair, eyes, mouth, and teeth for evidence of nutritional deficiencies or dehydration. In addition, muscle bulk, bone growth, presence of contractures, and presence of scoliosis are important to assess.

Biochemical indices. Generally evaluated include the biochemical indices relating to iron metabolism (hemoglobin, ferritin, and total iron-binding capacity), protein status (total protein, serum albumin, and pre-albumin), and immune function (white blood cell count or immunoglobulins). Other laboratory tests may include a vitamin D level, alkaline phosphatase, folic acid and B-6 levels, especially for adolescents receiving anticonvulsant medication.

The comprehensive nutritional assessment includes evaluation of all factors that affect intake, growth, and nutritional status. It is essential that this assessment be included as part of the comprehensive care plan for the child with developmental disabilities. Due to the complex and multifactorial aspects of feeding, it is recommended that an interdisciplinary team approach be used to fully assess feeding concerns/abilities for the adolescent with developmental disabilities. The team should include professionals experienced in the assessment of the following areas:

1. Oral-motor and swallowing function (speech/language therapist, occupational or physical therapist with a specialty in oral-motor functioning)
2. Optimum positioning for enhancement of oral-motor control (physical therapist, occupational therapist)

3. Needs for adaptive feeding equipment to meet oral-motor and self-feeding goals (occupational therapist, physical therapist)

4. Dietary modifications and supplements to meet nutritional requirements for optimal growth (dietitian, nurse, physician)

5. Knowledge of actual or potential impact that current medical status may have on intake and growth (physician, nurse)

6. Behavioral and psychosocial factors that impact feeding (psychologist, nurse)

The use of a comprehensive interdisciplinary team in assessing nutrition has been previously described.[8] Given the multiple factors that impact the health, growth, and nutrition of individuals with developmental disabilities, the use of a team approach is not only beneficial, but essential.

Specific Disabilities and Nutritional Status

Autism.   A developmental disorder characterized by a severe impairment of language, communication, and social skills. Ritualistic and obsessive/compulsive behavior is frequently seen. In one study, the overall adequacy of diets of 40 children with autism and 34 controls was similar when compared by a 7-d diet history; children with autism had greater intake of all nutrients with the exception of vitamins A and C, and fat; a higher incidence of food cravings and pica was seen in the children with autism.[17] Some children with autism also show significant texture/temperature/food preferences.[18]

Because of the occasional bizarre behavior of individuals with autism, nutritional concerns should be anticipated. One case report described an 8-year-old boy with autism who ate only French fried potatoes and water for several years.[19] He developed an abnormal gait and periorbital swelling with hypocalcemia and radiographic evidence of rickets consistent with vitamin A and D deficiency. Close attention to eating dysfunction in autism can avert serious nutritional deficiencies. Nutrition evaluation is warranted with consideration of multivitamin and mineral supplements, especially if eating habits result in the exclusion of entire food groups.

Epilepsy.   Common in persons with developmental disabilities and may occur at any time. Adolescence, in general, is associated with an elevated risk of onset of epilepsy. Seizures, when severe or frequent, can interrupt the intake of food, resulting in decreased nutrient intake, which can potentially impair growth and health. The child could also be at risk for aspiration if seizures occur during mealtimes.

The side-effects of anticonvulsant medications exert a profound effect on nutritional status. Nearly all anticonvulsants disturb vitamin D metabolism[20] and some increase the need for folic acid.[21] Adolescents receiving anticonvulsants should consume foods high in vitamin D, i.e., milk, sardines, and salmon. It is important to note that milk products such as yogurt and cheese are not fortified with vitamin D. Therefore, if milk intake is low, supplementation with a multivitamin is recommended. A multivitamin containing folic acid should be given with phenobarbital daily. Gum hyperplasia is seen with phenytoin and this can lead to periodontal disease, chewing difficulties, as well as poor lip closure resulting in loss of food and/or fluids. Carbamazepine and valproic acid can cause nausea, vomiting, abdominal pain, diarrhea or constipation, decreased appetite and dry mouth.

Attention-deficit hyperactivity disorder. Affects about 10% of school-aged children and is manifested by a short attention span, distractibility, fidgetiness, and impulsivity. This can impact the individual's ability to sit for a meal long enough to consume an adequate intake. Methylphenidate and dextroamphetamine are common medication treatments and can also impact intake by suppressing appetite. Dosing with a meal instead of before a meal minimizes appetite suppression. A child's height and weight should be followed carefully while on these medications so as to minimize drug effects on growth. If the adolescent begins to fall off the weight curve, an alternative medication such as a tricyclic antidepressant may be helpful. If medication cannot be substituted, drug "holidays" over weekends or other times when school is out of session may be helpful.

Behavior disorders. Adolescence is a time when behavior disorders may become apparent in children with developmental disabilities. At times, the behavior disorder itself may directly affect,nutrition with the adolescent either demanding or refusing food. A team approach to assessment of the behavior is necessary,including: (1) a medical assessment to rule out an emerging endocrine, psychiatric, or neurological disorder; (2) psychological evaluation to determine antecedents and consequences of behavior; (3) nutritional assessment to evaluate intake, actual nutrient requirements, and growth; and (4) family assessment to examine caretaker considerations.

Common behavioral treatment for adolescents with developmental disabilities may include either using food as a reinforcer or withholding food for medical or therapeutic reasons. Careful monitoring of parameters such as the adolescent's nutritional and dental status is necessary.

Psychotropic medications are used commonly in this population and have direct effects on nutrition. Neuroleptic medications (major tranquilizers) are associated with an increase in appetite and can lead to a weight gain of more than 100 lb. Many antidepressant medications are associated with constipation and anorexia. When in doubt, the drug insert should be consulted for potential side-effects.

Cerebral palsy. A nonprogressive motor impairment due to an injury to the developing brain. Spastic cerebral palsy involving one or more limbs is most common. Choreoathetosis (constant uncoordinated movements) is also seen. Associated problems affecting food intake include positional or motor difficulties, abnormal reflexes, pseudobulbar palsy, and seizures. Positional or motor difficulties occur when the child may not be able to feed him- or herself due to muscle tone abnormalities.[22] In addition, arching of the back is frequently seen. Scoliosis is common and can also significantly complicate optimal positioning for feeding. Abnormal reflexes occur due to the persistence of primitive reflexes such as an asymmetric tonic neck reflex or tongue thrusting that impairs intake. A hyperactive gag reflex can also impair swallowing and cause choking or vomiting. Pseudobulbar palsy refers to a lack of coordination of the muscles of the face and mouth that leads to swallowing difficulties and poor oral-motor control, especially drooling. Finally, seizure disorders are common if the child has spastic quadriplegia, i.e., tight muscles in all four extremities. Seizures can impair food intake by interrupting the alertness required for safe feeding and thus increase the risk of aspiration. Moreover, appetite can be decreased.

Growth failure is common in adolescents with cerebral palsy due to the frequent incidence of feeding difficulties and increased caloric needs of children with hypertonia. Severe malnutrition can also impair sexual maturation.[23] However, growth failure can be prevented when nutritional interventions occur early in the course of recovery. According to Sanders et al.,[24] "Children who were within one year of their injury evidenced an 82% average weight gain over a six-month period when given supplemental feeds, enterally if necessary; children between one and eight years of their injury evidenced a lesser response; children more than eight years beyond their injury evidenced little objective or subjective gain with supplemental feeds." It is therefore unlikely that growth failure will reverse in an adolescent with cerebral palsy. However, sexual maturation can be attained with proper nutritional support.

Dysphagia.   Difficulty with intake, chewing, and swallowing, or dysphagia can be due to pseudobulbar palsy in persons with cerebral palsy and can be seen in people with less severe neuromuscular disorders. A video fluoroscopic swallowing study is used to assess dysphagia and the safety of oral intake. Common criteria for referral for a comprehensive feeding and swallowing evaluation are found in Table 16.4. Recommendations regarding feeding position, food bolus size, and food consistency can then be made to optimize safe and efficient oral intake.

Duchenne muscular dystrophy.   A degenerative muscle disease only occurring in males. The natural history of the nutritional status of boys with Duchenne muscular dystrophy has been studied.[25] Obesity may occur from the age of 7 yr and it becomes quite common by early adolescence. Undernutrition occurs due to loss of oral-motor skills associated with muscle weakness, affecting

Table 16.4   Referral Criteria for Feeding and Swallowing Evaluation

An evaluation should be considered if the child shows any of the following conditions:
Child chokes, coughs, or gulps when eating or immediately after eating
Food remains in the mouth after the child has swallowed
Child has difficulty initiating a swallow
Child swallows repeatedly to clear food
History of chronic lung difficulties
Secretions build up during or shortly after feeding
Large amounts of oral secretions
Difficulty in gaining weight or weight loss
Aspiration
Head and neck anatomical abnormalities
Food suctioned out of the tracheostomy tube
Hoarseness or change in voice
Safety of introducing a new food texture is questioned

From L. Ernest and R. J. Young, in *Nutr. Focus*, **8**, 4 (1993). Reprinted with permission.

the majority of teens by 18 yr of age. Willig's study confirms the accuracy of a Duchenne muscular dystrophy ideal-weight chart.[26]

Mental retardation.   Commonly defined as having an intelligence quotient of less than 70 and corresponding deficits in adaptive behavior. There are various causes for mental retardation and most do not carry nutritional implications. Congenital infections causing mental retardation or prenatal toxins such as alcohol usually involve growth failure. Metabolic disturbances or enzyme deficiencies may necessitate a special diet.

It is estimated that 85% of individuals with mental retardation are living in the community, either in the parental home, group homes or variably supervised apartments. In a comparative study of the nutritional habits of persons with mental retardation, it was found that the diet adequacy scores of residents in an intermediate care facility were significantly higher than those of residents in group homes.[27] The authors also noted that 64% of the meals individually selected and prepared by residents in group homes consisted of foods from two or fewer food groups. Clearly, nutritional counselling is needed in group homes to increase a wider variety of food choices.

One problem seen in adolescents with mental retardation is rumination syndrome. This is a behavioral disorder where there is frequent regurgitation of previously ingested food into the mouth where it is chewed and either reswallowed or spit out. It occurs more commonly in persons who are institutionalized and has been reported in up to 10% of these patients. The behavior has been known to occur up to 100 times/d and is not always associated with mealtime. Physical causes such as gastroesophageal reflux and hiatal hernia must be suspected and investigated before treatment of the behavior. In addition, rumination can be seen in psychiatric disorders such as depression and/or epilepsy. Successful treatment of rumination will vary depending on the underlying cause.[28]

MANAGEMENT

Attention-Deficit Hyperactivity Disorder

In 1973, the Feingold diet was proposed to treat attention-deficit hyperactivity disorder, at that time called hyperkinesis. Low-molecular-weight chemicals were thought to cause hyperkinesis and the diet consisted of fresh meats, milk, vegetables, and homemade products and was low in salicylates and food additives. Food flavoring and food colors were to be avoided. The National Advisory Committee on Hyperkinesis and Food Additives of the Nutrition Foundation later found evidence to refute the claim that artificial food colorings, artificial flavors, and natural salicylates produce hyperactivity.[29] Thus, this diet has since been abandoned as a treatment. Another popular therapy for attention deficit hyperactivity disorder was massive doses of vitamins or orthomolecular therapy. In a placebo-controlled study of the use of megavitamins for minimal brain dysfunction, another term for attention-deficit hyperactivity disorder, no significant difference was found between placebo and vitamin groups.[30]

In 1994, a double-blind controlled trial found that diets high in sucrose did not affect children's behavior or cognitive functioning.[31] This same study also reported that diets high in aspartame also had no effect.

Autism

Niacin and vitamin B-6 have long been thought to have psychoactive properties. Vitamin B-6 continues to demonstrate effectiveness in a small percentage of patients with epilepsy. A review article examined 53 controlled studies on the effects of niacin, vitamin B-6, and multivitamins on the mental functioning of persons with a variety of diagnoses such as hyperactivity, Down syndrome, schizophrenia, and autism.[32] Only in children with autism were rare positive results found and these were associated with very high dosages of vitamin B-6 combined with magnesium. However, further evidence of efficacy is necessary before the use of high doses of individual nutrients can be supported as a treatment for people with autism. However, supplementation with a general multivitamin may be necessary for individuals with restrictive diet preferences. Behavior management strategies may be necessary for those with autism who have dangerously restrictive diet preferences.

Mental Retardation and Fragile X Syndrome

Adolescents with mental retardation have been assisted in their ability to learn by the use of behavior management therapy. This therapeutic approach may require the use of reinforcers and frequently food is used, such as candy and fruit. Although these food items may be quite powerful in modifying the adolescent's behavior, they can negatively impact on nutrition (weight gain, interference with more nutritious food intake, constant stomach acid secretion) and dental care (cavities).

The use of folic acid as a therapy for people with mental retardation became especially popular after it was discovered in the 1970s that fragile X syndrome could be diagnosed when chromosomes were grown in a medium deficient in folate. Fragile X syndrome accounted for many cases of mental retardation heretofore unexplained in males. In a review of 15 studies on the effect of folic acid in people with developmental disabilities or fragile X syndrome, only in prepubertal boys with fragile X syndrome was folic acid found to have some positive effect.[33] However, the number of subjects was so small that no conclusions about efficacy could be drawn. As in the case of autism and vitamin B-6, further evidence of efficacy is needed before any dietary supplements can be recommended for people with mental retardation or fragile X syndrome.

Seizures

Nutritional therapy for seizures in severe cases of intractable seizures has included the use of a ketogenic diet. Ketosis has an anticonvulsant effect. Use of medium-chain triglycerides (MCT) in the diet can lead to reduction or discontinuation of anticonvulsant medications.[34] However, compliance with the diet may be poor due to the unpleasant taste of some of the dietary components containing MCT oil. Because of this, there has been modification of the ketogenic diet that uses heavy cream in place of the MCT oil. In addition, the high level of MCT oil causes diarrhea in some individuals. Because of the dietary restrictions inherent in the ketogenic diet, multivitamin supplementation is essential. A detailed protocol for dietary management of the ketogenic diet is available.[35]

Magnesium therapy can sometimes improve seizure control. In a survey of 79 people with epilepsy and developmental disabilities, the authors measured serum magnesium levels.[36] Three people were noted to have a low level of magnesium associated with malabsorption or hyponatremia and were started on a replacement regimen of oral magnesium. The authors noted a significant improvement in seizure control attributed to treatment with oral magnesium.

Enteral Feeding

Enteral feeding refers to the use of tubes to bypass the oral route for nutrient and fluid intake. Adolescents with developmental disabilities often have difficulty maintaining adequate growth and nutritional status, as well as fluid requirements, by oral intake alone. Inadequate intake may be due to oral-motor difficulties resulting in food and/or fluid losses; decreased stamina for feeding due to increased cardio/respiratory, and/or motor effort required for feeding; and/or increased requirements combined with either oral motor difficulties or decreased stamina. For adolescents with these difficulties, support with a supplemental enteral feeding to help meet requirements for growth and adequate nutrition is indicated. In addition to weight gain and improved growth, improved nutritional status will result in better immune function and resistance to infection, increased energy level, and often decreased irritability. Supplemental feeding can also help alleviate constipation difficulties by providing adequate fluid intake. For some children at risk for choking or aspiration, i.e., those with dysphagia, tube feeding also provides a safer means of intake rather than oral feeding.

Enteral feeding includes the intermittent use of a naso-gastric tube or surgically placed gastrostomy or jejunostomy tubes that can permanently bypass the oral route. These procedures can be accomplished either with or without a fundoplication, a procedure that involves wrapping of the upper portion of the stomach. A fundoplication helps avoid gastro-esophageal reflux if it is present or becomes a problem after a tube is placed. The percutaneously placed gastrostomy has recently become a common means of achieving enteral feeding without the significant risk associated with surgically placed gastrostomies.

The decision to use enteral feeding is complex and often associated with uncertainty as to the potential benefits and harm. In order to counsel patients as to the use of enteral feeding, a number of issues must be reviewed (see Table 16.5).[37]

The choice of which type of supplemental feeding method to use depends on various factors including expected length of time that supplemental feeds will be required. Generally, oro- or naso-gastric tubes are used for short-term nutritional support, as long-term use of these tubes can adversely affect oral feeding by causing the development of oral aversion or esophageal irritation, making oral intake uncomfortable or even painful. Gastrostomy or jejunostomy tubes are

Table 16.5   Criteria for Consideration of Enteral Feeding in Children

1. Unable to meet 80% of caloric needs by mouth
2. No weight gain or weight loss for 3 mo
3. Weight/height ratio less than 5th percentile
4. Triceps skinfold less than 5th percentile for age
5. Total feeding time greater than 4–6 h/d

From Smith B and A. Pederson A., in *Nutr. Focus*, **5**, 5 (1990). Reprinted with permission.

used for longer-term supplemental feeding. See Table 16.6 for alternatives of delivery site.

Absolute indications for tube feeding may include severe oro-facial anomalies, uncorrected tracheo-esophageal fistula, or the absence of gag and other protective reflexes, as well as recurrent aspiration pneumonias. Several studies may be helpful prior to instituting enteral feeding.[38] An upper GI barium contrast study can rule out esophageal stricture, hiatal hernia, gastric outlet obstruction, and malrotation. Prolonged (24 h) esophageal pH monitoring has evolved as a standard for diagnosing gastroesophageal reflux. Upper endoscopy is done when poor appetite, excessive irritability with posturing, and hematemesis suggest esophagitis.

A common reason for starting enteral feeds would be poor fluid intake. Frequently, oral-motor skills are better for solids than liquids. Over time and

Table 16.6 Delivery Sites for Enteral Nutrition

Site	Advantages	Disadvantages	Physical Complications
Nasogastric	Surgery not required, short-term.	Nasal, esophageal, or tracheal irritation. May interfere with breathing.	Vomiting, reflux, delayed gastric emptying. Delay of oral-motor skills.
Gastrostomy	More stable. Greater patient mobility. More physiologic. Large tubes for viscous formulas. Doesn't interfere with breathing. Long-term. Able to continue oral food intake.	Surgery required. Local skin care is required. More equipment is required.	Risk of intraabdominal leakage with petitonitis.
Jejunal	Bypasses the stomach and pylorus, helpful for gastric reflux, delayed emptying, or hypomotility. Decreased risk of aspiration. Able to continue oral food intake.	Requires continuous drip feeds. Surgery required. May require elemental formula.	Distention, diarrhea, tube displacement.

From Smith B and A. Pederson , in *Nutr. Focus,* **5,** 5 (1990). Reprinted with permission.

especially during illness, poor fluid intake can affect hydration status. Constipation and urinary tract infections may occur as a result of inadequate hydration. Enteral supplementation of fluids can greatly improve dehydration symptoms during an acute illness.

Severe gastro-esophageal reflux and aspiration products can be a reason to bypass the lower esophageal sphincter by fundoplication of the stomach with a gastrostomy tube or jejunal tube feeding. Formula or fluid can be delivered either by bolus (intermittent) or continuous administration. See Table 16.7 for advantages and disadvantages of each route.

The choice of formula will depend on several factors including calorie, protein and nutrient requirements, fluid volume restrictions, volume tolerance, fiber requirements, and potential diet intolerances, i.e., milk protein intolerance or malabsorption concerns. The price of formula may also be a factor as well as parent preference (e.g., use of a "whole food" formula or even puréed food vs. a "synthetic" formula). Adult formulas are generally used for adolescents. There are multiple types of formulas available on the market today, allowing for greater choice and flexibility in selecting a formula to meet the specific needs of the individual.

Complications.   Although enteral feeds can vastly improve nutritional status and allow for the administration of life-saving fluid, some grave complications must be considered. In a large study of persons receiving services from the California Department of Developmental Services,[39] it was demonstrated that

Table 16.7   Administration of Formulas

Method	Advantages	Disadvantages
Bolus (intermittent). 4–8 times/d, lasting 15–45 min.	Physiologic, mimics normal feedings. Do not need pump. Allows freedom of movement/breaks from feeding.	Increased risk of aspiration. Poor tolerance of volume, may not be recomended with reflux, vomiting, or delayed gastric emptying.
Continuous. Given over 12–24 h.	Maximal nutrient absorption. Improved tolerance. Allows increased amount of formula to be given. Can be given at night while child sleeps. Recommended for jejunal feeds.	Requires pump, bag, and tubing. Child is tied to feeding equipment.

From Smith B and A. Pederson, in *Nutr. Focus*, **5**, 5 (1990). Reprinted with permission.

the presence of a feeding tube significantly increased the rate of mortality rate. This phenomenon may have been caused by overfeeding, which subsequently led to increased rates of aspiration pneumonia. In addition, the fundoplication procedure did not seem to reduce the risk of aspiration following placement of a gastrostomy for this population. Again, feeding techniques should be examined.

The method of formula administration also impacts the tolerance of enteral feedings. Rapid administration of formula can increase the risk of complications. Nausea and vomiting can occur. Frequently, the patient is nonverbal and cannot communicate the discomfort associated with rapid feeding. If green bile appears in vomitus, a small bowel obstruction may be present due to migration of the feeding tube. Placement of a tube that cannot migrate or a "button/stomate" device that keeps the gastrostomy site open for the administration of an external tube should be used. Tube placement should be checked prior to administration of each enteral feeding by listening to the infiltration of air.

Diarrhea can occur with too rapid enteral feeding as well as a hyperosmolar cold formula. It may also be an indicator of lactose or protein intolerance. Considerations of enteral feeding administration are listed in Table 16.8.

Excessive gas in the stomach or intestine can contribute to feeding intolerance. It may be due to swallowed air, forced air such as with CPAP (continuous positive airway pressure) or gas as an abnormal biproduct of digestion. The stomach should be emptied of air prior to administration of an enteral feed by venting the G-tube 10–15 min before each feeding. Some patients find that the administration of an antiflatulent prior to each feeding may reduce distention. Swallowing of mucus can also interfere with enteral feeding and the stomach should be emptied of mucus prior to feeding.

Constipation may occur as a complication of enteral feeding due to inadequate fluid or fiber intake. The fiber content of the formula administered should be

Table 16.8 Considerations for Enteral Feeding

Speed of administration (bolus, continuous)
Gravity vs. pump administation
Timing
Portability of feeding apparatus
Osmolarity of formula
Fiber content
Protein base
Carbohydrate base
Temperature of formula
Expiration of date of formula
Amount of concomitant water administration
Client preference
Caretaker preference

examined with supplementation if necessary. Also, concomitant water or other fluid intake should be examined and increased if necessary.

Delayed gastric emptying time can lead to prolonged residual of the enteral feed in the stomach. Modification of the amount or timing of the feed may then be necessary. The side-effects of concomitant medications should be examined. Medications to accelerate gastric emptying may be required. Fat content of formula should also be evaluated, as a high fat content in formula can also affect gastric emptying time.

A clogged feeding tube can be an irritating complication of enteral feeds. Frequently, this is due to medication administration rather than formula complications, notably, vitamins with minerals or other hard-to-crush medications. Formulas that have been supplemented with additional fiber may also clog tubes. All fiber-containing formulas should be well shaken before administration. Some have found diet ginger ale flushes to be useful in alleviating tube clogging, but corrosion of the tube should be monitored.

Leakage around the stoma site is common. This can lead to skin irritation, skin ulceration and granuloma formation. Changing the gastrostomy tube to a new one or larger size may help. Placement of a button/stomate device can eliminate the irritation of a long tube against the skin.

As mentioned earlier, gastroesophageal reflux leading to aspiration pneumonia is the most serious complication of enteral feeding. In general, it is recommended that the individual be kept upright with head and trunk at 30–45 deg for at least 20 min after a feeding to help prevent reflux. Placement of a gastrostomy tube can precipitate gastroesophageal reflux. In one study, 44% of patients who had a negative preoperative evaluation for reflux developed reflux after a gastrostomy tube was placed without fundoplication.[40] Incompetence of the lower esophageal sphincter is usually the cause, but an ineffective fundoplication of the stomach may also lead to reflux. As a result of these concerns, the percutaneous gastrostomy has emerged as a popular surgical procedure for the delivery of enteral feeding. However, in a study comparing percutaneous gastrojejunostomy against gastrostomy and Nissen fundoplication in children with gastroesophageal reflux, children who underwent a percutaneous procedure had higher rates of major complications, minor complications, and mortality.[41]

Enteral feeds provide the opportunity for significant caloric and nutrient administration. Prevention of excessive weight gain following the initiation of enteral feeding is essential. Excessive weight gain can strain other organ systems. For example, the pulmonary system must provide more oxygenation for the added weight and the skeletal system may be stressed so that scoliosis or other deformities may develop. Careful monitoring of weight gain to accommodate linear growth, if the child has not reached puberty, is necessary.

Enteral feeds and oral feeds.   Oral feeding can be combined with enteral feeding if it has been determined to be medically safe. There should be careful adjustment of enteral caloric intake to accommodate the oral intake. Oral intake should be offered first during a mealtime, with subsequent enteral supplementation. If oral feeding is unsafe, due to dysphagia and/or aspiration, the implementation of an oral motor stimulation program is recommended to help minimize oral motor defensiveness or aversion that frequently occurs in the prolonged absence of oral feedings. Early initiation of an oral-motor stimulation program is important for maximizing success. Oral-motor stimulation programs may include "tastes" of foods and flavors such as licks from a popsicle or lollipop with close supervision, oral-motor play with textured toys, with a nuk brush or toothette. The oral-motor stimulation program should be done with music or as a game to make it more enjoyable. Finally, a feeding program should be developed by a therapist with experience in oral-motor stimulation and feeding techniques.

CASE ILLUSTRATION

Kate was a normal, healthy baby until 8 mo of age, at which time crawling behavior stopped. Kate had been self-feeding biscuits and assisting with a spoon, but by 12 mo, she lost these skills and would only hold her bottle at times. In the next year of life, Kate's parents took her to many doctors until finally a diagnosis of Rett syndrome was made. Her growth was appropriate for age.

Kate subsequently developed a seizure disorder at the age of 4 yr and had an episode of aspiration during a seizure that required hospitalization for pneumonia. At that time, she was showing typical hand-wringing behavior and little purposeful movement of the hands was seen.

After her hospitalization, Kate's weight dropped two percentiles on the growth chart within 6 mo. In general, it took longer to feed Kate as she was alternately irritable and sleeping and sometimes had a seizure during meal time. Seizure medication was changed from phenobarbital to carbamezepine and Kate's irritability decreased, although she was initially very sleepy for 2 wk. With intensive occupational and speech/language feeding therapy, Kate was weaned from a bottle by 5 yr of age and was able to drink from a cup and use a straw with assistance. By this time, she could stand but not walk independently. Some muscle spasticity was present and at 6 yr, height and weight slipped well below the fifth percentile.

By the age of 9 yr, Kate's oral-motor skills deteriorated and she was constantly drooling. At times, she had bouts of hyperventilation and she frequently had aspiration episodes due to an abnormal breathing pattern. She had 10 hospitalizations by the time she was 14-years-old because of respiratory problems and aspiration pneumonia. Signs of puberty were absent. By this time, Kate was totally dependent for all activities of daily living and was listless in interactions. A feeding team evaluation found her to be undernourished and it was determined that Kate should have a G-tube inserted. Tastes of food could be continued to maintain oral-motor experiences. A 24-h pH probe study indicated that a fundoplication would be necessary to prevent gastroesophageal reflux. Parents initially refused any surgery and some family members thought that tube feeding would just prolong Kate's life. However, parents did agree to naso-gastric feeds. She received Ensure by continuous drip from 8 P.M to 8 A.M at 125 cc/h. Stools, which had been hard, continued so and formula was switched to Ensure with fiber and external water was given by bolus. Parents were pleased with a weight gain of 10 lb in 2 mo and an increased alertness. The weight gain proved too excessive for Kate's lungs, and she required a hospitalization for oxygen. Her feeds were adjusted to maintain weight until Kate was proportional to her height. The tube dislodged frequently, especially during seizures, which were becoming more frequent. Parents agreed to a percutaneous G-tube, but did not allow a fundoplication, as one doctor thought that it may not even help Kate's reflux, which was medically treated with an antacid. A percutaneous gastrostomy was done and continuous night-time feeds were actually continued the next day. Kate had an episode of bilious vomiting 1 mo after the gastrostomy and it was determined that the G-tube had migrated and obstructed her duodenum. A gastrostomy button was placed, which also lessened skin breakdown around the site.

After her G-tube feeds were started, Kate became more interactive and attentive in therapy sessions. In addition, pubertal changes became evident 11 mo after tube feedings were started.

REFERENCES

1. J. H. Rimmer, D. Braddock, and G. Fujiura, *Am. J. Ment. Retard.*, **98**, 510 (1994).

2. A. Dikovics, ed., *Nutritional Assessment Case Studies*, George F. Stickley Co., Philadelphia, PA (1987).

3. P. Pipes, ed., *Nutrition in Infancy and Childhood*, Times Mirror/Mosby Publishing Co., St. Louis, MO (1989).

4. A. R. Frischanco, *Am. J. Clin. Nutr.*, **34**, 2540 (1981).

5. W. Culley and T. Middleton, *J. Peds.*, **75**, 380 (1969).

6. W. Culley, *J. Peds.*, **66**, 772 (1965).

7. L. Bandini, D. Schoeller, N. Fukagawa, L. Wykes, and W. Dietz, *Ped. Res.*, **29**, 70 (1991).

8. K. A. Pesce, L. A. Wodarski, and M. Wang, *Res. Develop. Disab.*, **10**, 33 (1989).

9. S. Ekvall, ed., *Pediatric Nutrition in Chronic Disease and Developmental Disorders*, Oxford University Press, New York (1993).

10. Q. Spender, C. Cronk, B. Charney, and V. Stallings, *Develop. Med. Child Neurol.*, **31**, 206, (1990).

11. J. Krick, P. Murphy, J. Markham, B. Schapiro, *Develop. Med. Child Neurol.*, **34**, 481 (1992).

12. J. K. Nelson, K. Moxness, C. F. Gastineau, and M. D. Jensen, eds., *Mayo Clinic Diet Manual: A Handbook of Dietary Practices*, VII ed., C. V. Mosby, St. Louis, MO (1994).

13. P. Kreuther, ed., *Nutrition in Perspective*, Prentice Hall, Englewood Cliffs, NJ (1980).

14. H. Cloud and J. Bergman, *Nutr. Focus*, **6**, 1 (1991).

15. C. Griggs, P. Jones, and R. Lee, *Develop. Med. Child Neurol.*, **31**, 303 (1989).

16. T. E. Shaddix, *Nutr. Focus*, **6**, 2, (1991).

17. D. J. Raiten and T. Massaro, *J. Autism Develop. Dis.*, **16**, 133 (1986).

18. M. Coleman, *Infants Young Child.*, **1**, 22 (1989).

19. J. H. Clark, D. K. Rhoden, and D. S. Turner, *J. Parenteral Enteral Nutr.*, **17**, 284 (1983).

20. J. Silver, T. J. Davies, E. Kupersmitt, M. Orme, A. Petrie, and F. Vajda, *Arch. Dis. Child.*, **49**, 344 (1974).

21. J. R. Moore and E. W. Ball, *Arch. Dis. Child.*, **49**, 344 (1974).

22. L. H. Ernst and R. J. Young, *Nutr. Focus*, **8**, 4 (1993).

23. T. Feigelman, R. E. Frisch, M. MacBurney, and D. Wilmore, *J. Peds.*, **111**, 620 (1987).

24. K. Sanders, K. Cox, and R. Cannon, *J. Parenteral and Enteral Nutr.*, **14**, 23 (1990).

25. T. N. Willig, L. Carlier, M. Legrand, H. Riviere, and J. Navarro, *Develop. Med. Child Neurol.*, **35**, 1074 (1993).

26. R. D. Griffiths and R.H.T. Edwards, *Arch. of Dis. Child.*, **63**, 1256 (1988).

27. K. C. Mercer and S. W. Ekvall, *J. Am. Diet. Assoc.*, **92**, 356 (1992).

28. W. E. Whitehead, V. M. Drescher, E. Morrill-Corbin, and M. F. Cataldo, *J. Ped. Gastoenterol. Nutr.*, **4**, 550 (1985).

29. National Advisory Committee on Hyperkinesis and Food Additives, *Final Report to the Nutrition Foundation*, Nutrition Foundation, New York (1980).

30. L. E. Arnold, J. Christopher, R. D. Heustis, and D. J. Smeltzer, *JAMA*, **240**, 2642 (1978).

31. M. L. Wolraich, S. D. Lindgren, P. J. Stumbo, L. D. Stegink, M. I. Appelbaum, and M. C. Kiritsy, *N. Engl. J. Med.*, **330**, 301 (1994).

32. J. Kleijnen and P. Knigschild, *Biol. Psych.*, **29**, 931 (1991).

33. M. Aman and R. Kern, *J. Child Adol. Psychopharmacol.*, **1**, 285 (1990/1991).

34. D. A. Trauner, *Neurology*, **35**, 237 (1985).

35. J. Freeman, M. Kelly, and J. Freeman, *Epilepsy Diet Treatment*, Demos Publication, New York, (1994).

36. M. Vacanti, O. Merveille, J. Smart, and S. Sone, *Ment. Retard.*, **29**, 363 (1991).

37. B. C. Smith and A. L. Pederson, *Nutr. Focus*, **5**, 5 (1990).

38.   J. T. Boyle, *Ped. Surg.*, **6,** 76 (1991).

39.   H. Bui, C. V. Dang, R. Chaney, and L. Vergara, *Am. J. Ment. Retard.*, **94**, 16 (1989).

40.   J. L. Langer, D. E. Wesson, S. H. Ein, R. M. Filler, B. Shandling, R. A. Superina, and M. Papa, *J. Ped. Gastroenterol.*, **7**, 837 (1988).

41.   C. T. Albanese, R. B. Towbin, I. Ulman, J. Lewis, and S. Smith, *J. Peds.*, **123**, 371 (1993).

CHRONIC DISEASE

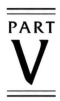

PART
V

Nutrition in the Primary Care Setting

Ellen S. Rome, M.D., M.P.H.,
Isabel M. Vazquez, M.S., R.D., and
Elizabeth R. Woods, M.D., M.P.H.

INTRODUCTION

Adolescence represents a period of physical, cognitive, and emotional changes in which the teenager gradually separates from the family and develops a sense of identity. Physically, as the teen progresses through puberty, he or she is faced with significant body changes, early on raising the question of "Am I normal?" Later, the questions change to a more external focus, with "Am I liked?" and "Am I loved?" Subjected to media imagery of "the perfect physique," peer pressure, and the influence of parents, teachers, or other adults, teenagers may manifest concerns over nutritional issues. Besides being of subjective importance to the teenager, nutrition plays a key role in growth and development and has been shown to aid in modulation of the immune system and the prevention of chronic diseases.[1-3] The primary care provider and dietitian can use the ambulatory office visit with the adolescent as a window of opportunity in which to anticipate, educate, and intervene with respect to nutritional choices, issues of both malnutrition and obesity, body image, and overall health.

Nutritional assessment and management have come under increasing national scrutiny, with more and more responsibility placed on the primary care clinician in consultation with the dietitian to provide nutritional services and counseling. The U.S. Preventive Medicine Task Force's *Guide to Clinical Preventive Services*[4] and the U.S. Department of Health and Human Services' *Healthy People 2000*[5] emphasize the need to improve the nutritional status of all Americans during the next decade. In the latter initiative, 21 of 298 objectives relate to nutrition, with the goals of health promotion through primary prevention and treatment of health problems. The American Medical Association has also put forth nutritional recommendations in its Guidelines for Adolescent Preventive Services (GAPS).[6] In GAPS, recommendations detail the need for annual guidance on dietary habits and safe weight management; emphasize the need for annual guidance on regular exercise; address hypertension; tackle hyperlipidemia and risks of adult coronary heart disease; and outline annual screening for eating disorders and obesity. Thus, the idea that nutrition affects the health of all patients from adolescence through adulthood is emphasized. Moreover, primary care providers can help their patients establish healthy behaviors at multiple points on this timeline.

ASSESSMENT

Obtaining a Nutritional History

The goal of the dietitian in obtaining a nutritional history is to identify problems that warrant further evaluation to educate teens and their parents regarding normal nutrition. Teens, as a group, are at high risk for nutritional problems. As adolescents spend more time outside of the home and away from the family dinner table, food choices frequently change. Featured prominently are items from vending machines, fast-food restaurants, concessions at movies or sporting events, and microwavable meals.[7]

Several studies have examined the nutritional choices and dietary behaviors of adolescents. The National Adolescent Students Health Survey (NASHS) analyzed questionnaires from 11,419 eighth and tenth grade students. Breakfast was eaten less than or equal to 2 d in the past week by 32% of the boys and 48% of the girls. Fried foods were consumed at least once a day by 18%. In the year prior to the survey, 61% of the girls and 28% of the boys had tried to lose weight. Of these, 16% had tried diet pills, 12% tried vomiting to lose weight, and 8% used laxatives.[8] In a study of urban, suburban, and rural high school students, laxatives (10% vs. 3%) and diuretics (5% vs. 2%) were used more frequently by African American girls than Caucasian girls. Vomiting was more commonly reported by Caucasian girls, with 8% vomiting monthly, as compared to only 1% of African American girls.[9] In a Minnesota study,[10] chronic dieting was reported in 12.1% of the girls and 2.1% of the boys, with no differences among urban, suburban, or rural Caucasian youth. Chronic dieters were more likely to report unhealthy weight-loss techniques, including self-induced vomiting and the use of laxatives, ipecac, or diuretics. Story et al.[10] conclude that chronic dieting may serve as a useful screen for unhealthy eating behavior or early eating disorders.

In obtaining a dietary history from the adolescent, the clinical dietitian begins with simple questions to assess usual intake. Frequency of meals, snacks, and the quantity of food consumed are useful starting points. Does the teen usually skip breakfast, lunch, or dinner? Does he or she eat a bagel on the run, or grab a quick lunch at McDonald's? Will he or she eat food from the school cafeteria? Also, where is the food consumed? Does the teen eat while performing other activities, i.e., watching television, at work, while walking to school? Does the teen eat alone, with family, or with peers? In what settings?

The dietitian can try to assess dietary intake by the method of 24-h recall. Although this technique is popular and easy to perform, its validity has been questioned.[11,12] Moreover, teens may not accurately remember what they ate or be embarrassed to admit to consumption of perceived nonnutritious foods. The previous day's meals may not be "typical"; just as adolescents tend to floss more the week before they see the dentist, the teen may eat in a more healthy fashion prior to visiting his or her clinician.

Another method of collecting nutritional data involves having the teen keep a food record for at least 3 d. Specific instructions on how to complete a food record usually improve the accuracy of the information. Ideally, the patient should quantify the food using standard measuring tools, such as in tablespoons or cups, to avoid misinterpretation resulting from measuring "by the mouthful." The patient should record food intake immediately after eating. Quality of the diet can be assessed by examining the amount and type of dairy products, fruits and vegetables, sources of protein, and junk foods recorded.

Several problems with this technique are immediately apparent. First, this method requires more time, understanding, and motivation on the part of the adolescent. Second, compliance can be an issue, as teens may forget to record information on foods consumed or may not wish to draw attention to themselves after mealtimes, especially in the presence of friends and/or family. Some patients will underestimate the amounts consumed, intentionally or unintentionally. In some instances, the desire to please the clinical dietitian or nutritionist will cause the teen to either avoid eating certain foods during the recording period or fill out the record incompletely.

The 3-d dietary journal also has its advantages. For patients with bulimia nervosa, the food record may help them identify foods or situations that trigger a binge. With obese patients, the dietary intake may not provide exact quantities, but it can serve as a useful means of information on which to base dietary recommendations. One example would be the observation that the teen consumes three cans of Coke per day; the clinician can suggest substituting diet soda, low-fat milk, or water for the sugar-containing beverage. Guenther[13] found that soft drinks are substituted for milk in many teenage diets and were negatively correlated with appropriate calcium intake. Overconsumption or deficits in protein, fat, iron, calcium, and other essential components can be targeted for change.

A food frequency questionnaire for adolescents has been developed in conjunction with the Bogalusa Heart Study.[14] The questionnaire was devised to provide a reliable and accurate method for describing eating patterns and to relate those patterns to physiologic and behavioral measures.[15] Although useful as a research tool, this method may be too time-consuming for the clinician practicing in an outpatient primary care setting. A shorter, validated screening instrument would be a useful addition. Having obtained a dietary history, the dietitian should screen for disturbances in body image and self-esteem (see Chapter 8 and Table 17.1). Family history of coronary heart disease, diabetes mellitus, hypertension, hypercholesterolemia, and obesity should also be assessed. Asking these questions can help the teen to begin thinking about the relevance of eating behaviors, and education can occur at multiple points in the process. As early-, mid-, and often late-stage adolescents may not have developed the ability for abstract thought, nutritional education should help the patient make direct and tangible changes. Dwelling on the risk of a heart attack at age 60 will have little influence on a 15-year-old in your office. Positive encouragement for small improvements may help the teen to make necessary changes.

Other relevant questions include menstrual history, onset of menarche, regularity of periods, duration of flow, and presence/absence of dysmenorrhea (pain with periods). Menstrual irregularities can be a sign of low and high estrogen states. The former can occur in the context of an eating disorder, with extreme exercise, and with stress.[16,17] Amenorrhea for more than 1 yr in duration can place the teen at risk for osteoporosis and increased risk of fractures.[18–20] In

Table 17.1   Screening Assessment of Body-Image and Self-Esteem

1. Do you feel you are underweight? Overweight? Just right?
2. What weight would you like to be?
3. What is the most you have ever weighed? The least?
4. Often, people would like to change their shapes in some ways. Do you have any "trouble spots" that you would like to change?
5. Do you have any "taboo foods," or foods that you just won't eat (useful in ascertaining whether the patient is consuming inadequate fat, protein, or other essential nutrients)?
6. Do you ever vomit to lose weight? Use laxatives? Ipecac? Diet pills? Diuretics?
7. Do you ever have binges or "pig outs," alone or with friends?
8. How much physical activity do you engage in? How often?
9. How do you feel about yourself?

polycystic ovary syndrome (PCO) and other states of androgen excess, obesity can lead to increased conversion of estrogen to androgens. This shift can result in increased acne, hirsutism, and increasing obesity, with ensuing anxiety to the teenage girl concerned with body image. The health care provider and dietitian should work simultaneously on the nutritional and medical issues.

Many aspects of the physical exam can point the clinician toward detection of underlying disease. Table 17.2 outlines particularly relevant aspects of the physical exam.

Office Tools for Evaluation

Weight. Patients should have their weight taken while in light indoor clothing with shoes off. A platform beam-balance scale can give an accurate estimate to the nearest ¼ pound or 0.1 kg. Patients with a suspected eating disorder should be weighed in a johnnie or hospital gown, as often they may try to manipulate the measured weight. Less sophisticated methods include hiding pennies in a pocket, heavy jewelry, or multiple layers of clothes. More elaborate means include placing weights or coins in various orifices, hiding a purse under the gown, or using a hand "resting" on a counter to apply pressure on the scale.

Height. Best obtained to the nearest ¼ inch using a Holtain stadiometer (Holtain Limited, Crosswell, Crymmych, Pembrokeshire, UK), which consists of a fixed vertical piece attached to the wall, on which rides a movable headboard maintained in a horizontal position, direct-reading dial, and footboard with a heel plate.[21] Since this piece of equipment is expensive, the office practitioner can instead use a meter stick(s) attached to the wall next to a bare floor with a movable headboard positioned perpendicular to the wall. Platform scales with attached sliding stick devices for measuring height are inaccurate and should be avoided. The patient should stand with shoes off and both heels flat and flush against the wall. Eyes should be directed ahead, with eyes and ears forming a horizontal plane. Care should be taken to keep the patient from assuming a lordotic stance, as a falsely low height can result.

Height and weight for age should be plotted on the same growth chart over time in order to highlight patterns of growth. The most commonly used growth charts come from the data collected by the National Center on Health Statistics (NCHS), shown in Figures 17.1 to 17.4. On the NCHS growth charts, the 50th percentile is used as a standard, with percentiles ranging from the 5th–95th percentile. The dietitian must remember that these charts represent cross-sectional data rather than longitudinal assessment of individual patients. Individual growth patterns through puberty follow a slightly different pattern. Tanner and Davies[22] have developed charts that portray height velocity as a function of age for average adolescents, early maturers, and those with delayed puberty. These charts are available form Serono Laboratories, Inc., 280 Pond St., Randolph, MA 02368.

Table 17.2   Aspects of the Physical Exam Useful in Detection of Underlying Disease

Body area	Disease process or missing nutrient
Skin:	
Dryness, flakiness	Hypothyroidism, essential fatty acids
Hyperkeratosis	Vitamin A deficiency
Easy bruising	Vitamin K deficiency
Petechiae	Vitamin C or K deficiency
Pallor	Iron-deficiency anemia
Xanthoma	Hyperlipidemia
Hair:	
Dull, dry, brittle	Protein-calorie malnutrition insufficient fat intake
Nails:	
Brittle, with frayed borders	Malnutrition, iron deficiency, calcium deficiency
Concave or eggshell	Vitamin A deficiency
Lips:	
Angular stomatitis (inflammation at corners of the mouth)	Riboflavin (B-2), niacin (B-3) deficiencies
Cheilosis (reddened lips with fissures at angles)	Riboflavin (B-2), pyridoxine (B-6)
Tongue:	
Glossitis	Niacin (B-3), folic acid, B-12, or B-6 deficiencies
Papillary atrophy	Riboflavin, niacin, folic acid, B-12, or iron deficiencies
Loss of taste	Zinc deficiency
Gums:	
Soft, spongy, or bleeding	Vitamin C deficiency (scurvy)
Teeth:	
Excessive caries	Diet high in refined sugar
Eyes:	
Pale conjunctivae	Anemia (iron, folic acid, B-12)
Bitot's spots (gray, yellow, or white foamy spots on the whites of the eye)	Vitamin A deficiency
Red conjunctivae	Bulimia nervosa (valsalva with emesis)
Cheeks:	
Enlarged parotid glands	Bulimia nervosa, chronic vomiting

continued on next page

Table 17.2 *Continued*

Body area	Disease process or missing nutrient
Thyroid:	
Enlargement	Hypo- or hyperthyroidism, iodine deficiency
Cardiovascular:	
Tachycardia, enlarged heart	Beriberi (vitamin B-1 deficiency), iron, folic acid, B-12 deficiency
Bradycardia, low-voltage ECG	Cardiac muscle wasting or functional hypothy roidism due to anorexia nervosa or other malnourished state
GI:	
Hepatomegaly	Protein-calorie malnutrition
Musculoskeletal:	
Wasting	Protein-calorie malnutrition
tender extremities	Scurvy (vitamin C deficiency)
Neuro:	
Confusion	Thiamine (B-1) deficiency, protein-calorie malnutrition
Peripheral neuropathy	Vitamin E deficiency (liver disease)
General:	
Edema	Protein-calorie malnutrition
Amenorrhea	Malnutrition, stress, intense athletics
Delayed puberty	Malnutrition

Review of the growth chart can alert the clinician to significant trends of weight loss or weight gain, giving clues to underlying disease processes that need to be pursued. Celiac disease, inflammatory bowel disease, hypo- and hyperthyroidism, and other medical disorders can be picked up by the astute clinician even before overt symptomatology has been reported by the patient or family. Ideally, eating disorders should be picked up before gross changes on the growth chart have occurred. All deviations from expected patterns of growth should be investigated, including rapid or significant weight change.

Measurements of Obesity and Overweight for Height

Overweight status can be measured directly or indirectly. "Direct" measures for estimating adiposity include measurement of body density using underwater

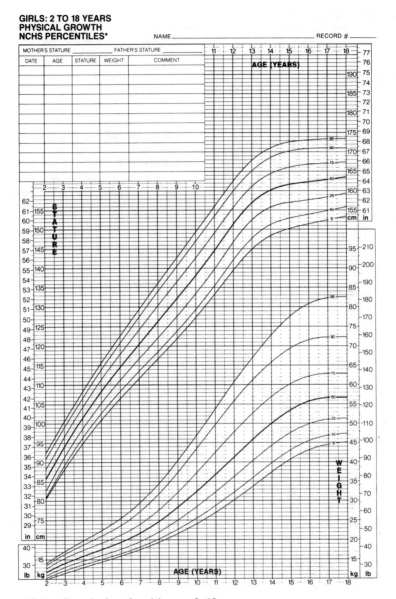

Figure 17-1.   Growth chart for girls ages 2–18 yr.

Used with pemission of Ross Products Division, Abbott Laboratories, Columbus, OH 43216 from NCHS Growth Chart. ©1982 Ross Products Division, Abbott Laboratories.

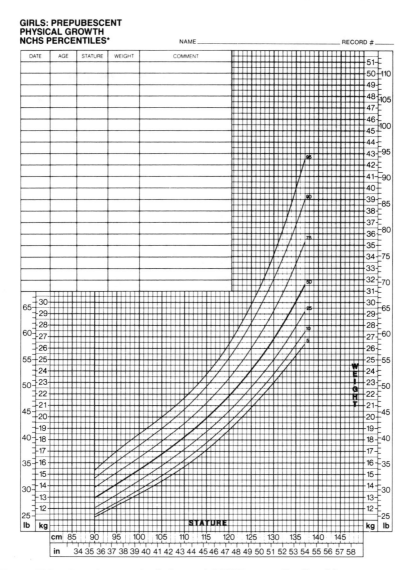

GIRLS: PREPUBESCENT PHYSICAL GROWTH NCHS PERCENTILES*

Figure 17-2. Prepubescent physical growth NCHS percentiles for girls.

Used with pemission of Ross Products Division, Abbott Laboratories, Columbus, OH 43216 from NCHS Growth Chart. ©1982 Ross Products Division, Abbott Laboratories.

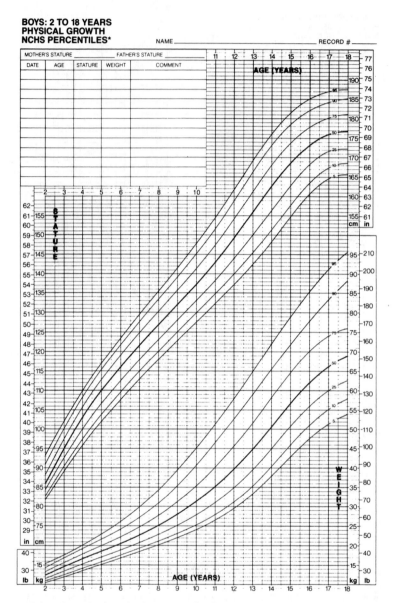

Figure 17-3. Growth chart for boys ages 2–18 yr.

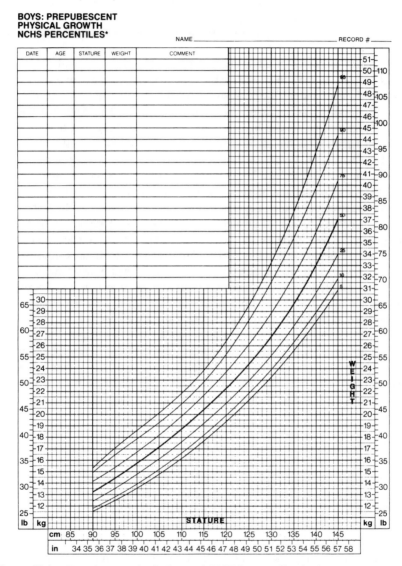

Figure 17-4. Prepubescent physical growth NCHS percentiles for boys.

Used with pemission of Ross Products Division, Abbott Laboratories, Columbus, OH 43216 from NCHS Growth Chart. ©1982 Ross Products Division, Abbott Laboratories.

weighing, estimation of lean body mass using deuterium distribution, and estimation of lean body mass by measurement of potassium 40 levels. Although these methods are considered to be the gold standard, they are expensive, inconvenient, potentially risky, and of questionable validity when applied to children and adolescents.[23,24]

"Indirect" measures of adiposity include skinfold thickness and weight-for-height indices. In the office, the easiest way to gauge obesity involves the use of the body mass index (BMI). Also known the Quetelet Index,[25] the BMI has often been used as an index of obesity in children.[26,27] The BMI is defined as weight in kilograms divided by height in meters squared (kg/m^2); this value can easily be calculated in the office setting, or extrapolated by using the nomogram found in Chapter 11. Percentile curves of BMI have been developed and can be used by the practitioner as a base reference.[23] Table 17.3 outlines the standard BMI's at various ages and heights, for office use. GAPS defines patients as "at risk for overweight" if they have a BMI between the 85th and 94th percentile. Obesity is defined by a BMI greater than or equal to the 95th percentile for age and gender.[6] These patients should have a comprehensive dietary and health assessment to determine psychosocial morbidity and risk for future cardiovascular disease. Adolescents also require a more intensive dietary assessment if they have (1) a family history of premature heart disease, hypertension, obesity, or diabetes mellitus; (2) elevated blood pressure; (3) hypercholesterolemia; or (4) demonstrate moderate to excessive concerns about their weight.

The BMI has less use in patients who are underweight for height. For instance, primary and secondary amenorrhea has been associated with having a body fat content below 19–21%. In the patient with anorexia nervosa or athletic amenorrhea, the BMI may be above the 5th percentile due to muscle mass despite the suboptimal level of body fat. Body weight represents the sum of lean body mass and fat.

Skinfold thickness.   Some investigators have used skinfold thickness as the standard in the clinical setting against which to judge other measures of obesity.[28] However, this method has its own limitations. First, skinfold thickness is usually measured at only a limited number of sites and reflects site-specific subcutaneous fat deposition.[29] Also, the distribution of subcutaneous fat varies widely by age, sex, race, and body habitus.[30,31] Clinical dietitians must also be comfortable with this technique (see Chapter 18), as there can be much interobserver error.[32] Our group prefers the Lange skinfold calipers (Cambridge Scientific Industries, Inc., Cambridge, MD) due to their potential enhancement of interobserver accuracy. Triceps skinfold thickness has a high correlation with percentage of body fat (%BF), with BMI showing less strong correlations with %BF.[33] Useful standards for skinfold thickness in boys and girls from prepuberty through postpuberty are provided in Tables 17.4 and 17.5.[34] Providers may find this technique especially useful in working with the undernourished teen with primary or secondary

Table 17.3   Reference Data on Percentiles of Body Mass Index (kg/m²) for Adolescents (based on smoothed percentiles from NHANESI, using BMI and triceps skinfold thickness)

| | Percentiles | | | | |
Age (yr)	5th	15th	50th	85th	95th
			MALES		
10	14.42	15.15	16.72	19.60	22.60
11	14.83	15.59	17.28	20.35	23.73
12	15.24	16.06	17.87	21.12	24.89
13	15.73	16.62	18.53	21.93	25.93
14	16.18	17.20	19.22	22.77	26.93
15	16.59	17.76	19.92	23.63	27.76
16	17.01	18.32	20.63	24.45	28.53
17	17.31	18.68	21.12	25.28	29.32
18	17.54	18.89	21.45	25.92	30.02
19	17.80	19.20	21.86	26.36	30.66
	Percentiles				
Age (yr)	5th	15th	50th	85th	95th
			FEMALES		
10	14.23	15.09	17.00	20.19	23.20
11	14.60	15.53	17.67	21.18	24.59
12	14.98	15.98	18.35	22.17	25.95
13	15.36	16.43	18.95	23.08	27.07
14	15.67	16.79	19.32	23.88	27.97
15	16.01	17.16	19.69	24.29	28.51
16	16.37	17.54	20.09	24.74	29.10
17	16.59	17.81	20.36	25.23	29.72
18	16.71	17.99	20.57	25.56	30.22
19	16.87	18.20	20.80	25.85	30.72

Adapted from A. Must, G. E. Dallal, and W. H. Dietz, *Am. J. Clin. Nutr.*, **54**, 773 (1991). Reprinted with permission.

amenorrhea. Measurements can be used to explain the composition of the patient's body and how suboptimal fat content may be associated with menstrual irregularities and the future risk of osteoporosis.

Laboratory assessment.   Useful measures of nutritional status include the hemoglobin level, hematocrit, and cholesterol level. GAPS recommends that

Table 17.4　Percentage of Body Fat Estimated from the Sum of Biceps, Triceps, Supra-iliac, and Subscapular Skinfold in Boys of Different Maturation Level

	Percentage of body fat (mean value and 95% confidence interval, CI)					
	Prepubertal 10.5 (SE 1.6) yr		Pubertal 13.2 (SE 1.3) yr		Post-pubertal 16.8 (SE 2.1) yr	
Sum of Skinfolds	Mean	95% CI	Mean	95% CI	Mean	95% CI
15	9.0	8.2–9.8	10.1	8.9–11.3	—	—
20	12.3	11.5–13.1	12.4	11.2–13.6	8.7	0.3–10.1
25	14.9	14.1–15.7	14.2	13.0–15.4	10.5	9.1–11.9
30	17.0	16.2–17.8	15.7	14.5–16.9	12.0	10.6–13.4
35	18.8	18.0–19.6	17.0	15.8–18.2	13.3	11.9–14.7
40	20.3	19.5–21.1	18.0	16.8–19.2	14.4	13.0–15.8
45	21.7	20.9–22.5	19.01	7.8–20.2	15.4	14.0–16.8
50	22.9	22.1–23.7	19.9	18.7–21.2	16.2	14.8–17.6
55	24.0	23.2–24.8	20.6	19.4–21.8	17.0	15.6–18.4
60	25.0	24.2–25.8	21.3	20.1–22.5	17.7	16.3–19.1
65	25.9	25.1–26.7	22.0	20.8–23.2	18.4	17.0–19.8
70	26.8	26.0–27.6	22.6	21.4–23.8	19.0	17.6–20.4
75	27.6	26.8–28.4	23.2	22.0–24.4	19.6	18.2–21.0
80	28.3	27.5–29.1	23.7	22.5–25.9	20.1	18.7–21.5
85	29.0	28.2–29.8	24.7	23.5–25.9	20.6	19.2–22.0
90	29.7	29.1–30.5	24.6	24.4–25.8	21.0	19.6–22.4
95	30.3	29.5–31.1	25.1	23.9–26.3	21.5	20.1–22.9

Adapted from P. Duerenberg, J. J. Pieters, and J. G. Hautvast, *Br. J. Nutr.*, **63**, 300 (1990). Reprinted with permission.

cholesterol be checked once in the adolescent period, with more frequent or comprehensive evaluation if there are specific risk factors.[6] Other laboratory tests can be used to help detect specific disease states, i.e., an erythrocyte sedimentation rate for suspected inflammatory bowel disease or other autoimmune process, specific vitamin assays with a high index of suspicion, or liver function tests with suspected hepatitis. Measurements of albumin (with a half-life of 14–20 d), prealbumin (with a half-life of 2–3 d), and transferrin (with a half-life of 8–10.5 d) can provide information about protein synthesis; however, each may be affected by certain disease processes. For instance, albumin is less useful in the context of acute or critical illness due to its long half-life, its distribution extensively both extravascularly and intravascularly, and the influence of the presence of circulating inflammatory mediators and liver function on its formation.[35] In protein malnutrition, the ratio of albumin to globulin may decrease. In such specialized patients, the nutritionist can work with the primary care provider and the gastroenterologist to pursue appropriate problem-specific evaluation.

Table 17.5 Percentage Body Fat Estimated from the Sum of Biceps, Triceps, Suprailiac, and Subscapular Skinfold in Girls of Different Maturation Level

Percentage of body fat (mean value and 95% confidence interval, CI)

Sum of Skinfolds	Prepubertal 10.5 (SE 1.6) yr		Pubertal 13.1 (SE 1.3) yr		Post-pubertal 16.8 (SE 2.1) yr	
	Mean	95% CI	Mean	95% CI	Mean	95% CI
15	9.2	8.3–10.1	9.3	8.6–10.0	—	—
20	13.0	12.1–13.9	12.3	9.6–13.0	—	—
25	15.9	15.0–16.8	14.6	13.9–15.3	11.1	9.9–12.3
30	18.2	17.3–19.1	16.5	15.8–17.2	14.1	12.9–15.3
35	20.2	19.3–21.1	18.1	17.4–18.8	16.8	15.6–18.0
40	22.0	21.1–22.9	19.5	18.8–20.2	19.0	17.8–20.2
45	23.5	22.6–24.4	20.7	20.0–21.4	21.0	19.8–22.2
50	24.8	23.9–25.7	21.8	21.1–22.5	22.8	21.6–24.0
55	26.1	25.2–27.0	22.8	22.1–23.5	24.4	23.2–25.6
60	27.2	26.3–28.1	23.7	23.0–24.4	25.9	24.7–27.1
65	28.2	27.3–29.1	24.5	23.8–25.2	27.2	26.0–28.4
70	29.2	28.3–30.1	25.3	24.6–26.0	28.5	27.3–29.7
75	30.1	29.2–31.0	26.0	25.3–26.7	29.7	28.5–30.9
80	30.9	30.0–31.8	26.7	26.0–27.4	30.8	29.6–32.0
85	31.7	30.8–32.6	27.3	26.6–28.0	31.8	30.6–33.0
90	32.5	31.6–33.4	27.9	27.2–28.6	32.8	31.6–34.0
95	33.2	32.3–34.1	28.5	27.8–29.2	33.7	32.5–34.9

Adapted from P. Duerenberg , J. J. Pieters, and J. G. Hautvast, *Br. J. Nutr.*, **63**, 300 (1990). Reprinted with permission.

MANAGEMENT

Anemia

Iron deficiency continues to be the most common cause of anemia in childhood and adolescence.[36] Iron-deficiency anemia is defined in adolescent girls as a hemoglobin (Hgb) level of less than or equal to 11.8 g/dL and hematocrit (Hct) of 35.5% at the ages 12–14.9 yr; in girls ages 15 yr and older, anemia is defined at a Hgb of 12.0 g/dL and Hct 36.0%. In boys, anemia is defined by a Hgb cutoff value of 12.3 g/dL and Hct 37.0% at ages 12–14.9 yr, with values of 12.6 g/dL and 38.0% for boys ages 15–17.9 yr, and at Hgb 13.6 g/dL and Hct 41% for boys over 18 yr.[37] Factors that place adolescents at risk include rapid physical growth, dietary insufficiencies, and blood loss in menstrual cycles in females.[38, 39]

Other causes of blood loss include occult loss from chronic analgesic use, peptic ulcer disease or another gastrointestinal problem, frequent blood donations, and intensive physical training. Anemia may also be a manifestation of underlying chronic disease. Regardless of origin, anemia can impair physical work capacity, lower endurance, increase fatigue, decrease maximum oxygen consumption, and generally make the teen feel bad.[40,41] Intense physical activity may predispose the adolescent to "sports anemia," which may represent an adaptive physiological response reflecting the body's attempt to meet increased needs for oxygen delivery to tissues during exercise without overly increasing the mass of red blood cells or blood viscosity.[42]

Along with the dietary history, the dietitian can aid the adolescent by discussing iron-rich sources of foods, such as dried fruits, whole grains, nuts and seeds, legumes, green leafy vegetables, and prune juice. Although these non-heme sources have substantial amounts of iron, they are less readily absorbable than iron in animal sources such as liver and red meat. Ingestion of Vitamin C aids absorption of nonheme iron. Iron deficiency anemia can be treated with ferrous sulfate 325 mg P.O. tid for 3 mo, with a repeat Hct done after 2–3 mo to assess compliance and correction of the deficit. Other nutritional insufficiencies may be corrected with dietary manipulation as well.

Malnutrition of Other Causes

Malnutrition in the adolescent can be due to a variety of etiologies. Primary causes include the inadequate consumption of appropriate calories or nutrients, as might occur in a third world country or any underprivileged area. Secondary causes include any illness that either impairs intake or utilization of nutrients or increases nutrient requirements or metabolic losses. In teenagers, secondary malnutrition most commonly occurs in the context of chronic disease, such as in patients with cystic fibrosis, chronic renal failure, inflammatory bowel disease, or acquired immunodeficiency syndrome. For instance, in cystic fibrosis, malnutrition develops due to a combination of exocrine pancreatic insufficiency, recurrent respiratory infections with increased caloric needs and total energy expenditure, and poor dietary intake due to chronic illness and malabsorption.[43]

Chronic diarrhea, celiac disease, and lactose intolerance can lead to a malabsorptive state with secondary malnutrition. The latter often does not show up until the second decade of life and can be suspected in patients with a history of watery diarrhea, bloating, crampy abdominal pain, and flatulence. The teenager may or may not be able to identify associated dairy products or foods causing symptoms. The breath hydrogen test allows for easy screening for lactose intolerance. It is noninvasive and can be done in the office or at home using a breath collection kit that can be packaged and mailed (Med Care Home Health Resources, Inc., Baltimore, MD).[44] Hospital-based testing sites are also readily available. Dietary restriction without testing for carbohydrate or lactose intolerance can further predispose the adolescent to calcium deficiency or lifestyle inconvenience through food avoidance. In most adolescents and adults with disease, the total elimination of lactose or dairy products is rarely necessary. Those patients who wish to drink milk or eat dairy products have several alternatives: They can delay gastric emptying by drinking milk with meals, use prehydrolyzed milk treated with microbial-derived lactase enzyme, or use commercial over-the-counter preparations prior to ingesting lactose (Lactaid, Lactrase, Dairy-Ease). For those patients on chronic lactose-restricted diets, a chewable calcium supplement should be considered in order to provide the 1200 mg RDA for adolescents. Teaching patients to read labels can help minimize their symptoms by restricting the intake of offending foods.

In newly arrived immigrants, marasmus and kwashiorkor can still be seen. Both disorders are caused by a deficiency in energy intake and are more common in infants and children. Kwashiorkor is associated with a disproportionately low-protein intake relative to overall caloric intake; it has been thought to represent edematous malnutrition due to low-serum oncotic pressure. It occurs most commonly in children ages 1–3 yr and is characterized by dependent edema, growth failure, and muscle wasting. Frequently associated symptoms include depigmentation and easily pluckable hair, hepatomegaly, hyperkeratosis, and mental apathy. Often preceded by or associated with infection (diarrheal disease, measles, respiratory infection), kwashiorkor may not be exclusively due to dietary deficiency. Multiple infections, parasitic diseases, abrupt weaning from the breast, aflatoxin, and ochratoxin may represent other causative factors.[45,46]

Marasmus is severe nonedematous malnutrition caused by a mixed deficiency of protein, calories, and other nutrients over a period of time. Patients may have diarrhea, anorexia, vomiting, and recurrent infections. Characteristics of marasmus include low body weight, loss of subcutaneous fat, and wasting of muscle tissue. Patients also may mimic hypothyroidism, with cold intolerance, dry skin with decreased turgor, thin, sparse hair, and listlessness. Serum protein and albumin levels are usually normal despite the muscle wasting and loss of adipose tissue.

Obesity

When working with the obese adolescent, the clinical dietitian should ask detailed questions about the meal and snack pattern (see Chapters 11 and 18) . Does the teen eat many fried foods or fast foods? The location of eating becomes more important, as teens tend to eat more while in front of the television or with peers. Food availability should also be assessed. Who buys and prepares the food in the home? What previous and/or current weight control methods have been tried? Many teens may feel hopeless or depressed by their inability to lose weight; the provider must be careful to give much positive reinforcement for *any* healthy behaviors with the goal of instilling confidence and a sense of self-efficacy in the teen.

Parental recruitment into weight-loss strategies can be useful. In one study, daughters of mothers who regularly attended nutritional group sessions lost more than twice as much weight as daughters of mothers with poor or no attendance.[47] Whether the mother attended sessions simultaneously or separately from the daughter did not produce significant differences in the amount of weight lost. Moreover, the more weight the mothers lost, the more weight their teenage daughters lost.[47,48] On the negative side, in patients and mothers with eating disorders, the primary care provider must be careful not to set up an atmosphere of competition over weight loss between mother and teen. Patient and parental attitudes about obesity can vary; Hispanic families tend to view obese children as healthier than nonobese children, and research suggests that African American families do not prefer the ultra-thin habitus sought by Caucasian females.[49,50]

For teenagers who are still in midgrowth spurt or early puberty, the goal should be maintenance of actual weight rather than weight loss. The dietitian may need to thoroughtly explain the rationale in order to persuade the teen to endorse the concept of weight maintenance. With older adolescents, a gradual weight loss of ½–2 lb/wk should be recommended. Youth-oriented group therapy may be available in the community and can be offered; most teens will have a definite preference on whether to try a group or individual approach. Work with a nutritionist can be vital; good rapport and knowing that *you care* can also be quite helpful in the teen's weight-loss efforts.

Hyperlipidemia

Once diagnosed, the teen with hypercholesterolemia (see Chapter 5) should be counselled on dietary changes designed to lower serum cholesterol. For patients requiring oral contraceptives (OCPs), selecting a pill with minimal impact on lipids is preferred. Some of the OCPs that contain the newer progestins (norgestimate and desogestrel) are associated with an increase in high-density lipoprotein levels (see Chapter 3). Patients with high cholesterol levels should be encouraged to start or continue an exercise plan, as in combination with caloric restriction, this method may obviate the need for drug therapy.[51] Details of dietary and pharmacological management are addressed elsewhere.[51]

Whom Should the Dietitian Evaluate in the Outpatient Setting?

In the office, dietitians and primary care providers should offer brief nutritional counseling for the teen with nutritional insufficiencies or excess in order to continually educate the patient, as well as the parents and to set short-term, realistic goals. As outlined above, many chronic diseases and conditions can be ameliorated with appropriate nutritional interventions using a registered dietitian. Medical conditions for which patients should be referred include inflammatory bowel disease, cystic fibrosis, acquired immunodeficiency syndrome, cancer, diabetes mellitus, hyperlipidemia, hypertension, obesity, eating disorders, chronic renal disease, malabsorptive syndromes, and inborn errors of metabolism.[52] Many of these patients have worked with nutritionists from time of diagnosis. However, in "stable" disease, the changes of puberty with respect to growth and body image may necessitate a revisit to the nutritionist for updated management. The American Diabetes Association recommends that any child or adolescent with diabetes mellitus should see a registered dietitian every 6 mo and more frequently as needed to monitor growth and changing eating patterns.[53] Patients who are significantly underweight for height may also benefit from referral to a nutritionist or clinical dietitian.

Several nutritional supplements are commercially available to complement intake for special dietary needs (see Tables 17.6 through 17.8). Patients with protein calorie malnutrition, dysphagia, or who are otherwise underweight for height can use supplements to provide extra calories and protein. Temporary use of supplements can be beneficial in patients who are unable to ingest sufficient calories with food alone due to lack of appetite or intolerance of sufficient quantities of food. In most cases, tolerance of food increases slowly with refeeding, and supplements can be weaned over time. Most teens will choose to add food back into their diets as quickly as possible. Supplements vary in flavor, calories, and cost, with milk-based supplements being the least expensive. Lactose-free formulas are also available (Tables 17.7 and 17.8). Many of the supplements can be used in tube feedings. Several of the milk-based supplements can be mixed with milk for added calories and calcium. For instance, 1 package of Carnation Instant Breakfast mixed with 8 oz of whole milk will give 280 kcal, 36 g carbohydrate, 14 g of protein, and 8 g of fat, a significant increase from the Table 17.6 numbers for that item as mixed with water.

The Role of Culture and Faddism

The dietitian should be sensitive to variations in food patterns of different cultures. Language barriers can mean that office recommendations cannot be followed through, and the clinician should ascertain whether the individual family member buying and preparing the food understands the advice given. Often, adolescent diets suffer when the teen eats fewer meals in the home, as they are more prone to eating foods higher in fat, sugar, and salt.[50] In general, teenagers may be very well informed on healthy nutrition, but their knowledge may not be easily translated into behavioral change. Barriers to dietary modification as identified by teens include lack of time, self-discipline, and a sense of urgency.[54] Poverty can also be an issue, as patients may lack fresh fruit and vegetables,

Table 17.6   Milk-Based Supplements

Formula	Size	kcal	CHO (g)	PRO (g)	FAT (g)	Flavor	Company
Ensure powder	½ cup mixed with 8 oz of water	250	34.3	8.8	8.8	Vanilla	Ross Labs
Sustacal powder	1 package	200	36	12.5	.3	Vanilla, chocolate	Mead-Johnson
Meritene powder	1.14 oz	116	19.1	9.4	.20	Plain, vanilla, chocolate, eggnog, milk chocolate	Sandoz
Meritene liquid	8.45 oz	240	14.4	27.6	8	Vanilla, chocolate, eggnog	Sandoz
Sustagen powder	1 tbsp	51	8	1.9	.3	Vanilla, chocolate	Mead-Johnson
CIB Carnation Instant Breakfast	1 package	130	28	4	1	Vanilla, chocolate, eggnog, strawberry	Clintec
Scandi Shake powder	3 oz	440	4	58	21	Vanilla, chocolate, strawberry	Scandi-pharm

cooking and refrigeration facilities. Lack of neighborhood safety may limit teens' ability to exercise outdoors.

Bringing It All Together

Most adolescents can begin to make dietary changes in small, progressive steps. Overwhelming them with too much information early on may reinforce their feelings of hopelessness and helplessness. Positive reinforcement remains a useful adjunct to any behavioral intervention. Dietitians can have a significant impact on their patients' lives through the formation of a trusting relationship with continuity over time. Reinforcement of the message on healthy behaviors can occur through appropriately placed posters and reading materials in the office. Dietitians and primary care providers can be strong advocates for change with respect to the nutritional information given on television, on the radio, and at the movies. Consistency, persistence, and an instilled sense of confidence can help teens make positive changes with respect to their nutrition and health.

Table 17.7 Lactose-Free Supplements

Formula	Size	kcal	CHO (g)	PRO (g)	FAT (g)	Flavor	Company
Ensure	8 oz	250	34.3	8.8	8.8	Vanilla, coffee, strawberry, chocolate, black walnut, eggnog	Ross Labs
Sustacal	8 oz	240	33	14.5	5.5	Vanilla, strawberry, chocolate, eggnog	Mead-Johnson
Resource	8 oz	250	34.3	8.8	8.8	Vanilla, strawberry, chocolate	Sandoz
Nutren 1.0	8.45 oz	250	31.8	10	9.5	Vanilla, strawberry, chocolate, unflavored	Clintec
Comply	8.4	375	45	15	15	Vanilla, banana, orange	Sherwood Medical
Ensure Plus	8 oz	355	47.3	13	12	Vanilla, strawberry, chocolate, eggnog, coffee	Ross Labs
Resource Plus	8 oz	355	47.3	13	12.6	Vanilla, chocolate	Sandoz
Nutren 1.5	8.45 oz	375	42.4	15	16.9	Vanilla, chocolate, unflavored	Clintec
Nutren 2.0	8.45 oz	500	49	20	26.5	Vanilla	Clintec
Ensure pudding	5 oz	250	32	6.8	9.7	Vanilla, chocolate, tapioca, butterscotch	Ross Labs
Sustacal pudding	5 oz	240	32	6.8	9.5	Vanilla, chocolate, butterscotch	Mead-Johnson

Table 17.8   Lactose-Free Supplements with Fiber

Formula	Size	kcal	CHO (g)	PRO (g)	FAT (g)	Flavor	Company
Ensure with fiber	8 oz	260	38.3	9.4	8.8	Vanilla, chocolate	Ross Labs
Sustacal with fiber	8 oz	250	33	10.8	8.3	Vanilla, chocolate, strawberry	Mead-Johnson
Nutren 1.0 with fiber	8.45 oz	250	31.8	10	9.5	Vanilla, chocolate, unflavored	Clintec

CASE ILLUSTRATION

Anna is a 17-year-old Hispanic teenager being seen for her annual physical. She also mentions that for the last 3 mo she has been trying to gain weight without success. Further history reveals that she lives at home with her mother, has been doing well in high school (grade 11), and has a boyfriend with whom she has been having unprotected intercourse. She states that they occasionally use condoms, but have stopped using them because she is thinking about trying to get pregnant. She has also thought about going to college or getting a better job.

Physical exam reveals a slender young lady in no acute distress. Height is 162 cm (5 ft, 3 ¾ in., 25%), weight is 48.2 kg (106 lb, 10%). HEENT is entirely normal, she has no thyromegaly, no adenopathy, with normal cardiac, lung, and abdominal exam. Breasts are Tanner 5 with no masses or discharge. Pelvic exam reveals Tanner 4 pubic hair, no clitoromegaly, normal external genitalia, no cervical motion tenderness, and no uterine or adnexal tenderness or masses. Thus, current concerns to health providers were unprotected intercourse and Anna's desire to gain weight.

Further history is needed and includes obtaining a dietary history by means of 24-h recall, meal patterns, list of "taboo" foods, and information on who does the cooking and shopping for food in her home. Anna reports typically skipping breakfast and lunch, stating, "I don't have time for breakfast, and school lunch is gross." She does eat most foods without major restrictions, drinks regular soda pop, some junk food, little fruits and vegetables, and eats dinner as prepared by her mother. Although finances and food availability are not big issues for her, other patients may have more difficulty in obtaining a balanced diet including fruits and vegetables, which tend to be more expensive than fast food.

Interventions for this patient could involve getting her to eat three meals a day plus two or three snacks, providing a high-calorie, high-protein diet. For Anna, suggestions for incorporating breakfast might include getting her to wake up earlier to provide adequate time for breakfast, having fruit or cereal with milk as a quick meal, or eating a bagel with cream cheese on her way out the door. Anna should be reassured that changes take time, with a focus on small increments that Anna can incorporate with minimal discomfort. She should be encouraged to bring her own lunch to school, packing well-balanced, high-calorie choices. For teens who refuse to bring their own lunch, one alternative would be to eat their snack at lunchtime and then lunch at 2 P.M. when they get home from school.

The dietitian might also suggest substituting whole milk for soda, as Anna is trying to gain weight and lacks adequate calcium in her diet per 24-h recall. Calories can be concentrated through the use of peanut butter, margarine or butter, mayonnaise, cheese, wheat germ, or other items. Milk shakes can also provide calcium and calories. Available handouts on calcium, healthy eating, or other topics can be useful office tools. Follow-up by the dietitian may be helpful for additional support. The dietitian could also ask Anna to complete a 3-d food record, to be brought to her next appointment.

With respect to her sexual activity, the prevention of sexually transmitted diseases and HIV should be discussed with her primary care provider, along with further questions to help Anna clarify why and when she truly wishes to become pregnant. If she will be trying to conceive in the immediate future, folic acid should be added with a daily multivitamin, as a dose of 0.4 mg orally/d prior to conception may decrease the risk of neural tube defects in the fetus. If she wishes to defer pregnancy, the dietitian can still encourage the use of a daily multivitamin and refer her for further counseling on contraceptive options, including the use of condoms.

Laboratory evaluation at this point might include a complete blood count to screen for iron-deficiency anemia or low hematocrit in a menstruating female. As mentioned above, keeping Anna healthy and happy will involve regular follow-up with her primary care provider, with close monitoring of intake and weight gain by the dietitian.

Acknowledgments.   The authors wish to acknowledge S. Jean Emans, M.D., and Clifford Lo, M.D., for their thoughtful critique of this chapter. This work has been supported in part by Project #MCJ-MA259195 from the Maternal and Child Health Bureau (Title V, Social Security Act), Health Resources and Services Administration, Department of Health and Human Services.

REFERENCES

1. R. K. Chandra, *Lancet*, **1**, 688 (1983).
2. National Research Council, National Academy of Sciences, *Diet and Health: Implications for Reducing Chronic Disease Risk*, National Academy Press, Washington DC (1989).

3. H. J. Walter, R. D. Vaughan, and E. L. Wynder, *J. Natl. Cancer Inst.*, **81**, 995 (1989).

4. U.S. Preventive Services Task Force, *Guide to Clinical Preventive Services: An Assessment of the Effectiveness of 169 Interventions*, Williams & Wilkins, Baltimore, MD, (1989).

5. U.S. Department of Health and Human Services.,Public Health Service, *Healthy People 2000, National Health Promotion and Disease Prevention Objectives*, Government Printing Office, Washington, DC, (1990).

6. A. B. Elster and N. J. Kuznets, eds., *AMA Guidelines for Adolescent Preventive Services*, Williams & Wilkins, Baltimore, MD, (1994).

7. M. C. Farthing, *Nutr. Today*, **26**, 35 (1991).

8. Results from the National Adolescent Student Health Survey, *MMWR*, **38**, 147 (1989).

9. L. Emmons, *J. Am. Diet Assoc.*, **92**, 306 (1992).

10. M. Story, K. Rosenwinkel, J. Himes, et al., *AJDC*, **145**, 994 (1991).

11. L. H. Eck, R. C. Klesges, and C.L. Hanson, J. Am. Diet Assoc., **89**, 784 (1989).

12. P. M. Howat, R. Mohan, C. Champagne, et al., *J. Am. Diet Assoc.*, **94**, 169 (1994).

13. P. M. Guenther, *J. Am. Diet Assoc.*, **86**, 493 (1986).

14. G. C. Frank, T. A. Nicklas, L. S. Webber, et al., *J. Am. Diet Assoc.*, **92**, 313 (1992).

15. T. A. Nicklas, L. S. Webber, B. Thompson, et al., *Am. J. Clin. Nutr.*,**49**, 1320 (1989).

16. Committee on Sports Medicine, *Pediatrics*, **84**, 394 (1989).

17. J. Benson, D. M. Gillien, R. D. Bourdet, et al., *Phys. Sports Med.*, **13**, 79 (1985).

18. S. J. Emans, E. Grace, F. A. Hoffer, et al., *Obstet. Gynecol.*, **76**, 585 (1990).

19. M. J. Davies, M. L. Hall, and H. S. Jacobs, *Br. Med. J.*, **301**, 790 (1990).

20. S. Dhuper, M. P. Warren, J. Brooks-Gunn, R. Fox, *J. Clin. Endocrinol. Metab.*, **71**, 1083 (1990).

21. G. B. Forbes, in *Textbook of Adolescent Medicine*, (E. R. McAnarney, R. E. Kreipe, D. P. Orr, and G. D. Comerci, eds.), Harcourt Brace Jovanovich, Inc., Philadelphia, PA, pp. 68–74 (1992).

22. J. M. Tanner and P.S.W. Davies, *J. Peds.*, **107**, 317 (1985).

23. L. D. Hammer, H. C. Kraemer, D. M. Wilson, et al., *AJDC*, **145**, 259 (1991).

24. T. G. Lohman, *Med. Sci. Sport Exer.*, **16**, 596 (1984).

25. W. Z. Billewicz, F. F. Kemsley, and A. M. Thomson, *Br. J. Prev. Soc. Med.*, **16**, 183 (1962).

26. S. J. Fomon, R. R. Rogers, E. E. Ziegler, et al, *Pediatrics*, **18**, 1233 (1982).

27. M. F. Rolland-Cachera, M. Sempe, M. Guilloud-Bataille, et al., *Am. J. Clin. Nutr.*, **36**, 178 (1982).

28. R. Michielutte, R. Diseker, W. T. Corbett, et al., *Am. J. Pub. Health*, **74**, 604 (1984).

29. D. S. McLaren, Z. A. Ajans, and Z. Awdeh, *Am. J. Clin. Nutr.*, **17**, 171 (1965).

30. D.A.W. Edwards, *Clin. Sci.*, **10**, 305 (1951).

31. S. M. Garn, *Hum. Biol.*, **27**, 75 (1955).

32. M. L. Pollack and A. S. Jackson, *Med. Sci. Sports Exer.*, **16**, 606 (1984).

33. A. F. Roche, R. M. Siervogel, W. C. Chumlea, et al., *Am. J. Clin. Nutr.*, **34**, 2831 (1981).

34. P. Deurenberg, J.J.L. Pieters, and J. G. Hautvast, *Br. J. Nutr.*, **63**, 293 (1990).

35. J. B. Mason and I. H. Rosenburg, in *Harrison's Principles of Internal Medicine*, 12th ed., (J. D. Wilson, E. Braunwald, K. J. Isselbacher, et al., eds.), McGraw-Hill, New York, pp. 406–411 (1991).

36. P. R. Dallman, in *Hematology of Infancy and Childhood*, 3rd ed., (D. G. Nathan and F. A. Oski, eds.), W. B. Saunders, Philadelphia, PA, p. 288 (1987).

37. CDC criteria for anemia in children and childbearing-aged women, *MMWR*, **38**, 400 (1989).

38. P. R. Dallman, R. Yip, and C. Johnson, *Am. J. Clin. Nutr.*, **39**, 437 (1984).

39. A. Ballin, M. Berar, U. Rubinstein, et al., *AJDC*, **146**, 803 (1992).

40. W. L. Risser, E. J. Lee, H.B.W. Poindexter, et al., *Med. Sci. Sports. Exer.*, **20**, 116 (1988).

41. R. A. Raunikar and H. Sabio, *AJDC*, **146**, 1201 (1992).

42. D. L. Carlson and R. H. Mawdsley, *Am. J. Sports Med.*, **11**, 109 (1986).

43. H. P. Chase, M. A. Long, M. H. Lavin, *J. Peds.*, **95**, 337 (1979).

44. R. G. Montes and J. A. Perman, in *Sem. Ped. Gastroenterol. Nutr.*, **2**, 2 (1991).

45. D. B. Jelliffe and E.F.P. Jellife, *Pediatrics*, **90**, 110 (1992).

46. A. H. Hallab and R. I. Tannous, in *Nutrition in the Community*, (D. S. McLaren, ed.), John Wiley, London, England, pp. 133–139 (1976).

47. T. A. Wadden, A. J. Stunkard, L. Rich, et al., *Pediatrics*, **85**, 345 (1990).

48. K. D. Brownell, J. H. Kelman, and A. J. Stunkard, *Pediatrics*, **71**, 515 (1983).

49. M. P. Stern, J. A. Pugh, S. P. Gaskill, et al., *Am. J. Epidemiol.*, **115**, 917 (1982).

50. E. Luder, *Adol. Med.: State Art Rev.*, **3**, 405, (1992).

51. E. A. Stein, *Am. J. Med.*, **87** (suppl. 4A), 20S (1989).

52. A. B. Lasswell, *Ped. Ann.*, **21**, 676 (1992).

53. American Diabetes Association Task Force on Nutrition and Exchange Lists, *Diab. Care*, **10**, 126 (1987).

54. M. Story and M. D. Resnick, *J. Nutr. Ed.*, **18**, 188 (1986).

CHAPTER	# Hypertension
18	*Shelley Kirk, M.S., R.D., L.D., C.D.E., and*
	Jennifer M. H. Loggie, M.D.

INTRODUCTION

Essential hypertension is a common disorder affecting adults in the Western world. Morbidity associated with it includes stroke, heart failure, and renal failure. In addition, it is an independent risk factor for coronary artery disease and therefore myocardial infarction.

The term "benign essential hypertension" was coined at the turn of the century when physicians believed that some individuals required higher blood pressure for adequate perfusion. The condition is neither benign nor essential, and it also seems likely that what is called essential hypertension may well be a collection of several pathophysiological entities that will eventually be identified with respect to their etiology, pathogenesis, and prognosis. Some prefer to use the term primary hypertension rather than essential hypertension, thus separating high blood pressure for which no organic cause can be found from hypertension secondary to renal and renal artery diseases and hormonal forms of hypertension.

Until about 30 yr ago, primary hypertension was a diagnosis of exclusion in children and adolescents. It was considered extremely rare, but is now considered the most common form of hypertension among adolescents. Why this change has occurred may be due to several factors, but three are immediately recognized. Prior to 1960, blood pressure was rarely measured during childhood and adolescence unless there were symptoms suggesting its presence or the young patient had a disease, such as acute poststreptococcal glomerulonephritis, that was known to be associated with hypertension. Adolescents presenting with symptoms thought to be due to hypertension, such as headaches, dizziness, and nosebleeds, or with complications of hypertension such as stroke, seizures, or heart failure, usually had severely elevated blood pressures and almost always an organic cause for hypertension was found. However, as is now known, primary hypertension is generally mild and asymptomatic in adolescence and because blood pressure was not routinely measured in this population, many young people with the disorder were probably overlooked until they became adults. Detection has improved as the concept has gained credence that primary hypertension is an inherited disorder that begins in childhood and blood pressure measurement has become fairly routine in the care of both children and teenagers.

A second factor that has led to increased recognition of hypertension in adolescence is that it is no longer diagnosed only when blood pressures $\geq$ 140/90 mm Hg are found. This measurement is the adult cut-point for defining blood pressure as high and was routinely used for children and adolescents. However, in industrial societies, blood pressure rises gradually from infancy, through childhood and adolescence, and reaches normal adult levels by 17–18 yr of age. Therefore, a different cut-point or definition was required for what should be considered hypertensive prior to this age. Londe in 1968[1] and the Task Force on Blood Pressure Control in Childhood in 1977[2] recommended that a child or adolescent considered hypertensive if the systolic and/or diastolic blood pressure were at or above the 95th percentile for age and sex on three separate occasions. This is because in adults, systolic hypertension is significantly associated with risk for cardiovascular disease irrespective of the level of diastolic blood pressure. It is presumed, but not proven, that this is also true for younger individuals.

The Second Task Force Report on Blood Pressure Control in Childhood,[3] published 10 yr after the first, also recognized a "high normal" level of blood pressure for children and adolescents. It was suggested that youngsters with blood pressures frequently between the 90th and 95th percentiles for their age and sex, unless tall for their age, should be kept under surveillance as perhaps being at risk for later hypertension (see Table 18.1). This is compatible with the notion that adults with high normal blood pressure[4] may also be at risk for eventual sustained hypertension.

The third factor is the established relationship between high blood pressure and obesity. Obesity in the teen years is a significant risk factor for the development of hypertension during adolescence[5,6] and also increases the probability of becoming hypertensive during adulthood.[7] During the past two decades, the proportion of obese adolescents (triceps skinfold $\geq$ 85th percentile) has risen 39%, with a

Table 18.1 Blood Pressure Levels for the 90th and 95th Percentiles for Youth 10–17 Yr of Age by Percentiles of Height

Age (yr)	Percentile	Systolic BP (mm Hg) by Percentile of Height							Diastolic BP (DBPS) (mm Hg) by Percentile of Height						
		5	10	25	50	75	90	95	5	10	25	50	75	90	95
MALES															
10	90th	111	112	113	115	117	119	119	77	77	78	79	80	81	81
	95th	115	116	117	119	121	123	123	81	82	83	83	84	85	86
11	90th	113	114	115	117	119	121	121	77	78	79	80	81	81	82
	95th	117	118	119	121	123	125	125	82	82	83	84	85	86	87
12	90th	115	116	118	120	121	123	124	78	78	79	80	81	82	83
	95th	119	120	122	124	125	127	128	83	83	84	85	86	87	87
13	90th	118	119	120	122	124	125	126	78	79	80	81	81	82	83
	95th	121	122	124	126	128	129	130	83	83	84	85	86	87	88
14	90th	120	121	123	125	127	128	129	79	79	80	81	82	83	83
	95th	124	125	127	129	131	132	133	83	84	85	86	87	87	88
15	90th	123	124	126	128	130	131	132	80	80	81	82	83	84	84
	95th	127	128	130	132	133	135	136	84	85	86	86	87	88	89
16	90th	126	127	129	131	132	134	134	81	82	82	83	84	85	86
	95th	130	131	133	134	136	138	138	86	86	87	88	89	90	90
17	90th	128	129	131	133	135	136	137	83	84	85	86	87	87	88
	95th	132	133	135	137	139	140	141	88	88	89	90	91	92	93
FEMALES															
10	90th	112	113	114	115	116	118	118	75	75	76	77	77	78	79
	95th	116	117	118	119	120	122	122	79	79	80	81	81	82	83
11	90th	114	115	116	117	119	120	120	76	77	77	78	79	79	80
	95th	118	119	120	121	122	124	124	81	81	81	82	83	83	84
12	90th	116	117	118	119	121	122	123	78	78	78	79	80	81	81
	95th	120	121	122	123	125	126	126	82	82	82	83	84	85	85
13	90th	118	119	120	121	123	124	124	79	79	79	80	81	82	82
	95th	122	123	124	125	126	128	128	83	83	84	84	85	86	86
14	90th	120	121	122	123	124	125	126	80	80	80	81	82	83	83
	95th	124	125	126	127	128	129	130	84	84	85	85	86	87	87
15	90th	121	122	123	124	126	127	128	80	81	81	82	83	83	84
	95th	125	126	127	128	130	131	131	85	85	85	86	87	88	88
16	90th	122	123	124	125	127	128	129	81	81	82	82	83	84	84
	95th	126	127	128	129	130	132	132	85	85	86	87	87	88	88
17	90th	123	123	124	126	127	128	129	81	81	82	83	83	84	85
	95th	127	127	128	130	131	132	133	85	86	86	87	88	88	89

B. Rosner et al., *J. Peds.*, **123**, 871 (1993). Reprinted with permision.

64% increase in the severity of overweightness. It is now estimated that approximately 21% of adolescents in the United States are obese,[8] with a disproportionate representation by African American adolescent females,[9] Hispanic and American Indian youth,[10] and those of lower socioeconomic status.[11] There is evidence to show that 70% of obese adolescents will continue to be obese as adults.[12] The proportion of obese adolescents with hypertension has increased according to analysis of data from the National Health Examination Surveys.[8] However, this conclusion was based on single blood pressure measurements made between 1967 and 1970 compared with single readings made between 1976 and 1980.

In a selected population, Becque et al.[13] reported in 1988 that 80% of 36 obese adolescents studied (weight and triceps skinfold > 75th percentile) had elevated systolic or diastolic blood pressure. In addition, 97% of these obese adolescents were found to have four or more of the following cardiovascular risk factors: hypertriglyceridemia, hypercholesterolemia, decreased serum levels of high-density lipoprotein (HDL) cholesterol, elevated systolic or diastolic blood pressure, reduced maximum oxygen uptake, and strong family history of cardiovascular disease. The broader definition of adolescent obesity used in this study did not alter the strong association found between excess weight, high blood pressure, and other cardiovascular risk factors.

The distribution of body fat, rather than the total amount, appears to be a stronger predictor for elevated blood pressures in obese teens,[14] a finding that is well established for adults.[15-7] Central obesity (excess body fat in the abdominal region or "apple-shaped") was found to be more highly correlated to blood pressure than peripheral obesity (excess body fat in the gluteal and thigh regions or "pear-shaped") during adolescence.[17] However, more research is needed to elucidate the effect of central and peripheral obesity in adolescence on later development of cardiovascular disease during adulthood.

Factors contributing to the increasing problem of adolescent obesity are both genetic and environmental. The tendency to become obese is, in part, inherited regardless of environmentally influenced eating habits and activity patterns. Adoption studies have shown that the adoptee's body weight is correlated with the relative weight of the biological parents, especially the biological mother, whereas no relationship was found to the body weight of the adoptive parents.[18]

Environmental influences affecting level of exercise and eating behaviors, however, can enhance one's genetic predisposition for obesity. Lifestyle factors strongly associated with obesity in youth include an increase in inactivity as influenced by television viewing habits,[19] a decline in regular physical activity,[20] a higher percentage of calories from fat in the diet as opposed to an increase in total caloric intake,[21] and persistent emotional overeating used as a coping mechanism in response to traumatic events or situations in the home environment, such as divorce, substance abuse, physical, or sexual abuse.[22,23]

Prevalence

The prevalence of persistent hypertension in the free living preadult population in the United States has been reported to be 1–2%.[24] However, this estimate may be inaccurate because few blood-pressure-screening programs have been undertaken in the young, especially those of low socioeconomic status. The Second Task Force on Blood Pressure Control in Children[3] did suggest that screening programs might be useful if targeted at high-risk populations such as teens living in inner-city neighborhoods. These individuals often have irregular contact with a primary care provider and hypertension in males is often detected during a presports physical examination. Hypertension in females is more likely to be identified because they are seen by health care providers more frequently, usually for gynecologic and obstetric reasons.

Another means of case-finding would be to routinely measure the blood pressure of the offspring of hypertensive adults who are seen in public health clinics or physician's offices, particularly when their children are adolescents or young adults. This is similar to that proposed for identifying youths with familial lipid disorders by screening the offspring of parents who have had premature myocardial infarction, angina, or coronary artery bypass surgery.[25]

The question has frequently been raised about whether hypertension and atherosclerosis can be prevented by lifestyle interventions beginning in childhood. The answer is not known and the logistics of changing the eating, smoking, and exercise habits of the entire population are formidable. Nonetheless, many families who are at increased risk for hypertension and coronary artery disease can be identified in childhood and adolescence by means of a meticulously detailed family history that includes all first-degree relatives. It is in such families that lifestyle intervention from an early age may be feasible, especially if the family is intact with adequate socioeconomic support. In single-parent families, most often with a father absent, there may be difficulty in role model identification by gender. In lower-socioeconomic-class families, it may be financially difficult to buy foods that are nutritious, filling, and also low in sodium, fat, and calories.

Although there are many causes of both acute and chronic hypertension in children, among teenagers these are limited. In this age group, particularly when the onset of hypertension has been acute, one has to consider the ingestion of drugs or substances such as amphetamines.[26] However, chronic hypertension can also be seen in individuals taking drugs such as glucocorticosteroids, anabolic steroids, and birth control pills. Although these agents may not cause hypertension in all who take them, they certainly may unmask in some a genetic or underlying organic reason for high blood pressure.

The vast majority of adolescents seen in the past, as well as those presently followed by us, have mild to moderate hypertension, associated with being overweight or obese, and with positive histories of hypertension in first-degree relatives. They often also have high triglyceride and low HDL-cholesterol levels. Their physical examinations are normal except for their weights and they have normal urinalyses, renal function studies, and renal ultrasound examinations. The most important component of their medical evaluation is the family history. One must ask about high blood pressure and its complications, such as heart failure, stroke, and renal failure. The family history of obesity or overweightness, premature coronary artery disease, and diabetes is of equal importance. As some endocrinopathies are familial, information about thyroid, parathyroid, and adrenal tumors should also be sought, but these conditions are rare.

There is a subset of adolescents, usually white males, who are of normal or lower than normal weight and have hypertension. Generally, they also have a relative tachycardia, an active precordium, and quite often cardiac flow murmurs. They are considered to have a hyperdynamic cardiovascular state, thought to be due to autonomic overactivity. They usually respond well to beta-blocking agents, but not dietary sodium reduction.

ASSESSMENT

In evaluating a hypertensive adolescent, after a good medical and family history has been taken, a general physical examination is required. Particular attention should be paid to the cardiovascular system, including the retinal vasculature. Although being overweight is the most common clinical finding, a thorough nutritional assessment of the patient usually also needs to be undertaken. This includes an assessment of food intake, physical activity, and various anthropometric measurements.

Anthropometrics

Due to the strong association between obesity and borderline or definite hypertension, and the evidence that weight loss can significantly lower blood pressure in overweight hypertensive youth,[27–28] it is important to assess adolescents with high blood pressure for the appropriateness of body weight for height. Objective anthropometric measurements can guide the clinician as to whether weight-control strategies are indicated as part of the treatment plan for the hypertensive adolescent and how effective those strategies will be over time.

Body mass index.   Screening hypertensive adolescents for being overweight can easily be done in a public health or clinical setting. Access is needed to a platform beam balance scale to measure body weight, and a stadiometer (wall-mounted stature-measuring board) or steel measuring tape attached to a wall without a baseboard for measuring height (see Chapters 1 and 17). The weight and height values obtained are then used to determine body mass index (BMI).

The BMI, also known as Quetelet's index, is the preferred method for determining whether an adolescent is at a healthy weight.[29] The BMI is defined as body weight (in kilograms) divided by the square of one's height (in meters), i.e., BMI = body weight (kg) / height $(m)^2$.

When weight and height are obtained in pounds and inches respectively, BMI is derived by using the metric conversion constants (0.4545 kg/lb; 0.0254 m/in.) as shown below:

$$BMI = \frac{Body\ weight\ (lb) \times 0.4545\ kg/lb}{[Height\ (in.) \times 0.0254\ m/in.]^2}$$

This calculation can be further simplified by combining the conversion constants and varying height values in inches [height factor (HF) = $0.4536/(height\ (in.) \times 0.0254)^2$] to generate a table of height factor (HF) values as shown in Table 18.2.

BMI can then be readily determined by multiplying body weight (in pounds) by the HF that corresponds to one's height in inches [BMI = body weight (lb) × height factor (kg/m²-lb)].[30] (see Table 18.2 for listing of HF values for height ranging from 4'4"–6'6".)

The preferred percentile rankings for age- and gender-based BMI values were generated from population data collected for the National Health and Nutrition Surveys (NHANES I) during the early 1970s.[31] With BMI percentile rankings (see Table 18.3), the currently accepted criteria for assessing the appropriateness of weight-for-height for adolescents[32,33] are as follows:

BMI ≥ 95th percentile, overweight

BMI ≥ 85th and < 95th percentile, at risk for being overweight

BMI < 85th and ≥ 15th percentiles, average weight

BMI < 15th and ≥ 5th percentile, at risk for being underweight

BMI < 5th percentile, underweight

Skinfold measurements. It must be kept in mind that an overweight adolescent may not necessarily be obese, defined as body fat >25% of total body weight for males and >30% for females.[34] The most accurate method for measuring body fat is hydrostatic or "underwater" weighing, but is usually not practical in a clinical or public health setting due to the cost of equipment and time constraints.

Skinfold measurements provide a relative measure of body fatness and can help distinguish those overweight adolescents who are obese from those with a large skeletal size or who are very muscular, such as is found in some athletes. Excess body fat is correlated with the sum of the triceps and subscapular skinfold measurements when the value obtained is greater than the 85th percentile of age-

Table 18.2 Height Factor*
[body mass index (kg/m^2) = (HF) × weight (lb)]

Height	HF	Height	HF	Height	HF	Height	HF
4'4" or 52"	0.260	4'11" or 59"	0.202	5'6" or 66"	0.161	6'1" or 73"	0.132
¼	0.258	¼	0.200	¼	0.160	¼	0.131
½	0.255	½	0.199	½	0.159	½	0.130
¾	0.253	¾	0.197	¾	0.158	¾	0.129
4'5" or 53"	0.250	5'0" or 60"	0.195	5'7" or 67"	0.157	6'2" or 74"	0.128
¼	0.248	¼	0.194	¼	0.155	¼	0.128
½	0.246	½	0.192	½	0.154	½	0.127
¾	0.243	¾	0.191	¾	0.153	¾	0.126
4'6" or 54"	0.241	5'1" or 61"	0.189	5'8" or 68"	0.152	6'3" or 75"	0.125
¼	0.239	¼	0.188	¼	0.151	¼	0.124
½	0.237	½	0.186	½	0.150	½	0.123
¾	0.235	¾	0.184	¾	0.149	¾	0.123
4'7" or 55"	0.232	5'2" or 62"	0.183	5'9" or 69"	0.148	6'4" or 76"	0.122
¼	0.230	¼	0.181	¼	0.147	¼	0.121
½	0.228	½	0.180	½	0.146	½	0.120
¾	0.226	¾	0.179	¾	0.145	¾	0.119
4'8" or 56"	0.224	5'3" or 63"	0.177	5'10" or 70"	0.143	6'5" or 77"	0.119
¼	0.222	¼	0.176	¼	0.142	¼	0.118
½	0.220	½	0.174	½	0.141	½	0.117
¾	0.218	¾	0.173	¾	0.140	¾	0.116
4'9" or 57"	0.216	5'4" or 64"	0.172	5'11" or 7"	0.139	6'6" or 78"	0.116
¼	0.215	¼	0.170	¼	0.138	¼	0.115
½	0.212	½	0.169	½	0.138	½	0.114
¾	0.211	¾	0.168	¾	0.137	¾	0.113
4'10" or 58"	0.209	5'5" or 65"	0.166	6'0" or 72"	0.136	6'7" or 79"	0.113
¼	0.207	¼	0.165	¼	0.135		
½	0.205	½	0.164	½	0.134		
¾	0.204	¾	0.163	¾	0.133		

Note: Height factors for 4'4" to 6'7" at ¼" increments.

*Height factor values are independent of age and gender.

Adapted from R. P. Abernathy, *J. Am. Diet. Assoc.*, **91**, 843 (1991). Reprinted with permission.

and gender-based population data.[35] Values at or above the 95th percentile occur with those more severely obese (see Table 18.4).

Skinfold measurements can also assess relative changes in body fat, particularly for adolescents trying to manage body weight through dietary modifications and increased physical activity. Obese adolescents seen in our clinic for weight management who achieve weight stabilization in this manner over a 3–6-mo period may also be experiencing desirable changes in body composition, i.e., preserving or increasing lean body mass while decreasing body fat. Baseline

Table 18.3 Percentile of Body Mass Index for the Adolescent Years

Age (yr)	5th	15th	50th	85th	95th
			MALES		
10	14	15	17	20	23
11	15	16	17	20	24
12	15	16	18	21	25
13	16	17	19	22	26
14	16	17	19	23	27
15	17	18	20	24	28
16	17	18	21	24	29
17	17	19	21	25	29
18	18	19	21	26	30
19	18	19	22	26	31
20–24	19	20	23	27	31
			FEMALES		
10	14	15	17	20	23
11	15	16	18	21	25
12	15	16	18	22	26
13	15	16	19	23	27
14	16	17	19	24	28
15	16	17	20	24	29
16	16	18	20	25	29
17	17	18	20	25	30
18	17	18	21	26	30
19	17	18	21	26	31
20–24	17	19	21	26	31

Adapted from A. Must, G. E. Dallal, and W. H. Dietz, *Am, J. Clin. Nutr.*, **53**, 839 (1991). Reprinted with permission.

skinfold measurements should be obtained for obese adolescents beginning a weight-management program and repeated every 3–6 mo. Knowledge of a relative decrease in body fat with either little or no change in body weight may provide the needed incentive for the adolescent to sustain the desired lifestyle changes adopted for weight control that ultimately may improve the blood pressure level as well.

The equipment and technique recommended for obtaining accurate and reproducible measurements for triceps and subscapular skinfold thicknesses follow the methods described in the *Anthropometric Standardization Reference Manual*[36] and are shown graphically in Figures 18.1 through 18.7. With the Lange skinfold caliper (Cambridge Scientific Instruments, Cambridge, MD), the general practice

Table 18.4 Sum of Triceps and Subscapular Skinfold Thickness (mm) at the 85th
and 95th Percentile for the Adolescent Years*

Age (yr)	Males		Females	
	85th	95th	85th	95th
10–10.9	27.0	42.0	34.5	51.0
11–11.9	33.0	53.5	37.0	55.0
12–12.9	34.0	53.0	37.0	57.0
13–13.9	29.0	48.0	43.0	56.0
14–14.9	27.0	45.0	44.5	62.0
15–15.9	27.0	43.0	42.5	62.5
16–16.9	27.5	44.0	47.0	69.5
17–17.9	27.0	41.0	49.0	67.4
18–24.9	37.0	50.5	52.0	70.0

Adapted from R. A. Frisancho, *Anthropometric Standards for the Assessment of Growth and
Nutritional Status,* The University of Michigan Press, Ann Arbor, MI, p. 56, (1991). Reprinted
with permission.

is to take the average of three measurements at the same skinfold site on the
right side of the body.

The clinician prepares the adolescent for the measurements by first explaining
what the skinfold values mean, where the measurements are taken, and how the
skinfold caliper works. The adolescent is also given the experience of how much
pressure the skinfold caliper can exert by placing the prongs of the caliper around
his or her index finger. This orientation will help enlist the teen's cooperation
and allay fears about the procedure. Since the positioning of the body and site
location do not allow the adolescent to see the skinfold measurement being taken,
it is important to continue explaining what is happening to the adolescent as one
proceeds with the actual measurement.

To further ensure comfort with the procedure and respecting the adolescent's
need for privacy, the adolescent is asked to wear or bring lightweight shorts to
change into when skinfold measurements are taken. In a private examining room
with the clinician absent, the adolescent disrobes from the waist up, with girls
leaving on their brassiere if it can be unfastened from the back so as not to
interfere with taking the subscapular skinfold measurement. The adolescent is
provided with a short-sleeved adult-sized hospital gown that is worn with the
opening to the back and left untied.

In preparation for the triceps skinfold measurement, the clinician can assist
the adolescent in removing the right arm from the sleeve of the hospital gown
and then tying the hospital gown in the back, with the empty sleeve placed under
the right armpit. This will allow complete exposure of the right arm while still
maintaining coverage of the front of the body. (see Figures 18.2 through 18.4).

On completion of the triceps skinfold measurement, the right arm is placed

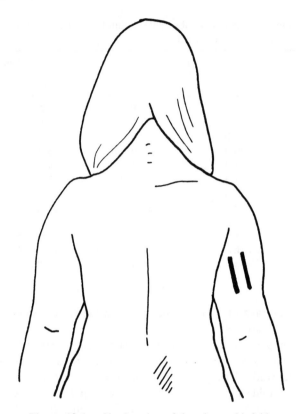

Figure 18-1.   Site location of the triceps skinfold.

back in the sleeve of the gown. The gown is left untied in the back, and if a brassiere is worn, the clasp is undone at this time in preparation for the subscapular skinfold measurements that follow.

TRICEPS SKINFOLD.   The triceps skinfold is measured at the midpoint of the right upper arm. To locate the midpoint of the upper arm, the right arm is bent at a 90-deg angle. By using a metric tape measure, the midpoint of the upper arm is located equidistant from the bony protrusion at the back of the upper shoulder (acromial process) and the tip of the elbow (olecranon process).

An insert tape designed for this measurement is also available. Identical numbers on the insert tape are aligned with the olecranon and acromial processes. With the insert tape in this position, the midpoint marking on the tape will correspond to that of the upper arm. The midpoint of the upper arm using either measuring device is then marked with a water-soluble ink pen (Figure 18.2).

The triceps skinfold measurement is obtained with the adolescent standing, fac-

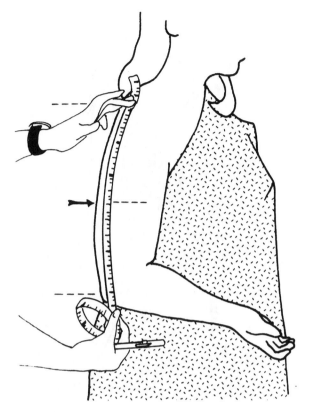

Figure 18-2. Locating the midpoint of the upperarm for the triceps skinfold measurement.

ing straight ahead, and with the right arm hanging loosely at the side of the body. Giving the adolescent a concrete image, such as "Imagine yourself as limp as a rag doll," may help to achieve a more relaxed and comfortable position of the arm.

With the left hand positioned approximately 1 cm above and the right hand 1 cm below the marked midpoint of the upper arm, the clinician standing behind the adolescent then gently, but firmly grasps with the thumb, index, and middle fingers of both hands a vertical pinch of skin and subcutaneous fat. This can be done repeatedly to ensure there is no involvement of the underlying triceps muscle (see Figure 18.3).

The Lange skinfold caliper is then picked up with the right hand, while the left hand continues to hold the skinfold. The prongs of the caliper are opened by pressing the caliper lever with the right thumb and then positioned around the skinfold approximately 1 cm proximal from the midpoint marking (Figure 18.4). The lever is then released by removing the right thumb. When the prongs

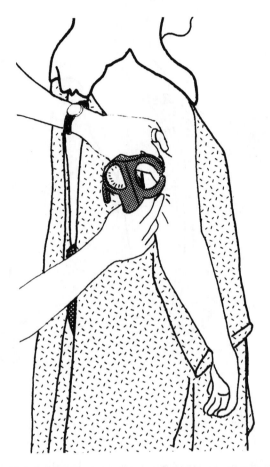

Figure 18-3. Two-handed grasp in preparation for triceps skinfold measurement.

of the caliper are exerting full pressure on the skinfold following the first rapid fall of the needle on the dial, a measurement in millimeters is read. The procedure is repeated three times and the average of the values obtained is the triceps skinfold measurement.

SUBSCAPULAR SKINFOLD. The subscapular skinfold measurement is obtained with the adolescent standing erect, shoulders relaxed, and arms hanging comfortably at the side (see Figure 18.5). The clinician locates the tip of the right shoulder blade (scapula). With the thumb, index, and middle fingers of both hands, the clinician gently, but firmly, grasps on a diagonal the layer of skin and subcutaneous fat located approximately 1 cm below the right scapula (Figure 18.6). With the left hand still holding the skinfold, the Lange skinfold caliper

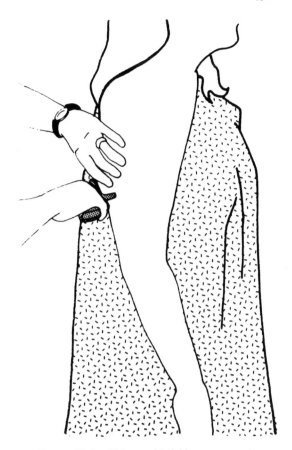

Figure 18-4. Triceps skinfold measurement.

is then picked up with the right hand. With the prongs of the caliper opened by pressing the lever with the thumb of the right hand, the caliper is placed on a diagonal approximately 1 cm away from the position of the thumb and index fingers of the left hand. The lever is then released by removing the right thumb (Figure 18.7). When the prongs of the caliper are exerting full pressure on the skinfold following the first rapid fall of the needle on the dial, a measurement in millimeters is read. The procedure is repeated three times and the average of the values obtained is the subscapular skinfold measurement.

Waist-hip circumference ratio. Due to the association between "central obesity" and increased cardiovascular risk,[17] measuring the waist-hip circumference ratio may help identify those overweight adolescents whose adiposity places them at higher risk for elevated blood pressure.[37] The waist-hip ratio (WHR) is

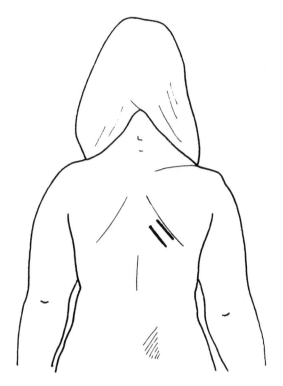

Figure 18-5. Site location of the subscapular skinfold.

derived by measuring the waist at its smallest circumference located midway between the lower rib margin and the iliac crests, and the hips at the largest circumference over the great trochanters. A tape measure is used as shown in Figures 18.8 and 18.9, and the ratio is then calculated, i.e., WHR = waist (inches or centimeters) / hip (inches or centimeters).

The adult values for defining central obesity (> 1.00 for males, and > 0.80 for females)[38] can be applied to adolescents who have a sexual maturity rating (SMR) of 4 or 5 (see Chapter 1). Currently there are no specific WHR values distinguishing central from peripheral obesity for adolescents at the earlier Tanner stages. However, the graph in Figure 18.10 can be used to determine whether there is a trend toward more central or peripheral obesity.[39] A WHR that is above the mean WHR for age, gender, and race indicates a tendency toward central obesity, and one below the mean WHR toward peripheral obesity.

Dietary Factors

Nutritional adequacy. A comprehensive dietary evaluation is needed to assess the overall adequacy of food and drink consumed when compared to the

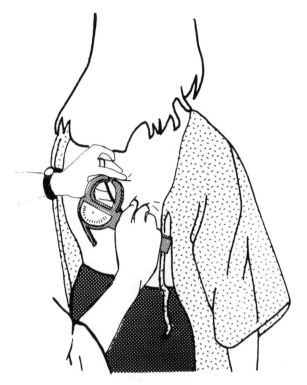

Figure 18-6. Two-handed grasp in preparation for subscapular skinfold measurement.

nutritional guidelines recommended for adolescence, as represented by the food guide pyramid (Figure 18.11).[40] As graphically shown, a well-balanced diet will include more servings of grain products, fruits, and vegetables in comparison to meat and dairy products, with moderation stressed for fats and sugars that are added to or occur naturally in foods.

When accounting for differences in gender, growth, weight status, or activity level, adolescents who eat the recommended number of servings from each food group as advised will meet the nutritional needs to support normal growth and development (see Table 18.5).

Adolescent males need more calories than females due to increased muscle mass, and for those teens involved in sports on a regular basis, caloric requirements are greater due to increased energy expenditure (see Chapter 12). A reduction in caloric needs is indicated for those who have completed their growth (SMR 4–5 for females and SMR 5 for males) and also are inactive or overweight.

Sodium and salt. Population studies have shown that a reduced intake of salt and sodium in the diet is associated with lower blood pressure levels.[41–3]

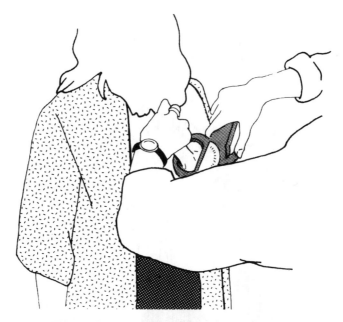

Figure 18-7. Subscapular skinfold measurement.

Short-term clinical trials done with hypertensive adults have reported that blood pressure can be lowered by following a sodium-restricted diet.[43,44] The blood-pressure-raising effect of a higher sodium intake is more pronounced for those who are regarded as "salt-sensitive."[4,27] This is reported to be characteristic of approximately 50% of those adolescents with essential hypertension.[5] Currently, there is no simple way to screen for salt sensitivity, so the prudent course is to advise those teens with essential hypertension to modify their intake of sodium and salt.

The results of dietary surveys conducted in the United States estimate sodium intake to range from 1800–5000 mg/d,[45,46] with some reporting sodium levels as high as 8000 mg/d.[3] This far exceeds the minimum daily requirement for sodium (500 mg/d) needed to support normal growth and development during adolescence, as well as health maintenance in adulthood.[47]

Potassium.   There is some evidence to show that changing the sodium-potassium ratio in the diet by increasing potassium intake may be as important in reducing blood pressure as restricting dietary sodium alone in adults with hypertension.[48,49] Therefore, assessing hypertensive adolescents for how regularly they consume low-sodium, potassium-rich foods such as fresh fruits and vegetables, milk and milk products, and lean meats and meat substitutes is another dietary factor to consider for lowering blood pressure. There is growing evidence

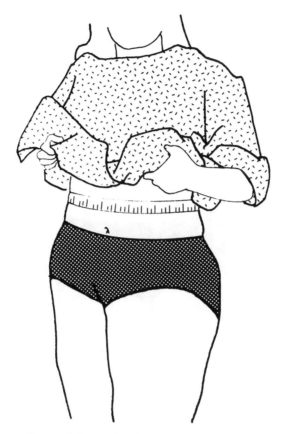

Figure 18-8. Waist circumference measurement.

to support the idea that a high dietary potassium intake may be a beneficial intervention for hypertension management,[48,50,51] but results reported are inconsistent, and research involving adolescents is limited.

Some studies with hypertensive adults have shown a modest decrease in blood pressure with potassium supplementation,[52,53] with African Americans reportedly having a more pronounced blood pressure reduction.[54,55] Other investigators have not found potassium supplementation in hypertensive adults to be effective in lowering blood pressure either alone,[56,57] or in combination with a sodium-restrictive diet.[58] However, some studies show that with adults, lowering the sodium-potassium ratio in the diet may be as effective in reducing blood pressure as restricting dietary sodium alone.[48,49] The results of one multiyear clinical trial with normotensive adolescents found potassium supplementation to lower blood pressure in girls, but not in boys, an effect potentially confounded by the lack of

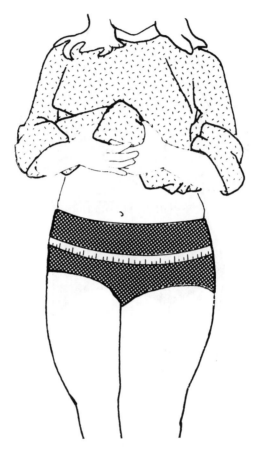

Figure 18-9.   Hip circumference measurement.

adherence by boys to a reduced sodium intake.[59] At this time, there is insufficient information to determine what effect potassium supplementation would have on hypertensive adolescents and much uncertainty about what would be an effective dose.

It has been reported that adults who consume large amounts of fruits and vegetables have potassium intake levels as high as 8000–11,000 mg/d.[60] Based on a national diet survey conducted in the early 1980s, the average intake of potassium for those aged 15–20 year-olds in the United States was found to be 3400 mg/d.[46] Other studies show considerably lower intakes of potassium for African Americans at 1000 mg/d[61] and urban whites at 2500 mg/d.[62]

A more recent diet survey of adolescents in the United States indicates that the intake of fruits and vegetables is significantly less than the recommended

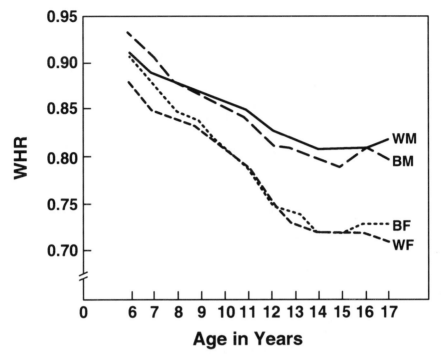

Figure 18-10. Mean ratio of waist-to-hip girth by age, sex, and race. *(WM=white males; BM=black males; WF=white females; BF=black females;WHR=ratio of waist-to-hip girth)* R. F. Gillum, *J. Chron. Dis.*, **40**, 413 (1987). Reprinted with permission.

levels, with only 8–18% of adolescents surveyed consuming five or more servings of fruits and vegetables the day preceding the survey.[63] Consumption of milk and milk products has also been shown to be inadequate during the teen years[64] and may further contribute to a less than desirable intake of potassium.

Calcium. Dietary calcium may have a role in blood pressure regulation, as is suggested by many observational studies with adults.[65–68] However, data are not available for normotensive or hypertensive adolescents.[5] The epidemiologic evidence for adults showing an inverse association of dietary calcium and blood pressure levels has been regarded with some skepticism because the confounding factor of sodium intake as best measured by urinary excretion was not accounted for in any of the investigations.[51] The finding that a reduced intake of calcium may enhance the blood-pressure-raising effect of a high sodium intake[69] further supports this criticism.

A pooled analysis of 23 clinical trials using calcium supplementation with either normotensive or hypertensive adults estimated no significant change in

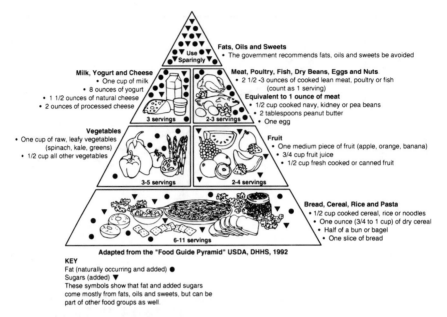

Figure 18-11.   Food guide pyramid.

U. S. Department of Agriculture, Human Nutrition Information Service, Leaflet no. 572, Hyattsville, MD, (1992).

systolic blood pressure, but a significant, although minimal, reduction (−0.29 mm Hg) in diastolic blood pressure.[51] Two of the adult intervention studies with the largest sample size and conducted for the longest period of time were unable to demonstrate a reduction in either systolic or diastolic blood pressures with calcium supplementation.[70,71]

The recommended daily intake of dietary calcium for adolescents is 1200 mg. This is met primarily from consuming the advised number of servings for milk and milk products, as represented in Figure 18.11 and Table 18.5. Adequate intake of dietary calcium is needed for skeletal growth and increasing bone density.

Whether dietary calcium is also a significant factor for regulating blood pressure for hypertensive adolescents has yet to be established, and the evidence for adults remains questionable. At this time, there is no convincing scientific basis to advise hypertensive adolescents to increase dietary calcium beyond the levels recommended for supporting normal growth and development.[4]

Dietary fat.   Hypertensive adolescents who are overweight or have elevated blood lipids are advised to modify their intake of dietary fat. Dietary fat is a

Table 18.5 Recommended Number of Servings by Food Groups for Adolescents at Differing Levels of Activity, Physical Maturation and Weight Status

	Older Overweight* or Inactive Teens*	Teen Girls	Teen Boys
Calorie Level[+]	About 1600	About 2200	About 2800
Food Group	Servings	Servings	Servings
Bread, cereal, rice, and pasta	6	9	11
Vegetables	3	4	5
Fruits	2	3	4
Milk, yogurt, and cheese	3	3	3
Meat, poultry, fish	2	2	3
Dry beans and peas, eggs and nuts	(Total=5 oz)	(Total=6 oz)	(Total=7 oz)

* Applies to adolescents who have completed their growth spurt as assessed by their sexual maturity rating (an SMR of 4 or 5).

[+] These are the calorie levels if low-fat, lean foods are chosen from the five major food groups, and fats, oils, and sweets are used sparingly.

Note: An additional 600–1200 cal is generally needed by those involved in sports on a regular basis. The increased energy needs for an athlete are best met by additional servings of complex carbohydrates such as bread, pasta, cereal, rice, potatoes, dry beans, or peas to replace lost glycogen stores depleted during exercise.

Adapted from M. Story and I. Alton, *Guidelines for Adolescent Nutrition,* Department of Health and Human Services, U. S. Public Health Service, Region V, Chicago, IL, p.14, (1993).

more concentrated source of calories and when consumed in excess, is more efficiently stored as body fat in comparison to carbohydrates and protein. A study of preadolescent children found that a higher percentage of fat in the diet was significantly correlated with excess body fat.[21] Reducing total fat and saturated fat in the diet has been shown to lower both total cholesterol and LDL-cholesterol levels in youth,[72] which may decrease the risk for developing atherosclerosis and coronary heart disease (CHD) in adulthood. This is an important consideration for obese adolescents with hypertension since most have hypertriglyceridemia, elevated serum LDL-cholesterol, and decreased HDL-cholesterol levels.[13] The occurrence of these multiple cardiovascular risk factors adds to the morbidity and mortality from CHD predicted in later years.

Analysis of dietary surveys from adolescent populations does not reflect a significant increase in caloric intake over time, but rather that a greater proportion of calories consumed come from fat. Adolescents in the United States are consuming on the average 35% of total calories from fat, with saturated fat representing 14% of caloric intake.[72] It was recently reported in a national survey that 66.2%

of adolescents aged 12–19 yr were characterized as having a high-fat diet because they were regularly consuming high-fat meats (hamburgers, hot dogs, and sausage), French fries, potato chips, and baked goods (doughnuts, cake, cookies and pie).[73]

Alcoholic beverages.   Alcohol intake should also be assessed given the well-documented positive correlation between blood pressure and alcohol intake of three drinks or more per day.[54] Regular use and abuse of alcohol is a common finding among youth in the United States. A national survey conducted in 1988 reported that 63.9% of high school seniors had consumed alcohol in the previous 30 d and 4.2% of those surveyed were drinking alcohol daily.[74]

Physical Activity

Regular physical activity is associated with improved cardiovascular health. Studies have consistently shown that youth who are more physically fit as measured by submaximal and maximal exercise testing have lower blood pressure levels.[51] There is evidence to show that hypertensive adolescents who exercise more can improve their blood pressure level, whether overweight or not, and decrease blood lipid levels, if the activity chosen is aerobic, done for a sufficient amount of time and on a regular basis.[75]

Unfortunately, there are now less opportunities and requirements for adolescents to engage in physical activities, particularly at school. Participation of adolescents in school physical education (PE) programs has declined by 17% (65% in 1984–48% in 1990) according to a 1992 report by the U.S. Centers for Disease Control and Prevention (CDC).[20] The CDC also found that only 21.5% of high school students nationally attend PE classes daily and almost half (47.8%) are not enrolled at all. This is consistent with the fact that 25 states in the United States require only 1 yr of physical education between 9th and 12th grades, and Illinois is the only state requiring daily PE classes for grades K–12.[76] Encouraging adolescents to elect for more physical education classes than required is difficult, and often not possible given class offerings and other scheduling constraints.

Level of inactivity is also an important factor to consider when evaluating energy expenditure. The hypertensive adolescents seen in our clinic, particularly those who are overweight, are typically leading very sedentary lifestyles, with the majority of leisure time spent watching television. Access to cable television with its additional programming and inexpensive rental videos for use with home VCRs has broadened television's entertainment appeal for adolescents. Those adolescents residing in urban communities where safety issues are a concern can lead families to discourage and, in some cases, prohibit them from being active outside in their neighborhoods and may inadvertently lead to more television use when restricted to the home. Our clinical experience has found that families seldom place limits on the amount of television viewed. According to a 1990

Neilsen Report, adolescents are watching television an average of 21 h/wk.[77] When figured on an annual basis, adolescents are spending more time watching television than at school, and it is second only to time spent sleeping. One study has shown that the prevalence of obesity increased by 2% for each additional hour of television viewed.[19]

Imaging and Laboratory Studies

In obese adolescents who are asymptomatic, who have a positive family history of hypertension and a negative physical examination, few diagnostic studies are needed. Urinalysis, serum electrolytes, blood urea nitrogen, serum creatinine, and fasting lipids usually suffice. An echocardiogram may give information concerning left ventricular muscle mass, but it is not usually possible to determine how much of an increase, if present, is due to high blood pressure and how much results from obesity. Renal ultrasound examinations are almost invariably normal.

In the presence of moderate or severe hypertension, a more extensive laboratory and radiological evaluation is indicated. The work-up is usually directed by clinical clues and the results of the simple laboratory tests noted above. For detailed discussions on evaluation for renal, renovascular, and endocrine forms of hypertension in adolescents, the reader is referred elsewhere.[78]

MANAGEMENT

Once it has been determined that hypertension is persistent and no curable cause has been found, some form of intervention has to be selected. Adolescents with blood pressures in excess of the 99th percentile will usually require antihypertensive drug therapy. However, the nonpharmacologic strategies of a sodium-restricted diet, weight management (if overweight), and an increase in physical activity constitute the preferred initial intervention for adolescents with essential hypertension.

Nonpharmacologic Interventions

Dietary factors.

NUTRITIONAL ADEQUACY. To begin the nutritional intervention, a typical food intake screening (see Appendix C) is obtained by the clinician through direct interview with the adolescent alone. Responses given will provide information about the variety of food and drink consumed, regularity and timing of meals and snacks, comparison of weekday vs. weekend eating, the extent to which meals or snacks are eaten away from the home, and whether the family is a recipient of government-funded food assistance programs (e.g., food stamps, WIC, or school breakfast or lunch).

Determining which member(s) of the household are responsible for food purchasing and meal preparation in the home is also important. The clinician can identify which family members need to be actively involved when diet modifications are presented. The dietary changes advised that impact on food buying habits and cooking methods can be better achieved when key family members receive this information directly.

DECREASING SODIUM INTAKE.   All hypertensive youth are usually instructed to reduce their dietary intake of sodium. It is not established how much sodium restriction should be advised in order to significantly lower blood pressure in teenagers with hypertension. Therefore, an arbitrary level for sodium intake has been selected that represents a significant reduction from the average intake of sodium, but provides a margin of safety to meet the daily sodium needs for adolescents and adults. A consensus has been reached that a moderate reduction in sodium could be achieved if hypertensive adolescents would consume 1500–2500 mg of sodium/d.[3,4] Hypertensive adolescents will exceed this advised level for dietary sodium if they are:

1. Regularly eating processed foods that are high in salt (sodium chloride) or other sodium compounds, e.g., salted snacks like chips, pretzels, popcorn, nuts, or crackers; processed cheeses; condiments like ketchup and mustard; cured meats such as bacon, sausage, hot dogs, or lunch meats; and commercially prepared main-course foods that are frozen, boxed, or canned.
2. Frequently eating out at fast-food restaurants where some items offered provide one-third or more of the daily sodium intake advised (see Appendix C).
3. Salting their food at the table. Adding salt and other seasonings with sodium when cooking at home can also be a significant contributor to a high-sodium diet.

Identifying those foods with a high sodium or salt content that are consumed on a regular basis will help formulate a targeted intervention to modify sodium intake. Relying exclusively on the typical food intake screening (see Appendix C) may inadvertently miss significant sources of sodium in the diet. However, with the addition of a food frequency questionnaire that targets foods high in sodium and salt, a more comprehensive assessment of dietary sodium intake can be obtained (see Appendix C). Also by having the adolescent designate his or her favorite foods from this listing, the clinician will become aware of how easily specific foods can be restricted, modified, or omitted.

The food frequency questionnaire for sodium and salt intake can be completed by adolescents on their own and then reviewed with the clinician, or administered by interview as time and resources permit. Any of the items listed that are consumed "frequently" (1–3 times/wk) or "regularly" (4–7 times/wk) are providing too much sodium in the diet. Additional screening questions can be included to determine the contribution of sodium from fast-food intake and use of table salt if this has not already been determined with completion of the typical food intake screening (see Appendix C). Responses to the food frequency questionnaire for sodium can serve as a guide for the clinician to assist the adolescent in modifying his or her intake of sodium.

However, it must be remembered that it is not easy to reduce sodium intake to a level sufficiently low to affect blood pressure. In fact, in one of the few controlled clinical trials of dietary sodium reduction among U.S. children, Sinaiko et al.[59] concluded that it was impossible to get boys to comply with a low-sodium diet for an extended period of time. Many of the so-called "fast" and "junk" foods that are staples of the adolescent diet are relatively high in sodium. It is often a significant imposition on lifestyle to ask teenagers to adhere to a low-sodium diet. This is particularly true when they are eating with their friends either socially or in the school setting where they do not want to appear to be different. Therefore, it is important at first to modify a limited number of foods that add significant amounts of sodium and salt to the diet, and gradually build toward additional changes over time as compliance is achieved.

INCREASING POTASSIUM INTAKE.   There is strong evidence from population studies associating long-term exposure to a higher potassium diet with lower blood pressures.[41] Thus, it is reasonable to encourage hypertensive adolescents to consume a potassium-rich diet.[3] Daily servings of fresh fruits and vegetables, lean fresh meats and meat substitutes, and low-fat milk and milk products selected in accordance with guidelines adapted from the food guide pyramid (Table 18.5) will significantly exceed the estimated minimum daily potassium requirement of 2000 mg/d for adolescents.[47] The higher intake of fruits and vegetables now advised was changed, in part, in recognition of the potential benefit dietary potassium may have on blood pressure control.[60] See Appendix C for a listing of foods high in potassium and low in natural salt content and fat.

Specific questions about intake of fruits, vegetables, milk, and yogurt are included on the typical food intake screening form to ensure that the adequacy of dietary potassium intake is assessed (see Appendix C).

DECREASING TOTAL FAT AND SATURATED FAT.   It is recommended that fat intake represent 25–30% of total calories consumed[79,80] and no more than 10% of calories should be as saturated fat.[81] Adolescents will typically exceed these levels if they are regularly eating the following:

1. Foods with a naturally high fat content: red meats such as hamburgers, steak, roast beef, sausage, and hot dogs, chicken with skin, luncheon meats such as bologna and salami, bacon, sunflower seeds, nuts, peanut butter, olives, or avocados

2. Fried foods: French fries, fried chicken or fish, hash browns. or fried onion rings

3. Processed snack foods with added fats: Potato chips and other snack chips, high-fat crackers, popcorn with added fat

4. Baked goods: Biscuits, croissants, danish, sweet rolls, doughnuts, cakes, cookies, muffins, brownies and pie

5. High-fat dairy products: Whole milk (3.5% fat), chocolate milk, ice cream, milk shakes, hard cheeses (American, Swiss, cheddar, etc.), cream cheese, or sour cream

6. Foods prepared or served with the following added fats: Mayonnaise, salad dressing, margarine, butter, or gravy

Many of the foods listed above are also high in sodium and salt. The food frequency questionnaire targeting foods high in fat (Appendix C) does not repeat those items already included with the food frequency questionnaire for sodium and salt (Appendix C). If the food can be prepared or processed without added salt, such as unsalted nuts or French fries, then it appears on both screening tools. Attention should be given to the consumption of high-fat foods of animal origin and foods processed with tropical oils (palm, coconut, and palm kernel oil) since they are high in saturated fats. Learning to read the nutrition labels of packaged products will help the teen and family members responsible for grocery shopping to identify those foods that can contribute significant amounts of total fat and saturated fat to their diet.

The typical food intake screening (see Appendix C) combined with a food frequency questionnaire targeting high-fat foods (Appendix C) will identify specific foods that the adolescent can elect to omit, reduce, or modify. The questionnaire assessing dietary fat can be completed by adolescents on their own and then reviewed together with the clinician, or administered by personal interview as time and resources permit. Any of the items listed that are consumed on a weekly basis, particularly in large quantities, are providing too much fat in the diet.

Abstaining from Alcohol.   Determining whether an adolescent is consuming alcohol on a regular basis can be difficult, given, that drinking alcohol is illegal for those underage. Adolescents who drink may not be comfortable revealing their own involvement with alcohol, but may more readily describe the drinking habits of their friends or other peers. This approach to questioning about alcohol intake may provide more valid information regarding an adolescent's own use of alcohol and is included as part of the typical food intake screening (see Appendix C). Developing a level of trust and meeting individually with the adolescent for some time may enable the adolescent to be more open about drinking habits.

If regular alcohol use or abuse is present, the clinician will need to discuss the problems this presents to the adolescent's physical and emotional health, and management of his or her hypertension. Therapeutic counseling for the adolescent and family is likely indicated to better understand the underlying reasons for the drinking behavior. Depending on the severity of alcohol use or abuse, the clinician may also advise involvement in a substance abuse treatment program available in the community.

Weight Control.   For obese adolescents, every effort should be made to help them lose weight through an appropriate diet and exercise program. Providing an effective weight-management program for overweight hypertensive adolescents is difficult when time and resources for long-term, interdisciplinary intervention are limited. A multifaceted, family-based, group approach has shown some success because it attempts to account for the varying contributions of physiological, behavioral, and psychosocial factors involved and offers peer support.[81]

The medical necessity for weight control is not disputed for those overweight adolescents with hypertension. However, unless the adolescent is motivated to adhere to needed lifestyle changes affecting food choices and activity level, and appropriate parental/guardian support is enlisted, efforts to control weight are unlikely to succeed. The extent to which chronic overeating occurs in response to emotional difficulties related to family dynamics, peers, or school performance determines the need for further psychosocial and/or educational evaluation. If therapeutic counseling for the overweight adolescent and/or family is indicated, delaying weight-management intervention may be advisable until some degree of resolution of identified psychosocial issues is achieved.

For the overweight hypertensive adolescent who is ready and interested in pursuing weight management, an individualized approach with clearly defined objectives for modifying food intake and increasing physical activity is undertaken. Dietary factors to consider as potential contributors for the accumulation of excess body fat include regular intake of high-fat foods, overconsumption of sweets and beverages with a high refined sugar content and frequent meal skipping (breakfast and/or lunch). Meal skipping can lead to chronic overeating later in the day of either snacks, dinner or both due to the onset of extreme hunger.

Other behaviors to review that can result in extra eating and a subsequent increase in body weight are routinely taking additional helpings of food at meals or taking large portions of food served, eating too fast, eating while watching television, eating whatever peers may offer, or eating large quantities of food at one sitting. Developing behavioral interventions to alter the external cues for extra eating in these circumstances may be indicated. Limiting meals and snacks to one area of the home that is away from the television set and keeping serving platters off the table to limit extra helpings are easily implemented strategies. Family members can create a more interactive atmosphere for meals and snacks eaten at home; this can help slow down the rate of consumption and, thus, decrease the quantity of intake. Discussing ways to refuse food offers from peers without negatively affecting friendships is important to ensure that weight-management efforts do not interfere with needed peer involvement and support. Determining which specific dietary or behavioral changes to begin with is negotiated with the adolescent, family members, and the clinician. The clinician summarizes those areas affecting food intake that need modification and strategies to reduce inactivity (i.e., less television viewing) and increase physical exercise. A combined diet and exercise plan that is sustainable for the foreseeable future offers the best opportunity for success at weight management. Ultimately though, the adolescent has to accept what is proposed, and family members have to be willing to assume a supportive role.

Keeping the initial intervention to a few targeted strategies will help gauge the potential for long-term adherence to weight management. Using a written contract (Appendix C) will help to reinforce and concretely state what dietary and behavioral changes were agreed on by both the adolescent and family for a specified period of time. Frequent follow-up sessions are scheduled every 2–3 wk during the beginning months of counseling. Sessions can be extended to monthly visits depending on the level of adherence achieved. Meeting with the adolescent individually, followed by the adolescent and involved family members together, can provide a more balanced perspective regarding issues of compliance. Additional changes in eating habits or activity patterns can be contracted as the adolescent and family demonstrate readiness to do so.

Expectations for determining a successful intervention should be discussed. For those adolescents who have not completed their growth, weight maintenance is advised. Even when body weight remains stable, body composition can change. A decrease in body fat can occur as lean body mass increases due to growth and/or adherence to regular physical activity. Periodic skinfold measurements can be used to monitor relative changes in body fat as previously discussed. Older adolescents defined as females with a SMR of 4–5 and males with a SMR of 5 are advised to lose weight at a modest rate (½–2 lb/wk) in order to maximize the loss of body fat while preserving muscle mass. This again is best accomplished when exercise is included as part of the intervention for weight management.

Achieving weight stabilization for older hypertensive adolescents who have been consistently gaining weight in the past is a significant initial accomplishment. Offering praise and encouragement for efforts to keep weight stable can help motivate the adolescent to incorporate further lifestyle changes that may ultimately result in weight reduction.

Physical Activity

Adolescents with uncomplicated hypertension, implying that no cardiac symptomatology or other serious health problems are present, can begin a regular aerobic exercise of moderate intensity without needing an extensive fitness evaluation. However, for monitoring long-term adherence to an endurance exercise program, having a baseline measure and periodic serial measurements of aerobic capacity obtained with exercise testing is still useful.[82] Intense isometric exercise characteristic of power lifting and some approaches to weight training can dramatically increase systolic blood pressure as well as diastolic pressure and should be discouraged.[3]

Counseling hypertensive adolescents to become more active, particularly those who are primarily sedentary and significantly overweight, can be very frustrating. When exercise is not a priority for the family or peers and participation in school-based physical education programs is limited, asking adolescents to be solely responsible for increasing their physical activity is unrealistic. Having a supportive home environment that recognizes the importance of physical activity, involving school physical education instructors when possible, and utilizing community recreational programs when available is critical for establishing long-term adherence to any exercise regimen.

Assessing hypertensive adolescents for their current level of physical activity and inactivity (i.e., time spent watching television) can be done using the self-administered physical activity screening form (see Appendix C.) followed by clarifying questions during the direct interview with the adolescent (see Appendix C). Responses from the physical activity screening will indicate the availability and extent of participation in school physical education classes, regular involvement and preferences for specific physical activities and sports, and perception of television viewing habits, and whether limits are imposed on television use at home. Additional questions by the clinician can clarify the frequency, duration, and setting (e.g., school-based sports teams, community recreational facility, neighborhood, etc.) for the activities checked, and how many hours per week are spent watching television.

Brisk walking is the type of endurance activity most commonly recommended in our clinic for hypertensive adolescents who are sedentary. To be effective in reducing blood pressure levels and controlling body weight, the adolescent is advised to start with brisk walking continuously for at least 20 min, three times weekly. This can be increased to 30 min, four to five times weekly as the adolescent becomes more accustomed to regular aerobic exercise.

When beginning an exercise program like brisk walking, the adolescent is instructed on how to monitor heart rate during the walk by stopping and taking his or her pulse at the wrist or neck for 6 sec using a watch with a second hand. For adolescents 20 yr of age or younger, a pulse count of 15 beats in a 6-sec period (target heart rate) will ensure the pace set is aerobic and can be sustained for at least 20 min. However, if the hypertensive teen is more than 30 lbs overweight or has been inactive for a long period of time, it is advisable to reduce the target heart rate by two beats (13 beats in a 6-sec period) until he or she is in condition to take on more. When the pulse count exceeds the recommended target heart rate for 6 sec, the adolescent is advised to walk at a slower pace, and conversely, if the pulse count is below what is expected, then the adolescent can safely walk at a faster pace. Checking one's pulse periodically during the walk will help the adolescent become familiar with the pace that is desired.

Stretching exercises done before and after a brisk walk are advised to help avoid injury. A "cool down" (walking at a slower rate) for about 5–10 min immediately following the end of the brisk walk is recommended so as to gradually bring the heart rate to a resting level.

Adolescents will often find walking for exercise more enjoyable if they can share the activity with a friend or family member who is willing to walk at their pace. A physical education instructor at school or staff member at a community recreational facility may be willing to help monitor or oversee a brisk walking program for a hypertensive adolescent and other peers who may also benefit from this activity. Involving school and community resources may help to resolve concerns for those who feel unsafe walking in their neighborhoods.

The motivation to exercise is minimal to nonexistent with some of the hypertensive adolescents seen at our clinic. Using a monthly calendar to keep track of exercise done between counseling sessions can be helpful with compliance. The completed calendar is brought to follow-up sessions for review. Establishing a reward system linked to the adherence to an exercise plan can also serve as positive reinforcement. The adolescent and family together negotiate appropriate rewards (e.g., time on telephone with peers, time spent watching television, time off from household chores, time out with peers, individual time with parent or guardian, a family outing, weekly allowance, etc.) for weekly compliance with an exercise routine.

Other endurance activities like swimming, soccer, basketball, stationary cycling, low-impact aerobic classes, or aerobic exercise videos can be selected as well. These activities are interchangeable with brisk walking when the same guidelines for the target heart rate and duration of exercise are used. Offering alternative aerobic activities can add variety and help to maintain interest in an exercise regimen.

Education About Hypertension

The entire management of hypertensive youths is made more difficult because they do not experience symptoms or relate to complications of hypertension that may occur in older adult life. Denial and nonadherence to both nutritional and pharmacologic interventions are common problems. Therefore, it is mandatory to make sure that blood pressure is truly abnormal before labeling an adolescent hypertensive. It is also important to recurrently educate about the serious effects of hypertension and how to avoid them, as well as teaching healthier lifestyles. A videotape entitled, "Taking Control: Adolescents & Hypertension" is available from Health Sciences Consortium, 201 Silver Cedar Court, Chapel Hill, North Carolina 27514–1517 (919–942–8731). It was made with a cast of teenage patients who have hypertension.

Practical Problems

Most patients with mild to moderate hypertension are asymptomatic so that it is difficult for them to believe that they have a potentially serious health problem. This is particularly true for teenagers who cannot relate to the target organ damage that manifests in midadult life. To them, the terms heart failure, kidney failure, and stroke may have little meaning. Theses are events that happen to old people. Even when given information repetitively, little is retained.

This leads to difficulties in motivating adolescents to keep regularly scheduled out-patient visits, to make serious lifestyle changes, and take prescribed medication, particularly if they feel less well on it than off of it. Reducing dietary sodium to a level low enough to affect blood pressure is difficult, especially in an age group accustomed to eating fast and junk foods frequently. They do not want their peers to identify them as sickly or different, so eating pizza is easier than refusing it. Likewise, it is less conspicuous to consume high-sodium foods at lunchtime than to bring a packed lunch from home, especially for males. It is also more difficult to stay on a low-sodium diet when away at college than at home.

All overweight adolescents, as well as their health care providers, know only too well the difficulties of losing weight and then maintaining that weight loss. Frequently, being overweight is a family problem and all family members may not be willing to participate in adopting a healthier diet and exercising more frequently. It is hard to do these things alone especially if one has low self-esteem, as many overweight teenagers do. Not infrequently they are teased by their peers, unable to exercise much because of poor conditioning, and depressed about their lot. Depression may lead to further eating and a vicious cycle begins that is hard to break. Furthermore, it is difficult to get many third-party payors to reimburse for nutritional advice, behavior modification, and exercise programs.

For those who come from families where the importance of regular exercise is not valued, it may be extremely difficult to even get started. The concept of walking for enjoyment and to improve health is a cultural one that may be entirely lacking. Similarly, cultural cooking habits may make it very difficult to eat a healthy diet. All these factors need to be considered in dealing with each adolescent as an individual. Furthermore, cost may be an important factor affecting the availability of healthy foodstuffs or even appropriate walking shoes. It certainly is a factor for some patients who have to buy expensive antihypertensive drugs if they have no health care coverage. Quite often, these youngsters are from families who are ineligible for public assistance, but without medical insurance.

Many of the antihypertensive drugs currently used to treat mild or moderate hypertension have fewer side-effects than those in common usage a decade or more ago. They also can often be taken once or twice a day at the most. These factors facilitate adherence to drug regimens, but it is still difficult for teenagers, who feel healthy, to take medication every day. Nor do the parents of many older adolescents feel obliged to supervise their drug taking.

Unfortunately, it is not yet clear which individuals with hypertension in adolescence will continue to have it as adults. Certainly, a proportion of hypertensive teenagers become normotensive and the uncertainty of prognosis does not help to convince young people of the seriousness of their problem. On the other hand, prematurely labeling adolescents as having hypertension may have future implications for their obtaining health care insurance, life insurance, and even certain careers. For example, the Marine Corps will not accept candidates who have a prior history of high blood pressure.

Much of the management of hypertension has to be the responsibility of the patient and his or her family. Rarely does anything catastrophic happen when there is lack of adherence to proposed interventions. These factors make it a frustrating condition for the clinician to treat and a difficult condition for the young patient to understand.

CASE ILLUSTRATION

Ken, an African American male, age 16 yr, was first referred for evaluation of hypertension at age 4 yr. He was found to have a significantly elevated blood pressure prior to surgery for an umbilical hernia. He was said to have gained about 25 lbs in the 4–5 months before being seen. Because of temper outbursts and discipline difficulties, he had also been seen at a local psychiatry facility for one year before coming to the hypertension clinic. Both parents had histories of hypertension and the father was said to have had a "mild stroke" at age 53 yr. The mother was overweight, as was the maternal grandmother.

At his initial visit to the hypertension clinic at age 4, Ken weighed 34 kg (74.8 lb) with a height of 115 cm (45 ¼"). These are above and at the 95th percentiles for age, respectively. His blood pressure averaged at 138/76 mm Hg supine and 122/86 mm Hg sitting. These values are well in excess of the 95th percentile for age and gender. A diagnostic evaluation was negative for an organic cause for hypertension. At age 5 yr, Ken was found to have a fasting cholesterol of 196 mg%, triglycerides of 100, an HDL of 52, and LDL of 124. Repeated 6 mo later, these values were 233, 132, 44, and 153, respectively. At that time, he weighed 40.3 kg (88.6 lb) and was 125 cm (49 ¼") tall. He was referred to the pediatric lipid clinic, to be seen every 3 wk by a clinical dietitian there. His caloric and sodium intake were targeted for reduction and he was encouraged to exercise. Eventually, because of an inability to improve his lipids with weight loss, he was placed on colestipol hydrochloride. At 7 yr of age, Ken stopped going to the lipid clinic and stopped seeing its clinical dietitian several months later. His mother said that going to the dietitian was too "time-consuming"; she complained that she was never given a written diet plan and could not remember what she was told. She also said that her low income made it difficult to buy the foods recommended. Around this time, Ken's father died, but the marriage had been dysfunctional for a prolonged period.

At age 9 yr, with a weight of 73.4 kg (161.5 lb), Ken was placed on a diuretic for management of his hypertension. About a year later, an ACE inhibitor was added. His blood pressure was under relatively good control (≤ 95th%) until age 14 yr. During this time, he gained 68.5 kg (150.7 lbs) without any periods of weight loss. His mother sporadically kept promising to work on their diets and increase their level of exercise, but was noncompliant. Unfortunately, Ken's only sibling could eat voraciously without gaining excess weight. The mother was often depressed and her mother died at age 58 yr of a heart attack.

In 1989, Ken developed symptoms suggestive of sleep apnea that was confirmed by a sleep study. A tonsillectomy and adenoidectomy were performed with relief of his snoring. He subsequently became less compliant with his antihypertensive medication and after age 13 yr his mother infrequently accompanied him to hypertension clinic. He admitted to not following either caloric or sodium restrictions and exercising infrequently. His academic performance was average to poor.

At the age of 15 ½ yr, for the first time Ken expressed an interest in getting help with his weight, which was 166.8 kg (367 lb). Funding for long-term outpatient nutrition counseling services was secured from the Bureau for Children with Medical Handicaps given the family's socioeconomic status. By the time nutrition counseling got underway, Ken was at his highest weight of 176 kg (387.5 lb) and was 174.5 cm (68.7") tall.

Following an initial nutritional assessment by a clinical dietitian who specializes in weight management for adolescents, Ken was enrolled in the weekly exercise component of the weight control program, SHAPEDOWN. Ken and his mother also contracted for specific dietary modifications to reduce his intake of sodium and fat, and Ken agreed to begin a brisk walking program on his own. Mother attended the initial session, but clearly current food purchasing and cooking habits did not reflect previous interventions to help mother modify the patient's diet. Ken and his mother may have benefited from more involvement with the peer group discussion and parent sessions offered with SHAPEDOWN, but time needed to travel by bus did not permit this.

Three weeks passed before Ken came to his first group exercise session of brisk walking, but his weight had dropped about 7 lb during that period. Attendance at the weekly group exercise sessions was sporadic. Ken managed to participate in a total of five exercise sessions during the 3-mo period when SHAPEDOWN was being offered. At the end of the program, Ken had lost 10 lb over a period of 13 ½ wk.

Individual family follow-up nutrition counseling was also scheduled on a monthly basis for Ken and his mother during the SHAPEDOWN phase and afterwards. After 9 mo since the initial assessment, Ken at age 16 ½ had lost a total of 23.8 lb on completion of the 10th grade. This represented the most significant weight loss he had ever experienced.

After the start of the next school year over a 4-mo period, Ken had regained about 11 lb. During the 13-mo involvement with Ken, his mother had attended only two of the ten follow-up sessions with him. Ken's adherence to diet changes advised was limited at home given mother's apparent inability and resistance to consistently alter types of food purchased and cooking methods. Ken understood he could manage his hypertension and weight better if he ate less canned vegetables, cheese, fried foods, and frozen or boxed food items high in sodium and fat. However, he had difficulty refusing what mother prepared for him given the effort mother made to cook for the family.

Ken was very aware of the stress his mother was experiencing with her own poor health, being a single parent, financial constraints, and coping with the behavioral problems of his younger brother. He passively accepted his mother's noncompliance, and was appreciative and protective of what she was capable of providing. Only recently has Ken acknowledged that he needs to take more responsibility for what he eats. He now is considering using his own money to buy food for himself in an effort to avoid eating mother's meals that are typically high in sodium and fat.

Ken's adherence on his own to a brisk walking program was variable and likely affected his ability to maintain weight lost. When the weekly group exercise sessions ended, it was more difficult for him to keep motivated to exercise without peer support. Ken also lacked the needed family support and role modeling at home for regular exercise. This significantly affected his ability to sustain an exercise regimen on his own.

In order to provide regular support to keep Ken active, his physical education teacher at school was contacted to explore substituting a brisk walking program for him in place of the regular activities offered in his gym class. Ken's high school could accommodate his needs because the school had an indoor track separate from the gym, and the PE teacher was willing to modify his PE program and oversee his progress. Ken was appreciative of the support received at school from his teacher and peers alike. In the last month based on the PE teacher's records, he had brisk walked at school 2–3 times/wk nonstop for at least 20 min each time out. With Ken's positive attitude and commitment shown, the PE teacher is willing to maintain this exercise program throughout the school year, and the patient wants to increase the frequency to 3–4 times/wk.

Despite the gains made with enlisting the school to promote regular aerobic exercise and Ken willingness to accept more responsibility for the types of food he consumes, he continues to struggle with weight management. Progress is slow considering that Ken is still about 200 lbs overweight. However, he has managed to sustain a net weight loss of 12.5 lb during his 13-mo involvement with nutrition counseling despite the lack of family support. Nutrition counseling services for Ken are still required to help maintain weight loss achieved and to support his efforts for further weight reduction.

REFERENCES

1. S. Londe, *Clin. Pediat.*, **7**, 400 (1968)

2. Report of the Task Force on Blood Pressure Control in Children, *Pediatrics*, **59**, 797 (1977).

3. Report of the Second Task Force on Blood Pressure Control in Children, *Pediatrics*, **79**, 1 (1987).

4. Joint National Committee on Detection, Evaluation and Treatment of High Blood Pressure, *Arch. Intern. Med.*, **153**, 154 (1993).

5. F. F. Jung and J. R. Ingelfinger, *Ped. Rev.*, **14**, 169 (1993).

6. L. K. Rames, et al., *Pediatrics*, **61**, 245 (1978).

7. R. M. Lauer, W. R. Clarke, L. T. Mahoney, and J. Witt, *Ped. Clin. N. Am.*, **40**, 23 (1993).

8. S. L. Gortmaker, W. H. Dietz, A. M. Sobol, and C. A. Wehler, *AJDC*, **141**, 535 (1987).

9. T. A. Wadden, A. J. Stunkard, L. Rich, C. J. Rubin, G. Sweidel, and S. McKinney, *Pediatrics*, **85**, 345 (1990).

10. R. M. Malina, *Crit. Rev. Food Sci. Nutr.*, **33**, 389 (1993).

11. R. Yip, K. Scanlon, and F. Trowbridge, *Crit. Rev. Food Sci. Nutr.*, **33**, 409 (1993).

12. National Institute of Child Health and Human Development, *Science*, **232**, 20 (1986).

13. M. D. Becque, V. L. Katch, A. P. Rocchini, et al., *Pediatrics*, **81**, 605 (1988).

14. A. J. Hartz, D. C. Rupley, and A. A. Rimm, *Am. J. Epidemiol..*, **119**, 71 (1984).

15. M. Krotkiewski, P. Bjorntorp, L. Sjostrom, and U. Smith, *J. Clin. Invest.*, **72**, 1150 (1983).

16. B. Larsson, K. Svardsudd, L. Welin, et al., *Br. Med. J.*, **288**, 1401 (1984).

17. C. L. Shear, D. S. Freedman, G. L. Burke, et al., *Hypertension*, **9**, 236 (1987).

18. A. J. Stunkard, T. I. Sorenson, C. Hanis, et al., *N. Engl. J. Med.*, **314**, 193 (1986).

19. W. H. Dietz and S. L. Gortmaker, *Pediatrics*, **75**, 807 (1985).

20. Centers for Disease Control, *MMWR*, **41**, 597 (1992).

21. J. M. Gazzaniga and T. L. Burns, *Am. J. Clin. Nutr.*, **58**, 21 (1993).

22. T. Mellbin and J. C. Vuille, *Acta Paediatr. Scand.*, **78**, 568 (1989).

23. V. J. Felitti, *South. Med. J.*, **84**, 328 (1991).

24. W. W. McCrory, in *Pediatric & Adolescent Hypertension*, (J.M.H. Loggie, ed.), Blackwell, Boston & Oxford, pp. 104–111 (1992).

25. B. A. Dennison, D. A. Kikuchi, S. R. Srinivasan, et al., *J. Peds.*, **115**, 186 (1989).

26. S. R. Daniels and J.M.H. Loggie, *Adol. Med.: State Art Rev.*, **3**, 551 (1991).

27. D. Grobbee, *J. Hyper.*, **7**, S25 (1989).

28. A. P. Rocchini, J. Key, D. Bondie, et al., *N. Eng. J. Med.*, **321**, 580 (1989).

29. H. H. Himes and W. H. Dietz, *Am. J. Clin. Nutr.*, **59**, 307 (1994).

30. R. P. Abernathy, *J. Am. Diet. Assoc.*, **91**, 843 (1991).

31. A. Must, G. E. Dallal, and W. H. Dietz, *Am. J. Clin. Nutr.*, **53**, 839 (1991).

32. A. B. Elster and N. J. Kuznets, eds., in *AMA Guideline for Adolescent Preventive Services (GAPS)*, American Medical Association, Chicago, IL, p. 7 (1992).

33. M. Story and I. Alton, *Guidelines for Adolescent Nutrition*, Department of Health and Human Services, U. S. Public Health Service, Region V, Chicago, IL, (1993).

34. M. H. Slaughter, T. G. Lohman, R. A. Boileau, C. A. Horswill, et al., *Hum. Biol.*, **60**, 709 (1988).

35. R. A. Frisancho, in *Anthropometric Standards for the Assessment of Growth and Nutritional Status*, The University of Michigan Press, Ann Arbor, MI, pp. 31–34 (1991).

36. T. G. Lohman, A. F. Roche, and R. Martorell, ed., in *Anthropometric Standardization Reference Manual*, Human Kinetics, Champaign, IL, pp. 55–58, 67–68, (1988).

37. T. N. Robinson, *Crit. Rev. Food Sci. Nutr.*, **33**, 313 (1993).

38. M. H. Rasmussen, T. Anderson, L. Breum, et al., *Int. J. Obes.*, **17**, 323 (1993).

39. R. F. Gillum, *J. Chron. Dis.*, **40**, 413 (1987).

40. *The Food Guide Pyramid*, U. S. Department of Agriculture, Home and Garden, Bulletin No. 252, Hyattsville, MD (1992).

41. INTERSALT Cooperative Research Group, *Br. Med. J.*, **297**, 319 (1988).

42. P. Elliot, *Hypertension*, **17** (suppl. I), 3 (1991).

43. M. R. Law, C. D. Frost, and N. J. Wald, *Br. Med. J.*, **302**, 811 (1991).

44. J. A. Cutler, D. Follmann, P. Elliott, and I. Suh, *Hypertension* , **17**(suppl. I), 1 (1991).

45. S. Abraham and M. D. Carroll, *Fats, Cholesterol and Sodium Intake in the Diet of Persons 1–74 Years: United States*, *Advance Data No. 54.*, U. S. Department of Health, Education, and Welfare, Washington, DC, (1981).

46. J.A.T. Pennington, D. B. Wilson, R. F. Newel, B. F. Harland, R. D. Johnson, and J. E. Vanderveen, *J. Am. Diet. Assoc.*, **84**, 771 (1984).

47. National Research Council. *Recommended Dietary Allowances, 10th ed.*, National Academy Press, Washington, DC, (1989).

48. S. L. Linas, *Kidney Int.*, **39**, 771 (1991).

49. J. Treasure and D. Ploth, *Hypertension*, **5**, 864 (1983).

50. F. P. Cappuccio and G. A. MacGregor, *J. Hyper.*, **9**, 465 (1991).

51. The National High Blood Pressure Education Program Working Group, *Arch. Intern. Med.*, **153**, 186 (1993).

52. G. MacGregor, N. Markandu, S. Smith, et al., *Lancet*, **2**, 567 (1982).

53. A. Siani, P. Strazzullo, L. Russo, et al., *Br. Med. J.*, **294**, 1453 (1987).

54. L. P. Svetkey, W. E. Yarger, J. R. Feussner, E. DeLong, and P. E. Klotman, *Hypertension*, **9**, 444 (1987).

55. S. M. Matlou, C. G. Isles, A. Higgs, et al., *J. Hyper.*, **4**, 61 (1986).

56. R. Grimm, J. Neaton, P. Elmer, et al., *N. Eng. J. Med.*, **322**, 569 (1990).

57. A. Richards, E. Espiner, A. Maslowski, et al., *Lancet*, **1**, 757 (1984).

58. F. Skrabal, J. Aubock, H. Hortnagi, *Lancet*, **2**, 985 (1981).

59. A. R. Sinaiko, O. Gomez-Marin, and R. J. Prineas, *Hypertension*, **21**, 991 (1993).

60. National Research Council, *Diet and Health: Implication for Reducing Chronic Disease Risk*, Report of the Committee on Diet and Health, Food and Nutrition Board, National Academy Press, Washington, DC, (1989).

61. K. T. Khaw and E. Barrett-Connor, *N. Eng. J. Med.*, **316**, 235 (1987).

62. C. E. Grim, F. C. Luft, J. Z. Miller, G. R. Meneely, H. D. Battarbee, et al., *J. Chron. Dis.*, **33**, 87 (1980).

63. Centers for Disease Control, *MMWR*, **41**, 597 (1992).

64. L. H. Eck and C. Hackett-Renner, *Prev. Med.*, **21**, 473 (1992).

65. J. A. Cutler and E. Brittain, *Am. J. Hyper.* , **3**, 137S (1990).

66. D. A. McCarron, C. D. Morris, E. Young, et al., *Am. J. Clin. Nutr.*, **54**, 215S (1991).

67. D. McCarron, *Kidney Int.*, **35**, 717 (1989).

68. J. Witteman, W. Willett, M. Stampfer, et al., *Hypertension*, **80**, 1320 (1989).

69. P. Hamet, E. Mongeau, J. Lambert, et al., *Hypertension* , **17** (suppl. 1), 1 (1991).

70. The Trials of Hypertension Prevention Collaborative Research Group, *JAMA*, **267**, 1213 1992).

71. N. E. Johnson, E. L. Smith, and J. L. Freudenheim, *Am. J. Clin. Nutr.*, 42, 12 (1985).

72. National Cholesterol Education Program, *Report of the Expert Panel on Blood Cholesterol Levels in Children and Adolescents*, NIH Pub. no. 91–2732, USDHHS, Bethesda, MD (1991).

73. Centers for Disease Control, *MMWR*, **43**, 129 (1994).

74. L. Johnston, J. Bachman, and P. O'Malley, *Drug Use, Drinking and Smoking: National Survey Results from High School, College, and Young Adult Populations 1975–1988*, U. S. Department of Health and Human Services, Rockville, MD, (1989).

75. J. M. Hagberg, D. Goldring, A. A. Ehsani, et al., *Am. J. Cardiol.*, **52**, 763 (1983).

76. National Association for Sport and Physical Education., *Shape of the Nation: A National Survey of State Physical Education Requirements*, National Association for Sport and Physical Education, Reston, VA, pp. 1–32 (1993).

77. A. C. Nielsen Company, *1990 Nielsen Report on Television*, Nielsen Media Research, New York, (1990).

78. J.M.H. Loggie, ed., in *Pediatric & Adolescent Hypertension*, Blackwell, Boston & Oxford, pp. 112–118 (1992).

79. *Nutrition and Your Health: Dietary Guidelines for Americans*, U. S. Departments of Agriculture and Health and Human Services, Washington, DC, (1990).

80. E. L. Wynder, J. H. Weisburger, and S. K. Ng, *Am. J. Public Health*, **82**, 346 (1992).

81. L. M. Mellin, L. A. Slinkard, and C. E. Irwin, *J. Am. Diet. Assoc.*, **87**, 333 (1987).

82. J.M.H. Loggie and S. R. Daniels, *The Phys. Sports Med.*, **20**, 121 (1992).

Diabetes

Nancy A. Held, M.S.,R.D.,C.D.E.

INTRODUCTION

Diabetes is a heterogeneous group of disorders with distinct genetic patterns, etiology, and pathophysiologic mechanisms resulting in impaired glucose tolerance. The various types of diabetes are indicated in Table 19.1.[1]

Type I diabetes or insulin-dependent diabetes (IDDM) is a chronic disorder caused by a deficiency of insulin. The onset and progression of early IDDM can be variable. In some patients, the disease progresses rapidly with definite clinical symptoms and others have minimal or no symptoms at diagnosis. Common symptoms at presentation are polyuria, polydipsia, occasionally polyphagia, and weight loss. Lethargy and weakness are common as well. Polyuria results from hyperglycemia-induced osmotic diuresis. Increasing fluid intake then attempts to compensate for the fluid loss. Electrolytes are also lost along with fluids. Weight loss results from fluid and glucose losses through the urine, as well as muscle wasting.

If children are not diagnosed at an early stage, diabetic ketoacidosis (DKA) can develop. Over-production of ketone bodies lowers serum pH and causes abdominal pain and vomiting. Once vomiting starts, the patient cannot keep up

Table 19.1 Summary of Classification of Diabetes Mellitus in Children and Adolescents.

Category	Criteria
Diabetes mellitus	
1. Insulin-dependent (IDMM, type I)	Typical symptoms: glucosuria, ketonuria; random plasma glucose (PG) >200 mg/dL
2. Noninsulin-dependent (NIDDM, type II)	Fasting PG >140 mg/dL with 2 h + intervening value >200 mg/dL on OCTT[*] more than once and in the absence of precipitating factors
3. Other types	Type I or II criteria with genetic syndrome, drug therapy, pancreatic disease, or other known causes or associations
Impaired glucose tolerance (IGT)	FPG<140 mg/dL with 2 h >140 mg/dL on OGTT[1]
Gestational diabetes (GDM)	Two or more abnormal fasting of FPG >105 mg/dL, 1 h >190 mg/dL, 2 h >165 mg/dL, 3 h >145 mg/dL on OGTT
Statistical Risk Classes	
1. Previous abnormality of glucose tolerance (prev. AGT)	Normal OGTT with previous abnormal OGTT, spontaneous hyperclycemia, or GDM
2. Potential abnormality of glucose tolerance (pot. AGT)	Genetic propensity (e.g., identical twin with DM); islet cell antibodies

[*]Oral glucose tolerance testing - 1.75 mg/kg body weight, to a maximum of 75 gm

Adapted from National Diabetes Data Group, *Diabetes*, 28, 1039 (1979). Reprinted with permission.

with the ongoing osmotic diuresis and dehydration rapidly ensues. Signs of DKA are fruity breath, Kussmaul respirations (rapid, shallow breathing), and decreased level of consciousness. In DKA, the blood glucose level is above 300 mg/dL, and ketonemia, acidosis (pH 7.3 or less and bicarbonate <15 mEq/L), glycosuria, and ketonuria are present.[2] The treatment of DKA is fluid and electrolyte replacement, as well as insulin to correct the underlying metabolic disturbance.

Sometimes, asymptomatic IDDM is diagnosed in school children or adolescents during a routine physical exam for sports or school. The need for insulin in these children is debatable. On one hand patients can be closely followed and glucose levels monitored without insulin therapy. Alternatively, it may be beneficial to initiate insulin treatment to help preserve beta-cell function.

Type II diabetes or noninsulin-dependent diabetes (NIDDM) comprises 80–90% of those with diabetes.[3] In type II diabetes, insulin levels may be normal, occasionally low, and often increased. Those with NIDDM are not dependent on insulin for survival, but may require insulin for the control of hyperglycemia.

In most cases, onset is after 40 yr, but can occur at any age. There is 90–100% concordance rate among identical twins, implying that type II diabetes is inherited.[3] Eighty–85% of individuals with NIDDM are obese and insulin-resistant, which helps explain the elevated glucose levels in the face of increased insulin concentrations. Presenting symptoms of NIDDM may be fatigue, weakness, dizziness, blurred vision, or mild polyuria and polydipsia.

Abnormal carbohydrate tolerance with symptoms similar to NIDDM can occur in children with a strong family history of type II diabetes and is termed maturity-onset diabetes of the young (MODY). It affects multiple family members and is dominantly inherited. Individuals with MODY may or may not require insulin.

A variant of type II diabetes with clinical manifestations between type I and II occurs in African American youth. These patients present with symptoms of acute insulin deficiency such as hyperglycemia, polydipsia, polyuria, weight loss, and ketonemia or ketoacidosis. They differ from the typical patient with IDDM in their ability to go off insulin or have drastically reduced insulin needs for prolonged periods. This atypical diabetes also differs from classic insulin deficiency in that it is nonprogressive, nonautoimmune and dominantly inherited.[4]

Individuals who have glucose levels higher than normal, but lower than that which defines diabetes have impaired glucose tolerance (IGT). IGT does not lead to the complications of diabetes, but approximately 25% eventually go on to develop type II diabetes.[5] The onset or recognition of glucose intolerance during pregnancy is classified as gestational diabetes. There is an associated increased risk of perinatal complications and progression to diabetes within 5–10 yr after parturition. Hyperglycemia may also be associated with diseases such as pancreatic disease, endocrine disorders or administration of drugs.

Epidemiology

The prevalence of type I diabetes in the United States varies according to different sources, but studies place the incidence between 1–2/1000 (0.1–0.2%) population.[6–9] Type I diabetes is three to four times more common than other chronic childhood diseases, such as cystic fibrosis, peptic ulcer, juvenile rheumatoid arthritis, or leukemia. The incidence varies throughout the world, with the highest rate in Scandinavia, the lowest in Japan, and intermediate in the United States. Prevalence in the United States is similar to that in Great Britain, Sweden, and Australia. In the United States prevalence of type I diabetes is lower in African, Mexican, and Asian Americans than Caucasians.[10]

The incidence appears to be low early in life, and peak between 8–12-years-old and declines after 12 yr.[11] This may be due to exposure to viral illness at school triggering onset in a predisposed child. There appears to be a seasonal effect, with more cases presenting in the fall and winter months.[11] This may be explained by marginal beta-cell function compounded with the added stress of illness in winter-producing insulin resistance.

Etiology

The primary defect in type I diabetes is the loss of insulin secretion by pancreatic insulin producing beta-cells. The causes of beta-cell failure are not well understood, but probably result from a combination of factors. Genetic, environmental, and autoimmune factors together result in the selective destruction of beta cells.

Genetic predisposition. Although all the genes linked to IDDM have not been identified, a gene cluster on chomosome number 6 is most likely involved. Ninety % of individuals with type I diabetes have this particular gene cluster,[12] and inheritance of this cluster places an individual at greater risk for developing diabetes. However, because many in the general population also exhibit these genes, it is thus difficult to use as a screening test for diabetes.[12]

Precipitating events. It appears that the susceptibility to develop diabetes is inherited, not the disease itself. If heredity was the only factor, then identical twins would have a 100% concordance rate, rather than the 30–40% concordance rate that is actually observed.[12] Thus, certain environmental factors appear necessary to initiate the disease process. Virus and drug initiators as well as cow's milk protein have been proposed, but not universally accepted.[13] The evidence for virus-induced diabetes stems from both experimental animals and some studies in humans and implicates congenital rubella, cytomegalovirus, and particularly, coxsakie virus.[14,15]

Autoimmune destruction of beta-cell. A number of factors point to immunologic abnormalities in the etiology of diabetes. The presence of islet cell antibodies (circulating antibodies against islet cells) and GAD antibodies (glutamic acid decarboxylase, a constituent in beta-cells) have been identified at diagnosis and in first-degree relatives who later developed IDDM.[16]

The earliest abnormality in insulin secretion is a progressive reduction of the immediate first-phase plasma insulin response during intravenous glucose tolerance testing. At this stage, no clinical abnormality is evident. Overt diabetes emerges when the majority (80–90%) of beta cells have been destroyed after a silent process of beta-cell destruction of months to year (see Figure 19.1). Nevertheless, some endogenous insulin may remain for 1 or 2 yr and a substantial fraction of patients diagnosed at older ages appear to have evidence of insulin production (C-peptide positive) for up to 5 yr or longer.[17]

Prognosis

Diabetic complications. Adolescents with diabetes should be encouraged to live as normal a life as possible and enjoy the usual activities of youth. Complications are seen infrequently among youth. However, diabetes is a serious disease

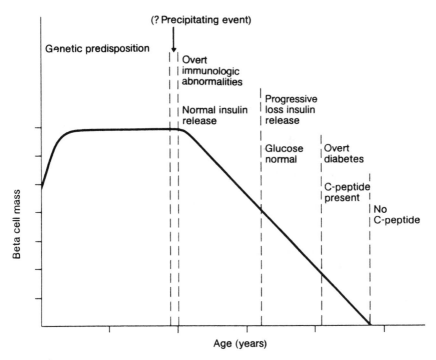

Figure 19-1. Stages in the development of type 1 diabetes (listed from left to right).

G. S. Eisenbarth, *Triangle*, **23**, 4 (1984). Reprinted with permission.

associated with the development of retinopathy, nephropathy, neuropathy, and macrovascular complications. Retinopathy is usually not evident until 5yr after diagnosis, but by a duration of 20 yr nearly all individuals with IDDM have some retinopathy.[18] In most (80%), it is background retinopathy that does not progress. The years prior to puberty do not appear to contribute to the development of retinopathy.

Nephropathy or end-stage renal failure develops in approximately 30–40% of patients with IDDM by a duration of 20 yr.[19] The earliest sign of this complication is small amounts of protein in the urine (microalbuminuria). This may be caused by abnormal permeability of the glomerular membrane, increased glomerular perfusion pressure, or a combination of these two factors. Micoalbuminuria occurs in children and adolescents with IDDM as well as adults.[19]

Neuropathy can occur after a duration of 5 yr and occurrence increases with duration and uncontrolled blood glucose levels. Neuropathy can affect all regions of the body, especially in the periphery of the feet and hands; and autonomic neuropathy occurs in the gastrointestinal system and heart. Coronary heart disease, peripheral vascular disease, and cerebrovascular disease are more common and occur at an earlier age in those with diabetes. Patients with diabetes are 11 times more likely to die of cardiovascular disease than individuals of the same age without diabetes.[20]

Control: DCCT results.   The DCCT (Diabetes Control and Complications Trial) was a 9-yr multicenter, randomized clinical trial designed to assess whether near-normalization of blood glucose control prevents or delays diabetes complications. Exactly 1441 individuals with IDDM, 13–39-year-old, participated in the trial from 1983–1993; 715 were randomized to the experimental group and 726 to the standard group. The experimental group treatment consisted of intensive insulin therapy, utilizing either continuous subcutaneous insulin infusion (CSII) via an insulin pump or multiple insulin injections. The standard treatment group was asked to perform conventional care that included two insulin injections per day. Intensive treatment in the adolescent subset ($n=195$), as well as the larger group, was associated with significant reductions in the risk of retinopathy, nephropathy, and neuropathy.[21,22]

Medical Management

The primary goals of treatment for insulin-dependent diabetes is to facilitate a feeling of well being and minimize symptoms of hypoglycemia and hyperglycemia. Another goal of diabetes management is to prevent, delay, or arrest vascular complications. The former can be attained with a moderate degree of effort. The latter can be achieved through intensive efforts to obtain near-normalization of blood glucose levels. It involves a commitment of time and energy, as well as increases the risk of hypoglycemia.

Treatment goals should be agreed on by the teen, health care team, physician, and family. A team that encourages tight control for an adolescent who is not interested or motivated feels frustrated because they are providing suboptimal care. A motivated, inspired teenager, on the other hand, who desires tight control similarly will feel frustrated if a physician or treatment team does not have interest or skill in intensive therapy.

Insulin preparations.   Exogenous insulin replacement attempts to mimic the normal endogenous physiologic insulin secretion. Normal insulin secretion can be broadly divided into two categories: continuous basal secretion that regulates the body's own production of glucose when the individual is not eating and, augmented secretion that occurs in response to food.

Insulin preparations can be classified by the duration of action and species. The time course of action can be short-acting or rapid onset (Regular insulin), intermediate-acting (NPH or Lente), and long-acting (Ultralente). Absorption rates vary depending on injection sites. Peaks and duration of action do not always fall neatly into a category. Using SBGM will help establish an individual's blood glucose response to different types of insulin (see Tables 19.2 and 19.3).[23]

Insulin regimens.   There are various insulin regimes that difffer in sophistication. Most patients with IDDM take at least two injections of insulin a day. A split-mix regimen is commonly used. This is a mix of NPH/Lente and Regular in the morning before breakfast and then again presupper. An individual can use SBGM to adjust the insulin doses in an effort to produce better glucose control. Three injections a day may be selected if hypoglycemia during the middle of the night occurs. In this regimen, short-acting insulin is used for supper and the intermediate insulin is delayed until bedtime. Another approach is to use short-acting insulin before each meal and longer-acting insulin at bed. Three or more injections a day is called "multiple daily injections" or MDI therapy.

Continuous subcutaneous insulin infusion (CSII) or insulin pump therapy delivers basal short-acting insulin and allows the patient to administer boluses of insulin before each meal. MDI and CSII are designed to provide intensive treatment. SBGM must be used in conjunction with these regimens to work toward the goal of intensive therapy, near-normalization of blood glucose levels.

Target blood glucose levels will vary depending on the philosophy of the clinic, and of course, the adolescent. In our center, glucose goals are as follows: fasting 70–120 mg/dL, 2-h postprandial 120–180 mg/dL, 3 A.M. >65 mg/dL.

Adolescents require more insulin than prepubertal children or adults to achieve the same glucose levels and glucose values fluctuate much more widely in this age group. This is not due solely to erratic and poor eating and lifestyle habits, but also insulin resistance evident in puberty.[24] Puberty is associated with an impairment of insulin-stimulated glucose metabolism and thus insulin resistance is accentuated by the diabetic state. Adolescents generally receive insulin in doses much greater per kilogram of body weight than prepubertal children. In children, insulin needs may be on average 0.5 U/kg/d. The insulin dose in adults usually averages about 0.6 U/kg/d; in adolescents, the average dose often exceeds 1.0 U/kg/d.

Assessment of diabetes control.   Biochemical tests provide an overall picture of blood glucose control, as well as indicate the degree of complications related to diabetes. Blood glucose can be assessed in a lab or measured by the patient. Individuals can perform capillary blood glucose testing or SBGM using a lancet to obtain blood from their finger and a portable blood glucose reflectance meter. Patients are encouraged to keep a record of blood glucose levels in a log book in order to identify patterns of changing glucose levels across time. This is especially important in growing children and adolescents because their insulin needs usually increase. Glucose records also aid the teen, dietitian, and physician in adjusting the appropriate insulin doses for variations in exercise or food intake. The frequency of SBGM depends on treatment intensity and goals. For intensive

Table 19.2   Insulins Sold in the United States

Product	Manufacturer	Strength
Short-acting		
(usual onset 0.5–2.0 h; usual duration 3–6 h)		
Human		
Humulin Regular	Lilly	U-100
Humulin BR (only external insuline pumps)	Lilly	U-100
Novolin R (regular, formerly Actrapid human)	Squibb-Novo	U-100
Velosulin Human (Regular)	Nordisk-USA	U-100
Novolin R Penfill (Regular)	Squibb-Novo	U-100
Pork		
Iletin II Regular	Lilly	U-100, U-500
Purified Pork R (Regular, formerly Actrapid)	Squibb-Novo	U-100
Purified Pork S (Semilente,		
formerly Semitard)	Squibb-Novo	U-100
Regular	Squibb-Novo	U-100
Beef/Pork		
Iletin I (Regular)	Lilly	U-40, U-100
Iletin I (Semilente)	Lilly	U-40, U-100
Intermediate-acting		
(usual onset 3–6 h; usual duration 12–20 h)		
Human		
Humulin L	Lilly	U-100
Humulin NPH	Lilly	U-100
Novolin L (Lente, formerly Monotard human)	Squibb-Novo	U-100
Novolin N (NPH)	Squibb-Novo	
Pork		
Iletin II Lente	Lilly	U-100
Iletin II NPH	Lilly	U-100
Purified pork Lente (formerly Monotard)	Squibb-Novo	U-100
Purified Pork N (NPH, formerly Protaphane)	Squibb-Novo	U-100
Beef/Pork		
Iletin I Lente	Lilly	U-40, U-100
Iletin I NPH	Lilly	U-40, U-100
Long-acting		
(usual onset 6–10 h; usual duration 18–36 h)		
Human		
Humulin U (Ultralente)	Lilly	U-100
Beef		
Purified Beef U (Ultralente,		
formerly Ultratard)	Squibb-Novo	U-100
Beef/Pork		
Iletin I PZI	Lilly	U-40, U-100
Iletin I Ultralente	Lilly	U-40, U-100

continued on next page

Table 19.2 *Continued*

Product	Manufacturer	Strength
Premixed Combinations		
Human		
Novolin 70/30	Squibb-Novo	U-100
Humulin 70/30	Lilly	U-100
Humulin 70/30	Lilly	U-100

treatment, continuous subcutaneous insulin infusion pumps (CSII) or multiple daily injections ($\geq$ 3 insulin injections per day), frequent blood glucose monitoring is essential (three to seven times per day). Awareness of the blood glucose levels allows self adjustment of insulin. Patients on a less rigorous treatment regimen require less frequent monitoring (two or three times per day). The treatment goal may be to simply avoid hypoglycemia. Adolescents, especially older teens, often omit monitoring their glucose levels or only occasionally test. As a compromise with the health care professional, teens may agree to check their blood glucose once per day (varying the times) or, alternatively, monitor two or three times a day for 2 wk prior to their next clinic visit. In this way, the health care professional has more accurate data on which to base modifications of insulin doses.

Long-term glycemic control can be assessed by the glycated hemoglobin assay (HbA$_1$C or HbA$_1$). Glucose binds to hemoglobin and an index of the average blood glucose over the preceding 2 mo, i.e., the higher the blood glucose the higher the glycated hemoglobin. The normal range depends upon the lab; HbA^{1}C is 3–6% and HbA^1 is 4–8%.

Table 19.3 Insulins by Relative Comparative Action Curves

Insulin	Onset (h)	Peak (h)	Duration (h)	Duration (h)
Animal				
Regular	0.5–2.0	3–4	4–6	6–8
NPH	4–6	8–14	16–20	20–24
Lente	4–6	8–14	16–20	20–24
Ultralente	8–14	Minimal	24–36	24–36
Human				
Regular	0.5–1.0	2–3	3–6	4–6
NPH	2–4	4–10	10–16	14–18
Lente	3–4	4–12	12–18	16–20
Ultralente	6–10	?	18–20	20–307

Adapted from American Diabetes Association, in *The Physician's Guide to Type 1 Diabetes*, (M. Sperling, ed.), ADA, Alexandria, VA, pp. 33, (1988). Reprinted with permission.

Fructosamine is a relatively new assay to measure glycosylated albumin that reflects glucose control over a 2–3 wk period, because the half-life of albumin is much shorter than that of red blood cells. It is most often used during pregnancy when changes in glycemic control over the short term are important.

Urine glucose provides an inaccurate measure of glycemic control and is not recommended for patients with type I diabetes. However, patients still need to be taught how to check their urine for ketones. Urine ketones do not routinely need to be checked, but should be monitored when the youth is sick or if blood glucose levels are consistently over 300 mg/dL. The presence of ketones indicates a breakdown of fatty tissue and, if untreated, leads to ketoacidosis.

Assessment of diabetes complications.   There are numerous tests that assess kidney damage including protein excretion and glomerular filtration rate. Measurements of creatinine clearance can be used to estimate the glomerular filtration rate (GFR) that may be elevated during the first few years of diabetes (hyperfiltration). A GFR that then drops below the normal range indicates deterioration of kidney function. Microalbuminuria detects small amounts of protein (albumin) in the urine, suggesting very early kidney damage to the glomerular capillary basement.

An elevated serum creatinine level indicates more advanced diabetic nephropathy. Frank proteinuria precedes elevation of serum creatinine levels, but implies further damage (>300 mg of albumin/24 h) than microalbuminuria.

The risk for developing coronary heart disease in those with diabetes is at least twice that of those without this disease.[25] Thus, it is important to assess and monitor blood lipid levels that are associated with the development of heart disease. Since lipids tend to be elevated at diagnosis, it is more accurate to assess them when blood glucose stabilizes. Total cholesterol, HDL, LDL, and triglyceride levels should be measured yearly thereafter. The cause of abnormal lipid metabolism in patients with IDDM is probably primarily due to hyperglycemia and/or hypoinsulinemia.

Hypertension increases the risk of macrovascular and microvascular complications of diabetes. Blood pressure above 160/90 mm Hg is generally the point where treatment is initiated in the general population. There is a general agreement that in diabetes a blood pressure of 135/85 requires treatment. However, the optimal blood pressure in diabetes is unknown.

ASSESSMENT

Nutritional Interview

Nutrition assessment for an adolescent with diabetes is similar to youth without diabetes. The assessment usually includes biochemical data, medical history, physical examination, and anthropometric measurements. These accumulated data provide an indication of nutrition status and help determine the extent of nutrition education and counseling required. Additionally, this information lets the dietitian select the appropriate meal planning method and educational approach for the teen.

Information may be obtained from the medical record, the adolescent, parents, and other health care team members. It is helpful to obtain diabetes-related history, including age of onset, prior diabetes education, and previous diabetes-related hospitalizations, if any. Current insulin regimen is important data to help match insulin dose to food intake. Exercise and activity habits provide additional information that help to formulate the meal plan.

For an adolescent who is newly diagnosed with diabetes, information such as history preceding onset and severity of symptoms at the time of presentation are additional data to help determine the family's readiness for education. A patient who was extremely sick will be in a different frame of mind than one who had mild symptoms.

Diabetes-specific questions should be included in the nutrition history. The time and frequency with which meals and snacks are usually eaten will help establish a schedule for a meal plan. Are any meals missed or is the timing of eating erratic? Are snacks eaten on a regular basis and when are they consumed? The teenagers' school and usual activity schedule are other useful pieces of information to obtain. For example, lunch hours may vary between 10:40 A.M. to 1:00 P.M. in a given week. On days with an early lunch, a morning snack is generally not necessary, but on days when lunch is later, a morning snack may be appropriate. Time span between meals is also a critical variable. There is not a definite time span between meals when a snack is required; snacking instead depends on an individual's insulin regime.

The nutrition counselor should gather information about activity patterns, including time of gym class and time and type of after-school exercise. Thus, data should include questions of duration, frequency, and intensity. Modified food intake in conjunction with activity can also provide useful insights into a teen's management pattern. Often, adolescents involved in team sports have practice schedules that vary from day to day. The dietitian should ask about eating-out patterns, including frequency, type of restaurant, and whether the individual eats with friends or relatives. It is helpful to understand the home environment, including who shops and prepares meals. Does the family have a routine or is eating haphazard? It is helpful to gain insight into the adolescent's values and peer environment. Is there a preoccupation with dieting or particularly strong peer pressure to be thin?

Recent appetite and thirst can provide information about hyperglycemia. Reports of napping after school and frequent fatigue are a cue to elevated blood glucoses. On the other hand, a short attention span before lunch or ravenous appetite after school may indicate low blood glucose at these times. Frequency of self-blood glucose monitoring must be assessed. How the adolescent treats hypoglycemic reactions will reveal whether an appropriate or excessive amount of calories and carbohydrate are consumed.

The nutritional adequacy of the diet should be assessed, including both macronutrient and micronutrient consumption, especially iron and calcium intake among female adolescents. The evaluation of the macronutrient composition of the diet determines caloric intake as well as the proportion of protein, carbohydrate, and fat (including type of fat). The frequency of caloric and noncaloric sweetener use and consumption of foods high in simple sugar are also evaluated.

Anthropometric Measurements

Weight, height, and blood pressure measurements provide additional useful data. These can be accessed from the patient's chart or easily obtained by the dietitian or nurse. At diagnosis, a substantial amount of weight loss suggests insulin deficiency, glycosuria, and dehydration. Weight and growth history gathered from the primary physician, the patient, or parents provide a background for premorbid nutritional status.

Serial measurements for weight and height plotted on a standardized growth chart assess overall growth (see Chapter 17). Unintended weight loss is often an early indicator of poor glycemic control that can be confirmed by glycated hemoglobin measurements. Intervention to improve glucose control should be quickly initiated. Continued poor glucose control can cause a decline in height percentile because of a caloric deficit and negative nitrogen balance. A deceleration in growth may be short-term and height may return to its expected percentile when improved glucose control is achieved. On the other hand, if poor control continues over an extended period of time, adult height can be permanently affected.

Excessive weight gain in the face of poor diabetes control strongly suggests excessive energy intake. In either case, reduction in food intake or increased exercise are probably more important than simply increasing insulin doses. Conversely, weight gain may be observed with an improvement in glycemic control. Data from the DCCT suggest that weight gain occurs with intensive treatment and may be due to a reduction in glycosuria and excess calories consumed to treat hypoglycemia.[26] Patients embarking on an intensive treatment program should be warned of the possibility of excessive weight and preventive measures should be instituted before increases in weight occur.

Although the growth charts are essential for assessing growth, they are not an accurate tool for assessing ideal body weight in adolescents.[27] It is not necessarily correct to recommend that weight and height should be in the same percentile channel. The curves only describe the distribution of heights and weights of a representative sample of teenagers of each age. There is a wide distribution of weights at any age, particularly in adolescence. The subjects in the survey included overweight as well as lean teens, since data were meant to reflect the demographics of the population.[28]

Ideal weight for height for children and adolescents taller than 137 cm (girls) and 145 cm (boys) can be assessed by referring to the original data from which the percentile charts were derived.[29] There is a range of weights given for a particular height and age. The 50th percentile weight for the height is the median. An appropriate weight for height can be defined as the weight between the 25–75th percentile.

Adolescents 18 yr and older are considered adults with respect to weight standards. Commonly used standards to assess ideal body weight are the revised Metropolitan Life Insurance Company tables (1983) and the Fogarty Conference table.[30,31]

Psychological Concerns

A number of factors influence how an adolescent adapts to diabetes. These include age of onset, chronologic age and developmental stage, relationships with parents and peers, self-image, as well as his or her relationship with health care professionals. The demands of the diabetes regimen stand in conflict with normal adolescent struggles such as independence from parents and the desire to conform. Unfortuately, many aspects of diabetes management force a teen to be different, such as testing blood glucose levels, injecting insulin, eating extra snacks, and eating at specified times. Of course, there are many adjustments that can be made in diabetes management to minimize feeling different. The dietitian must be sensitive to these issues and adjust the management plan accordingly. Adolescents have concerns about their own sexuality, alcohol, drug use, and interaction with diabetes. It is important to provide them with information about these issues so they can make informed choices.

MANAGEMENT

Nutrition research on adolescents with IDDM is sparse. The ideal composition of the diet for this population is not even known. A meal plan that supports the individuals' lifestyle, promotes goals of management and optimal adherence is essential, regardless of age.

Energy requirements are those appropriate for the normal growth and development of adolescents. Although an estimation of energy needs can be calculated using various methods, there is tremendous variation in actual energy intake in adolescents depending on the stage of development and activity level. Because of this, it may be difficult to calculate the appropriate energy requirement. An inappropriate calorie level could result in a teen feeling hungry or overfed. It is more accurate to estimate caloric needs based on usual intake by obtaining a careful diet history. A teen who is newly diagnosed with IDDM often presents with weight loss. Additional calories are needed for the repair of negative energy balance and catch-up weight gain. These additional calories should be provided based on appetite. Adolescents who were overweight prior to diagnosis may be pleased with the weight loss and often state that they plan to keep off the weight. However, weight invariably returns to premorbid levels within a short time due to re-hydration, insulin replacement, and increased appetite. Realistic expectations should be honestly discussed and explained to the teenager. Frequent follow-up by the dietitian is necessary after diagnosis to monitor appetite and weight gain and help parents and adolescents modify the meal plan as appropriate.

Adequate energy for normal growth and development is of primary importance and insulin can then be adjusted based on the pattern of glucose levels. Parents sometimes withhold food when glucose levels are high. Others may tell their teen to go run around the block to try to bring down the glucose. However, it is more appropriate to note the high reading. If a pattern of high readings at this time are apparent, then the appropriate insulin can be subsequently adjusted. On the other hand, if glucose levels are low, parents may try to force food on a satiated teen. There are situations when this may be unavoidable. However, force feeding is usually not necessary and can be remedied with a reduction of insulin. Older teenagers who have completed their longitudinal growth can be more flexible and adjust their food intake based on blood glucose levels.

Meal Plan Composition

Protein.   The primary function of protein is for tissue growth and maintenance. The currently accepted recommendation is at least 0.8 g/kg or 10–20% of calories for those with and without diabetes. The optimal level of protein for diabetics is unknown. A high-protein intake may be involved in kidney deterioration. Recent studies suggest that restricting protein delays the progression of renal failure.[32] However, a number of questions still remain about the efficacy and practicality of protein-restricted diets. Most studies have been short-term and therefore the long-term effects of low-protein intake are unknown. Recently, IDDM patients on a low-protein diet for 2 yr were investigated and found to have a decrease in microalbuminuria.[33] Unfortunately, adherence to very-low-protein diets is difficult and no studies have been conducted with adolescents. Since many adolescents eat excessive quantities of protein, decreasing protein closer to the RDA theoretically might help to reduce glomerular changes. Recent studies suggest that it is animal rather than vegetable protein that is the important determinant in the progression of renal disease.[34] Further research is needed to determine the degree of protein restriction necessary to prevent renal damage without resulting in adverse effects (such as malnutrition), the type of protein, and the stage in nephropathy when protein restriction is effective.

Carbohydrate.   A high-carbohydrate, low-saturated-fat diet is recommended for individuals with IDDM. The American Diabetes Association (ADA) does not currently specify the amount of calories that should be derived from carbohydrates.[35,36] A high carbohydrate diet necessitates low-fat intake, which is important in promoting overall health and reducing cardiovascular risk factors. Controversy exists regarding the general recommendation that all diabetics consume a high-carbohydrate, low-fat diet. High-carbohydrate diets have been shown to increase triglyceride levels, reduce HDL, and increase postprandial glucose levels.[35] In type II diabetes, a prevalent lipid abnormality is hypertriglyceridemia and it may be prudent for these individuals to consume a more moderate-carbohydrate and moderate-fat diet. For adolescents taking exogenous insulin, high-carbohydrate intake is appropriate.[35]

At one time, individuals with IDDM were instructed to eliminate sucrose from their diet, based on the belief that sugar is more rapidly absorbed and causes greater glycemic excursions than other carbohydrates. It is currently thought that sucrose can be included in the context of an otherwise balanced meal plan.[37] When grams of carbohydrate are equal, the source of carbohydrate, sugar vs. starch, is not the major factor in determining the effect of the food on blood glucose levels. In many controlled studies using sucrose fed as a single nutrient and substituting sucrose for other carbohydrates, no adverse effects were shown on glycemic control.[36,38] The crucial point is to maintain consistent total carbohydrate intake regardless of source. Sucrose-containing foods should remain limited because of the association with dental caries and foods high in sucrose are often high in total fat as well. Currently, there is not a definitive amount of sucrose that is accepted as reasonable, although 10 % of total calories has been suggested, particularly in NIDDM.[36]

Fiber.   Soluble fiber has been implicated in improving glycemic control, as well as reducing blood lipids. However, the positive effect of dietary fiber on plasma glucose is not thought to be significant.[35,37,38] In studies examining high-fiber foods, it is difficult to ascertain whether the improved glucose levels were due to the fiber component or changes in macronutrient content, such as increasing carbohydrate or decreasing fat. Adherence to high-fiber diets is not practical for many individuals, especially adolescents. Diets high in soluble fiber have been shown to modestly reduce total and LDL cholesterol when consumed with a diet of at least 50% carbohydrate. Dietary fiber appears to be associated with the prevention of gastrointestinal disorders and colon cancer. In fact, the optimal amount of fiber for adolescents with IDDM is not known. The recommended fiber intake is the same as for those without diabetes, 25–30 g/d.[37]

Sodium.   There is an association between hypertension and diabetes. It is not clear whether hypertension is secondary to kidney damage or precedes it.[39] In general, individuals show a variable response to sodium restriction. It is not known whether sodium restriction specifically in adolescents will reduce hypertension. However, it is probably a good dietary habit to avoid the excessive use of salt.

Alcohol.   Although alcohol consumption is generally inappropriate for adolescents, as well as illegal, many experiment with this substance. It is essential to provide teens with accurate information regarding the relationship of alcohol and diabetes. Hypoglycemia is a significant danger when combining alcohol and insulin, especially if the teen has not eaten for a number of hours. Alcohol blocks gluconeogenesis in the liver. It also enhances the action of insulin by interfering with the release of counter-regulatory hormones that promote glycogenolysis, thereby impairing the body's ability to raise its own blood glucose levels. If an adolescent has recently eaten, alcohol may produce hyperglycemia due to the breakdown of glycogen stores in the liver. The quantity of alcohol consumed and amount of glycogen stores determine the extent of the blood glucose rise. Symptoms of low blood glucose can easily be mistaken for intoxication. Alcohol should be consumed with food to avoid potential hypoglycemia. If they choose to drink, teens should be advised to limit their intake to one or two drinks in an evening and in combination with food. Additionally, SBGM should be performed before and after drinking.

Alternative sweeteners.   Sweeteners can be categorized as caloric and noncaloric. Fructose is a monosaccharide with 4 kcal/g and is found primarily in fruits and honey. It appears to have a lower glycemic index than sucrose and other starches.[37,38] However, studies in individuals with and without diabetes have shown that a high-fructose diet increases serum cholesterol, albeit in relatively small increments. These studies generally used much more than the usual intake of fructose. Thus, teens with diabetes do not need to avoid naturally occurring fructose. Due to the potential adverse effects of fructose in large amounts on serum lipids, the use of added fructose as a sweetening agent is not advised.

The sugar alcohols are monosaccharides that contain alcohol. Sorbitol is derived from glucose, mannitol from mannose, and xylitol from xylose and all are found naturally in a variety of plants. They are also used as sweeteners in reduced-calorie or dietetic products. These polyols are absorbed slowly and do have a lower glycemic response than sucrose.[40] However, these sweeteners contain calories and are usually combined with fat. Foods sweetened with sugar alcohols therefore may have more calories than those they are meant to replace. Additionally, they produce diarrhea and flatus, with tolerance varying among individuals. Polyols offer no substantial advantage over other nutritive sweeteners.

Hydrogenated starch hydrolysates are being used more commonly by manufactures to sweeten candies and gums. They have no adverse effect in individuals with IDDM; however, they too offer no advantage over the other nutritive sweeteners.[41]

The three FDA-approved noncaloric or nonnutritive sweeteners are saccharin, aspartame, and acesulfame K. Intake at expected levels of use of all three is considered safe. Current approval is being sought for sucralose, alitame, and cyclamates.

Timing and Consistency

Meals and snacks should be eaten at approximately the same time every day to be coordinated with the insulin injections. Insulin should be injected at consistent times to prevent under-or overinsulization. Teenagers who have a haphazard daily routine make regulating blood glucose levels difficult.

There is not a recommended standard distribution of food or calorie distribution throughout the day, as was promoted in the past. Every effort should always be made to accommodate usual eating styles and choose an appropriate insulin regimen and dose on that premise. Ideally, good nutrition is a goal, but may have to be attained gradually.

Another basic guideline in meal planning is that amounts of food eaten at each meal and snack should be consistent.[42] Consistency should be a goal, but is not always practical since fluctuations in appetite occur. Exercise or increased activity level usually require extra caloric intake. Teenagers can be taught how to continue to eat at fast-food restaurants and parties and still maintain adequate glycemic control. It is recommended to eat consistent types of food day to day. This infers that each daily meal and snack should include the same proportion of protein, fat, and carbohydrate. Carbohydrate has the greatest impact on blood glucose levels postprandially.[43] Thus, it is critical for carbohydrate intake to be consistent. The author has found that incorporating flexibility improves adherence and small variations in protein and fat intake probably have little impact on glucose levels.

Snacks are usually needed in midafternoon and before bed on a two-injection, split-mix regimen. Snacks provide some caloric intake to counterbalance insulin action peaks. Compliance with eating a snack is not usually a problem among teens. However, an adolescent trying to lose weight may intentionally omit snacks and have resultant hypoglycemia.

Meal Planning Approaches

There are a number of meal planning strategies available.[44] The exchange system for meal planning is the one most commonly utilized by dietitians.[45] This tool is useful as it teaches food composition and food density as well as how to provide balanced and consistent meals. Unfortunately, this approach does not work with all teens because many feel it is too complicated and cumbersome. Carbohydrate exchange counting is somewhat simpler and may make it easier for some adolescents to adhere to a meal plan. There are other methods of varying sophistication. These include healthy food choices, calorie counting, total available glucose (TAG), and carbohydrate gram counting. Realistically, there are teens who do not adhere to any particular meal plan. It is then important to prioritize the critical eating behaviors and not alienate the teenager with what is perceived as superfluous information.

Eating Disorders

Anorexia nervosa and bulimia are clearly serious eating disorders with significant psychological and physical sequelae (see Chapters 9 and 10). In diabetes, an eating disorder can wreak havoc on blood glucose levels. Diabetes has been suggested as a risk factor for the development of an eating disorder since diet takes on a strong focus in diabetes. Recent studies, however, have failed to show increased prevalence of eating disorders in diabetes.[46-48] Health professionals should nevertheless be aware of the potential risk of eating disorders. This malady should be considered with unexplained poor diabetes control (skipping or reducing insulin) and frequent hypoglycemia (restrictive dieting).

Obesity

There exists sparse research in the literature regarding the prevalence of obesity in adolescents with IDDM.[49] It may become a growing problem as glucose control is intensified. Moreover, improvement in metabolic control is associated with weight gain.[26] The weight gain is probably due to better utilization of calories with reduction a in glycosuria, overtreatment of hypoglycemic reactions, and the perceived freedom to eat more that may come with the ability to adjust preprandial insulin doses. The adolescents in the DCCT who were intensively treated with insulin had a 2-fold greater risk of becoming overweight, as determined by body mass index.[22] There may be other causes of weight gain in diabetes. Children with diabetes may grow up with the idea that they must finish all their exchanges or they will get sick. Food becomes viewed as medicine. An inappropriate calorie prescription can also promote excessive intake. This necessitates follow-up visits between the dietitian and patient to clear up misconceptions about meal management and alter the prescribed caloric intake.

Exercise

Exercise should be encouraged in adolescents with diabetes. It is important to emphasize exercise for adolescents who have a sedentary lifestyle, are overweight, or manage their diabetes with intensive therapy (to combat a tendency to gain weight). Regular exercise reduces risk factors for coronary heart disease and aerobic exercise decreases the incidence of heart disease. Exercise decreases both systolic and diastolic blood pressure, promotes weight control by increasing energy expenditure, and most important for the teen, improves self-image, enhances well-being, and promotes a healthy lifestyle. For example, exercise helps to control blood glucose levels in NIDDM. However, in IDDM exercise may not improve overall control, but it can decrease insulin doses. Acute exercise increases glucose utilization and chronic training improves sensitivity to insulin and thus a smaller amount of insulin is needed.

As important as it is to exercise, it is also essential to be aware of the risks of exercise with IDDM. The foremost concern regarding exercise is the increased risk of hypoglycemia. Exercising, especially when insulin action is at its peak, can result in a fall in blood glucose unless counteracted with carbohydrate. Insulin absorption from an injection site in an exercising limb is accelerated when exercise is begun too soon after an injection. If an injection is given in the legs and then a teen goes for a walk or run there is a good chance of hypoglycemia occurring without additional carbohydrate. Exercise 40 min after regular insulin or 2 ½ h after intermediate-acting insulin will have less of an effect on insulin absorption.

Glucose levels can be affected for many hours after exercise is completed, and it is essential to monitor blood glucose levels postexercise to assess the need for extra carbohydrate. For example, strenuous exercise or exercise over an extended period in the afternoon may require a decrease in the presupper insulin dosage in order to avoid a late fall in plasma glucose in the middle of the night. Food intake often needs to be increased with exercise. However, many teens tend to overeat before exercise due to fear of hypoglycemia. The most effective way to determine how much food is needed is to monitor blood glucose before, during, and after exercise. Some physicians advise their patients not to exercise if their blood glucose level is over 300 mg/dL. Presumably, in the very underinsulinized patient, exercise can actually increase rather than decrease blood glucose levels. However, plasma glucose values often exceed 300 mg/dL in adolescent patients even in the face of adequate diabetes control. Consequently, in our clinic there is no restriction in exercise unless the patient is not feeling well and is ketotic. SBGM is an essential component to exercise with IDDM. A fast-acting carbohydrate should always be readily available and water should always be consumed to prevent dehydration, particularly in those less well-controlled.

Psychosocial

Diabetes is more than a medical condition. Many aspects of life are affected by diabetes. Self-perception and the perceptions of peers and lifestyle are all affected by the diagnosis of diabetes. Diabetes adds to the normal stress of adolescence and problems can become magnified. Teens naturally strive to conform, but they may perceive diabetes as a constant reminder that they are different. A teenager hanging out with his friends will have a difficult time saying "no thanks" when everybody else is snacking at 5 P.M. (shortly before his scheduled mealtime). Parents may worry as their teen engages in the risk-taking behavior normal in adolescence. In addition to these concerns are those related to diabetes. Parents are concerned about hypoglycemia, hyperglycemia, compliance with the meal plan, appropriate insulin doses and ultimately long-term complications. Obtaining a driver's license symbolizes freedom to a teen, but produces anxiety in a parent. Precautions need to be taken to avoid hypoglycemia, such as monitoring blood glucose prior to driving or keeping a fast-acting carbohydrate in the car. For some adolescents with IDDM, rebelling may take the form of not communicating with their parents, staying up late, and noncompliance with dietary restrictions. A teen may skip meals that results in hypoglycemia or snack on large quantities of food at haphazard times during the day that also produce erratic glucose levels. A more serious behavioral concern is skipping insulin doses, which causes hyperglycemia and the accompanying symptoms and, if continued, DKA.

There are a number of factors that will make working with adolescents more effective. Initially, the dietitian should build a rapport and develop a sense of trust with the adolescent. Talking to the teen about the things that interest him or treating her like an adult with something worthwhile to say facilitates this process. Most important, a relationship separate from the parent is also needed to facilitate autonomy. Diabetes-management goals, by necessity, must be adjusted for adolescents with IDDM. Even when adolescents are intensively managed with insulin, the glycated hemoglobin is higher than that of intensively treated adults.[22] The clinical dietitian needs to be flexible in his or her expectations. Dietary goals may be modified, e.g., for a teenager who consumes a high-fat diet and does not adhere to a meal plan and eats "almost continuously" between 3 P.M. and 6 P.M. Ideally, nutritionally related goals are to decrease fat intake and eat three meals and two discreet snacks. However, that may involve more changes than the teen is willing to make. Realistically, small changes would be more reasonable. Negotiating with the teen to only eat one large afternoon snack would probably control blood glucoses more effectively.

Choosing an appropriate insulin regime for the particular lifestyle can help to promote overall adherence. Ultralente in the morning instead of NPH may control predinner glucose levels for the individual who eats a large snack in the afternoon. Eliminating Regular in the evening for a teen who swims or plays soccer may reduce the need to eat extra calories to prevent hypoglycemia. Generally, simple treatment regimens are usually the most effective. Adolescents do not want to use a complex meal planning approach or insulin regimen that requires frequent SBGM. There are some adolescents who do find intensive insulin treatment with frequent SBGM acceptable, as evidenced by the success of the adolescents who participated in the DCCT.[22]

Behavioral modification techniques can also be successfully employed. For those adolescents who are receptive, behavioral changes can be promoted by simplfying treatment, shaping, or making a series of small changes to reach a desired goal. Additionally, behavioral contracts (see Chapter 7 and Appendix C) can be used as well as teaching the adolescent to anticipate and plan ahead. Self-management skills are techniques to help individuals gain greater control over their own behavior. For example, cues or reminders can be used to remember to eat a snack or take a third injection. In addition, substituting positive behaviors for those that do not support the treatment plan, e.g., influencing a teenager to go bike riding instead of eating excessive calories with a snack. Self-monitoring and goal setting can help an individual focus and examine one's patterns. Daily food and blood glucose records can assess calorie intake and glucose patterns.

CASE ILLUSTRATION

Alice is a 14-year-old girl who presents to the diabetes clinic.

PHYSICAL INFORMATION

Height, 163 cm (5'4"), 50–75th percentile of height for her age

Weight, 63.6 kg (140lb), 75–90th percentile of weight for her age

75–90th percentile of weight for height for age

Appropriate weight range for height, 53–59.7 kg (117–132lb), which is determined by the weight at the 50–75th percent of weight for height for her age

Weight goal, 130 lb

Blood pressure, 120/75 mm Hg

USUAL DIETARY INTAKE

Breakfast, small bowl of unsweetened cereal with 2% milk and 4 oz of orange juice

Lunch, sandwich (turkey and cheese or tuna with mayonnaise), fresh fruit, and whole milk

Snack, (time and amount varies), may include varying combinations of chips, cookies, bagel, cheese and crackers

Dinner, approximately 4 oz meat (lean beef, chicken without skin, baked fish, ½–1 cup of rice,potatoes, or vegetables, 1 cup 2% milk

Night snack, eats throughout evening, foods are similar to those eaten in afternoon

Caloric intake varies due to variable snack intake, between 2100–2400 cal

DIABETES HISTORY

10-yr duration, HbA^{1}C 12.5% (nl, 4.0- 8.0)

SBGM, 1–2 times/d

Insulin regimen, 10 Regular, 20 NPH in morning, 12 Regular,18 NPH before dinner

LIPIDS

Total cholesterol, 200 mg/dL, triglycerides, 150 mg/dL, HDL 40, LDL 130 mg/dL.

EXERCISE

Plays soccer with town recreation department and softball after school seasonally. Enjoys exercise, but participates only to a limited extent.

PSYCHOSOCIAL

Until recently Alice's mom had primary control of her daughter's diabetes having done so since the initial diagnosis when Alice was 4. She maintained fairly strict discipline and diabetes management and consequently good control. She used the exchange system for meal planning. She made sure that Alice checked her blood glucose at least three times a day. At present, Mom is very upset with her daughter's diabetes management and concerned about her health.

Alice thinks she is doing fine. She reports feeling physically well. She thinks she is a little overweight and wants to lose weight. Alice recognizes that some blood sugars are high, but she thinks her mom is overreacting and is strict and unreasonable. Alice thinks an occasional candy or cookie is not so bad. She counters her mother's complaints with the fact that she checks her glucose every day, eats a nutritious diet, and in general feels ok.

CALCULATED ENERGY NEEDS

47Kcal/kg $\times$ 53–60kg = 2500–2800 kcal
(Using the RDA for energy for her age and IBW range)

Approximately 2000 kcal needed for weight loss. A 500-cal deficit will promote a weight loss of approximately 1 lb/wk. These are calculated or theoretical needs and are to be used as a general guide. Alice's actual intake is more important.

MEAL PLANNING

Trying to reinstruct Alice on the exchanges seemed futile since she was rebelling against her mothers' structured management. It is more appropriate to use a more flexible approach, but one that still promotes goals of diabetes management. Alice didn't realize there are ways to meal plan other than the exchange system. We chose to work on specific written guidelines with which she agreed to go along.

NUTRITION AND BEHAVIORAL GOALS

Short-term, facilitate Alice's "ownership" of her diabetes and taking responsibility for her diet, help her see what behaviors will improve her diabetes management

Long-term, implement appropriate diet changes or adjustments

EDUCATIONAL SESSIONS

Initially identify and address the things that are important to Alice that will help to reach her and have a greater chance of success. Her weight is something she wants to change. She verbalized that sports are an enjoyable activity. Develop a rapport with Alice, find out what else is important to her. An additional goal is to work with Alice's mother and social worker to discuss realistically how teenagers eat, consider realistic expectations of diabetes control in an adolescent, and assess Alice's present level of diabetes control.

The ongoing sessions, allow Alice to talk about her frustrations with diabetes and the diet. It is important to be empathic and understanding. Explain that you will work with her on present eating habits in the context of good diabetes management and will not prescribe major changes..

Explain a few of the meal planning approaches. Together, discuss behavioral goals that will improve blood glucose levels and reach her goals of weight reduction. Jointly, select and systematically work on these making these changes.

SPECIFIC MODIFICATIONS

Decrease fat in the diet, a switch to 1% or skim milk.

Decrease high-fat snack foods being particularly careful with cheese and cookies (appropriate low-fat snacks are pretzels, rice cakes, low-fat crackers, fruit, sugar-free popsicles, air-popped popcorn).

Reduce the size of snacks and frequency of eating snacks between meals.

Eat afternoon and evening snacks at regular times (same time every day).

Snacks should be approximately the same size.

To increase flexibility, Alice can be taught how to take extra insulin for extra carbohydrate, especially for concentrated sweets that are high in total carbohydrate. Also, explain why sweets are not appropriate more than occasionally since these foods are high in fat and calories.

REFERENCES

1. National Diabetes Data Group, *Diabetes*, **28**, 1039 (1979).

2. M. A. Sperling, in *Clinical Pediatric Endocrinology*, (S. A. Kaplan, ed.), W. B. Saunders Co., Philadelphia, PA, pp. 127–164 (1990).

3. American Diabetes Association, in *The Physician's Guide to Type II Diabetes (NIDDM)*, (H. Rifkin, ed.), ADA, Alexandria, VA, pp. 1–12 (1994).

4. W. E. Winter, N. K. Maclaren, W. J. Riley, D. W. Clarke, M. S. Kappy, R. P. Spillar, *N. Engl. J. Med.*, **316**, 285 (1987).

5. American Diabetes Association, *The Physician's Guide to Type I Diabetes (IDDM)*, (M. Sperling, ed.), ADA, Alexandria, VA, pp. 1–12 (1988).

6. L. J. Melton, P. J. Palumbo, and C. P. Chu, *Diab. Care*, **6**, 75 (1983).

7. C. J. Kyllo and F. A. Nutall, *Diabetes*, **27**, 57 (1978).

8. G. Holmgren, G. Samuelson, and B. Hermansson, *Clin. Gen.*, **5**, 465 (1974).

9. M. Calnan and C. S. Peckham, *Lancet*, **1**, 589 (1977).

10. Diabetes Epidemiology Research International Group, *Diabetes*, **37**, 1113 (1988).

11. F. M. Fleegler, K. D. Rogers, A. Drash, A. L. Rosenbloom, L. B. Travis, and J. M. Court, *Pediatrics*, **63**, 374 (1979).

12. J. P. Palmer and D. K. McCulloch, *Diabetes*, **40**, 943 (1991).

13. F. W. Scott, *Am. J. Clin. Nutr.*, **51**, 489 (1990).

14. G. S. Eisenbarth, *N. Engl. J. Med.*, **5**, 1360 (1986).

15. T. Tuvemo, G. Frisk, G. Friman, J. Ludringsson, and H. Diderhalm, *Diab.Res.*, **9**, 125 (1988).

16. M. Salimena and P. DeCamilli, *Nature*, **366**, 15 (1993).

17. The DCCT Research Group, *J. Clin. Endocrinol. Metab.*, **65**, 30 (1987).

18. ADA Position Statement, *Diab. Care*, **16**, 16 (1992).

19. J. J. Cook and D. Daneman, *AJDC*, **144**, 234 (1990).

20. J. S. Dorman, R. E. Laporte, L. H. Kuller, K. J. Cruickshanks, T. J. Orchard, D. K. Wagener, D. J. Becker, and D. E. Cavender, *Diabetes*, **33**, 271 (1984).

21. The DCCT Research Group, *N.Engl. J. Med.*, **329**, 977 (1993).

22. The DCCT Research Group, *J. Peds.*, **125**, 177 (1994).

23. American Diabetes Association, in *The Physician's Guide to Type I Diabetes (DM)*, (M. Sperling, ed.), ADA, Alexandria, VA, p. 33 (1988).

24. S. A. Amiel, R. S. Sherwin, D. C. Simonson, A. A. Lauritano, and W. V. Tamborlane, *N. Engl. J. Med.*, **315**, 215 (1986).

25. American Diabetes Association, in *The Physician's Guide to Type I Diabetes (IDDM)*, (M. Sperling, ed., ADA, Alexandria, VA, pp. 130 (1988).

26. R. R. Wing, R. Klein, and S. E. Moss, *Diab. Care*, **13**, 1106 (1990).

27. L. K. Mahan, R. H. Rosebrough, in *Nutrition in Adolescence*, (L. K. Mahan and J. M. Rees, eds.), C.V. Mosby Co., MO, pp. 40–73 (1984).

28. P.V.V. Hamill, J. A. Drizd, C. H. Johnson, R. B. Reed, A. F. Roche, and W. M. Moore, *Am. J. Clin. Nutr.*, **32**, 607 (1979).

29. National Center for Health Statistics, in *Vital and Health Statistics, Series 11, no. 124*, U. S. Government Printing Office, Washington, DC, (1973).

30. *Obesity in America, Guidelines for Body Weight*, NIH Pub. no. 79–359, Public Health Service DHEW, Washington, DC, (1979).

31. Society of Actuaries and Association of Life Insurance Medical Directors of America , *1979 Build Study*, Metropolitan Life Co., New York, (1983).

32. M. J. Wiseman, E. Bognetti, R. Dobbs, H. Keen, and G. G. Viberti, *Diabetologia*, **30**, 154 (1987).

33. R. P. Dullaart, B. J. Beusekamp, S. Meijer, J. J. van Doormaal, and W. J. Sluiter, *Diab. Care*, **16**, 483 (1993).

34. M. M. Jibani, L. L. Bloodworth, E. Foden, K. D. Griffiths, and O. P. Galpin, *Diab. Med.*, **8**, 949 (1991).

35. Technical review: Nutrition principles for the management of diabetes and related complications, *Diab. Care*, **17**, 490 (1994).

36. G. M. Reaven, *Am. J. Clin. Nutr.*, **47**, 1078 (1988).

37. American Diabetes Association Position Statement, *Diab. Care*, **17**, 519 (1994).

38. J. P. Bantle, *Diab. Care*, **12**, 56 (1989).

39. R. Nosadini, P. Fioretto, R. Teveisan, and G. Crepaldi, *Diab. Care*, **14**, 210 (1991).

40. M. A. Powers and D. C. Laine, in *Handbook of Diabetes Nutritional Management*, (M. A. Powers, ed.), Aspen Publishers, Rockville, MD, pp. 281–300 (1987).

41. M. L. Wheeler, S. E. Fineberg, R. Gibson, and N. Fineberg, *Diab. Care*, **13**, 733 (1990).

42. M. A. Powers, ed., *Nutrition Guide for Professionals*, American Diabetes Association and American Dietetic Association, pp. 1–5 (1988).

43. P. Halfon, J. Belkhadir, and G. Slama, *Diab. Care*, **12**, 427 (1989).

44. J. A. Green and H. J. Holler, eds., *Meal Planning Approaches for Diabetes Management*, ADA, Alexandria, VA, (1994).

45. J. Green, M. L. Wheeler, and J. W. Rosett, *Diabetes*, **35** (suppl.), 44A (1986).

46. T. Stancin, D. Lintz, and J. Reuter, *Diab. Care*, **12**, 601 (1989).
47. R. Striegel-Moore, T. J. Nicholson, and W. V. Tamborlane, *Diab. Care*, **15**, 1361 (1992).
48. R. Birk and M. D. Spencer, *Diab. Ed.*, **15**, 336 (1989).
49. S. Billion, *On the Cutting Edge*, **10**, 1 (1989).

Renal Disease

Jean Stover, R. D., and
Polly Nelson, R. D.

INTRODUCTION

Adolescents, as well as individuals in any age group, can develop either acute or chronic renal failure. Acute renal failure (ARF) may be secondary to nephrotoxins (antibiotics, chemotherapeutic agents, accidental poisoning), shock, infection, or complications associated with other disease states, but can be a reversible process in which normal kidney function is restored.[1] Chronic renal failure (CRF) results in the eventual permanent loss of normal kidney function and, in its end stages, requires dialysis and/or renal transplantation for survival.

Specific causes of CRF more peculiar to younger children include hemolytic uremic syndrome, cortical necrosis, renal malformations, and obstructive uropathy with infection. Renal hypoplasia, certain hereditary nephropathies (such as Alport's syndrome) and glomerular diseases are more frequent etiologic factors in older children and adolescents.[2] The cause of CRF, how advanced it has become, the specific modality of dialytic therapy, or whether transplantation has been performed will all determine which specific dietary restrictions are necessary. Growth and development during adolescence will be influenced by age at onset of CRF.

In the adolescent population, the clinical dietitian may be caring for those who have been on dialysis and/or had a renal transplant for several years, or those who have developed renal disease suddenly after their pubertal growth spurt. Each of these two groups will have different physiologic, nutritional, and emotional impacts of renal disease.

When an adolescent is diagnosed with CRF, regular follow-up to evaluate biochemical parameters, growth, and the need for medical, nutritional, and psychosocial intervention is necessary. If dialysis is not immediately required, regular physician office visits should be scheduled with the inclusion of the dietitian, social worker, and other health care team members as needed.

When renal function is impaired, hypertension, edema, elevated blood urea nitrogen (BUN), creatinine and electrolyte, mineral, fluid, and hormonal imbalances may exist. Some or all of these conditions may be present for each individual at various times during the course of CRF. It is important to determine which of these factors requires treatment with medication, diet, and/or dialysis. Not all factors must be addressed simultaneously due to their potential for development in the future and priorities must be set to promote compliance. It is important to remember that the adolescent is likely to be experiencing a period of adjustment due to hormonal and behavioral changes prior to the impact of discovering he or she has a chronic disease. Thus, adjustments in lifestyle with regard to medical treatments and dietary restrictions should be made gradually whenever possible.

Once dialysis is imminent, ideally the various modalities of dialytic therapy are discussed with the teen, caretakers and renal health care team. The two general types of dialysis are hemodialysis and peritoneal dialysis.

Hemodialysis is generally an in-center outpatient treatment for 3–4 h at a time, three times per week. A vascular access, such as an arterio-venous graft (a synthetic tubelike piece of material that connects an artery to a vein) or arterio-venous fistula (an internal connection of the individual's own artery and vein), must be surgically created in order to access the blood to the "artificial kidney" or dialyzer.[3] The blood is exposed to dialysate within the dialyzer and filtered for removal of waste products and excess fluid not adequately excreted by the impaired kidneys. A temporary subclavian or femoral catheter may be used if dialysis must be done immediately and there is not yet a more permanent access created or ready for use. Vascular access grafts and fistulas take time to "mature."

Peritoneal dialysis (PD) involves the removal of waste products in the blood as well as excess fluid by using the individual's peritoneal membrane as a filter. Dialysis occurs by instilling 1–2 L of dialysate into the peritoneal cavity through a surgically placed catheter. This fluid dwells for a period of time while the dextrose in the dialysate increases the osmolality of the solution and pulls fluid from the blood into the peritoneal cavity. Waste products also diffuse across the peritoneal membrane into the peritoneal cavity. The dialysate solution is then drained from the body through the dialysis catheter and discarded.[4]

There are different forms of PD that may be chosen by the adolescent and/ or his or her caretaker(s) once this general modality of dialysis is selected. These various forms include continuous ambulatory peritoneal dialysis (CAPD) that involves manual exchanges performed daily at home, continuous cycling perito- neal dialysis (CCPD) that involves a cycler that automatically performs exchanges nocturnally (usually) at home while the individual sleeps, and tidal PD that is a variation of CCPD. Intermittent peritoneal dialysis (IPD) involves an individual receiving approximately 10 h of PD three times per week in an outpatient center. This form of PD is rarely utilized due to time and financial constraints. IPD may also refer to 48–72 h of dialysis done intermittently a few times on an inpatient basis prior to the individual receiving training to perform PD at home.

The peritoneal dialysis catheter must be cared for at home to prevent exit site infection, and the patient or caretakers must also be taught to perform the dialysis procedure with an aseptic technique. An inflammation of the peritoneum that can result from bacteria entering the peritoneal cavity is called peritonitis. This can cause serious illness if not treated immediately with intraperitoneal antibiot- ics. Many forms of peritonitis can be successfully treated at home.

The adolescent is usually taught to do the dialysis procedure, unless significant mental or physical impairments are present. In these instances, a caretaker may require training.

Renal transplantation is also a modality of care for adolescents with CRF in addition to dialytic therapy. Many nephrologists feel this is the treatment modality of choice for teens. A well-functioning kidney usually provides the best opportu- nity for adequate physical, psychological, and social development.

Living related, living unrelated, or cadaveric transplantation are all options depending on available donors. Donors must have compatible blood and tissue type with the recipient. If cadaveric donation is the plan, the recipient is ultimately placed on a computerized transplant list. Depending on blood and tissure typing, the wait for a kidney may be from a few months to a few years.

Medical evaluation for renal transplantation may take place prior to the adoles- cent requiring dialysis, and transplantation may even occur before the adolescent is ever dialyzed. The social worker or psychologist also play an important role in evaluation of the recipient and potential living donors for this modality of therapy.

ASSESSMENT

Nutritional assessment of the adolescent with CRF includes the collection of anthropometric data, evaluation of biochemical parameters, and dietary intake, as well as the formulation of the dietary prescription.

Anthropometric data include height, weight, and, in some centers, skinfold measurements and arm muscle circumference. Weight should be carefully evaluated because initially, it may include edema. A nonedematous weight or "estimated dry weight" (EDW), as well as the other measurements, are compared to standardized tables and charts for age in a healthy population. Ideal body weight (IBW) can be determined by using 50th percentile weight for height grids (NCHS growth charts).[5]

Because there are no specific norms for children and adolescents with chronic renal disease, normal values for healthy adolescents are used to evaluate anthropometric data. These measurements are most useful as baseline values to which the individual can be compared to him- or herself on an ongoing basis.[6] Measurements should be obtained regularly (monthly except for weight that will be more frequent if the individual is undergoing dialysis) and by one consistent practitioner if possible. Skinfold and arm circumference measurements should be taken after dialysis and/or when the adolescent is close to his or her EDW, as excess fluid in the tissues may affect obtained results.[7,8]

If CRF develops after the pubertal growth spurt, the adolescent may be at a reasonable height for age. However, if renal function becomes significantly impaired in childhood or early adolescence, growth may be stunted during conservative management and even while undergoing dialytic therapy. If renal transplantation cannot be performed early in the course of treatment for CRF, treatment with growth hormone, which has recently been utilized successfully in clinical trials, may be a consideration.[9]

Regardless of potential surgical or pharmacologic treatment as mentioned above, the adolescent with chronic renal failure needs adequate calories and protein to promote growth and the maintenance of adequate weight for height. At the same time, biochemical parameters and volume status must be maintained within reason. Nutrient needs are calculated during various phases and modalities of treatment of CRF as follows (see Table 20.1).

MANAGEMENT

Predialysis

Kilocalories. Caloric intake can be calculated by one of two methods. It is based on the Recommended Dietary Allowances (RDA) for IBW for chronological age for the adolescent at close to ideal height for age (50th percentile height for age on standard NCHS growth charts).[5,10] If the adolescent developed chronic renal failure in childhood or early adolescence, however, he or she may be significantly growth-retarded. For this group, kilocalories based on the RDA for IBW for "height age" may be used. Height age is the age at which the actual height of the individual crosses the 50th percentile for height on standardized growth charts.

Table 20.1   Daily Nutrition Recommendation for Adolescents with Renal Disease.

| | Predialysis | Hemodialysis (HD) | |
	Chronic Renal Insufficiency	Peritoneal Dialysis (PD)	Transplantation
Kilocalories	Females, 11–14 yr: 47 kcal/kg Females, 15–18 yr: 40 kcal/kg Males, 11–14 yr: 55 kcal/kg Males, 15–18 yr: 45 kcal/kg	HD: Same as for predialysis. PD: Same as for predialysis, decrease if excess weight gain.	Same as for predialysis after ideal weight for height is achieved.
Protein	11–14 yr: 1.0 g/kg 15–18 yr: 0.9 g/kg Protein losses in the urine should not be replaced by diet.	HD: min. 1.3–1.5 g/kg. PD: min. 1.5 g/kg.	2 g/kg initially; RDA after approximately 3 mo.
Sodium	Generally unrestricted; 1–3 mEq/kg if edema or HTN is present (1–4 g/d).	HD: Restricted in conjunction with fluid to attain 1–2 kg of interdialytic weight gain. PD: 3–4 g/d.	2–4 g/d initially; unrestricted when HTN and edema present.
Potassium	Generally unrestricted; 1–3 mEq/kg if needed.	HD: Restricted appropriately to maintain serum levels < 5.5 mEq/L.	Unrestricted unless indicated.
Calcium	1200 mg/d provided; hypercalcemia does not occur and Ca/P product does not exceed 70.	Same as predialysis.	Unrestricted; supplement if indicated.
Phosphorus	600–800 mg/d when serum levels are elevated; diet used in conjunction with phosphate binders.	600–800 mg/d; diet used in conjunction with phosphate binders.	Unrestricted; supplement if indicated.
Vitamins	Use a multivitamin or B-complex plus C in deficient; vitamin D metabolite, if needed, based on Ca/P/PTH levels.	HD: Same as predialysis. Vitamin D, if indicated given orally or intravenous with HD treatment. PD: Same as predialysis.	Vitamin D as indicated to promote bone growth; other supplementation usually not necessary beyond RDA.

continued on next page

Table 20.1   *Continued*

	Predialysis	Hemodialysis (HD)	
	Chronic Renal Insufficiency	Peritoneal Dialysis (PD)	Transplantation
Trace Mineral	Supplement zinc and iron, if indicated.	HD: May need iron with EPO; zinc if indicated. PD: Same as HD.	Supplementation usually not necessary beyond RDA; iron if indicated.
Fluid	Unrestricted unless indicated, then provide insensible losses plus urinary output.	HD: Insensible losses plus urinary output; if no urine output, approximately 1 L/d. PD: Unrestricted unless indicated.	Unrestricted; encourage min. of 1.5– 2.0 L/d.

Adapted from P. Nelson and J. Stover, in *A Clinical Guide to Nutrition Care in End-Stage Renal Disease*, (J. Stover, ed.), The American Dietetic Association, Chicago, IL, pp. 81–85, (1994).

Protein.   These are also calculated based on the RDA for either chronological or height age. Generally, individuals in our society consume much more protein than the RDA; thus, the RDA becomes a restriction in itself. The use of severely restricted protein diets (less than the RDA) to retard the progression of renal disease is not advised for this youth due to possible negative effects on growth potential.

Elevated blood urea nitrogen (BUN) levels will always be present with renal insufficiency, and it is possible that protein restriction may help reduce the toxic effects of extremely high BUN levels in the predialytic period. If adolescents are receiving glucocorticoid (steroid) therapy for their renal disease or other reasons, these catabolic drugs may produce even higher BUN levels.[11] Protein should not be restricted to less than the RDA in efforts to compensate.

Serum proteins such as albumin, prealbumin, and transferrin levels may be used to evaluate nutritional status with regard to protein intake in the adolescent population, but they may be falsely low in overhydrated states. Also, transferrin may fluctuate depending on iron deficiency or overload.[12] Albumin may also be very low when "nephrotic syndrome" is present with the adolescent's renal disease. This syndrome is identified by greater than 3 g albuminuria per 24 h.[13] Excess protein is not generally given beyond the RDA with nephrotic syndrome, due to reported cases of excessive protein intake increasing proteinuria.[14]

Sodium.   The serum sodium level is not a reliable indicator of actual sodium intake. Fluid retention can dilute a normal level, making it appear low. Thus, when hypertension and/or edema are apparent, a dietary sodium restriction is prescribed. The diet must still remain palatable for the adolescent; therefore, priority is generally given to limiting, but not necessarily eliminating, preferred high-sodium foods. The judicious use of diuretics in combination with a mild sodium restriction may help to keep the diet acceptable, while still preventing hypervolemia and subsequent related hypertension.[15]

Potassium. A potassium restriction may not be necessary during the predialytic period because as renal function decreases, the potassium excretion of each nephron increases until the glomerular filtration rate (GFR) reaches 10% of normal. At this level of GFR, the potassium secreted into the bowel also increases. Some diuretics that may be prescribed, such as furosemide, may increase urinary potassium excretion as well.[16] Sometimes, high-potassium foods or potassium supplements may even be required! Generally, a restriction should only be instituted when the serum potassium level is consistently greater than 5.0–5.5 mEg/L (after the correction of metabolic acidosis).

Calcium and phosphorous. The maintenance of normal serum calcium and phosphorous levels in adolescents with chronic renal failure is extremely important to prevent the development of bone disease and promote growth. When chronic renal insufficiency exists, the kidney does not excrete excess phosphate or produce adequate amounts of active vitamin D. Thus, phosphorus levels may be elevated, calcium levels decreased, and subsequently alkaline phosphatase and parathyroid hormone elevated.[15] Serum levels of calcium, phosphorus, alkaline phosphatase, and parathyroid hormone are closely monitored even in the predialysis period in efforts to prevent renal osteodystrophy and soft tissue calcifications. Radiographic studies and/or bone biopsies are done to diagnose the presence of renal osteodystrophy.

Elevated serum phosphorus levels are treated with both a phosphorus-controlled diet in which dairy products and other phosphorus-rich foods are limited, as well as phosphate-binding medications. Calcium carbonate and calcium acetate are frequently used and should be given immediately after meals to prevent maximum phosphorus absorption from food. These medications also contribute calcium intake, as calcium ingestion from food sources is limited due to those foods high in calcium also having a high phosphorus content. Aluminum-containing binders (aluminum hydroxide or aluminum carbonate) are not recommended for long-term use, as the potential for aluminum toxicity exists.[15] They may be used initially to lower serum phosphorus levels, however, when these levels are greater than 6.0–6.5 mg/dL or the calcium-phosphorus product (serum calcium × phosphorus) is greater than 70.[12] Calcium citrate is not used as a phosphate binder or calcium supplement due to its potential to increase aluminum absorption from the gut.

Low serum calcium levels are also treated with active vitamin D metabolites (calcitriol). However, it is important to note that when serum albumin levels are low, the calcium level must be "corrected" due to a substantial portion of total calcium being protein-bound. A decrease in albumin results in a decrease in total calcium (but not ionized calcium). A helpful way to calculate "corrected" calcium levels is to add 0.8 mg/dL for every g/dL decrease in serum albumin from 4.0 g/dL to the serum calcium laboratory value reported.[17] Ionized calcium levels are also helpful.

Vitamins and other minerals.   A regular multivitamin or water-soluble vitamin supplement may be given in the predialysis period if oral intake is inadequate due to dietary restriction or poor appetite. Vitamin D is not well utilized unless given in its active form, 1.25 dihydroxycholecalciferol, as the activation takes place in the kidney. This process is impaired in poor-functioning kidney tissue.[18] Supplements of active vitamin D are often started early in the treatment of renal failure on the basis of serum parathyroid and alkaline phosphatase levels above normal for age.

Iron supplementation is required for adolescents in the predialysis period when the depletion of iron stores is documented by iron studies. Individuals receiving recombinant human erythropoietin (Epogen®) usually require iron for red blood cell formation.[19] Erythropoieten is a hormone normally produced in healthy kidneys to stimulate red blood cell production and is not produced in adequate amounts with CRF. This is the primary reason for anemia associated with declining renal function.[20]

Serum iron and transferrin (to calculate iron saturation or available iron) as well as ferritin (to determine iron stores) should be monitored regularly.[21] Also, the adolescent should be advised to take oral iron supplements apart from meals and calcium or aluminum phosphate-binding medication to promote better absorption. If nausea develops, iron supplements can be taken with a few crackers or another small nondairy snack.

Zinc supplementation is not routinely administered to adolescents in the predialysis period, but may be required (RDA for age or height age) if there is reason to suspect deficiency.[15]

Fluid.   During the predialysis period, fluid requirements are dependent on the type of renal disease and level of GFR. Increased urine output dictates increased fluid intake. Maintenance fluid needs may be estimated by the following formula: 100 mL for the first 10 kg of body weight, 50 mL for each additional kg between 11 and 20 kg and 20 mL for each additional kilogram.[22] For example, a 50-kg adolescent would require 1000 mL for the first 10 kg, plus 500 mL for 11–20 kg, and 30 times 20 mL (600 mL) for the remaining 30 kg, for a total of 2100 mL/24 h. If fluid limitations become necessary due to edema, the prescribed amount is based on insensible fluid needs (fluid required for oxidation, respiration, perspiration, etc.) plus measured urine output. Insensible needs are estimated at 1500 mL/m^2/24 h.[22] However, for adolescents receiving outpatient services, insensible fluid needs may be increased with physical activity, requiring increased fluid allowance.

Hemodialysis

Kilocalories. Caloric needs for the adolescent undergoing hemodialysis are calculated by the same methods as in the predialysis period. The potential for adequate caloric intake is enhanced by minimizing the number of dietary restrictions to those that are absolutely necessary. Food preferences are honored as much as possible based on the need for other diet restrictions. Regular food items will generally have better acceptance than commercially available caloric supplements. Beverages such as fruit drinks should be encouraged as the preferred fluid, rather than water. Periodic 3-d intake records and ongoing skinfold measurements may be helpful to evaluate caloric adequacy of the diet as well as EDW changes. When skinfold measurements are done, they should be performed after a dialysis treatment when the individual is close to his or her EDW, as previously mentioned, and the arm without a vascular access (or at least a functioning access) should be used to perform these measurements.[7,8,12]

When necessary, caloric supplementation may be done by utilizing carbohydrate and/or fat modules such as Polycose® or Microlipid®, corn syrup or vegetable oil. Commercial supplements utilized for both caloric and protein supplementation, such as powdered breakfast drinks, Ensure®, and Sustacal®, are often appropriate, but may be impractical due to their expense and limited reimbursement from third-party payors. Lower cost recipes for low electrolyte "renal" shakes and drinks can be given to those who are motivated to make them. When commercial supplements are used, the electrolyte and mineral content must be evaluated, and potassium levels monitored closely.

Protein. Requirements for protein are slightly greater than those in the predialysis period to account for amino acid losses during each hemodialysis treatment.[3] Predialysis BUN levels greater than 100 mg/dL are generally considered too high, but may result for a variety of reasons. Thus, reducing protein intake in the diet is usually not the first method of treatment for this biochemical abnormality. The technical aspects of hemodialysis including type of dialyzer and blood flow rates, as well as time on dialysis and residual renal function, all need to be evaluated. Adequacy of dialysis studies (Kt/VURR) is done routinely in many centers to prompt assessment of these factors. Also, recirculation of blood secondary to the condition of the individual's vascular access may be considered. Catabolism resulting from infection or gastrointestinal bleeding may also be a reason for excessive azotemia, and if all of the above are ruled out, dietary aspects including quantity of protein intake and sufficient ratio of nonprotein to protein calories must be assessed. Verbal recall and food records may be helpful to assess overall dietary intakes.[15]

Kinetic modeling involving the protein catabolic rate (PCR), which calculates the urea generation rate, may also aid in assessing protein status for adolescents undergoing hemodialysis. In nutritionally stable individuals, PCR equals dietary protein intake.[23] For the unstable individual, the calculation of PCR is done so that dietary strategies can be planned and effects monitored. Different formulas and kinetic modeling programs are used in different hemodialysis centers; thus, the practitioner should be aware of these and his or her role in calculating or obtaining kinetics as an assessment tool.

Persistently low BUN levels may not necessarily indicate inadequate nutrition, and again, kinetic modeling information in conjunction with food intake recalls and diaries are most helpful for assessment. Also, arm anthropometry (as previously described) may document prolonged inadequate protein ingestion as well as caloric intake.

Serum protein levels have the same limitations as discussed in the predialysis period, except that proteinuria often decreases as the adolescent's renal function declines with time. Serum protein levels may not be decreased unless inadequate food ingestion has occurred for prolonged periods of time.

Sodium.   Allowances for sodium for adolescents undergoing hemodialysis are similar to those in the predialysis period. Edema as noted by excessive interdialytic weight gains and hypertension, as well as urinary output, will influence the amount of sodium prescribed. Interdialytic weight gains of 1 kg (2.2 lb) between short-interval treatments and 2 kg for long intervals (Friday to Monday) are generally acceptable and need not require strict sodium restrictions. If sodium must be restricted, reasonable efforts are made as in the predialysis period to include some favorite high-sodium foods.

Potassium.   Dietary potassium allowances for individuals undergoing hemodialysis are based on serum levels. Residual renal function, especially if urine output is $\geq$ 1000 mL/24 h, will often permit unrestricted intakes. If serum levels are persistently greater than 5.5 mEg/L after the longest interdialytic interval, a restriction is required.

When initiating a potassium restriction, the first step is to eliminate concentrated sources of this mineral, such as citrus fruit and juices, dark green leafy vegetables, and dried fruits. Altering methods of food preparation, such as soaking potatoes and other vegetables in large volumes of water several hours before cooking, may help "leach out" some of the potassium. Other foods such as those containing chocolate may need to be limited, but since they are a good source of calories, they can be used sparingly in the diet.

When serum potassium levels are repeatedly elevated despite dietary counseling, either a lower potassium hemodialysis dialysate solution or sodium exchange resin, polystyrene sulfonate (Kayexalate®, may need to be prescribed.[24]

Calcium and phosphorus. The guidelines for dietary restrictions and medications are similar to those for adolescents in the predialysis period. If phosphorus levels are persistently high, perhaps the type of phosphate binder needs to be changed to promote better compliance. The adolescent may not like the chewable form and desire a tablet, liquid, or capsules. If hypercalcemia develops when aggressively using calcium-containing medications and active vitamin D therapy to prevent or treat bone disease, the use of lower calcium dialysate solutions may be a consideration.

Vitamins and other minerals. Water-soluble vitamins should be routinely prescribed for adolescents on hemodialysis. These are now essential because they are somewhat dialyzable, in addition to diets often being inadequate in vitamin content secondary to diet restrictions or poor intakes. Generally, a specialized vitamin developed for adults with renal disease is prescribed. These vitamin preparations contain 10 mg OF pyridoxine, 0.8–1.0 mg of folate, 60–100 mg of ascorbic acid, and the RDA for other B-complex vitamins.[24] Vitamin A is not recommended due to the potential for toxicity in renal failure with its impaired clearance.[25]

An intravenous form of calcitriol is frequently given at the end of the dialysis treatment when significant hyperparathyroidism is apparent. It is believed that the intravenous form may provide a more direct suppressive effect of parathyroid hormone, in order to prevent osteodystrophy.[26]

Iron and zinc supplementation is also prescribed as noted during the predialysis period. However, in some cases, when iron studies are significantly decreased despite the prescribed oral iron therapy, intravenous iron dextran can be given in five to ten doses at the end of the hemodialysis treatment.[21]

Fluid. Restrictions are based on the principles of fluid management as previously described in the predialysis period. Also, they are often prescribed based on the amount of interdialytic weight gain (see "Sodium").

Peritoneal Dialysis

IPD requires dietary restrictions between treatments similar to those for hemodialysis. Thus, the following recommendations will use the term PD as referring to CAPD, CCPD or tidal PD.

Kilocalories. Caloric intake for adolescents undergoing PD may be inadequate, especially for those doing CAPD, due to a feeling of fullness from the indwelling dialysate exerting pressure on the stomach. Also continuous glucose absorption from the dialysate solutions that contain 1.5, 2.5, 3.5, or 4.25%

dextrose may play a role in appetite suppression. Both of these problems are somewhat resolved by doing CCPD or tidal PD, due to these modalities being performed at night, with only one daytime dwelling exchange. Nevertheless, caloric supplementation may be necessary for the adolescent undergoing PD as it is with hemodialysis.

Caloric needs for individuals undergoing PD are similar to those for hemodialysis. They are based on the RDA utilizing IBW. However, there is glucose absorption to be considered, with 50–80% of the glucose in the total number of 1.5–2 L PD exchanges utilized in 24 h being absorbed.[4] Due to this glucose absorption, obesity may develop in some adolescents with CRF who may already be overweight when initiating PD (often due to previous steroid therapy).[15] Methods to control unwanted solid weight gain include more strict control of sodium and fluid intake in order to use less concentrated dextrose solutions and the limitation of fast foods and snacks.

Elevated serum levels of cholesterol and triglycerides are also sometimes seen in adolescents undergoing PD. The rationale for these lipid abnormalities is due in part to increased protein losses into the dialysate, as well as the continuous infusion of glucose from the dextrose in PD solutions.[27] Thus, monounsaturated fats, polyunsaturated fats, and complex carbohydrates are encouraged as much as possible.

Protein. Requirements for protein for those undergoing PD are even higher than for those on hemodialysis due to protein losses with each exchange. Current recommendations are adapted from those for adults undergoing PD and based on the RDA for IBW (as for predialysis) plus added requirements to replace 24-h losses into the peritoneal dialysate.[15]

Assessment of adequacy of PD and PCR can be done with urea kinetics for the adult population.[28] Although these may be applicable to older adolescents, standards for children are now being developed that may become more appropriate for younger and smaller adolescents.[15]

Protein intake may need to be supplemented with commercial protein modules or protein-calorie supplements due to daily protein losses with this dialytic modality. Those on PD should better tolerate the potassium content of these supplements since PD also removes potassium daily. Homemade shake or drink recipes may still be utilized, however, due to cost.

Sodium. The amount of sodium intake for adolescents undergoing peritoneal dialysis can usually be greater than for those on hemodialysis due to daily sodium and fluid removal.[15] It is usually not unlimited, however, and the presence of edema and/or hypertension despite efforts to remove excess fluid by adjusting the dialysis regime will dictate the need for greater restrictions. A palatable diet containing less than 2 g/d, however, is difficult to achieve for most adolescents.

Potassium. Frequently can be unrestricted or may even need to be encouraged for those undergoing PD due to the amount removed daily. However, restrictions of dietary potassium are indicated when the serum level exceeds the upper limit of normal and other reasons for hyperkalemia are ruled out. It must be noted also that improved protein and calorie intake, in general, may alleviate the high potassium levels caused by catabolism.[15]

Fecal excretion of potassium plays an important role in the maintenance of normal serum potassium levels; thus, questioning about bowel habits must be components of the initial and ongoing assessments. A higher-fiber diet and adequate, but not excessive, fluid intake should be encouraged. If these recommendations do not suffice alone, a stool softener may be needed on a regular basis.[15]

Calcium and phosphorus. The calcium content of diets prescribed for those undergoing peritoneal dialysis remains low due to continued need for phosphorus restriction with this dialytic modality. As previously mentioned, high-phosphorus-containing foods are also those with significant calcium content. Thus, calcium-containing medications and active vitamin D preparations are used for this population to prevent or treat hypocalcemia and bone disease.

Although controlled, phosphorus intake must be slightly higher for those undergoing peritoneal dialysis due to the need for increased amounts of dietary protein. A daily milk limitation of 4–8 oz usually continues to allow ingestion of more meat, fish poultry, and eggs. Cheese products are often permitted, but also in small quantities depending on individual food preferences.[15]

Vitamins and other minerals. Recommendations for vitamins and minerals are the same as for those undergoing hemodialysis. Intravenous forms of iron and calcitriol are not administered as routinely with this dialysis modality. However, they can be prescribed as a part of the patient's home medication regime or given during outpatient visits in a clinical setting.

Fluid. Intake of fluid should not need formal restriction under most circumstances as long as the individual's ultrafiltration capacity is adequate and dialysis is performed as prescribed. When edema and/or hypertension are present, the adolescent or caretakers are taught how to manipulate the use of more highly concentrated dextrose PD solutions to increase fluid removal. The sodium content may also need to be reduced in conjunction with dialysis modification.

Transplantation

The nutritional needs following transplantation will depend on how well the kidney is functioning. The following recommendations will be for a well-functioning allograft. When there is suboptimal function (either acute or chronic rejection), nutrient recommendations are similar to those during the predialysis and dialytic phases of treatment for CRF. Some immunosuppressive medications may cause anorexia, nausea, vomiting, and/or diarrhea, which should be treated symptomatically.[15]

Kilocalories. Goals after renal transplantation are to achieve and maintain an ideal body weight. Treatment with corticosteroids is part of the immunosuppressive regime, but can increase appetite and cause unwanted weight gain.[29] Control of total calorie intake and increased exercise are emphasized. The RDA for age or height age is used as a guideline, with adjustments made as needed.

Corticosteroids affect carbohydrate metabolism by increasing insulin secretion causing glucose uptake by fat cells, impaired glucose tolerance, glycosuria, and relative resistance to insulin.[30] Suggestions have been made to restrict carbohydrate to as low as 1 g of carbohydrate/kg of body weight/d in efforts to overcome some of these steroid side-effects and reduce cushingoid appearance.[31] This is not practical for most adolescents; however. Thus, sugar and other concentrated sweets may be eliminated from the diet instead for a period of time after transplant surgery. Complex carbohydrates are permitted, with a goal of approximately 40–50% of total calories as carbohydrate.

As hyperlipidemia has been reported after transplantation, ongoing nutrition education recommendations must include monounsaturated and polyunsaturated fats, lean meats, and a fat intake of 30–35% of total daily calories.[32]

Protein. Immunosuppressive medications alter protein metabolism, causing decreased anabolism through decreased uptake of amino acids in muscle tissue and increased liver uptake of amino acids. Also, azathiaprine has been shown to inhibit DNA and RNA synthesis.[33] As a result, protein intake is recommended to be approximately 2 g/kg of IBW daily in the immediate posttransplantation period, tapering to the RDA after 3 mo.[15]

Sodium. Some immunosuppressive medications (corticosteroids and cyclosporine) can cause hypertension and/or edema due to increased sodium retention. Sodium is usually restricted in the immediate posttransplantation period, while the highest doses of these medications are utilized to prevent rejection. Sodium intake can often be liberalized once these medications are tapered and hypertension and fluid retention are no longer present.[15]

Potassium. Cyclosporine can cause transient hyperkalemia, apparently from the suppression of renin and aldosterone levels.[34] This occurs mainly when cyclosporine blood levels are very high and resolves as this medication is decreased.[15] Potassium intake is restricted as necessary, depending on serum levels.

Calcium and phosphorus. Calcium metabolism is affected by corticosteroids, causing decreased absorption from the intestine and increased calcium reabsorption. If serum levels of calcium decrease, a supplement may be required.

Phosphorus content of the diet is liberalized and supplements of this mineral may also be required due to its impaired reabsorption in the renal tubules.[32]

Vitamins and other minerals. Supplements of vitamins and other minerals are not generally given, but active vitamin D may be supplemented if hypocalcemia is present. Also, a magnesium supplement may be necessary initially after transplantation due to cyclosporine therapy, and iron may need supplementation for individuals with continued low iron stores.[15]

Fluid. Often encouraged after transplantation, with a minimum of 2 L/d. To prevent unwanted weight gain, water rather than calorie-containing beverages is encouraged.

Psychosocial and Practical Concerns

There are definite emotional and social aspects of chronic renal disease because of its multifaceted alteration of lifestyle. The adolescent must follow a regime including medications, diet restrictions, and eventually dialysis and/or renal transplantation. The goal of the health care team is to promote a normal lifestyle given all of these therapeutic issues.

During the various phases of treatment of chronic renal disease, the adolescent should be given as much control as possible based on his or her ability to understand and comply with needed care. It is almost always best to discuss plans for treatment with both the patient *and* caretakers simultaneously to promote consistency in communication. However, the adolescent also requires time alone with various team members. The ability to cope with disease while in a very "peer group conscious" phase of life emphasizes the potential for difficulty in adjusting to a complicated medical regime. The social worker and/or psychologist are important resources for the adolescent, as well as other health care team members. They are trained to care for adolescents and their families in addition to communicating with other team members about the overall approach to care.

Nutritional management of the adolescent with chronic renal disease must therefore take into consideration practicality with regard to care of the individual as a whole. For example, favorite and popular foods must be a part of the diet so that the individual can socialize with peers at preferred eating establishments. The rationale for various diet restrictions, such as sodium and fluid control vs. edema and hypertension, is provided. Thus, occasional limited amounts of pizza or other fast-foods are allowed as long as the adolescent is able to control his or her intake.

Compliance with medications is also a concern in the adolescent population with chronic renal disease. There are often many medications prescribed, including vitamins, antihypertensives, calcium and iron supplements, and phosphate binders. In efforts to avoid seeming different from peers, the adolescent may not want to take medications that must be taken with meals for maximum effectiveness in the presence of others. It can be suggested that these medications be taken at home just before going out to eat if the meal or snack will be consumed within one half-hour. Also, taking these medications in the rest room just before or after meals is an option.

Compliance with dialysis treatments can be problematic for many teens. Although peritoneal dialysis that is done at home allows more freedom with time schedules, some adolescents do skip exchanges for social or other reasons, resulting in inadequate biochemical and fluid balance. It may be necessary for members of the health care team to meet with the adolescent separately and then the caretakers to discuss a change in dialysis modality. Sometimes, a trial for improved compliance may be an option, but if this fails, a change to hemodialysis may be required. This change should not be presented as punishment, but as an aid to help the adolescent better comply with the needed dialysis therapy. Underdialysis can cause more uremic symptoms, including a decrease in appetite and irritability.

The nutritional status and overall well being of the patient may improve when he or she is receiving more adequate dialysis once a change in modality is made. If there is a change in dialysis modality from peritoneal to hemodialysis, dietary restrictions will likely need modification as well. The diet is usually more strictly controlled in regard to sodium, potassium, and fluid.

All of the above concerns associated with chronic renal failure plus coping with short stature often impact on adolescents who developed end-stage renal failure in childhood. A 16-year-old may be the average height of an 8-year-old! This certainly makes peer group acceptance even more difficult, and more comprehensive psychosocial support from the health care team is often needed. It is hoped that with growth hormone therapy and advances in the pharmacological management of renal transplant recipients, growth potential for this group of adolescents will improve.

CASE ILLUSTRATION

Will is a 22-year-old male who was diagnosed with congenital obstructive uropathy at 8 mo of age. He had ureterostomies created at an early age to allow proper urination. Due to renal hypoplasia resulting from this urologic abnormality, however, he developed chronic renal failure and progressed to its end stages by the time he was 16. He did have sufficient renal function through puberty so that he was able to attain a height of 5'6".

Will and his mother met with the health care team when dialysis was imminent and decided peritoneal dialysis was the best option to allow him as normal a lifestyle as possible. Will would be responsible for dialyzing himself overnight via the cycler machine.

Initially, with residual renal function including a urine output of greater than 1000 cc/d, Will required only a mild sodium limit. He was taught to adjust the concentration of the dialysate to remove fluid as needed based on his weight. Thus, a fluid limit was not necessary. Will's potassium level was low-normal due to residual renal function combined with nightly dialysis. High potassium foods were actually encouraged in his diet.

Due to high serum phosphate levels, Will was instructed to limit dairy products in his diet as well as to take calcium carbonate tablets with all meals and snacks to bind phosphorus.

Will's weight was 53 kg on the initiation of dialysis, but his caloric needs were based on an ideal body weight of 54.5 kg (50th percentile weight for age 14.5 yr, which is the age at which his height met the 50th percentile on NCHS growth charts). He was calculated to need 45 kcal/kg of IBW, or 2450 kcal/d.

Protein needs of 80–85 g/day were calculated for Will based on 1.5 g/kg of IBW.

Monthly clinic visits were scheduled once training for home peritoneal dialysis was complete. Will seemed to be doing fairly well during the first year after training except for only mild edema and elevated phosphate levels.

Persistently high serum phosphate levels despite a review of diet and change in medications indicated probable noncompliance with one or both of these regimes. The risk of renal osteodystrophy and its consequences were repeatedly explained to Will and his mother together, as well as to Will alone. However, he was rarely able to attain desired goals for phosphate control.

Will completed his medical work-up for renal transplantation after 1 yr on dialysis and was placed on the cadaveric transplant list. There were no compatible living donors available for him at the time.

During the second year of undergoing peritoneal dialysis, Will's residual renal function began to decline and he was often volume-overloaded and hypertensive. His weight was now 65–68 kg at clinic visits. Will was felt to have gained some solid body weight during the first year on dialysis, but his EDW was still only considered to be 60 kg.

Although renal function was declining, it was believed Will was not taking his medications properly, following his diet, or doing all of his dialysis as prescribed. He had received instructions on medication, diet, and dialysis prescription adjustments for the loss in his residual renal function. He repeatedly denied noncompliance, and his mother indicated only that he missed an occasional night of dialysis.

During his first hospitalization for severe hypertension and volume overload, antihypertensive medications were further adjusted, dietary sodium and fluid restrictions were reviewed, and the dialysis prescription was again altered. Will left the hospital in good volume status and with reasonable blood pressure control, but soon returned to the clinic volume-overloaded and hypertensive again. Will's physician suggested that he switch to hemodialysis because he was not adequately managing his health care with peritoneal dialysis at home. Will did not want a change in dialysis modality, promising to be more compliant with his whole medical regime. His physician agreed to let him try again.

Finally, after the third hospitalization for volume overload and hypertension, Will, with the assistance of the social worker, realized that he needed to change to hemodialysis. He did admit that peritoneal dialysis was a "burden" and he would rather give up 5 h three times a week to go to an outpatient hemodialysis unit, than to have to worry about doing his own dialysis in addition to schoolwork and other school and social activities.

A permanent access (arterio-venous fistula) was placed along with a temporary subclavian catheter so that hemodialysis could begin immediately. Will dialyzed in the evening so that he could attend high school regularly during his senior year.

Although a dietary potassium restriction was now necessary with hemodialysis and very little residual renal function, Will adapted after some review. Elevated serum phosphate levels and occasional high interdialytic fluid weight gains were still problems, but Will seemed to be feeling better mentally and physically with this change in dialysis modality.

After 3 mo on hemodialysis, Will received a cadaveric renal transplant. He did well initially, following only a mild sodium-restricted diet. After 3 mo and repeated hospitalizations for antirejection therapy, it was evident that he had developed chronic rejection and would probably need dialysis again soon. Will started back on hemodialysis 5 mo after receiving his transplant, requiring dietary sodium, potassium, and fluid restrictions. Exactly, 1 mo later, the kidney was removed due to pain and fever.

Will was placed back on the cadaveric renal transplant list 6 mo after going back on dialysis. Unfortunately, he is still waiting for a suitable kidney after 3 yr. He is, however, doing fairly well with hemodialysis while working full time. He still has problems with hyperphosphatemia and now hyperparathroidism, in addition to high interdialytic fluid weight gains. These are common problems for adults undergoing hemodialysis as well as for adolescents. Diet and medications continue to be reviewed with Will on a regular basis in efforts to keep him in the best condition possible for his next kidney transplant.

REFERENCES

1. N. M. Wolfish and A. Fish, in *Care of the Renal Patient*, (D. Z. Levine, ed.), W. B. Saunders, Philadelphia, PA, pp. 107 (1991).

2. M. Broyer, in *Pediatric Nephrology*, (P. Royer, R. Habib, H. Mathieu and M. Broyer, eds.), W. B. Saunders, Philadelphia, PA, pp. 364 (1974).

3. P. Harum, in *A Clinical Guide to Nutrition Care in End-Stage Renal Disease*, (J. Stover, ed.), The American Dietetic Association, Chicago, IL, pp. 25–36 (1994).

4. L. McCann, in *A Clinical Guide to Nutrition Care in End-Stage Renal Disease*, (J. Stover, ed.), The American Dietetic Association, Chicago, IL, pp. 37–55 (1994).

5. National Center for Health Statistics Growth Curves for Children 0–18 Years, *U. S. Vital and Health Statistics*, series II, no. 165., Health Resources Administration, U. S. Government Printing Office, Washington DC (1977).

6. R. A. Frisancho, *Am. J. Clin. Nutr.*, **27**, 1052 (1974).

7. P. Nelson and J. Stover, in *End-Stage Renal Disease in Children*, (R. N. Fine and A. Gruskin, eds.), W. B. Saunders, Philadelphia, PA, pp. 209 (1984).

8. M. Massie, K. Niimi, W. Yang, et al., *J Ren. Nutr.*, **2**, 2 (1992).

9. R. N. Fine, O. Yadin, L. Moulton, et al., *J. Ped. Endocrinol.*, **7**, 1 (1994).

10. Food and Nutrition Board, National Academy of Sciences, National Research Council, *Recommended Dietary Allowances, X ed.*, National Academy Press, Washington DC (1989).

11. J. L. Stark, *Nursing*, **80**, 33 (1981).

12. K. Norwood, P. Thayer, CRN of Upstate New York, and J. Stover, in *A Clinical Guide to Nutrition Care in End-Stage Renal Disease*, (J. Stover, ed.), The American Dietetic Association, Chicago, IL, pp. 5–15 (1994).

13. D. Gillit and CRN of New Jersey, in *A Clinical Guide to Nutrition Care in End-Stage Renal Disease*, (J. Stover, ed.), The American Dietetic Association, Chicago, IL, pp. 1–4 (1994).

14. G. A. Kaysen, *Am. J. Kid. Dis.*, **12**, 461 (1988).

15. P. Nelson and J. Stover, in *A Clinical Guide to Nutrition Care in End-Stage Renal Disease*, J. Stover, ed.), The American Dietetic Association, Chicago, IL, pp. 79–97 (1994).

16. M. A. Holliday, K. McHenry-Richardson, A. Portal, et al, *Med. Clin. N. Am.*, **63**, 945 (1979).

17. A. Grant and S. DeHoog, in *Nutritional Assessment and Support*, (A. Grant and S. DeHoog, eds.), Grant and DeHoog, Seattle, WA, pp. 99–152 (1991).

18. P. Wright-Harris, in *A Clinical Guide to Nutritional Care in End-Renal Disease*, (J. Stover, ed.), The American Dietetic Association, Chicago, IL, p. 136 (1994).

19. I. Muth, *J. Ren. Nutr.*, **1**, 2 (1991).

20. K. R. Tuttle, R. A. DeFonzo, and J. H. Stein, *Sem. Nephrol.*, **2**, 220 (1991).

21. H. Combs-Peacey, in *A Clinical Guide to Nutrition Care in End-Stage Renal Disease*, (J. Stover, ed.), (The American Dietetic Association, Chicago, IL, pp. 195–197 (1994).

22. J. W. Eschbach and J. W Adamson, *Am. J. Kid. Dis.*, **11**, 203 (1988).

23. J. W. Eschbach, J. C. Egrie, M. R. Downing, et al., *N. Engl. J. Med.*, **316**, 73 (1987).

24. *The Harriet Lane Handbook, XII ed.*, (M. D. Greene, ed.), Mosby Year Book, St. Louis, MO, p. 271 (1991).

25. J. Levine and D. B. Bernard, *Am. J. Kid. Dis.*, **15**, 285 (1990).

26. E. Slatapolsky, C. Weerts, J. Thielan, et al., *J. Clin. Invest.*, **74**, 2136 (1984).

27. M. J. Blumenkrantz and W. R. Schmidt, in *Peritoneal Dialysis*, (K. D. Nolph, ed.), Martinus Nijhoff, The Netherlands, p. 295 (1981).

28. B. P. Teehan, J. M. Brown, C. R. Schleifer, in *Clinical Dialysis*, (A. R. Nissenson, R. N. Fine and D. E. Gentile, eds.), Appleton and Lange, Norwalk, CT, pp. 319–325 (1990).

29. R. B. Ettenger, T. Rosenthal, J. Marik, et al., *C. Clin. Transplant*, **5**, 197 (1991).

30. C. M. Hill, J. F. Douglas, K. V. Kumar, et al., *Lancet*, **2**, 490 (1974).

31. F. C. Whittier, D. H. Evans, S. Dutton, et al., *Am. J. Kid. Dis.*, **6**, 405 (1985).

32. S. E. Weil, in *Handbook of Kidney Transplantation*, (G. M. Danovich, ed.), Little, Brown and Co., Boston, MA, p. 395 (1992).

33. V. R. Liddle, P. J. Walker, H. K. Johnson, et al., *Dial. Transplant*, **5**, 9 (1977).

34. J. L. Pagenkemper and C. J. Foulks, *J. Ren. Nutr.*, **1**, 119 (1991).

Inflammatory Bowel Disease

Edwin Simpser, M. D. and
James F. Markowitz, M.D.

INTRODUCTION

Inflammatory bowel disease (IBD) is the term utilized for conditions known as Crohn's disease and ulcerative colitis. Although each represents distinct clinical pathological entitles, in practice these diseases are often indistinguishable. The chronic, relapsing nature can be particularly difficult for adolescents afflicted with these disorders. Both result in a variety of debilitating symptoms that interfere with daily activities, linear growth, sexual maturation, and psychosocial development.

Epidemiology

There are limited data on the incidence and prevalence rates for IBD in pediatric and adolescent populations. The disease appears to be most common in North America, Europe, and Scandinavia. The annual incidence of IBD has been estimated to range between 2–16/100,000 population. In 1971, an analysis from a database at the University of Chicago revealed that approximately 45% of all newly diagnosed patients with IBD presented by age 20 yr. Seventy-five %

of these presented between the ages 10 and 30 yr.[1] By contrast, data from our current clinical database based on referrals to a Pediatric Gastroenterology Center reveal that over half of the newly diagnosed IBD cases occur in children less than 10 yr of age. Pediatric prevalence rates have been estimated at 10–100/100,000.

There are a number of genetic factors that appear to predispose the development of Crohn's disease and ulcerative colitis. For example, anywhere from 5–25% of children newly diagnosed with IND have first relatives with IBD. Siblings of patients with Crohn's disease have a 17- to 35-fold increase risk over the general population of developing Crohn's disease. In addition, the offspring of parents with Crohn's disease have a reported 9% chance of developing IBD.[2] Interestingly, concordance rates from monozygotic twins appear to be higher for Crohn's disease (40%) than ulcerative colitis (6%). Finally, racial and ethnic factors also appear to be important, with Caucasians more often afflicted than African Americans, and certain ethnic groups such as Ashkenazi Jews having an increased frequency of IBD. Although the gene has yet to be identified, recent reports have linked HLA subtypes B-44, Cw5, and a DQ-beta allele to Crohn's disease.[3] Likewise, segregation analysis suggests but has not yet identified, a gene underlying certain familial cases of ulcerative colitis.[4]

Clinical Features

IBD can present either suddenly or insidiously. Occasionally, acute onset can mimic gastrointestinal infection or appendicitis. However, it is just as likely to wax and wane for an extended period of time, even years, prior to being recognized, especially in young patients with Crohn's disease or ulcerative proctosigmoiditis.

The site and extent of the intestinal inflammation often are reflected in the patient's symptomatology. Children with extensive colonic involvement commonly present with cramps, rectal bleeding, and watery diarrhea. In Crohn's disease that is isolated to the large intestine, symptoms may be indistinguishable from those of ulcerative colitis. Severe hemorrhage requiring multiple transfusions is rare and more likely to be seen in ulcerative colitis. Tenesmus and urgency suggest active proctitis, which may also occasionally be manifested by constipation. In some patients, a mild increase in the number of daily stools, a change toward a loose stool consistency, or occasional blood per rectum may be the only symptoms.

Small intestinal involvement in Crohn's disease frequently presents with different symptomatology such as severe abdominal cramps with or without diarrhea. Frank bleeding is uncommon, although stools may be positive for occult blood. Systemic symptoms such as fevers and arthralgias are common, as are tender abdominal masses. Dyspeptic symptoms including nausea, heartburn or even vomiting may arise from upper gastrointestinal tract Crohn's disease that may be present in up to 40% of children initially diagnosed with Crohn's disease.[5] Some patients may have this symptomatology without signs of upper intestinal tract disease. These symptoms may be related to a more distal gastrointestinal obstruction, or some interrelationship of lower GI tract disease with upper GI tract motor function that is, as yet, not understood.

Extraintestinal manifestation can be seen in the IBD, again more commonly in Crohn's disease than ulcerative colitis. These include transient arthralgias, asymmetric arthritis, and rashes including erythema nodosum, cutaneous vasculitis, and pyoderma gangrenosum. A variety of "autoimmune disorder" have also been described, as well as uveitis and spondylitis. The most common extraintestinal manifestation of Crohn's disease are chronic perianal fissures and tags, that occur in approximately 50% of children and adolescents with Crohn's disease. There are also occasional patients who develop severe perianal fistulas and abscesses that are often quite resistant to medical therapy.

Medical Evaluation

Since the presenting signs and symptoms of IBD are nonspecific, a high degree of suspicion is often necessary in making the initial diagnosis of either Crohn's disease or ulcerative colitis. The initial evaluation requires a thorough history, comprehensive physical examination, and appropriate studies as outlined in Table 21.1. These studies will invariably include contrast radiography and endoscopy in addition to a biopsy to confirm the suspicion of IBD. Once the diagnosis is made, the treatment has begun, and frequent follow-up examinations assessing the success of medical therapy and evaluation of nutritional status as well as growth are essential. The effects on the growth of the disease process itself or of medications such as corticosteroids, must be carefully monitored.

Medical Treatment

Therapy of both Crohn's disease and ulcerative colitis in adolescents is primarily supportive, since there are no curative medical treatments. Treatment aims include suppression of symptoms, promotion of normal growth and sexual development, control of unavoidable complications, and the avoidance of excessive or inappropriate therapy. Symptoms can rarely be completely eliminated. Therapeutic options include the range of pharmacologic and nutritional modalities generally available for the adult with IBD, including corticosteroids, 5-aminosalicylates, metronidazole, and cyclosporine. Nutrition support also plays an important therapeutic role. For patients with intractable symptoms or who have developed significant complications such as intraabdominal abscesses unresponsive to medical therapy, surgery is an option. Although surgery is curative only in

Table 21.1   Initial Evaluation of the Adolescent with Suspected Inflammatory Bowel Disease

---

History
Physical examination (include height, weight, anthropometrics, pubertal staging)
Growth records (include growth velocity)
Dietary evaluation (3-d record)
Laboratory
  Complete blood count, differential, erythrocyte sedimentation rate
  Electrolytes, serum chemistries (especially total protein, albumin)
  Serum iron, total iron-binding capacity, ferritin
  Serum B-12, folate
If indicated (i.e., malnourished)
  Vitamins A, D, E, PT/PTT, prealbumin, magnesium, zinc
  24-h urinary mg
Microbiology
  Stools for enteric pathogens
  Stool examinations for ova and parasites, Charcot-Leyden crystals, white blood cells
  Stools for *Clostridium difficile* toxin
Radiology
  Upper gastrointestinal series with small bowel follow-through
  Barium enema (?)
  Bone age (if indicated)
Endoscopy
  Flexible colonoscopy or sigmoidoscopy with mucosal biopsies
  Esophagogastroduodenoscopy and mucosal biopsies (if indicated)

---

ulcerative colitis, there are often benefits related to the improved quality of life and possible improved growth in Crohn's disease patients who undergo surgery.

Nutritional Considerations

Malnutrition and growth failure.   Weight loss is a very common presenting feature of IBD with approximately 85% of children with Crohn's disease and 65% of children with ulcerative colitis showing significant weight loss at the time of diagnosis.[6] Growth failure and delays of sexual maturation are features of IBD in the preadolescent and adolescent that most distinguish it from the adult with IBD. Children with Crohn's disease are primarily at risk, although those with ulcerative colitis can also be affected. Studies have suggested that anywhere from 30–60% of children who develop IBD prior to ordering puberty will undergo a period of marked impairment of linear growth during adolescence.[7–10] Permanent impairment of linear growth is seen in 20–30% of young adults whose IBD (especially Crohn's disease) is diagnosed in childhood or early adolescence.[11] The primary reason for poor weight gain, growth failure, and delayed development is often inadequate nutritional intake, whereas malabsorption and maldigestion of ingested nutrients are often less significant factors.[12,13] For adolescents to manifest growth spurts and puberty to progress, the older child and teen with IBD must consume a diet containing 75–90 kcal/kg/d. These amounts are often impossible for the child with IBD to consume on a regular basis. Eating often initiates symptoms of cramps and diarrhea that can ultimately result in patients avoiding food. Likewise, there appears to be a component of anorexia seen even in patients with isolated colonic disease. Whether this anorexia is related to dysmotility in the gastrointestinal tract or inflammatory mediators produced by the disease process remains unclear.

Inadequate dietary intake also occurs because of self-imposed or iatrogenically prescribed dietary restrictions that lack sound scientific or clinical basis. Inappropriate restrictions often further reduce both caloric value and the palatability of the food provided. Losses of macro-and micronutrients related to extent of disease, bacterial overgrowth, or bowel resection can also contribute to malnutrition.

Protein loss from an inflamed bowel is common and contributes to the catabolic state of patients. Fat malabsorption is less common, but can be seen in patients with significant ileal disease or following ileal resection. Carbohydrate malabsorption (e.g., lactose intolerance from small bowel Crohn's) is rarely of major nutritional significance, although it may contribute to symptoms and aggravate the "fear of eating" seen in some patients. Studies are conflicting as to whether children with IBD have increased energy expenditure.[14,15] Various manifestations including fistulae, fevers, and drugs such as corticosteroids may contribute to the increased nutritional requirements in adolescents with IBD (see Table 21.2).

MICRONUTRIENTS. These deficiencies are common in IBD. Although much data are gleaned from studies involving adults, these deficiencies are also seen among adolescents. The reasons that micronutrient deficiencies develop are similar to those responsible for growth failure and protein energy malnutrition.

Low serum folate occurs in 40–60 % of patients with IBD.[16,17] Deficiency is due to poor intake, small bowel disease, and the use of sulfasalazine, that interferes with folate absorption. Vitamin B-12 deficiency is seen most commonly in patients who have had ileal resections and occasionally in patients with significant ileitis. Other water-soluble vitamins, in general, are not significantly diminished although the poor intake of B-6, B-2, and pantothenic acid has been found.[18] Vitamin D deficiency is common in Crohn's disease, often related to the severity of the disease. Thus, patients with significant fat malabsorption and bile acid loss from ileal resections are at highest risk. The use of oral antibiotics contributes to vitamin K deficiency, but this is rarely clinically significant.

There is controversy surrounding trace element deficiencies, particularly zinc. Zinc deficiency in normal controls has been shown to cause retarded growth, delayed sexual development, and delayed bone age.[19,20] Serum zinc levels are

Table 21.2   Etiology of Malnutrition in Inflammatory Bowel Disease

Poor Caloric Intake
  Disease-induced
  Dietary restrictions (iatrogenic, parental, or self-imposed)
Malabsorption/intestinal losses
  Decreased surface area (disease, resection)
  Bacterial overgrowth
  Bile acid deficiency (ileal resection, severe ileitis)
  Protein-losing enteropathy
  Blood loss
  Micronutrient losses (diarrhea, fistulae)
Increased requirements
  Infection, fever
  Inflammatory process (?)
  Need for catch-up growth
Drugs
  Sulfasalazine (folate)
  Steroids (calcium, protein catabolism)
  Cholestyramine

often low in children with IBD and growth failure, but the levels usually can be shown to correlate with serum albumin.[21,22] However, there are reports of patients with excessive stool losses of zinc and diminished absorption.[21,23,24] Zinc loading tests and urinary excretions are low in some growth-retarded IBD patients, but similar findings were also present in controls with IBD and those with normal growth.[22] There are patients who have abnormal calcium metabolism related to fat malabsorption or steroid use that may predispose them to renal calcium oxalate stones. Occasionally, the inappropriate institution of dairy-free diets may contribute to poor calcium intake. Although magnesium deficiency can occur, it is not common. It has been suggested that measuring urinary magnesium is a better indicator of magnesium status in patients with IBD.[25] Other trace element deficiencies are rare, except as would be expected in the use of long-term parenteral nutrition without trace element supplementation.

ASSESSMENT

Macronutrient Status

In assessing the growth, energy, and protein status of an adolescent with IBD, the dynamic evaluation of changes over time is more valuable than single time-point measurements. This is true both at the time of initial evaluation and subsequent follow-up examinations.

Height and weight measurements can be expressed in a number of two ways to assess growth and nutritional status. Weight-for-age and height-for-age percentiles are useful indicators of acute and chronic malnutrition. This is especially helpful when percentiles can be compared to those obtained in the years prior to the onset of IBD (Figure 21.1). Follow-up of changes along these growth curves after diagnosis can be a measure of the efficacy of medical and nutritional therapies. Weight-for-height curves are also useful. However, caution must be used in their evaluation, as stunting can result in severely growth-retarded individuals with normal weight-for-height percentiles.

A corollary to the use of percentile curves is the evaluation of growth expressed as height and weight velocities. When measured sequentially, these serve as sensitive indicators of the adequacy of growth. Velocities are commonly expressed per year since growth is known to occur in spurts and rates derived for a period of time shorter than a year may be inaccurate. We commonly expect prepubertal girls to have a minimum growth of 4 cm/yr and prepubertal boy 3.7 cm/yr. Velocity curves may illustrate significant slowing in growth for an individual patient and unmask growth failure more quickly than height-for-chronological-age curves. Height velocity must also be interpreted in the context of the stage of sexual maturation and bone age is opposed to chronological age alone. This is because many adolescents with IBD have both pubertal and bone age delays. Bone age determination is, therefore, a useful measurement to help predict and monitor the (potential for) future growth. For example, a Tanner III, 15-year-old male with a bone age of 12 should have nutritional and medical intervention to treat his growth failure even if he is asymptomatic. This teen can expect to attain catch-up growth because the gap in bone age vs. chronological age. On the other hand, the same patient with a bone age of 15 yr is at high risk for permanent growth failure.

Protein and energy stores can be assessed by standard anthropometric measurements, including midarm circumference and triceps skinfold thickness. Since interobserver variability often causes significant error in these measurements, it is best to attempt to have these measurements taken by the same staff member. Other methods for measuring body composition, including bioelectrical impedance, stable isotopes, under water weighing, CT scans, TOBEC, and Dexa, are at this time mostly research tools and not readily available nor clinically validated.

Laboratory measurements are rarely helpful in the assessment of macronutrient status. Low serum albumin is very common and often reflects the severity of the inflammatory process. Hypoproteinemia is suggestive of chronic protein depletion in an adolescent with IBD and is a parameter that is often followed as an indicator of the efficacy of therapy. Prealbumin, tranferrin, and retinol-binding protein are somewhat more useful in documenting acute protein depletion. Nitrogen balance studies done utilizing urinary urea or urinary nitrogen alone are usually inaccurate given the protein loss in the stool. However, an estimate of

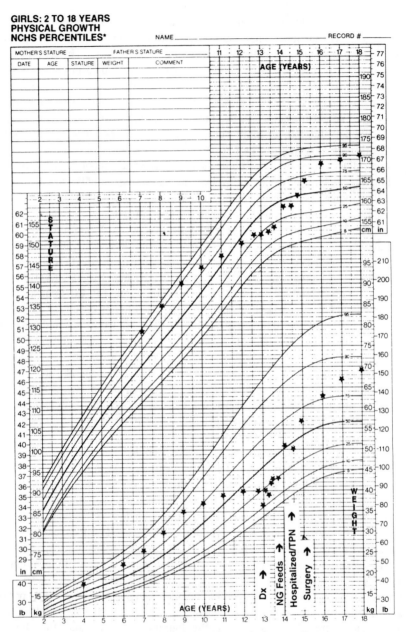

Figure 21-1. Height and weight growth curve of the illustrated patient. Note poor growth for 3 yr prior to diagnosis and response to different interventions.

the severity of protein loss in IBD can be obtained by measuring stool antitrypsin levels, that have been shown to correlate with enteral protein losses.

Assessment of the patient's caloric intake is often useful in managing the nutritional consequences of IBD. A written 3-d diet record is preferable to a 24-h recall, especially among adolescents. The dietician needs to enlist the teen patient as a partner in this process since parental involvement in the diet of adolescents if often minimal.

Micronutrient Status

Micronutrient assessment is most commonly performed by measuring serum levels of micronutrients based on the deficiencies discussed above. These include folate, vitamin B-12, serum iron, TIBC, and ferritin. Whereas low levels of the water-soluble vitamins reflect a need for supplemental therapy, measuring serum iron alone is not sufficient. The vast majority of IBD patients who do not have significant bleeding will have anemia and low serum iron, yet have a normal or high level of serum ferritin. This reflects the anemia of chronic inflammation, whereby iron stores are normal, but are unable to be utilized secondary to the inflammatory process. Supplementation with iron is these patients is generally ineffective. There are, as yet, no large-scale studies of erythropoietin levels or therapy in IBD. One study, of many adults, showed that 33% of patients with IBD had low erythropoietin levels. Three of these were treated and responded within 2–3 mo, but their anemia recurred on cessation of the erythropoietin.[26] More data are needed before widespread measurement and therapy with erythropoietin can be recommended. Measurements of fat-soluble vitamins and trace elements such as zinc are not routinely performed and often are reserved for the patient with evidence of severe malnutrition or growth failure. Table 21.1 summarizes the recommended assessment of the individual patient with IBD.

MANAGEMENT

Nutritional therapies in adolescents with IBD have dual roles. Clearly, patients suffering from malnutrition and concomitant growth failure will require nutritional support to reverse these situations. In addition, nutritional therapies, either alone or as an adjunct to medications, can also be used to induce a remission of disease activity.

General Considerations

As part of the routine management of any adolescent with IBD, nutritional counseling to assure adequate nutrition and growth is essential. All teens, even those without overt signs of malnutrition or growth failure, should receive counseling either from the treating physician or a dietician well versed in the disease process. Our approach is designed to insure adequate caloric intake, since very often these patients require 75–85 kcal/kg/d for adequate growth. Thus, we discourage any dietary restrictions unless there is a clear medical indication. We do not routinely restrict lactose, even in patients with small bowel Crohn's disease, unless the adolescents are symptomatic, diagnosed as lactose-intolerant with a lactose breath hydrogen test, and intolerant of dairy following exogenous lactase supplementation. Low-residue diets are not routinely pre-scribed, unless the adolescent has evidence of intestinal structures. Parental desires for a "good diet" and restriction of high-calorie "junk food" often is a stumbling block to the adolescent's ability to maintain appropriate caloric intake. Given the discomfort and anorexia associated with this illness, it is our policy to encourage teens to eat foods they enjoy while trying to maintain good micronu-trient balance with either certain foods or with supplemental vitamins. Nutritional supplementation with high-calorie liquid formulas or other products can be uti-lized for the teen who is at risk for nutritional problems based on his or her caloric intake or disease state. One needs to be prophylactic and not wait for significant growth failure and malnutrition to set in before recommending these supplements. However, the majority of these products have only fair palatability and only the highly motivated adolescent will continue to use them long term.

Nutritional Therapy of Malnutrition and Growth Failure in IBD

In the prepubertal adolescent, the potential for catch-up growth is limited in time because of bone maturation and eventual epiphyseal fusion.[6] Early aggressive intervention in patients with growth failure is imperative. The goal of the nutri-tional therapy is to allow for the reversal of growth arrest and catch-up growth, returning, it is hoped, to the individual teen's premorbid growth channel. The reversal of growth arrest requires an appropriate body weight for height, whereas catch-up growth may require additional calories over and above those necessary to maintain weight for height. Thus, caloric intake for catch up growth should be estimated according to the teen's ideal weight for age rather than his or her actual weight.

Initially, the most common approach is the use of orally ingested high-calorie supplements. These will result in weight gain and catch up growth only if utilized for a sustained period of time that may be difficult. Thus, many centers employ nocturnal nasogastric feedings as a standard therapy for malnutrition and growth failure in adolescents with IBD. Utilizing overnight nasogastric feedings, with the tube placed nightly by the teen, rarely interferes with normal daily activities. This intervention has been shown in a number of studies to effectively reverse growth failure.[27,28] Supplementation, whether oral or NG, may need to continue for a period of a year in order to maximize growth. However, a number of these patients even after a year or more of supplementation may manifest permanent growth impairment, possibly related to their need for corticosteroids.[11]

The type of formula used, whether polymeric or monomeric, should be tailored to the patient's clinical status, extent of disease, and previous surgery. However, for the purposes of growth failure, polymeric formulas have been shown to be quite effective. Some groups utilize a intermittent approach, i.e., once a month for 4 mo or for 3–4 mo over a 1-yr period.[6,28] We have tended to continue the NG feeds for longer consecutive periods, because of it additional therapeutic benefit as will be discussed.[27] Certainly, if the time for catch-up growth is limited as evidenced by the patient's bone age, then a more aggressive approach should be taken.

There are rarely contraindications to enteral nutritional support. The most significant problem is noncompliance. However, the most motivated patients are those with the most growth retardation and pubertal delay who have become increasingly embarrassed by comparison with their healthy teenage friends.

Parental nutritional support, also given overnight, can achieve weight gain and reverse growth failure in IBD. Many adolescents who are unable or unwilling to self-intubate for nocturnal nasogastric feeds are willing to utilize an indwelling catheter and administer nocturnal parental nutrition. Cost, potential infectious, metabolic complications, and difficulty of administration make parenteral nutritional support less preferable than enteral feedings. However, parenteral nutrition is an efficacious alternative that, if managed by a team well versed in its use and risks, can be quite a safe approach.

There are a group of patients, especially those that have short-segment bowel Crohn's disease with growth failure, who benefit from surgical resection of the diseased segment. However, not all patients achieve improved growth postoperatively and the risk of recurrence must be considered before this decision is made.[29,30] In general, a surgical should be reserved for the teen who has exhausted medical and nutritional therapies without success.

Nutrition as Therapy for IBD

Although classically nutritional therapy has been considered an adjunct to medical and surgical therapy for IBD, over the last 10–15 yr there has been considerable interest in nutrition as a primary therapy, especially in patients with Crohn's disease. Initial studies utilized parenteral nutrition, but more recently there have been a number of studies exploring enteral nutrition as a primary therapy.

Induction of remission.   There have been a number of controlled trials evaluating nutritional therapy for the induction of short-term remission in acute Crohn's disease. These studies have either compared enteral feedings to corticosteroids, enteral feedings to corcicosteroids, enteral feeding to parenteral malnutrition, or different types of enteral nutrition to each other. These studies are summarized in Table 21.3. The majority of these reports suggest that nutritional therapy can induce remission in Crohn's disease comparable to steroid therapy in both efficacy and time. One large European study, however, found that steroids were more efficacious than a semielemental diet.[31] Some feel that elemental diets may be more efficacious than polymeric diets[31–42] in inducing remission, but this remains unclear (Table 21.3).

Table 21.3   Induction of Remission with Nutritional Support in Inflammatory Bowel Disease

Prospective Randomized Controlled Trials		
Number of patients with short-term remission (<30 d)		
Author	Steroid Therapy	Monomeric Diet
O'Morain[33]	8/10 (80%)	9/11 (82%)
Saverymuttu[34]	16/16 (100%)	15/21 (71%)
Seidman[35*]	6/9 (66%)	8/10 (80%)
Gorard[36]	17/20 (85%)	10/13 (77%)
	Steroid Therapy	Oligomeric Diet
Malchow[37]	32/44 (73%)	21/51 (41%)
Sanderson[38*]	6/7 (86%)	7/8 (88%)
Lochs[31]	41/52 (79%)	29/55 (53%)
Lindor[39]	7/10 (70%)	3/9 (33%)
	Monomeric Diet	Polymeric Diet
Giaffer[32]	12/16 (75%)	5/14 (36%)
Park[40]	2/7 (29%)	5/7/ (71%)
Raouf[41]	9/13 (69%)	8/11 (73%)
Rigaud[42]	10/15 (67%)	11/15 (73%)
	TPN/NPO	Enteral Nutrition
Alun Jones[44]	14/19 (88%)	11/17 (85%)[†]
Greenberg[45]	12/17 (71%)	11/19 (58%)[‡]
Wright[46]	4/5 (80%)	3/6 (50%)[**]
Gonzalez-Huix[47]	10/20 (50%)	12/22 (55%)[†]

[*] =Pediatric studies
[†] =Monomeric diet/PO feeding.
[‡] =Polymeric diet/NG.
[**] =Oligomeric diet/PO.
Note: Numbers in parentheses are short-term remission rates.

In general, if one intends to induce remission in IBD without utilizing medications, then nasogastric infusions, usually nocturnal, are considered by most centers to be the least invasive and most efficacious approach. Many centers also recommend an elemental diet, but a firm recommendation based on good comparative data cannot yet be made. Unfortunately, there is considerable relapse when the diet is discontinued. Protocols investigating long-term intermittent elemental diets are currently under way. One preliminary report suggests that continuing nasogastric supplemental feeds with a semielemental diet diminishes the relapse rate (over a 12-mo period) and increases height velocity.[43]

Parenteral nutrition has been shown in many uncontrolled studies to induce a clinical remission, especially in patients with Crohn's disease who have failed other forms of medical therapy. "Bowel rest" along with the use of parenteral nutrition has not been shown to be more effective in inducing remission of disease activity than either enteral nutrition or steroid therapy. It may play a small role in helping to close postoperative fistulae. Long-term parenteral nutrition can maintain remission for extended periods of time.[44-50] However, given the risks and costs, we prefer nocturnal nasogastric feeding of either a polymeric or elemental diet to parenteral nutrition to induce and maintain remission. In our practice, parenteral nutrition is utilized either as an adjunct to medical therapy or to reverse growth failure only in those patients who have either failed or refused enteral nutrition support.

Research Considerations

Short-chain fatty acids.   It has been observed that patients with acute colitis may do better when they are fed enterally. It is well known that the anaerobic fermentation of carbohydrates that are delivered to the colon will produce short chain fatty acids including acetate, butyrate, and propionate. These compounds have been shown to be utilized by the colonic mucosa as a source of energy. Children with Crohn's ileocolitis and ulcerative colitis have been shown to have increased fecal concentration of n-butyrate, possibly related to an abnormality of colonocyte butyrate utilization.[51] Short-chain fatty acids have been utilized as a therapy for diversion colitis when used in an enema preparation.[52] A recent uncontrolled study in adults with refractory ulcerative colitis found a 60% response rate with butyrate enemas[53]. Consideration of the use of fiber inenteral diets for colitis patients of SCFA in enema preparations will require further study.

Polyunsaturated fatty acids.   There has been much recent interest in examining the effects of dietary polyunsaturated fatty acids (metabolized to eicosanoids) on modifying various autoimmune disorders. EPA (eicosapentenoic acid) has been studied in systemic lupus erythematosus, rheumatoid arthritis, diabetes mellitus, and in asthma. There are a number of preliminary studies suggesting the therapeutic efficacy of EPA in IBD.[54,55]

GLUTAMINE AND ARGININE.   Glutamine is the preferred metabolic fuel for the small intestinal mucosa. The most abundant amino acid is plasma; it represents over half the amino acids in skeletal muscle and stimulates lymphocytes and other rapidly dividing cells. Many nutrition researchers now consider glutamine a "conditionally essential" amino acid in catabolic and stressed patients. In these patients, low muscle and serum glutamine levels have been shown to occur fairly rapidly and some improvement in outcome has been noted in patients with glutamine supplemented parenteral nutrition. As yet, there are no methodologically sound studies demonstrating the effect of glutamine supplemented parenteral nutrition or enteral nutrition in IBD. Likewise, arginine has been considered a conditionally essential "amino acid" in stress individuals. Its role seems related to its stimulatory effect on immune function, but does seem to increase nitrogen retention and wound healing in a select group of patients. Studies on the role of these two amino acids in IBD are necessary.

Practical Considerations

To adequately care for chronically ill adolescents with IBD and their families, an integrated team approach is required to provide medical, surgical, psychological, and nutritional therapies. Our team includes pediatric gastroenterologists, a GI nurse clinician as well as a nutrition support nurse clinician, a pediatric nutritionist, and ancillary services such as child psychiatry, pediatric pathology, pediatric surgery, and pediatric radiology, all with a special interest in the gastrointestinal tract.

Members of the nutrition team must work in tandem with each other to best understand each individual teen's unique needs and tendencies so as to maximize his or her nutrition. Very often, decisions about the type of nutritional therapy will be made by the attending gastroenterologist following the evaluation and recommendations of the nurses, nutritionist, and psychiatrist. The nutritionist's role is that of evaluating both initially in an ongoing fashion the adequacy of the teen's diet as well as counseling for intensive oral nutritional supplementation as needed. Once nutrition support is indicated, then the nurse clinician begins the process of teaching the patient self-intubation. This can be done on an outpatient basis in the office setting supervised by the nurse clinician and then with follow-up at home by the home care staff. The current availability of sophisticated high-tech home care companies makes these arrangements quite simple. However, appropriate communication between the physician, nurse clinician (who acts as the coordinator), the family, and home care company is essential.

In general, we have found that most adolescents are willing to attempt nasogastric intubation. For those youth who fail, we then will begin nocturnal parenteral nutrition. This will often require a short hospital stay in order to place an indwelling central venous catheter (Broviac/Hickman) and initiate the parenteral nutrition. Given the risks of parenteral nutrition, there is considerable teaching time necessary to ensure proper care and handling of the catheter, site, equipment, and parenteral nutrition solutions. Adolescents are usually monitored on a regular basis by our nutritionist, nurse clinician, and a dedicated nutrition support physician. As the patient's clinical status improves and his or her oral intake increases, parenteral nutrition is weaned. Teams are usually seen monthly, but more frequent laboratory tests can be obtained by the home care company an communicated to the team.

Ongoing monitoring of the efficacy of treatment on weight gain and growth is essential in deciding the duration of both enteral and parenteral therapy. If the adolescent is otherwise well and has progressed over time to reach what it felt to be his or her final height, or there is radiographic evidence of closed epiphyses, then the nutrition support can be discontinued.

Education for teens and their families involves a variety of modalities, including audiovisual presentations. Adolescents who have learned the technique for inserting a nasogastric tube for nutritional supplementation often meet with others about to embark on such a program. In a similar fashion, self-help support groups for parents and other family members of adolescents with IBD can be of enormous benefit. Volunteers whose children suffer from IBD help counsel other parents, especially during critical periods such as time of diagnosis, initiation of nutrition support, or recommendations for surgery. Seminars and written educational materials on a variety of subjects including general good nutrition, nutrition support, self-image, quality of life, sexuality, and marriage are quite helpful.

CASE ILLUSTRATION

A 13-year-old girl, Chris, was referred to the Division of Pediatric Gastroenterology and Nutrition for evaluation of recurrent abdominal pain. diarrhea, and an 8-lb weight loss. The teen, who had been well until 3 mo prior to referral, noted the gradual onset of crampy, right lower quadrant, and suprapubic abdominal pains. This discomfort frequently awakened her about 6:00 A.M., and persisted on and off throughout the morning hours. She felt that the pains worsened after eating, so she had begun skipping breakfast. The discomfort would occasionally be relieved by having a loose, nonbloody bowel movement, but because eating often led to the development of cramps and the urge to defecate, she also refused to eat lunch in school. Chris's parents were particularly concerned about the weight loss because they had noted poor weight gain and growth in the 4 yr prior to the consultation (Figure 21.1) that they had attributed to the child being a "picky" eater. There were no other overt complaint, but review of systems revealed that the child often had unexplained fevers to 100.5°F.

A review of the Chris's growth records (obtained from the child's pediatrician and school nurse) revealed a gradual decline in weight percentile for age from >75th percentile at the age 9 yr to the 10th percentile at the time of presentation. A similar decline in height percentile for age (from 90–25th) was also evident (Figure 22.2). Height velocity curves were dramatically abnormal in the 3 yr prior to presentation.

Physical examination revealed a prepubertal teen whose height and weight percentiles were at the 25th and 10th percentiles for age, respectively. An ill-defined tender mass of bowel was palpable in the right lower quadrant. There were no perianal lesions, rectal sphincter tone was normal, and the rectal vault contained a small amount of loose stool that was positive for occult blood. Laboratory findings included WBC 12,600/cc with 72% polymorphonuclear leukocytes, 10% bands, and 18% lymphocytes, 8.5 g/dL of hemoglobin, hematocrit 26%, mean corpuscular volume of 63.2 m^3 (normal, 87 ± 5 m^3), mean corpuscular hemoglobin of 20.3 g (normal, 29 ± 2 g), mean corpuscular hemoglobin concentration of 32.1 g/dL (normal, 34 ± 2 g/dL), reticulocyte count 1%, erythrocyte sedimentation rate of 34 mm/h (normal <15 mm/h), total serum protein of 6.0 g/dL, 3.2 g/dL of serum albumin (normal >3.6 g/dL), 20 g/dL of serum Fe (normal, 60–160 g/dL), 220 g/dL of total iron binding capacity (normal, 180–480 g/dL), 70 g/dL of serum ferritin (normal, 10–150 g/dL), 500 pg/mL of vitamin B-12 (normal, 300–1100 pg/mL), 8 ng/mL of serum folate (normal, 4–14 ng/mL). Stool culture for bacterial pathogens, examinations for ova and parasites, and assay for *Clostridium difficile* toxin were negative.

An upper gastrointestinal series with small bowel follow-through revealed spiculation and ulceration of the terminal 10 cm of the ileum. Colonoscopy revealed scattered aphthous ulcerations extending from the rectum to the proximal transverse colon. The right colon and cecum had marked ulceration, with shaggy exudate and increased friability of the mucosa. The ileocecal valve was edematous and ulcerated, and the distal 5 cm of the ileum revealed marked nodularity, exudate, and ulceration. Endoscopic biopsies of the ileum, cecum, transverse colon, and rectosigmoid revealed patchy, active inflammation and crypt abscesses. A noncaseating granuloma was present in the biopsy from the cecum.

Dietary analysis of a typical 3-d food record demonstrated that Chris was consuming only 65% of her RDA for total calories. Protein intake was 105% of the RDA, but total caloric intake was inadequate. Micronutrient intakes ranged from 85–20% of the RDA; calcium and vitamin D intakes were particularly deficient.

Chris was hospitalized and placed on a continuous nasogastric infusion of a semielemental formula. The rate was increased over the first 5 d until the total daily caloric requirement was delivered. She was then discharged, and with the

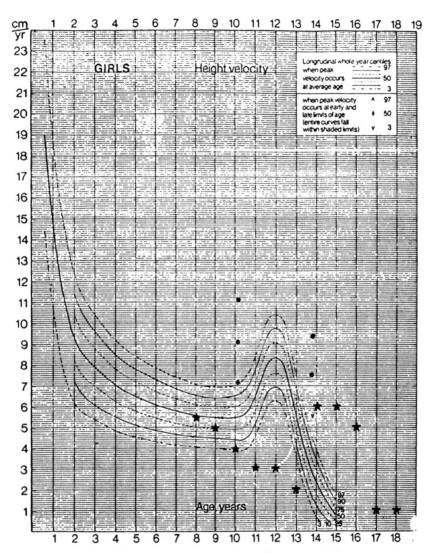

Figure 21-2. Height velocity curve of patient depicting diminished height and velocity from age 9 with recovery after diagnosis and treatment.

assistance of a local home care company, she was maintained on the continuous enteral infusion as her sole source of nutrition and therapy for 4 wk. Within 10 d, the patient reported remission of symptoms. Cramps disappeared, and Chris reported only 1–2 soft stools/d. She gained 8 lb.

After 1 mo, enteral nutrional support was discontinued, and Chris was allowed to eat an unrestricted diet. However, after 3 wk, crampy abdominal pain and more frequent loose stools recurred. Appetite decreased and the patient lost 2 lb. She refused reinstitution of enteral feedings, and so was treated with oral nutritional supplements and prednisone, 40 mg/d. Symptoms remitted, and weight gain resulted.

Over the following 6 mo, sulfasalazine was added and the prednisone gradually weaned to 10 mg/d. However, symptoms flared with each attempt to decrease the corticosteroid below this dose. Appetite diminished, weight gain stopped, and no height growth occurred. The patient agreed to begin nocturnal nasogastric infusions of a nonelemental formula to supplement her dietary intake. Approximately 1200 cal/night were delivered and after 6 wk, symptoms were again in remission and weight gain had resumed. Over the following 6 mo, while remaining on nocturnal nasogastric infusions, the patient was gradually weaned off prednisone. Chris gained weight, grew 2 in. and noted the development of breast buds and scant pubic hair.

However, at the age of 14.5 yr, the teen began, once again, to complain of diminished appetite, crampy abdominal pain, frequent loose stools, and weight loss despite continued use of nocturnal nasogastric feedings. A tender mass became palpable in the right lower quadrant. Partial relief of symptoms resulted with the reinstitution of corticosteroid therapy, but could not be maintained, even when the teen was hospitalized for a course of intravenous antibiotics. Repeat small bowel series revealed extensive distal and terminal ileal inflammation and stricture formation with evidence of partial small bowel obstruction. Surgery was advised, but was refused by the patient and her parents. Persistent symptoms led to the institution of total parental nutrition as a means of allowing the total "bowel rest."

The teen improved symptomatically over a period of 3 wk, and was able to begin eating a low-residue diet. However, despite ongoing corticosteroid therapy and TPN, she could only eat about 1200 kcal/d. Given the parents' refusal to consent to surgery, she was eventually sent home with a deep line for central venous access. She was maintained on 2500 kcal/d via TPN delivered between the hours of 8 P.M. and 6:30 A.M., while she continued to consume about 1200 kcal during the day by mouth. Daily prednisone was continued, but over a period of 3 mo, it was gradually tapered to 10 mg every other day. Chris gained 15 lb and grew 2.5 cm in 4 mo. She attended school, but did not participate in any extracurricular activities.

After 4 mo of home TPN, Chris was nearly 15-years-old, yet still only Tanner

II. There had been no progression in her sexual development since the onset of her heightened disease activity and signs of chronic partial small bowel obstruction. The teen was increasingly unhappy with her lifestyle and had taken an active part in discussions regarding the possibility of surgery. However, prior to the parents coming to a final decision about surgery, the child was hospitalized for line sepsis. After removal of the central venous catheter and an appropriate antibiotic course, a resection of the terminal ileum and right colon was performed. A primary reanastomosis was possible and the child recovered uneventfully. Chris was discharged consuming adequate diet by mouth and required no medications.

The patient's course remained uneventful throughout the remainder of her teenage years. Her disease remained in remission, growth and full pubertal development ensued, and the patient reached her ultimate adult height by the age of 18.5 yr.

REFERENCES

1. B. H. Rogers, L. M. Clark, and J. B. Kirsner, *J. Chron. Dis.*, **24**, 743 (1971).
2. R. G. Farmer, W. M. Michner, and E. A. Mortimer, *Clin. Gastroenterol.*, **9**, 271 (1980).
3. D. Neigut, R. Proujansky, M. Trucco, et al., *Gastroenterol.*, **102**, A671 (1992).
4. U. Monsen, L Iselius, C. Johmssom, et al., *Clin. Gen.*, **36**, 411 (1989).
5. M.N.L. Mashako, *J. Ped. Gastro. Nutr.*, **8**, 442 (1989).
6. E. Seidman, N. LeLeiko, M. Ament, et al., *J. Ped. Gastro. Nutr.*, **12**, 424 (1991).
7. B. S. Kirschner, *Acta Ped. Scand.*, **336** (suppl.), 98 (1990).
8. K. J. Motil and R. J. Grand, *Ped. Clin. N. Am.*, **32**, 447, (1985).
9. J. Markowitz and F. Daum , *Am. J. Gastro.*, **89**, 319 (1994).
10. E. G. Seidman, *Gastro. Clin. N. Am.*, **18**, 129 (1989).
11. J. Markowitz, K. Grancher, J. Rosa, et al., *J. Ped. Gastro. Nutr.*, **16**, 373 (1993).
12. D. G. Kelts, R. J. Grand, G. Shen, et al., *Gastroenterology*, **76**, 720 (1979).
13. K. J. Molti, R. J. Grand, C. J. Maletskos, et al., *J, Peds.*, **101**, 345 (1982).
14. M. Azcue, A. Griffiths, and P. Pencharz, *Ped. Res.*, **33**(4), 98A (1993).
15. K. J. Motil, R. J. Grand, C. J. Maletskos, et al., *J. Peds.*, **101**, 345 (1982).
16. A. D. Harries and R. V. Heatley, *Postgrad. Med. J.*, **59**, 690 (1983).
17. L. Elsborg and L. Larsen, *Scand. J. Gastro.*, **16**, 1019 (1979).
18. P. Hodges, M. Gee, M. Grace, and A. B. Thomsom, *J. Am. Diet. Assoc.*, **84**, 52 (1984).
19. N. W. Solomon, R. L. Rosenfield, R. A. Jacobs, et al., *Ped. Res.*, **10**, 923 (1976).
20. V. Caggiano, R. Schnitden, W. Strauss, et al., *Am. J. Med. Sci.*, **257**, 305 (1969).

21. G. C. Sturniolo, M. N. Molohhan, R. Shields, and L. A. Turnburg, *Gut*, **21**, 387 (1980).

22. Y. Nishi, F. Lifshitz, M. A. Bayne, et al., *Am. J. Clin. Nutr.*, **33**, 2613 (1980).

23. C. McClain, C. Soutor, and L. Zieve, *Gastroenterology*, **78**, 272 (1980).

24. N. W. Solomons, I. H. Rosenburg, H. H. Sandstead, and K.P.V. Khacter, *Digestion*, **16**, 87 (1977).

25. M. A. LaSala, F. Lifshitz, M. Silverberg, et al., *J. Ped. Gastro. Nutr.*, **4**, 75 (1985).

26. J. Hornia, W. Petritsch, C. Schmid, et al., *Gastroenterology*, **104**, 1828 (1993).

27. H. Aiges, J. Markowitz, J. Rosa, and F. Daum, *Gastroenterology*, **97**, 905 (1989).

28. D. C. Belli, E. Seidman, L. Bouthillier, et al., *Gastroenterology*, **603**, 610 (1988).

29. R. G. Castile, K. L. Telander, D. R. Cooney, et al., *J. Ped. Surg.*, **15**, 462 (1980).

30. G. Alperstein, F. Daum, S. E. Fisher, H. Aiges, et al., *J. Ped. Surg.*, **20**, 129 (1985).

31. H. Lochs, H. J. Steinhardt, B. Klaus-Wentz, et al., *Gastroenterology*, **101**, 1127 (1991).

32. M. N. Giaffer, G. North, C. D. Holdsworth, *Lancet*, **335**, 816 (1990).

33. C. O'Morain, A. W. Segal, and A. J. Levi, *BMJ*, **288** 1859 (1954).

34. S. Saverymuttu, H.J.F. Hodgson, and V. S. Chadwick, *Gut*, **26**, 994 (1985).

35. E. G. Seidman, L. Bouthillier, A. M. Weber, et al., *Gastroenterology*, **90**, 1625A (1986).

36. D. A. Gorard, J. B. Hunt, J. J. Payne-James, et al., *Gut*, **34**, 1198 (1993).

37. H. Malchow, H. J. Steinhardt, H. Lorenz-Meyer, et al., *Scan. J. Gastro.*, **25**, 235 (1990).

38. I. R. Sanderson, S. Udeen, P. D. Davies, et al., *Arch. Dis. Child.*, **62**, 123, (1987).

39. K. D. Lindor, C. R. Fleming, J. U. Burnes, et al., *Mayo Clin. Proc.*, **67**, 328 (1992).

40. R.H.R. Park, A. Galloway, B.J.Z. Danesh, and R. I. Russell, *Eur. J. Gastro. Hepatol.*, **3**, 483 (1991).

41. A. H. Raouf, V. Hildrey, H. Daniel, et al., *Gut*, **32**, 702 (1991).

42. D. Rigaud, J. Cosnes, Y. Le Quintrec, et al., *Gut*, **32**, 1492 (1991).

43. M. Wilschanski, P. Sherman, P. Pencharz, et al., *J. Ped. Gastro. Nutr.*, 19, 356 (1994).

44. V. Alun Jones, *Dig. Dis. Sci.*, **32**, 100S (1987).

45. G. R. Greenberg and C. R. Fleming, *Gut*, **29**, 1309 (1988).

46. R. A. Wright and O. L. Adler, *J. Clin. Gastro.*, **12**, 396 (1990).

47. F. Gonzalez-Huix, F. Fernandez-Banares, Esteve-Comas, et al., *Am. J. Gastro.*, **88**, 227 (1993).

48. R. J. Dickinson, M. G. Ashton, A. T. Axon, et al., *Gastroenterology*, **79**, 1199 (1980).

49. R. E. Kleinman, W. F. Balisterri, M. B. Heyman, et al., *J. Ped. Gastro. Nutr.*, **8**, 8 (1989).

50. H. Lochs, S. Meryn, L. Marosi, et al., *Clin. Nutr.*, **2**, 61 (1983).

51. W. R. Treem, N. Abson, M. Shoop, and J. Hyams, *J. Ped. Gastro. Nutr.*, **18**, 159 (1994).

52. J. M. Harig, K. H. Soergel, R. A. Komorowster, and C. M. Wood, *N. Engl. J. Med.*, **23**, 320 (1989).

53. A. H. Steinhart, A. Brezinslu , and J. Baker, *Am. J. Gastro.*, **89**, 179 (1994).

54. P. Salomon, A. A. Kornbluth, and D. Janowitz, *J. Clin. Gastro.*, **12**, 157 (1990).

55. R. Lorenz, P. C. Weber, P. Szimman, et al., *J. Intern. Med.*, **225** (suppl.), 225 (1989).

Cystic Fibrosis and Malabosorptive Disorders

CHAPTER

22

Amy Kovar M.S., R.D., C.S., L.D., C.N.S.P.,
and Alan M. Lake M.D.

INTRODUCTION

Cystic Fibrosis

Cystic fibrosis(CF), the most common genetic disease affecting Caucasians, is characterized by multisystem ductular obstruction. Of autosomal recessive inheritance, mutations in a single gene located on chromosome 7 result in defective ability of epithelial cells throughout the body to transport chloride anions. The resultant thickened mucus secretions obstruct the respiratory tree, reproductive tract, and pancreatic, intestinal, and hepatobiliary systems. Although 70% of affected individuals have a three-base pair deletion producing loss of a single amino acid, phenylalanine (ΔF508), CF may result from one of many mutations that cause varying degrees of the clinical symptoms.[1,2]

In 1960, the median life expectancy was 10 yr. However, today, persons affected with CF are living to 29 yr and beyond. The life-span will continue to improve, as more is learned about this disease, its optimal treatments, and anticipated potential cure through genetics and/or transplantation.

Clinical presentation of CF can take many forms: meconium ileus in the newborn (15%), abnormal stooling pattern or steatorrhea that results from pancreatic insufficiency (25%), failure to thrive (34%) and respiratory symptoms (40%). Patients generally succumb to progressive pulmonary disease and associated complications such as recurrent infections, pneumothorax, hemoptysis, and respiratory failure.[1,3] Although this accounts for more than 90% of mortality, a direct association between the degree of undernutrition and the severity of pulmonary disease is thought to exist. The importance of nutritional status for CF patients is emphasized by results of recent studies, that support better outcomes for individuals with normal growth and nutritional parameters.[4–7]

Pancreatic insufficiency. Approximately 85% of patients with CF are pancreatic enzyme insufficient, a condition marked by malabsorption, steatorrhea, and poor growth. Unlike other clinical aspects of CF, pancreatic insufficiency strongly correlates with the ΔF508 defect. Essentially all individuals with either two ΔF508 mutations, or a ΔF508 mutation accompanied by another pancreatic insufficient CF mutation present with this most common GI manifestation of CF.[1,2,4] Enzyme preparations used today significantly correct the pancreatic exocrine deficiency, but improvement is often not able to fully normalize absorption.[8]

The 85% of patients with pancreatic insufficiency have varying degrees of maldigestion, ranging from 10–80%. Thus, individuals have problems maintaining or gaining weight. To counteract the maldigestion, oral pancreatic enzymes are prescribed to be taken before consuming foods containing protein or fat.[8–11] The usual dose for treating pancreatic insufficiency is 1500–3000 units of lipase/kg/meal. The nonenteric-coated pancreatic enzyme replacement products, such as Cotazym® and Viokase®, are largely inactivated prior to reaching the duodenum. Although they are still employed in infants due to their ability to be mixed directly with formula, larger doses are needed to compensate the degree of inactivation. Additionally, one must remember that these preparations can cause contact skin excoriation.[9,12]

With the development of enterically coated microspheres, digestion and subsequent absorption improved. In these products, an acid-resistant microsphere coats the pancreatic enzyme powder. The microspheres are then encapsulated in a semiacid-resistant medium. These enzymes can more effectively pass through the lower pH of the stomach without deactivation, as the enteric coating remains intact. This protective layer then dissolves in the basic environment of the duodenum, supplying active pancreatic enzyme.[12–14] Although adolescents with CF commonly swallow these capsules, an individual with difficulty swallowing medications may open the capsule and mix the microspheres in a nonbasic medium such as strained fruits, applesauce, jam, or ketchup. It is imperative that the mixture containing the microspheres be swallowed whole because chewing this mixture may crack the enteric coating and leave the enzyme open to deactivation.

Ideally, fecal fat analysis should be routinely performed at the time of diagnosis and whenever enzyme dosages are manipulated. This analysis confirms the appropriate level of supplementation.[9,13,15] The collection can be cumbersome, and teens may not always be cooperative. Thus, planning for collections during scheduled school breaks may improve cooperation. It is important to prescribe pancreatic enzymes only when maldigestion is present. Fifteen % of individuals with CF are pancreatic sufficient, a characteristic often associated with lower severity and improved outcome. However, pancreatic insufficiency may develop in patients initially found to be pancreatic sufficient.[1]

Enzyme preparations now range from 4000 units/capsule up to 20,000 units/capsule. The use of higher-dose capsules may improve compliance[8] and nearly normalize absorption.[16] Flexibility in dose change is, of course, limited.

More than 20 patients have recently been described to develop right colonic strictures while on very-high-dose enzyme replacement. Clinically, all patients were assumed to have developed distal ileus obstructive syndrome, a condition that responds to higher lipase and hydration.[17] The risk factor for fibrosis and colonic stricture development is lipase intake in excess of 10,000 units/kg/meal, especially in children 2–10 yr of age, with a prior history of neonatal meconium ileus. To minimize inadvertent excessive dose therapy, no products with greater than 20,000 units/capsule are now on the market.

Approximately 10% of patients on appropriate pancreatic enzyme supplementation fail to adequately respond to intakes of 3000 units of lipase/kg/meal, and growth failure and steatorrhea may continue. In these situations, one must assess whether this results from insufficient enzyme supplementation (noncompliance or need for increased dosage), inappropriate technique (mixing with high-pH foods or chewing enzymes), or acidic intestinal pH. The pH-sensitive coating of the microspheres dissolves above pH 5.75. Occasionally, an individual's intestinal pH is lower than this, and in such situations antacids or histamine receptor antagonists may be used to alkalinize the intestine.[8,13,18] Typically, pancreatic endocrine function is spared, yet approximately 5% of older CF patients develop insulin-dependent diabetes mellitus. Glucose intolerance is more common. Dietary manipulation for both complications is less stringent than in an adolescent without the CF.[15]

Lactose Intolerance

Intestinal lactase, a brush border surface oligosaccharidase, hydrolyzes lactose to its monosaccharides, glucose and galactose, that can be absorbed through the luminal surface. Unlike other brush border enzymes involved in carbohydrate digestion, lactase exists in rate-limiting amounts in the intestine. Thus, diminishing amounts of available lactase more readily produce clinical signs and symptoms of carbohydrate malabsorption than other carbohydrases, since in the cases of different carbohydrates, hydrolysis in excess of what can be absorbed and utilized occurs.[19,20]

Intestinal hypolactasia, commonly referred to as lactose intolerance (LI), is the most common mucosal enzyme deficiency state and results from recessive inheritance. Unlike CF, LI at birth (congenital hypolactasia) is extremely uncommon. It usually develops over time, as the production of lactase declines (primary hypolactasia). Although symptoms may present as early as age 5–7 yr, typically LI is identified during adolescence and young adulthood.[21–23] The mechanism behind the genetic maturational decline remains unknown.[19] A third category of hypolactasia is secondary to intestinal mucosal injury, i.e., acute rotavirus diarrhea, in that case lactase sufficiency returns once the injury is healed.

Symptoms of those experiencing carbohydrate malabsorption may include osmotic diarrhea, crampy abdominal pain, bloating, and flatulence, usually occurring following ingestion of the non-digested sugar (in this case lactose). Figure 22.1 illustrates the mechanisms associated with lactose malabsorption.

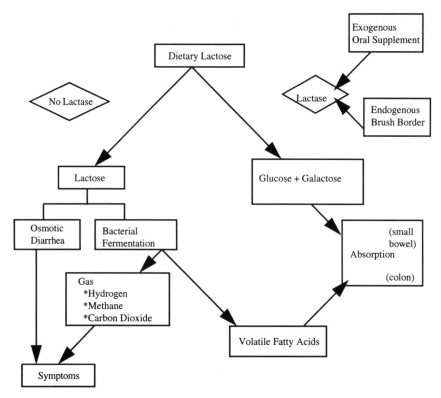

Figure 22-1.   Nutritional implications of lactase deficiency.

The unabsorbed carbohydrates enter the small bowel and colon, where significant osmotic pressure is exerted. The result, secretion of fluid and electrolytes into the lumen, is often coupled with a watery diarrhea. Some of the lactose, on the other hand, is fermented by colonic bacteria, producing lactic acid, as well as other short-chain fatty acids. The acids, being osmotically active, may exacerbate symptoms. The colonic mucosa has the capacity to absorb some of the volatile fatty acids, and thereby may salvage both calories and fluid. Those acids not absorbed pass into the fecal matter and explain the presence of acidic stools associated with carbohydrate malabsorption. Other byproducts resulting from the fermentation process include gaseous forms of hydrogen(H^2), methane, and carbon dioxide. These culprits account for the bloating and flatulence experienced by malabsorbers. In addition, they enter the portal circulation and eventually are expired in breath. The presence of H^2 in the exhaled air forms the basis for measurement and correlation of lactose intolerance within the diagnostic breath test.[21–23]

It has been realized that many who are symptomatically lactose-intolerant maintain the ability to digest some quantities of lactase-containing foods.[38] Many factors influence carbohydrate intolerance and thus exist as variables, determining that symptoms, if any, will prevail due to the malabsorption.[18]

Much inconsistency exists if the diagnosis of LI is confirmed based on symptom presentation alone. Those individuals consuming and tolerating a small amount of lactose-containing foods might not meet such diagnostic standards. Further, evidence exists confirming that symptoms of LI do not provide accurate predictive confirmation for this syndrome. Since treatment mandates a large degree of long-term diet modification, confirmation of LI needs to occur objectively.[21–24]

Celiac Disease

Celiac disease (CD), also known as gluten-sensitive enteropathy or celiac sprue, is a condition affecting the intestinal mucosa. Although the intestine normally has a "fingerlike" appearance that allows maximal absorptive area, those affected with CD often damage their villi as a result of consuming grains. The damage, thought to be caused by an immune response to the protein (gluten) within specific grains, causes the villous projections to shorten and eventually flatten. This, in turn, significantly decreases the available absorptive surface area and eliminates needed digestive enzymes normally found within the intestinal villi.

Gluten, the offending protein, is composed of several parts. Gliadin, one component, is thought to be the entity that causes the intestinal reaction. When removed from the diet, clinical symptoms resolve, and intestinal mucosa eventually returns to normal with expected villous projections.[25–27] Thus, growth delays and deficiencies are reversed, surface area is significantly increased, and digestive enzymes are once again available in appropriate proportion within the villi.[26]

The classic presentation of CD is that of the infant who presents with anorexia, weight loss, and diarrheal stools following the introduction of cereal within the diet. Although approximately 90% of cases of CD are diagnosed in infancy, some are not revealed until later in life.[26-28] During adolescence, atypical presentation of CD has become more common. Rather, adolescents frequently present with growth failure of unknown cause. Moreover, growth failure is not associated with any gastrointestinal symptoms. On further evaluation of history, it is not unusual to find that these youth were plagued with either frequent bouts of diarrhea during their first 2 yr of life, or constipation along with poor appetite.[29,30] Other vague complaints that should raise suspicion for CD include iron-deficiency anemia, rickets, and recurrent abdominal pain.[26,27]

Complications of malabsorption. Several of the clinical symptoms seen on presentation of CD directly result from malabsorption. First and foremost is that of micronutrient deficiencies. Perhaps the most common, vitamin D deficiency, presents in the form of osteomalacia or rickets. Vitamin D is malabsorbed due to a flattened mucosa. This, in turn, decreases calcium absorption. Calcium is further malabsorbed as a result of steatorrhea, because the increased fat binds calcium within the fecal matter.[26-34] Osteomalacia has been associated with CD and recognized as the sole symptom of an adolescent diagnosis of CD.[33] Practitioners have also found that vitamin D treatment alone is sufficient to reverse the problem.[31,32] Moreover, researchers examining the bone mineral content of CD patients found a significant improvement after initiation of a gluten-free diet.[31]

Folate deficiency may occur within the CD population, and megaloblastic anemia results. This deficiency contributes in worsening malabsorption, as folate plays a key role in intestinal turnover, a process believed to occur every 2–5 d. Without adequate folate, this renewal cannot occur. Treatment of the megaloblastic anemia with supplemental folic acid corrects the anemia, but the intestinal absorption site does not fully improve. Perhaps altered metabolism and not lack of folate alone cause the malabsorptive lesion.

Hypokalemia and inadequate magnesium levels may also present in CD. Like calcium, these may bind with malabsorbed fat, eliminating them from the absorptive pool.[34]

Finally, zinc has occasionally been reported to become deficient within the CD population. This deficiency may play a more striking role, as another complication and presenting symptom of CD in adolescence is failure of adequate growth response. One study documented that CD individuals not on a gluten-free diet generally weighed than less their peers following the gluten-free regimen.[35] Several investigators have reported the use of a gluten-free diet in promoting growth where previous stagnation occurred. Lack of weight gain is the first sign that linear growth may delay. During adolescence, this delay causes a later onset of puberty, and if CD is not diagnosed until late adolescence, may interfere with the individual's potential to reach maximum height. Treatment with zinc supplementation may improve growth when response of growth following initiation of a gluten-free diet is not seen.[34,35]

Anorexia may be present as well. For the individual who already is marked by growth failure, lack of intake from poor appetite will only create a more vicious cycle. Decreased consumption enhances the likelihood of inadequate intake, that in turn causes weight loss or growth stagnation. The malnutrition that results further exacerbates the anorexia.

ASSESSMENT

Cystic Fibrosis

Although it may be easy to observe poor growth due to a lack of adequate macronutrient intake, micronutrient deficiencies must not be overlooked. Malabsorption adversely affects retention of minerals, despite that they are water-soluble. This may be due to malabsorption (lack of digestive enzymes) or inadequate amounts of the nutrient within the diet, alteration of intestinal transport resulting from steatorrhea, or binding of the mineral within fecal losses because of excess fat content of the stool. Most often, micronutrient deficiencies are accompanied by growth failure, thus alerting the practitioner. Zinc is one of the more common deficiencies observed.[36,37] One study suggested that 33% of infants 6–8 wk of age already had suboptimal zinc levels.[38] Moreover, it was found that CF patients had a higher endogenous zinc loss without correlation to the amount of absorbed zinc.[39] Zinc deficiency in the adolescent may cause altered taste, further hampering an already deficient intake and thus exacerbating growth failure, and perhaps delaying the onset of puberty.

Selenium is another trace mineral that presents interest of concern. Studies have shown that serum selenium often is below desired limits among this population. However, glutathione peroxidase levels have provided conflicting results, suggesting that the serum levels alone, as a marker for deficiency, may not be accurate. Caution needs to be taken when supplementing selenium in the CF patient, as toxicity occurs at lower levels in vitamin-E-deficient patients, and vitamin E, being fat-soluble, poses a high risk of deficiency.[36,40]

It is well known that sodium losses are in excess within the CF population, and this is the basis for diagnosis. Previously, salt tablets were prescribed, but today, supplementation is encouraged by salting foods and including high-sodium content choices.[15,41] However, society has become salt-phobic and optimal choices for the individual with CF may be diminishing. Family habits are also more likely to be in opposition of CF needs; thus, careful attention must be given to this area.

Vitamin and mineral supplementation are routine therapy for the individual with CF, and specific guidelines are addressed. One needs to monitor serum levels for anyone receiving supplements to assure that toxicity does not occur. A newer preparation combining vitamins A, D, E, and K (ADEK, Scandipharm®) is now available for CF patients.

Nutritional impact on growth. Inadequate growth was so common within the CF population that, at one time, malnutrition was accepted as a consequence of this disease. However, this is no longer acceptable. Growth retardation results from excessive reliance on exogenous body fuels. Studies document that malnourished CF patients present in either a chronically catabolic state, a state of starvation, or both. Additionally, intercurrent pulmonary infections combine with the aforementioned state, causing further energy imbalance.[5] This deficit, illustrated in Figure 22.2, forms a vicious cycle, incorporating reduced intake and increased losses, in the context of increased need.

Individuals with CF can and do grow within normal parameters, and this is the goal. To assess the nutritional status of the CF patient, the clinical dietitian should collect anthropometric measurements and compare these over time. Height and weight for age should continue to follow usual growth curves, or show evidence of catch-up gains, where wasting and/or stunting was noted at the initial presentation. Growth potential during adolescence must not be ignored because foregoing this pubertal growth spurt will have lasting consequences for the teen. Much documentation exists supporting the notion that energy adequacy need be present for linear gains to occur. Assessment of midarm muscle circumference and the arm fat area may be helpful in documenting ongoing nutritional status. Many CF centers collect these data several times per year. The dietitian must also closely evaluate dietary compliance. A "routine dietary intake record" will provide insight regarding approximate caloric intake, use of appropriate foods, and supplements, and identify the risk for nutrient deficiency. Further, the clinician needs to investigate stool pattern as well as adequacy and compliance with enzymes regimens. Comparing the results of growth progress, usual intake, and enzyme adequacy with expected nutrient needs and usual gains for same-age peers will provide an overall picture of nutritional status.[4,6,41] Acceptance of emaciation as a consequence of CF is no longer appropriate and aggressive enteral or parenteral nutrition therapies are advised when oral intake alone fails. Studies have shown that nutritional status improves and growth returns to that of nonCF peers and declining lung function may stabilize or even improve.[5-7]

Lactose Intolerance

Nutritional assessment for the teen with LI should include checking to assure that growth is progressing adequately. Macronutrient and micronutrient intake recommendations for youth with LI are consistent with same-age peers.

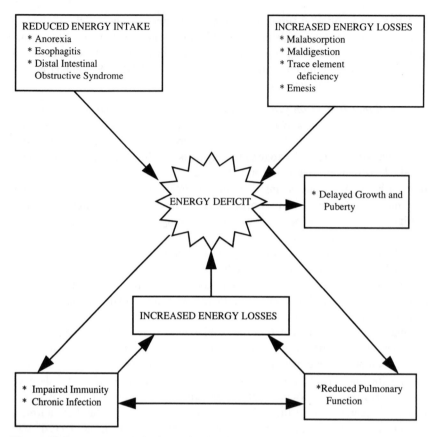

Figure 22-2.   Energy deficits in cystic fibrosis.

Adapted from L. D. Levy, P. R. Durie, P. B. Pencharz, and M. L. Corey, *J. Peds.*, **107**, 225 (1985). Reprinted with permission.

The dietitian must also evaluate the diet history, in order to help individualize the diet teaching. By doing so, he or she can more easily suggest substitutions in areas where lactose-containing foods are typically included.[42]

Celiac Disease

When CD is suspected, one should evaluate the past and current growth parameters, since growth delays often occur. In the presence of wasting and/or stunting, guidance for caloric supplementation is appropriate. However, one must be careful to include gluten-free choices. Many of the commercial, polymeric products are gluten-free. Nutritional recommendations for individuals with CD are the same as those for non-affected peers.

The dietitian must be attentive in evaluating the diet history because all traces of gluten must be eliminated. In the case of one previously diagnosed with CD, the dietitian's assessment of usual dietary intake may provide an explanation of whether or not continued discomfort is a result of hidden sources of gluten.

MANAGEMENT

Cystic Fibrosis

Adolescents with CF require larger amounts of energy to facilitate the same growth as their peers. This results from a combination of factors including pancreatic insufficiency, malabsorption (losses from energy consumed), energy cost of chronic lung disease, and recurrent infections.[4,8,41,43] As recently as 10–15 yr ago, a low-fat diet was typically advocated for these patients, to minimize fat malabsorption. Unfortunately, this created difficulty in meeting energy demands within the volume typically consumed. The low-fat diet compromised the caloric intake because fat provides 9 cal/g vs. the 4 cal/g supplied by carbohydrate and protein.

This revision of allowing a liberal fat inclusion in the diet of the CF patient has demonstrated growth mimicking nonCF peers, although enzyme therapy is a key component in nutritional management. However, this must be coupled with dietary manipulations to supply additional nutrients required (see Table 22.1) because of malabsorption, increased pulmonary involvement, and specific micronutrient repletion, especially if additional complications exist. The enzyme therapy available today aids in control of digestion such that control of steatorrhea via diet in these patients is no longer necessary.[44–46] Instead, individuals with CF should consume a liberal fat diet, containing approximately 40% fat. Although this is sometimes referred to as a high-fat diet, one must understand that the

Table 22.1 Cystic Fibrosis Diet Guidelines

Goal: Achieve a high-calorie, liberal fat dietary pattern. *Include pancreatic enzymes when malabsorption is present.*	
Allow	**Avoid**
All foods	Skipping meals
Modify diet by increasing calories, where able	Low calorie foods
Include fried foods	Reduced-fat milks
Frequent snacking	

inclusion of the higher percentage of fat within the diet serves as a vehicle to provide energy within a reasonable volume of food. It is thought that essential fatty acids will be provided with the provision of 5% total energy intake from fat sources.

Total caloric intake should initially approach 130–150% of recommended dietary allowances. The actual need varies according to complications such as the presence of lung infections, gastrointestinal function, or anorexia and mandates close growth monitoring. Individual variation should be adjusted as a result of growth outcomes. Protein needs are usually set at 50% above expectations of non-CF peers.[4,8,41,45,47–50] Carbohydrate is generally not restricted, and even with the complication of diabetes mellitis (DM) requiring insulin, dietary management with regard to carbohydrate is liberal.

The diabetic meal pattern restrictions often work in direct opposition to the guidelines offered to someone with CF. Whereas the former requires caloric restriction, the latter often aims to provide high-energy goals. With DM alone, one would restrict foods such as concentrated sweets, eliminating sugar, honey, and corn syrup. A teen with CF complicated by DM is allowed concentrated sweets within his or her diet, and glucose is controlled using insulin, rather than diet. The clinical dietitian should advise the avoidance of foods containing primarily concentrated sweets when not consumed with a meal in order to avoid large fluctuations in serum glucose. However, these foods may be strategically consumed along with a meal, when the mix of protein and fat from other foods consumed at that time will slow the serum glucose rise.[47,50]

Individuals who are pancreatic insufficient are also at risk for fat-soluble vitamin deficiency, and supplementation is advised (see Table 22.2). Fat-soluble vitamins, when prescribed, should be given in a water-miscible form. In an attempt to reduce expenses, some providers are following serum levels of nonsupplemented patients to assure adequacy, rather than prescribing prophylactic supplementation. It is important to tailor the treatment similarly to that of patients

Table 22.2   Vitamin and Mineral Supplementation in Cystic Fibrosis

Vitamins	
A	500–1000 IU/d
D	400–800 IU/d
E	5–10 IU/kg/d, up to 400 IU/d
K	5 mg/wk
Multivitamin	1–2 times RDA/d
Salt	¼tsp/d added to infant formula, *or* liberal use of salt and salty foods
Trace Minerals	
Zinc	As documented by deficiency
Selenium	

with liver disease because a complication of CF is the increased need for supplemental fat-soluble vitamins.[51]

Sodium depletion presents as a risk for CF patients, as a result of increased losses via sweat. Although salt tablets were prescribed in the past, currently CF teens are instructed to include high-salt foods within their diets. Adolescents must be cautioned regarding exercise and hot weather, when their sodium replacement needs are likely to increase. Keeping salty snacks available at these times often is sufficient.[4,8,15,41,45,47,50]

Despite aggressive nutritional intervention and wide dietary choices, some teens may remain malnourished. This is especially true for adolescents who did not benefit from early diagnosis or aggressive nutritional therapy in early childhood. Supplemental enteral feedings exist as an option and should be considered. The high incidence of sinusitis or nasal polyps may preclude nasogastric feeds, so a gastrostomy tube should be examined. However, caution should be exercised when considering this option with a teen who has portal hypertension liver disease, as varices may develop around the tube site. Supplemental enteral feedings have proven to enhance growth and reduce malabsorption, as well as stabilize if not improve lung disease. Nocturnal delivery of calories can maximize nutrition with minimal inconvenience.[5,6,52,53]

The choice of formulas to use via enteral feedings is controversial. One option is the use of polymeric formulations, that are less expensive, and to supplement with increased enzymes. This option has a lower osmolarity, and advancement to higher caloric density may be more achievable. Including choices that contain some medium-chain triglycerides within the fat to enhance absorption is recommended. Alternatively, elemental feedings can be used, precluding the need of enzyme therapy.

Enzyme therapy in conjunction with the enteral feedings may also be managed in several ways. One may choose capsules of enterically coated microspheres, but these cannot be mixed into the enteral formula due to the basic pH of the supplements. When this choice is prescribed, adolescents must be instructed to swallow the enzyme when enteral feedings are initiated. It is important to note that the benefit of this enzyme will last only about 90 min. Asking a teen to swallow more enzyme at some point midway through the enteral feed cycle is often not practical because supplemental feedings frequently occur when he or she sleeps. However, patients may take a second enzyme dose in the morning when they wake and stop the supplemental feeding. The authors recommend this only in the case where a patient's resultant growth is not progressing as desired when just the initial enzyme dose is taken. The alternative method allows mixing the enzyme directly into the enteral formula. The older, nonenterically coated enzymes serve this purpose, as they may be mixed directly into the product. One should be aware that mixing the enzyme directly into some products may cause thickening of the enteral formula and clog narrow tubes. Larger doses are often required to compensate when this option is employed because much of the enzyme is lost to inactivation.[4,41,45]

Adolescent specific guidelines must address several concerns (see Tables 22.1 and 22.3). First, realistic weight goals must be set. Adolescents are usually quite weight-conscious and often may diet with peers. This should be recognized and discouraged. Second, most adolescents' schedules leave little time for sitting down and eating a meal. Thus, the clinical dietitian must focus on how caloric goals can be met within a hectic schedule. Adolescents often frequent fast-food restaurants. Although the food generally violates guidelines for most Americans, the high-fat and high-sodium content is a perfect match for someone with CF. If enteral feeding therapy is needed, adolescents often have concerns about how this may affect relationships. It is important to address this concern honestly and openly, placing an emphasis on education to the adolescent and family. Enteral feedings should be adjusted so that they do not interfere with usual activities.

Maintaining the nutritional status of the CF patient becomes more important as more is learned about how improved nutritional status improves prognosis. Furthermore, well-nourished teens are better able to handle the stress and healing should they opt for transplantation.

Lactose Intolerance

Some concern exists regarding adequacy of nutritional intake because LI requires reduction or avoidance of a major group of food. Specifically, calcium poses the most risk, and osteoporosis correlated with LI is in question. Inadequate calcium intake is likely since sources rich in calcium are often eliminated, yet foods containing calcium but not lactose do exist and remain unlimited within the diet. Paradoxically, many of these sources, vegetarian in nature, also contain phytates that bind calcium, thus decreasing absorptive capacity. The role lactose plays in calcium absorption further complicates this issue. Although some studies confirm decreased calcium absorption because of dietary lactose elimination, others contradict those results. These studies suggest no significant difference in calcium absorption when diets containing lactose and those lacking lactose were compared. Thus, the risk of inadequate calcium intake must be addressed, especially for adolescents about to enter a critical period for linear growth. If inadequate dietary calcium is suspected, calcium supplementation should be suggested.[54-59]

Initially, LI is treated with a lactose-free diet (see Table 22.4). This includes elimination of all foods containing lactose—milk and dairy products, and foods containing these within their ingredients. The teen must be instructed to carefully read labels, in order to uncover hidden sources of lactose.

Substitutes for milk include soy milk, but many adolescents may reject the taste of that and nondairy creamers, and lactase-containing milk. The pre-hy-

Table 22.3   Tips on Increasing Calories

Food Additive	Suggested Uses
Butter/margarine/oil	Add to bread, crackers. Toss into pasta, even if adding other sauces. Add to hot cereals. Use over pancakes, french toast, and waffles, in addition to syrup. Use regularly over vegetables.
Jam/jelly/honey/syrups/sauces	Use on crackers, toast, bread. Add to hot cereal. Serve over ice cream. Use with pancakes, waffles, and french toast.
Salad dressing/mayonnaise/sour cream	Use as dips for vegetables or crackers. Use liberally on salad. Use liberally on sandwiches. Use over potatoes.
Gravy	Serve over meat and poultry. Serve over potatoes.
Cheese	Add to eggs, salads, sandwiches, and pasta. Serve as a snack. Make sauces and serve over vegetables and pasta. Use with crackers. Make a dip for vegetables, crackers, and snack chips.
Peanut butter/peanuts	Use to top crackers. Use on fruit (bananas, apples), or vegetables (celery). Use nuts as a snack.
Cream/yogurt	Add to whole milk to increase calories. Add to cereal. Serve as a snack (yogurt, ice cream). Use whipped cream with fruit. Use to make sauces.
Supplements	Use as needed. Can include, but are not limited to milkshakes, Carnation Instant Breakfast, Scandishake, Ensure Plus, Nutren 2.0, etc.

Table 22.4   Lactose-Free Diet Guidelines

Food Group	Foods Allowed	Foods Avoided
Bread/cereal/ rice/pasta	French, Italian, Vienna, and Syrian breads, bagels, English muffins, and others with allowable ingredients. French toast made without milk, saltines, graham, oyster, soda, Triscuit, Wheat Thins, Ritz crackers. All bread products and cereals containing no milk or milk products. Pasta (except as listed in avoid column), plain rice, rice pilaf with allowable ingredients.	Bread, rolls, biscuits, English muffins, muffins made with/ enriched with milk solids, pancakes, waffles, doughnuts, Pop-Tarts, Zwieback, Quaker 100% Natural, Special K, Cocoa Krispies, Captain Crunch's Crunchberries, Golden Grahams, canned spaghetti, ravioli with cheese filling, macaroni and cheese, rice pilaf with cheese.
Vegetables	All unless listed in "foods avoided" column.	Vegetables in butter, cheese, or cream sauces, potatoes mashed with milk.
Fruit	All are allowed.	None.
Milk/cheese/ yogurt	None.*	All types.*
Meat/fish/ poultry/eggs	Plain beef, poultry, fish, pork, lamb, bacon, kosher frankfurters, kosher cold cuts, tofu, peanut butter without added milk, other cold cuts and processed meats without milk and milk product fillers.	Creamed meats, gravies, sausage, hash, frankfurters, commercial hamburgers, peanut butter with added milk, pizza. Check labels on processed, canned, and luncheon meats.
Fats	Pareve margarine, Weight Watchers diet margarine, unsalted Mazola margarine, unsalted Fleishman's stick margarine, lard, vegetable oil, mayonnaise.	Butter, margarine containing milk/milk products, sour cream, whipped cream, salad dressing containing milk, cream or cheese, commercial gravy.
Soups	Broth-based soups with allowable ingredients.	Cream soups, chowders, bisque, other soups containing milk/milk products.

continued on next page

Table 22.4 *Continued*

Food Group	Foods Allowed	Foods Avoided
Desserts	Tofutti, Tofu Light, Jello, fruit sorbet, water ice, milk-free popsicles, fruit pie, pie crust made with Crisco shortening or allowed margarines, tapioca, homemade pudding cooked with fruit juice or milk substitute, angel food cake (made without milk), milk-free cookies (gingersnaps, graham crackers), Nature Valley Oats 'n Honey granola bars.	Cakes, cream pies, cookies made with milk, ice cream, frozen yogurt, sherbet, custard, commercial pudding mixes, whipped cream.
Sweets	Sugar, jam, jelly, syrup, honey, gum drops, other candy made without milk/milk products, Bakers unsweetened or semisweet chocolate.	Candy made with milk, chocolate, butter or butterscotch, caramel, toffee.
Beverages	Milk substitutes such as Isomil, Prosobee, Lactofree, Nursoy; fruit juices; carbonated beverages; Kool-Aid; cocoa without added milk solids; Coffee Rich, Ensure, Sustacal.	Milk, drinks containing milk and milk products.
Miscellaneous	Mustard, relish, catsup, salt, pepper, spices, soy sauce, cocoa powder, carob powder, potato chips, pretzels, pickles, olives, peanuts, popcorn (without butter), corn chips.	Corn curls, cheese-flavored corn chips, cheese-flavored popcorn, pretzel/cheese bites.

*Some amount of lactose is usually tolerated by lactose-intolerant individuals. Thus, milk and dairy products containing the lactase enzyme, aged cheeses, yogurt, and foods containing small quantities of lactose may be added back to the diet at the physician's discretion.

drolyzed milks should initially be avoided as they are not fully lactose free. However, those sold in liquid form are generally 70–99% lactose free. Adding 12–15 lactase drops/qt of milk will also reduce the lactose content by 90–99%.[42]

Adolescents with LI often tolerate varying amounts of lactose within their diets. Once the initial symptoms have been resolved, foods containing small amounts of lactose should slowly be added and subsequently hydrolyzed milks may be used. Thus, lactose is titrated back into the diet until the threshold is reached.[19]

Tolerance to dairy products may be increased by including yogurt (with active cultures) and aged cheeses. The fermentation process that occurs within these products reduces the lactase, and they are better tolerated by malabsorbers. However, this is not the case for the frozen yogurt products, or yogurts that lack active cultures. Interestingly, chocolate milk has been observed to be more tolerable by those affected with LI. In addition, tolerance may improve by delaying gastric emptying with the use of high fat. Lactose-containing foods taken in combination with other high-fat choices may improve tolerance. For those maintained via enteral tube feedings, most products are lactose-free. Changing the regimen from bolus feedings to continuous ones controls gastric emptying and may further decrease symptoms, should they persist.

As already mentioned above, enzyme preparations exist that prehydrolyze lactose (Lact-Aid, Lactrase, Dairy Ease), to allow more diet variability. The availability of these products takes several forms: within the food prior to purchase, liquid, tablets, or capsules.[42]

Celiac Disease

Treatment via diet is the primary therapy for those affected with CD. As discussed, gliadin (a component of gluten) appears to be the causal agent, and treatment is directed at removing all sources of gluten from the diet. It is believed that even the slightest trace of this protein within the diet of an affected teen may induce symptoms. As a result, patients are advised to eliminate any food ingredients that do not clearly identify all components.[26,28,60–62]

Wheat, barley, oats, and rye are universally accepted as significant offenders, and all teens are advised to eliminate all sources of them from their diets (see Table 22.5). Unfortunately, this affects a large number of foods and thus makes dietary management difficult at times. The teen and his family must understand what foods are permitted and relearn to cook using appropriate ingredient substitutions. Acquiring these special foods requires more effort, but often health food stores and mail supply houses carry allowed products and aid in returning variety to the diet. The above-mentioned offenders fall primarily within the bread/starch food group; however, these may be contained in much smaller quantities as food fillers, derivatives within oils, food additives, and stabilizers. Examples include wheat starch (a thickening agent) and malt flavoring (malt is derived from barley). When evaluating these food ingredients, the dietitian must obtain as much information as possible. Malt flavoring may actually be allowed, as the flavoring can be derived from either corn or barley. If derived from corn, the individual with CD will tolerate the food. However, the flavoring with barley as the source may exacerbate symptoms. Those following gluten-free diets are encouraged to communicate with individual food companies, in order to obtain the most precise information. In cases where the exact information cannot be uncovered, it is advisable to eliminate that food from the diet. One also should periodically

Table 22.5 Gluten-Free Guidelines

Food Group	Foods Allowed	Foods Avoided
Breads/ cereals/ pasta/grains	Products containing rice, corn, soy, arrowroot, and tapioca. Breads containing flour from rice, potato, tapioca, arrowroot, pea, corn, or bean. Cereals from corn meal, millet, buckwheat, hominy, puffed rice, crisp rice, and cream of rice. Malt or malt flavoring derived from corn. Oriental rice and bean noodles.	Products containing wheat, barley, rye, and oats. Breads and cereals containing wheat starch, wheat bran, oat bran, graham, wheat germ, and bulgur. Products containing malt flavoring derived from malt/barley, or unspecified origin. Regular spaghetti, macaroni, and noodles. Many packaged rice pilaf mixes.
Vegetables	Fresh, frozen, and canned products that are free of thickening agents, unless specified as an allowable source.	Products containing thickeners derived from wheat, barley, rye, or oats. Products containing stabilizers unless derived from allowed sources. Unspecified sources should be avoided.
Fruit	All unless listed in "foods avoided."	Prepared fruit containing thickening agents (i.e., pie filling).
Meat/ poultry/fish	Fresh and frozen products, canned meats, unless containing ingredients not allowed.	Prepared meats, luncheon meats, sausages, frankfurters, and canned meats containing grain and starch fillers, self-basting turkey and other poultry that often contain fillers with gluten.
Dairy products	All aged hard cheeses, pasteurized processed cheeses including cottage cheese and cream cheese, ice cream free of gluten-containing stabilizers. Products containing lactose (milk sugar) are often tolerated following initiation of the gluten-free diet.	Cheese food, including spreads, soft cheeses, and dips; ice cream with gluten-containing stabilizers or those of unspecified sources.

continued on next page

Table 22.5 *Continued*

Food Group	Foods Allowed	Foods Avoided
Beverages	Freshly brewed coffee, tea, chocolate made from powdered cocoa, carbonated drinks, and juices made from fresh fruit.	Some brands of instant coffee, tea, and cocoa mixes; beverages including malt/ malted milk, grain-derived drinks such as Postum and Ovaltine.
Fats	Butter, margarine, vegetable oil, hydrogenated vegetable oil, nuts, salad dressing with allowable ingredients (apple and wine vinegars are generally acceptable), mayonnaise with allowable ingredients.	Salad dressings containing grain vinegars (including distilled, white vinegar, or if unspecified vinegar), salad dressings containing emulsifiers and stabilizers derived from products containing gluten. Margarine and butter containing gluten.
Miscellaneous	Soy sauce that does not contain wheat or barley. Spices, alcohol-free extracts, FDA-approved food colorings, monosodium glutamate (MSG), hydrolyzed or textured soy and corn vegetable protein, corn malt, starch (raw or modified from arrowroot, corn, maize, potato, and tapioca). Vegetable gum from carob, locust bean, cellulose gum, guar gum, gum arabic, gum acacia, gum tragacanth, xanthan gum.	Soy sauce containing gluten, products with grain vinegar (including catsup and mustard), soups or broths containing bouillon, unspecified texturized or hydrolyzed vegetable protein, vegetable gum from oats and any other product containing an unspecified flour or cereal additive, barley malt, wheat starch, caramel candy containing gluten, flavorings made with alcohol.

*Product ingredients often change, and thus it is best to verify acceptability by reading labels and calling manufacturers for information regarding unspecified ingredients.

reevaluate if foods with additives like malt flavoring are allowed, as a food company may, at any time and without notice, change the type or brand of additive, thus affecting whether or not a food is allowed.

Other additives that may contain offending sources include textured vegetable protein, hydrolyzed vegetable protein, starch, modified starch, vegetable gum, and unspecified flour or cereal additives. When appearing within the ingredient list in this fashion, it is not clear what the actual source is. Although it may be corn and perfectly acceptable, oats or wheat present a different picture. Direct communication with the manufacturer may reveal the specific source of each questioned ingredient, but if undetermined, the teen may need to exclude the food.[28,62]

The importance of obtaining special, allowable flours and grains cannot be overly emphasized. Learning to substitute these products within the diet adds variety, increases the chances of a balanced nutrient intake, allows for more ease with meeting caloric goals, and presents a psychological advantage to the affected youth. This is especially true during adolescence, where peer pressure often plays such a great role, as does the need for acceptance. By using flours and grains derived from rice, corn, potato, etc., some foods mimicking those eliminated may be returned to his or her diet. This allows the CD teen to eat with friends and it provides the family an opportunity to share this diet. Accepting the gluten-free diet for the family, as much as possible, allows the affected teen to be seen as a part of the group, rather than an outsider posing difficulties related to food.

Finally, the dietitian should address the impact of this diet with regard to eating out. Although the many restrictions make this difficult, it is not impossible. The teen and his or her family should be prepared to speak with the restaurant management in advance, to assure that allowable foods exist. This often requires discussing food preparation and reading ingredient lists. Although timely, if the option of eating out becomes a reality, many positive outcomes may result, for the CD teen who can be an active participant.

CASE ILLUSTRATION

A 16-year-old female, Sally, with CF diagnosed in infancy presents with progressive growth failure and delayed purbertal development. Respiratory function is relatively stable, with no significant right heart failure, distal bowel disease, or biliary cirrhosis. She is exerting increased control of her diet and has been quite compliant in enzyme replacement therapy. Both the patient and her family seek your nutritional counsel.

On examination, her weight is 42 kg with a height of 150 cm, both below the 3rd percentile for Sally's age. She is Tanner II in sexual development, with a height age of 12 yr. Anthropometric evaluation reveals a midarm circumference of 218 (5th percentile) and triceps skinfold of 12 (10th percentile). Sally has gained only 1 kg and 2 cm in the past year.

Review of a 5-d diet history reveals an average energy intake of 2600 kcal/d with 38 g of protein and 28% of calories from fat. Her enzyme therapy has been 80,000 units of lipase/meal and 40,000 units of lipase snack that is documented to reduce fecal fat excretion to 15% of that ingested. Sally has been taking a daily multivitamin as well as a supplement of vitamins A, D, E, and K.

The slow rate of growth despite appropriate enzyme therapy and stable cardiopulmonary disease mandates an increase in total energy delivery. With a goal of 150% of energy RDA for height age, a caloric intake of 3500 kcal/d is desired. A meal plan is thus customized to achieve this goal with 40% of calories from fat and 50 g of protein daily. Oral high-energy milkshake supplements are included. The option of night infusion tube feeding is discussed, but not implemented until the response to oral supplements can be documented over the next 3 mo.

REFERENCES

1. P. R. Durie, *Int. Sem. Ped. Gastro. Nutr.*, **2**, 3 (1993).

2. M. R. Knowles, *New Insights Into Cystic Fibrosis*, **1**, 1 (1993).

3. D. V. Schidlow, L. M. Taussig, and M. R. Knowles, *Ped. Pulmonol.*, **15**, 187 (1993).

4. P. B. Pencharz and P. R. Durie, *Ann. Rev. Nutr.*, **13**, 111 (1993)..

5. R. W. Shepherd, T. L. Holt, B. J. Thomas, B. J. Kay, A. Isles, P. J. Francis, L. C. Ward, *J. Peds.*, **109**, 788 (1986).

6. L. D. Levy, P. R. Durie, P. B. Pencharz, and M. L. Corey, *J. Peds.*, **107**, 225 (1985).

7. G. Steinkamp, I. Ruhl, and H. von der Hardt, *Ped. Pulmonol.*, **8** (suppl.), 267 (1992).

8. K. J. Gaskin, *Int. Sem. Ped. Gastro. Nutr.*, **2**, 9 (1993).

9. *Clin. Cour.*, **11**, 1 (1993).

10. J. Bouquet, M. Sinaasappel, and H. J. Neijens, *J. Ped. Gastro. Nutr.*, **7** (suppl. 1), S30 (1988).

11. D. Castantini, R. Padoan, L. Curcio, and A. Giunta, *J. Ped. Gastro. Nutr.*, **7** (suppl. 1), S36 (1988).

12. N. Ansaldi-Balocco, B. Santini, and C. Sarchi, *J. Ped. Gastro. Nutr.*, **7** (suppl. 1), S40 (1988).

13. D. Y. Graham, *J. Ped. Gastro. Nutr.*, **3** (suppl. 1), S120 (1984).

14. J. M. Littlewood, J. Kelleher, M. P. Walters, A. W. Johnson, *J. Ped. Gastro. Nutr.*, **7** (suppl. 1), S22 (1988).

15. E. Luder, *Top. Clin. Nutr.*, **6**, 39 (1991).

16. D. V. Schidlow, R. J. Fink, and M. S. Brady, *Clinician*, **9**, 2 (1991).

17. R. L. Smyth, D. van Velzen, A. R. Smyth, D. A. Lloyd, and D. P. Heaf, *Lancet*, **343**, 85 (1994).

18. B. J. Boyle, W. B. Long, W. F. Balistreri, S. J. Widzer, and N. Huang, *Gastroenterology*, **78**, 950 (1980).

19. G. M. Gray, *Gastroenterology*, **105**, 931 (1993).

20. M. L. Lloyd and W. A. Olsen, *Viewpoints Dig. Dis.*, **23**, 13 (1991).

21. R. G. Montes and J. A. Perman, *Int. Sem. Ped. Gastro. Nutr.*, **2**, 2 (1991).

22. J. M. Saavedra and J. A. Perman, *Ann. Rev. Nutr.*, **9**, 475 (1989).

23. R. G. Montes and J. A. Perman, *MMJ*, **39**, 383 (1990).

24. R. E. Kleinman, E. F. Bell, T. F. Hatch, W. J. Klish, N. Kretchmer, V. Tolia, and J. J. Udall, *Pediatrics*, **86**, 643 (1990).

25. R. Troncone and A. Ferguson, *J. Ped. Gastro. Nutr.*, **12**, 150 (1991).

26. J. S. Trier, *N. Engl. J. Med.*, **325**, 1079 (1991).

27. M. F. Kagnoff, *Gastro. Clin. N. Am.*, **21**, 405 (1992).

28. J. S. Trier, *Hosp. Practice*, 41 (1993).

29. E. Cacciari, S. Salardi, R. Lazzari, A. Cicognani, A. Collina, P. Pirazzoli, P. Tassoni, G. Biasco, G. R. Corazza, and A. Cassio, *J. Peds.*, **103**, 708 (1983).

30. Y. Rosenbach, G. Dinari, I. Zahavi, and M. Nitzan, *Clin. Ped.*, **25**, 13 (1986).

31. S. Mora, G. Weber, G. Barera, A. Bellini, D. Pasolini, C. Prinster, C. Bianchi, and G. Chiumello, *Am. J. Clin. Nutr.*, **57**, 224 (1993).

32. G. W. Hepner, J. Jowsey, C. Arnaud, S. Gordon, J. Black, M. Roginsky, H. F. Moo, and J. F. Young, *Am. J. Med.*, **65**, 1015 (1978).

33. W. A. DeBoer and G. N. Tytgat, *J. Intern. Med.*, **232**, 81 (1992).

34. H. E. Harrison, R. R. Tompsett, and D. P. Barr, *Proc. Soc. Exp. Biol. Med.*, **53**, 314 (1943).

35. Y. Naveh, A. Lightman, and O. Zinder, *J. Peds.*, **102**, 732 (1983).

36. M. VanCaillie-Bertrand, F. DeBieville, H. Neijens, K. Kerrebijn, J. Fernandes, and H. Degenhart, *Acta Paediatr. Scand.*, **71**, 203 (1982).

37. N. F. Krebs, F. J. Accurso, and K. M. Hambidge, *Ped. Pulmonol.*, **9** (suppl.), 163 (1993).

38. N. F. Krebs, K. M. Hambidge, and M. Bronstein, *Ped. Pulmonol.*, **5**, 269 (1990).

39. N. F. Krebs, L. V. Miller, and P. V. Fennessey, *Ped. Res.*, **27**, 126 (1993).

40. R. Castillo, C. Landon, K. Eckhardt, V. Morris, O. Levander, and N. Lewiston, *J. Peds.*, **99**, 583 (1981).

41. B. J. Ramsey, P. M. Farrell, and P. B. Pencharz, *Am. J. Clin. Nutr.*, **55**, 108 (1992).

42. K. Y. Warman, *Int. Sem. Ped. Gastro. Nutr.*, **2**, 9 (1991).

43. S. A. Wootton, J. L. Murphy, S. A. Bond, J. E. Ellis, and A. A. Jackson, *J. Roy. Soc. Med.*, **84** (suppl. 18), 22 (1991).

44. E. Luder, M. Kattan, J. Thornton, K .M. Koehler, and R. J. Bonforte, *AJDC*, **143**, 458 (1989).

45. P. R. Durie and P.B. Pencharz, *J. Roy. Soc. Med.*, **82** (suppl. 16), 11 (1989).

46. L. Bell, P. R. Durie, G. G. Forstner, *J. Ped. Gastro. Nutr.*, **3** (suppl. 1), S137 (1984).

47. A. MacDonald, C. Holden, and G. Harris, *J. Roy. Soc. Med.*, **84** (suppl. 18), 28 (1991).

48. V. S. Hubbard and P. J. Mangrum, *JADA*, **80**, 127 (1982).

49. R. M. Buchdahl, C. Fulleylove, J. L. Marchant, J. O. Warner, M. J. Brueton, *AJDC*, **64**, 373 (1989).

50. B. M. Winklehofer-Roob, D. H. Shmerling, M. G. Schimek, and P. E. Tuchschmid, *Am. J. Clin. Nutr.*, **55**, 100 (1992).

51. R. J. Sokol, M. C. Reardon, F. J. Accuroso, C. Stall, M. Narkewicz, S. H. Abman, and K. B. Hammond, *Am. J. Clin. Nutr.*, **50**, 1064 (1989).

52. J. M. Bertrand, C. L.Morin, R. Lasalle, J. Patrick, and A. L. Coates, *J.Peds.*, **104**, 41 (1984).

53. E. K. Bowser, *Top. Clin. Nutr.*, **5**, 55 (1990).

54. J. C. Debongnie, A. D. Bewcomer, D. B. McGill, and S. F. Phillips, *Dig. Dis.*, **24**, 225 (1979).

55. I. Birlouez-Aragon, *Reprod. Nutr. Develop.*, **28**, 1465 (1988).

56. M. Griessen, B. Cochet, F. Infante, A. Jung, P. Bartholdi, A. Donath, E. Loizeau, and B. Courvoisier, *Am. J. Clin. Nutr.*, **49**, 377 (1989).

57. S. C. Miller, M. A. Miller, and T. H. Omura, *J. Nutr.*, **118**, 72 (1988).

58. M. Horowitz, J. Wishart, L. Mundy, and B.E.C. Nordin, *Arch. Intern. Med.*, **147**, 534 (1987).

59. W. T. Tremaine, A. D. Newcomer, B. L. Riggs, and D. B. McGill, *Dig. Dis.*, **31**, 376 (1986).

60. M. Hernandez, J. Argente, A. Navarro, N. Caballo, V. Barrios, F. Hervas, and I. Polanco, *Horm. Res.*, **38** (suppl. 1), 79 (1992).

61. N. G. McElvarey, R. Duignan, J. F. Fidding, *Ulster Med. J.*, **61**, 134 (1992).

62. K. Mormon, *G-I Nutr. News.*, **2**, 4 (1989).

Cancer

Cameron K. Tebbi, M.D., and
Ann Erpenbeck, R.D.

INTRODUCTION

Adolescence is a dynamic phase of life marked by profound changes in physical, biochemical, emotional, social, psychological, and spiritual development. Included in these changes are rapid growth and a significant tissue deposition in a relatively brief period of time. This so-called "growth spurt," along with the increased physical activity characteristic of this age group, results in a substantial increase in the nutritional requirement. With this background, it is apparent that cancer and its therapy, which often alter nutrition and nutrient requirements in all age groups, have a greater impact in adolescents.

At diagnosis, the nutritional state of the cancer patient often does not substantially differ from that of patients with benign tumors.[1-3] However, the incidence of undernutrition substantially increases during the treatment and course of the disease, especially in advanced and complicated cases. This can be caused by either increased energy expenditure or decreased intake, or both. Periods of "semistarvation" due to required lack of intake in preparation for surgery or tests, decline in appetite, emesis after chemotherapy or radiation therapy, infections, blood loss for laboratory tests, malabsorption, and renal damage may be contributing factors.[4-7] Increased resting energy expenditure has also been implicated. However, in a group of newly diagnosed patients with acute lymphoblastic leukemia, resting energy expenditure was similar to that of age- and sex-matched controls.[8] Alteration of smell and taste perception, which is seen with some chemotherapy regimens,[9] can contribute to diminished food intake.[10] In addition, increased intestinal permeability, reduction in nutrient absorption, and small bowel dysfunction in patients receiving chemotherapy can lead to malnutrition.[11]

To provide adequate nutritional support in cancer patients, a number of factors should be considered. These include the type of tumor and its metabolic effects, medical and surgical treatments, complications of therapy, including reduced appetite, emesis, and required restrictions of the teen's diet. In addition, the psychological, if not physical, effects of periodic hospitalization and removal from the family setting and foods to which one has been accustomed can impact on appetite. An unfamiliar hospital environment, regimented time, and changes in eating habits can avert the desire to eat. Furthermore, the psychological effects of the disease and separation from a peer group may significantly suppress appetite and decrease the food intake necessary for recuperation from the disease and support of rapid growth.

Metabolic Changes

Weight loss and malnutrition in adolescent cancer patients are usually multifactorial. Factors so far identified probably include only a fraction of the elements involved (see Table 23.1). The tumor, its metabolites, body defenses, and chemotherapy affect virtually every function of the digestive system. For example, an elemental, but important alteration is taste change, which is frequently seen among cancer patients. As a rule, sweet-tasting foods are better tolerated. This may be due to the heightened ability to taste urea, which manifests itself as a dislike of meat and protein-containing foods.[12] Decreased protein intake, coupled with utilization of nitrogen for malignant growth, results in the alteration of protein metabolism. Degradation of host skeletal muscle then becomes a nitrogen source and results in depletion of the host muscular structure and ultimately weight loss and anorexia.[13,14] Moreover, tumor metabolism places an undue burden on the host relative to substrate demand, metabolism, and disposal of the toxic and waste products, especially in cachectic patients. The prevalence and degree of malnutrition and the effect on organs and systems depend on the type of tumor, stage of the disease, and response to therapy. Some tumors have a higher incidence of protein-energy malnutrition. For example, Ewing's sarcoma and neuroblastoma have a 67 and 47% probability of malnutrition, respectively.[15,16] In contrast, the same risk for acute leukemias is 6% and for non-Hodgkin's lymphoma and osteosarcoma is 10–15%. Of course, these statistics depend on the tests employed and prevalance of malnutrition in the geographic area where the report is generated. For example, the incidence of malnutrition

Table 23.1 Causes of Cachexia in Adolescent Cancer Patients

Cause	Examples
Tumor-related	Type of tumor
	Mechanical effect
	Substrate consumption
	"Tumor-produced factors"
Chemotherapy	Nausea and vomiting
	Stomatitis
	Malaise
	Diarrhea
	Renal damage
Radiation	Nausea and vomiting
	Ostomatitis/xerostomia
	Esophagitis
	Ileus
Surgery	Requirement for lack of food intake
	Pain
	Ileus
	Energy needed for recovery
"Antibiotics"	Mineral and nutrient losses
	Diarrhea and vomiting
	Renal damage
Iatrogenic	Blood loss for laboratory tests
	Postsurgical intestinal obstruction
	"Short gut" syndrome
Host effect	Cytokine production IL-1, TNF, IFN-γ, IL-6
	Psychological effects
	Altered taste and smell
	Hospitalization/changes in environment
	Food aversion
Growth and development	Growth requirement
	Altered metabolism

in standard-risk acute lymphoblastic leukemia patients in Mexico was reported to be 37%.[17] The 5-yr disease-free survival correlated with the degree of nutrition, i.e., 83% for well-nourished and 26% for malnourished patients.

Alterations in amino acid and protein metabolism can be measured in cancer patients before the onset of anorexia or weight loss; thus, nitrogen depletion probably is not exclusively caused by reduced oral intake and, at least in part, is due to changes brought on by the cancer itself.[13,18] For example, amino acids are released at a lesser rate from extremity sarcomas, possibly due to consumption by the tumor.[19] Metabolism of carbohydrates may be altered in cancer patients.

Experimentally, the alteration of glucose generation turnover, pool size, and half-life in tumor-bearing animals has been documented.[20,21] In experimental models, some of the changes can be measured during the early stage of the tumor growth prior to the development of cachexia.[20] Alteration of carbohydrate metabolism, especially during cachectic states, may include reduced blood glucose, elevation of lactic acid due to tumor metabolism, elevated blood lactate, abnormal glucose tolerance, changes in glucose turnover and pool. Studies using 18F-2 deoxyglucose and positron emission tomography (PET) scanning to quantitate glucose consumption by large extremity sarcomas have found rates from 6–15 mg/100 g/min.[22] Likewise, brain tumors consume large amounts of glucose commensurate with the histologic grade of the tumor. Some chemotherapy agents widely used for the treatment of lymphomas and leukemias can substantially alter carbohydrate metabolism. The prime examples are L-asparaginase and corticosteroids. Adjuvant and support treatment may also influence such a metabolism. For example, in the adolescent age group, iatrogenic lactic acidosis in teens receiving parenteral or enteral hyperalimentation is reported.[23] Abnormalities of lipid metabolism have been observed. Hyperlipemia, along with the depletion of lipid stores, can occur. Increased mobilization and rate of turnover of fatty acids may be among the reasons for this paradoxical finding.[24] In the serum of some experimental animal models, a lipid-mobilizing factor and lipolytic agent have been identified.[25,26] The role of other abnormalities of the metabolism of protein, carbohydrate, and fat, including increases in the energy-wasteful Cori cycle that results in an increase in recycling of lactate, has been subject to discussion and debate.[27] Nevertheless, substrate consumption by the tumor cannot always explain the teen's weight loss.[28] Thus, other factors mediating distant tumor effects have been sought. Effects of increased levels of tryptophan and serotonin have been suggested, but remain unproven at this time.[29-31] Likewise, altered central control of food intake by the hypothalamic center remains doubtful.[32]

Tumor necrosis factor (TNF/cathectin) and other cytokines such as interleukin-1 (IL-1), interleukin-6 (IL-6), and interferon γ(IFN-γ),[33] have also been implicated in cachexia associated with cancer. TNF, a product of mononuclear phagocytes, can be produced in a significant quantity after exposure to lipopolysaccharides.[34] Experimentally, animals exposed to sublethal doses of TNF by injection or genetically-engineered TNF-producing cells develop cachexia.[35,36] Clinically, the determination of TNF levels in cancer patients has produced mixed results.[37,38] This agent can induce the biosynthesis and release of specific proteins, including interleukin-1.[34,39] Production of TNF can be greatly enhanced through priming with various agents, such as bacterias or defensive functions like interferon γ, and inhibited by others, e.g., glucocorticoid hormones.[34] These changes explain some, but not all, of the effects seen in tissues and organ systems. They also may shed light on the lack of correlation of symptomatology observed and the tumor size detected.

Psychological Effects

The psychological effects of cancer and its therapy on the adolescent's appetite cannot be discounted. The significant changes brought about by cancer and its treatment, which require exposure to the unfamiliar surroundings of the hospital and clinic, deprive adolescents of their normal family life, peers, and desired food. These can have a detrimental effect, ranging from withdrawal to occasional depression, and potentially decrease the individual's appetite and cause weight loss.[40] Food aversion in patients receiving chemotherapy is a relatively common phenomenon and can cause anorexia and reduced weight loss.[41] This may play a major role in tumor-induced anorexia, with cancer chemotherapy agents acting as stimuli. Clinically, and in experimental models, taste aversion is found to be a learned behavior.[41,42] In adolescents, the dislike of a previously preferred food is common. To decrease such a phenomenon, it is suggested that the patient's favorite food not be given during chemotherapy when gastrointestinal adverse effects are expected. Anticipatory vomiting, which is frequently seen among adolescent patients, is also a part of learned aversion. This conditioned phenomenon can be triggered with most sights or sounds reminding the teen of prior treatment experiences and can be a reason for inadequate nutrition and weight loss.

Adolescence is a period in which one attempts to become independent of parents. The process is gradual, but continues through the teenage years. It is graded, causing a decreased reliance on the parents for preparation and serving of foods. Unfortunately, this process may be interrupted by cancer and its therapy. It is a natural instinct of parents to feed their offspring and, in general, the degree of food intake is considered a measure of one's health. After the diagnosis of cancer and especially early during the course of the disease, parents can become preoccupied with the care and feeding of their adolescent.[43] The offer of food and care becomes an additional force on the side of the parents and can provoke resentment on the part of their child. Parental enforcement may further suppress the teen's appetite, resulting in food refusal[44] and thus further weight loss and deterioration in the adolescent's condition.

Psychological issues and food intake are significantly intertwined in the adolescent cancer patient. These effects, at times, can resemble disease-related symptomatologies and the finding may not be differentiable from those of somatic origin. Consideration of psychological effects of cancer on the patient and family must be an integral part of care for the adolescent oncology patient.

ASSESSMENT

The nutritional assessment should be an ongoing process tied to the adolescent's changing needs. The assessment should include a complete history and physical examination, psychosocial evaluation, and anthropometric, biological, and metabolic measurements. Although most aspects of the nutritional assessments are the same as those of normal adolescents, special attention should be paid to the age; gender; stage of development; activity and duration; type and site of malignant disorder; surgical interventions; treatments used; areas of irradiation; required dietary modifications, if any; food idiosyncrasies; food intolerances; patient's and family's prior food habits; religious restrictions; and cultural beliefs. Attention to the composition of food in a typical day or week can provide a better understanding of the teen's dietary habits. In the physical examination, special attention should be given to the patient's general appearance, condition of skin, subcutaneous tissues, hair texture, eyes, mouth (including gums and teeth), thyroid gland, and musculoskeletal system. Examination of the oral cavity is especially important since some of the complications of chemotherapy and radiation may include painful lesions of mucous membranes and dry mouth, which can severely affect appetite and oral intake. In addition, dental caries at the site of irradiation also need to be considered.

Anthropometric measurements at diagnosis and follow-up can reveal the degree of growth failure and undernutrition.[45] Reports of anthropometric measurement are relatively scarce in cancer patients. In one study of 277 children with benign and malignant tumors, 32% had less than normal measures for at least one of the three anthropometric indices evaluated.[3] Weight and height should be measured and plotted on the appropriate National Center for Health Statistics (NCHS) growth chart and remeasured at least every 3 mo. Visual observation also is essential in detecting obesity, wasting, and dehydration. Weight-for-height ratio is considered to be a reliable indicator of nutritional status in adolescents.[3] This compares weight to height, whereas height and weight for age are compared with those of other children of the same age. For those adolescents whose height values exceed the measurements indicated on the growth grid, an equation may be used to compare the patient with standard values. Ideal body-weight grids may be obtained from postpubertal weight/height tables such as those published by NCHS.[45a]

Weight for height below the 5th percentile may signify acute weight loss indicative of acute protein-energy malnutrition. Those whose height and weight for age plot below the 5th percentile may be experiencing chronic malnutrition, resulting in growth stunting. When the body is undernourished, one of the first values to decrease is weight. If this deficiency is not corrected, height could also be affected.

Midarm muscle circumference (MAMC) and triceps skinfold (TSF) measurements may be obtained to assess body composition and help detect muscle and fat depletion (see Chapter 18). Serial measurements are crucial in assessing nutritional status. Edema and obesity may skew accuracy and are contraindications for the use of this technique. Prior growth curves should continue to be used during the cancer therapy to evaluate changes in the patient's rate of growth status. A measurement below the 10th percentile should be further investigated for protein-energy malnutrition (PEM). Acute weight changes greater than 2% of body weight/d may suggest dehydration rather than actual weight loss.[46] The best long-term indicator for adequate energy intake is growth. Overall anthropometric measurement, while not accurate, can provide a gross estimation of body compositions.

Biochemical measurement can provide some insight to the teen's state of nutrition. Although the values can be influenced by other factors such as infections, timing of blood drawing, meals, stress, degree of hydration, treatments used, etc., the biochemical data are objective and measurable parameters. A host of biochemical profiles, including serum albumin, transferrin, prealbumin, retinol-bending proteins, total proteins, acute-phase reactants (α_1-acid glycoprotein, c-reactive protein, ceruloplasmin), vitamins, and creatinine, have been utilized.[47-51] Although these measurements cannot detect mild to moderate states of malnutrition, they should be considered as a part of a complete assessment of the youth's nutritional state. However, as a single parameter, these do not constitute a definitive measure of the patient's nutrition.

Serum albumin is most commonly used to assess protein status. Although a concentration less than 3.0 gm/dl may indicate PEM, it must be considered cautiously. It has a half-life of 14 d, making it inaccurate in detecting acute malnutrition. Albumin may also reflect an acute metabolic change in response to fever and infection, as opposed to visceral protein depletion.[52] Other factors that may alter albumin levels include liver dysfunction, overhydration, IV albumin, GI protein-losing enteropathy,[53] and zinc deficiency.[54] Prealbumin is a more accurate reflection of nutritional status and has a half-life of only 2 d.[55] However, it may be depressed in the presence of severe liver dysfunction, vitamin A or zinc deficiency.[54]

Hematologic parameters such as hemoglobin, hematocrit, and total lymphocyte count, while useful for the assessment of nutrition of normal undividuals,[56] are not valid parameters for assessing nutritional status. These reflect the disease state and effects of therapy, rather than nutrient status.[3,57] Virtually every aspect of the body's defense and immune system is damaged by malnutrition.

Treatment Effect

In some respects, malnutrition in adolescent cancer patients receiving multimodal therapy is iatrogenic.[58] Therapeutic agents can potentially alter the patient's metabolism. An example of such effects[59] is provided in Table 23.2.

Antibiotics are frequently used on a "prophylaxis" basis or treatment in cancer patients, such as ametoptrine with sulfametaxazole, can produce folate deficiency and changes in intestinal flora. Other broad-spectrum antibiotics can cause altered

Table 23.2   Nutritional Losses and Side-Effects of Medication Used in Cancer Patients

Drug	Nutrient Loss	Side-Effects
Alkylating agents, e.g., nitrogen, mustard, cyclophosphamide, myleran	Glucose malabsorption	Decreased wound healing, gastrointestinal disturbances, weight loss, cheilosis, glossitis
Antimetabolite, e.g., methotrexate, aminopterin, fluorouracil, cytosine arabinoside	Folate antagonist, glucose and xylose malabsorption	Stomatitis, gastrointestinal injury, macrocytic anemia, diarrhea
Plant alkaloids, e.g., vincristine		Adynamic, ileus, constipation, mucosal cell atrophy
Antibiotic chemotherapies, e.g., actinomycin D	Fat calcium, iron malabsorption	Nausea, vomiting, anorexia, mucositis, glossitis, diarrhea, cheilosis
Alkylating-like agents, e.g., cisplatinum	Magnesium waste	Nausea, vomiting, muscle cramps
Enzymes, e.g., L-asparaginase	Hypoproteinemia	Anorexia, weight loss
Steroids, e.g., prednisone	Muscle-protein, calcium loss, reduced glucose tolerance	Suppression of growth, loss of bone matrix, poor wound healing

Adapted from C. G. Neuman, D. B. Tellife, A. J. Zefras, et al., *Cancer Res.*, **432** (suppl.), 699s (1982).

taste, decreased appetite, nausea, vomiting, diarrhea, anorexia, glossitis, hypokalemia, and depletion of vitamin-K-producing intestinal bacteria.[60] Antifungals such as amphotericin-B can result in a loss of magnesium and potassium, which may have grave consequences. Narcotics and antiemetics may cause drowsiness and xerostomia, resulting in decreased intake. These effects can potentially result in hematological, metabolic, physiopathological and psychological changes, including anemia, with far-reaching results. The major gastrointestinal effects of chemotherapy agents are summarized in Table 23.3.

Mechanism of Chemotherapy-Induced Vomiting

The most common effects of chemotherapy agents used in the treatment of adolescents with cancer are nausea and vomiting. Various reflex pathways are involved in the initiation of emesis caused by chemotherapy. Mechanisms under-

Table 23.3 Agents and Adjuvants Used in Chemotherapy

Drug Groups/Examples	GI Side-Effects
Alkylating agents	
Busulfan	Dryness or oral mucosa, glossitis
Chlorambucil	N/V
Cyclophosphamide	N/V, anorexia, colitis, stomatitis
Ifosfamide	N/V
Melphalan	N/V, stomatitis
Nitrogen mustard	N/V, anorexia, diarrhea
Thiotepa	N/V, anorexia, stomatitis
Alkylating-like agents	
BCNU	N/V
CCNU	N/V, diarrhea, anorexia, stomatitis
Carboplatin	N/V, pain, diarrhea
Cisplatin	Severe N/V, anorexia, diarrhea
DTIC	N/V, anorexia, diarrhea, stomatitis, metallic taste during infusion
Procarbazine	N/V, diarrhea, anorexia, stomatitis
Antimetabolites	
Cytarabine	N/V, anorexia, diarrhea, oral and anal ulcers, esophagitis, abdominal pain
Hydroxyurea	N/V, anorexia, diarrhea, stomatitis
Methotrexate	N/V, anorexia, stomatitis, glossitis, gingivitis, pharyngitis, enteritis, diarrhea, ulcers
6-Mercaptopurine	N/V, anorexia, stomatitis, mucositis, ulceration, epigastric distress, abdominal pain
6-Thioguanine	N/V, anorexia, stomatitis, diarrhea
5-Azacytidine	N/V, diarrhea
5-Fluorouracil	N/V, stomatitis, diarrhea, esophagitis, proctitis
DNA-binding agents	
AMSA	N/V, diarrhea, mucositis
Bleomycin	N/V, anorexia, stomatitis, mucositis
Daunorubicin	N/V, diarrhea, stomatitis, esophagitis, abdominal pain
Doxorubicin	N/V, anorexia, stomatitis, esophagitis, diarrhea
Idarubicin	N/V, stomatitis, diarrhea, mucositis
Mitoxantrone	N/V, stomatitis, mucositis, diarrhea
Plant alkaloids	
Etoposide	N/V, anorexia, diarrhea, abdominal pain
Teniposide	N/V, diarrhea
Vincristine	Constipation, ileus, abdominal pain
Vinblastine	N/V, constipation, ileus, abdominal pain, anorexia, stomatitis

continued on next page

Table 23.3   *Continued*

Drug Groups/Examples	GI Side-Effects
Hormones	
Decadron	Abdominal distention, increased appetite, weight gain, esophagitis, peptic ulcer, GI hemorrhage
Hydrocortisone	Increased appetite, weight gain, peptic ulcer
Prednisone	Abdominal distention, increased appetite, weight gain, esophagitis, peptic ulcer, GI hemorrhage
Enzymes	
L-asparaginase	Mild N/V, anorexia, weight loss, abdominal cramps
Antimicrotubular agents	
Paclitaxel	N/V, diarrhea, mucositis, stomatitis, pharyngitis, ischemic or in farcted GI tract, neutropenic enterocolitis
Topotecan	N/V, mucositis, diarrhea
Biological response modifiers	
Alpha interferon	N/V, anorexia, diarrhea, abdominal pain, weight loss
IL_2	N/V, diarrhea, mucositis, xerostomia, anorexia
TNF	Malaise, cachexia
IL_6	Liver damage, cachexia
G-CSF	N/V, diarrhea, anorexia
GM-CSF	N/V, anorexia, weight loss
Erythropoietin	N/V, diarrhea
Antibiotics	
Actinomycin-D	N/V, anorexia, stomatitis, esophagitis, pharyngitis, diarrhea, abdominal pain
Enzyme inhibitor	
Allopurinol	N/V, anorexia, diarrhea, gastritis
Vitamins	
Leucovorin	N/V
Detoxifying agents	
MESNA	N/V, diarrhea, bad taste in mouth

N/V = Nausea and vomiting.

lying this reaction are poorly understood. Control of vomiting involves two anatomically and functionally distinct components. These are a vomiting center and chemotherapy trigger zone (CTZ). The exact location of the vomiting center in humans has not yet been identified. Thus, most data on vomiting are based on animal studies.[61–63] Current evidence suggests that the vomiting center is located within the lateral reticular formation adjacent to the medulla oblongata areas. This area is excited by visceral afferent nerve impulses arising in the gastrointestinal tract and elsewhere. The CTZ is responsive to the chemical agents in blood and cerebrospinal fluid. However, proper response will require an intact vomiting center, as the direct electrical stimulation of the CTZ does not result in vomiting.[64] Thus, chemotherapy-induced emesis is produced primarily by impulses originated by humoral stimulation of the CTZ and processed by the vomiting center, which also receives signals from the GI tract, vestibular nuclei and limbic system. After direct stimulation of the vomiting center or via the CTZ, efferent pathways cause the act of vomiting by phrenic, vagus, and spinal nerves connected to respiratory and abdominal musculature and organs.

Neurochemical mechanisms involved in chemotherapy-induced emesis are poorly understood. Evidence suggests compamine (D_2) receptors in the CTZ-mediated vomiting. D_2 agonists such as apomorphine bromocriptine and L-dihydroxyphenylanine can cause vomiting, whereas antagonists such as metoclo-pramide, control the emesis. The CTZ is also sensitive to stimulation by endogenous transmitters and neuropeptides such as norepinephrine, serotonin, 5-hydroxytryptamine (5-HT), substance P, enkephalin, and g-aminobutyric acid.[65,66]

Serotonin receptor antagonists can prevent chemotherapy-induced nausea and vomiting. Experimentally, the direct injection of 5-HT_3 receptor antagonists to the CTZ results in dose-dependent vomiting inhibition.[67] Of four receptors for serotonin, 5-HT_3 that, in addition to the peripheral nerves, is found to be concentrated in the cortical and limbic areas and area postrema is the main target.[61,62,68] The 5-HT_3 receptors are known to be agonized by several agents, including serotonins, 2-metaclopramide and cocaine.[69] Administration of cisplatin in animal models results in increased serotonin and 5-hydroxy indoleacetic acid levels in the intestinal mucosa.[70] It appears that chemotherapeutic agents release serotonin from enterochromoffin cells in gastrointestinal mucosa, resulting in CTZ activation.[71] This triggers a cascade of events, resulting in the stimulation of chemoreceptor zones located in the postrema aspect of the 4th ventricle.

Although the present generation of antiemetics, especially antiserotonins including ondansetron and granisetron that are selective antagonists of 5-HT_3, are highly effective in the control of drug-induced nausea and vomiting, their effects vary. Often, a combination of agents is used to prevent or control emesis.[72–76] Some agents used as antiemetics, such as chlorpromazine, have a sedative effect and thus decrease the patient's activity, including oral intake.[76] Nausea and vomiting are usually accompanied by anorexia, which also has a similar effect.

The psychological aspects of nausea and vomiting should not be ignored and must be considered as a part of therapy.[77]

Other Effects of Chemotherapy on GI System

Mucositis can be seen after the administration of a number of anticancer medications. Many chemotherapeutic agents are cell-cycle-specific and, as such, are active in certain phases of the cycle. Often, the lining cells of the gastrointestinal tract, which have rapid turnover, are unintended targets of these medications. Among the most vulnerable are epithelial cells of the buccal mucosa and gastrointestinal tract. Continued mucosal toxicity results in ulceration, diarrhea, and, in severe cases, proctitis and bleeding. Constipation due to neurotoxicity is seen with several agents, including vincristine. Fungal infections, especially with candida species, are common in the oral cavity and esophagus. Retrosternal pain in an immune-suppressed patient may be the first sign of candida infection. Good dental and oral hygiene and use of soft brushes and mouthwash can minimize these complications. Liver damage occurs after treatment with a number of chemotherapy medications, including folate antagonists, and anorexia may follow. Long-term therapy with purine synthesis inhibitors, antifolate, and other agents likewise may result in hepatic fibrosis and failure. Asparaginase can also induce damage to the liver and pancreas. Corticosteroids are often used in the treatment of leukemia and lymphoma or as an adjuvant to decrease intracranial pressure, or prevent adverse reaction to drugs, or as antiemetics to prevent reaction or vomiting. These agents can result in hypoglycemia, hyperphagia, hyperglycemia, glycosuria electrolyte disturbances, hypokalemic alkalosis, fluid retention, muscle wasting, abnormal fat deposition, gastric ulceration, etc.[4,78]

Corticosteroids can also increase prealbumin, retinol-binding proteins, and α_1-acid glycoprotein. Peptic ulceration and other organ and system damages can occur. As with most chemotherapy agents, the damage is proportional to the dose used, and in low doses, the functions are often returned to normal and compensation occurs after the insult is stopped. Nevertheless, high doses and repeated damage may result in permanent damage to organs, such as hepatic fibrosis and failure.

Common side-effects of therapy such as nausea, vomiting, anorexia, stomatitis, mucositis, diarrhea, constipation, bacterial and fungal infection, and malabsorption contribute to nutritional deterioration.[4] However, it should be noted that, at least in adults, appetite improves after the first 4 wk of therapy and GI functions improve.[79]

Radiation therapy. Radiotherapy can have significant short- and long-term nutritional consequences among adolescents.[80] Adverse effects of radiation therapy can be greatly enhanced by some chemotherapy agents such as cisplatinum and daunomycin. Furthermore, some cancer treatment agents such as actinomycin-D may cause a recall reaction at the site of prior irradiation. These phenomena may further increase the side-effects of irradiation. A summary of these effects is provided in Table 23.4. Consequences of irradiation depend on the site of irradiation. After radiotherapy of the head and neck, acute side-effects may include anorexia, loss of taste, xerostomia, and mucositis. Nausea, vomiting, weight loss, dysphagia, and acute gastroenteritis may be seen after irradiation of the thorax and abdomen/pelvis. The late effects described in Table 23.4 have further reaching effects. During head and neck radiation, good oral hygiene and protection of teeth are necessary to minimize side-effects.[80] Supportive care, including antiemetics, is also often required. A low-residue, low-fat diet free of gluten, milk, or milk products may reduce immediate gastrointestinal side-effects.

Consequences of Malnutrition

In cancer patients, PEM can have detrimental effects on the various organs and systems, as well as the overall prognosis of the patient. Malnourished adolescents generally lack the energy necessary to participate in activities appropriate for their age. Loss of sense of well-being will often result in apathy, which is counterproductive in coping with the disease and the teen's daily tasks. In animal studies, dietary protein restriction is shown to be associated with susceptibility to infection, especially pneumocystic carinii pneumonia. A similar pattern is seen in clinical medicine.[81] Cell- and humeral-mediated immunities are less than

Table 23.4 Effects of Radiotherapy on Nutrition

Site of Radiation	Early Effects	Later Effects
Central nervous system	Nausea and vomiting	Lethargy and somnolence
Head and neck	Xerostomia	Xerostomia
	Mucositis	Dental caries
	Odynophagia	Osteoradionecrosis
	Dysosmia	Trismus
	Hypogeusia	Hypogension
	Anorexia	Ulcer
Thorax	Dysphagia due to esophagitis	Fibrosis
		Stenosis
		Fistula
Abdomen and pelvis	Anorexia	Ulcer
	Nausea	Malabsorption
	Vomiting	Chronic diarrhea
	Acute gastroenteritis	Chronic gastroenteritis
	Acute colitis	Chronic colitis
	Weight loss	Bowel obstruction
	Hepatitis	

fully functional in malnourished cancer patients.[82] Phagocytosis of leukocytes in malnourished cancer patients is less than optimal.[83] The total granulocyte reserve may also be lower in malnourished cancer patients.[84] Zinc deficiency can decrease cell-mediated immunity.[85]

Cancer patients require adequate nutrition and energy to recover from surgery and infection, combat catabolic effects of the disease perform host defenses, and provide for body functions and growth. Protein-energy malnutrition may be present at diagnosis or develop during the course of the disease.[56,86] Although there is no agreement, depending on the measure used, 7–27% of pediatric oncology patients have been found to have some degree of malnutrition.[87,88] Patients with intraabdominal tumors are more likely to be malnourished than others.[88] Nutritional status at diagnosis may have a significant bearing on the patient's response to treatment.[1,89] In a retrospective study of 455 pediatric oncology patients, nutritional status had a significant effect on the patient prognosis.[1] In another study, pediatric patients who were well nourished at diagnosis tended to have a longer time interval to relapse than those who had poor nutritional status ($P=0.08$).[89] Likewise, in adult cancer patients losses up to 5% of body weight prior to therapy were found to be associated with poorer prognosis.[90] Some types of treatment place the patient at a higher risk for PEM. These include intense, frequent chemotherapy; radiation therapy to the head, neck, esophagus, abdomen, or pelvis; and surgery of the head, neck, or intestine. Additionally, patients with advanced disease at diagnosis, poor response to treatment, and those who relapse are placed at high risk for developing PEM.[60]

MANAGEMENT

As with all adolescents with a chronic disease, the importance of nutrition intervention in the adolescent oncology patient cannot be overemphasized. Nutrition goals include promoting normal growth, decreasing morbidity and mortality, and maximizing quality of life.[86] Nutrient depletion must not only be corrected in the malnourished, but prevented in the well-nourished. Cancer location, type of treatment, and nutritional status before, during, and after treatment must be examined in choosing the most appropriate nutrition treatment.

Guidelines for nutrition intervention include more than 5% preillness weight loss, weight for height below the 10th percentile, serum albumin less than 3.2, skinfold thickness less than the 5th percentile, and a drop in two percentile channels on the growth grid.[4]

Once energy and protein needs have been determined and an individual care plan has been formulated, the route of providing nutrients must be determined. Oral intake is always the preferred route, but it may be necessary to boost calories and protein in order to meet the increased needs of the cancer patient (see Table

23.5). Favorite foods should be avoided prior to therapy, due to the risk of developing aversion to a food that may be one of the adolescent's primary sources of nourishment.[53] It is beneficial to discuss the importance of nutrient intake with the patient and family, and the potential side-effects of therapy that may decrease the desire or ability to consume adequate nourishment. A summary of strategies to maintain nutritional status with selected side-effects can be seen in Table 23.6. Dietary intake should be monitored to detect inadequate intake before weight loss occurs and make quick changes in the diet to prevent PEM. Oral nutrition supplements may be incorporated into the diet if the teen is unable to take in enough with regular nutrient-dense foods alone. The major problem with liquid nutrition supplements in the adolescent oncology patient has been found to be acceptance.[91] Oral feeding programs should include food preferences and variety. Meals and snacks should be served when intake aversion is least likely to occur during antineoplastic therapy. For hospitalized adolescents, foods and beverages should be available when the kitchen is closed.[4,92] If the diet appears inadequate in vitamins or minerals, i.e., an entire food group eliminated, multivitamins should be given, if indicated. Care should be taken not to use vitamin compounds that include antagonistic agents which may alter desired chemotherapeutic medication given for the patient's cancer therapy. A prime example is the use of folate-containing multivitamins in patients receiving methotrexate. Iron supplementation is controversial. Iron can induce free radicals, which can cause DNA

Table 23.5   Calorie and Protein Boosters

Cheese	Melt on meats, vegetables, eggs, and bread.
Cream cheese	Mix with fruits and vegetables; add to casseroles and eggs.
Cottage cheese	Spread on fruit or crackers.
Milk or cream	Use in place of water in food preparation.
High-protein milk	Blend 1 qt whole milk with 1 cup powdered milk; substitute this for regular milk and water in food preparation.
Powdered milk	Add to drinks, casseroles, soups, and pudding.
Eggs	Add extra to French toast, pancake, and waffle batter; add to salads and casseroles.
Ice cream	Use in sodas, shakes, desserts, and with fruit.
Peanut butter	Spread on toast, crackers or fruit; add to cookie, muffin, or pancake batter; swirl through soft ice cream.
Wheat germ	Add to casserole and bread recipes; sprinkle on cereal, yogurt, and ice cream.
Nuts	Add to ice cream, cookies, meatloaf, and hamburgers.
Meat or fish	Add to salads, omelettes, casseroles, and soups.
Legumes	Add to pasta and grain dishes.
Yogurt	Add to fruit and desserts; use on cereal, pancakes, and waffles; add to milk-based beverages and gelatin dishes.

Table 23.6   Common Side-Effects with Suggested Nutrition Treatment

Side-Effect	Coping Suggestion
Nausea	Small, frequent meals.
	Serve sweet high-calorie liquids.
	Serve foods at room temperature or cooler.
	Encourage rest after meals.
	Serve low-fat, dry, salty, or cold foods.
	Avoid high-fat, overly sweet, and strong-odored foods.
Vomiting	Avoid tight clothing.
	Once vomiting is controlled, provide small amounts of clear liquids.
	Progress to full liquids as tolerated.
	Provide small amounts, frequently.
Diarrhea	Provide small amounts, frequently.
	Provide clear liquids for at least 12 h.
	Advance to full liquids, then a soft, low-residue diet as tolerated.
	Serve liquids at room temperature.
	Provide plenty of fluids throughout the day, between meals.
	Temporarily, avoid lactose.
	Avoid high-fat, acidic foods and fruit juices.
	Avoid high-osmolality beverages (carbonated beverages).
Constipation	Provide increased fluids.
	Encourage activity/exercise.
	Provide a high-fiber diet.
Mouth sores	Provide soft and tender foods.
	Puree or chop foods.
	Provide drinks and liquids with a straw.
	Add butter, gravies and sauces to ease swallowing.
	Serve foods cold or at room temperature.
	Avoid acidic, spicy, salty, rough, coarse and dry foods.
Dysgeusia	Serve tart foods.
	Provide foods cold or at room temperature.
	Use strong seasonings/marinades.
Xerostomia	Provide very sweet or tart foods.
	Provide hard candy/gum.
	Serve foods soft or puréed.
	Use gravies and sauces to moisten foods.

double-strand breaks and oncogene activation.[94–96] Also in vitro, iron can enhance the growth of some malignant cells.[97] Moreover, the association of iron and cancer is supported by epidemiological data.[96,98] If oral intake is suboptimal during treatment, but is only for a short duration (1–3 d), it may be beneficial to encourage weight gain between treatments and expect a slight weight loss during treatment. If treatment causes poor oral intake for more than 3 or 4 d and nutrient-dense supplements are routinely used, alternate forms of nutrition support must be considered. Although periods of starvation, irregular feeding, low animal protein and fat diet, and iron deficiency probably can decrease the incidence of cancer, they should not be utilized as a part of therapy in oncology patients. To date, no conclusive data have been presented to indicate that adequate general nutrition will enhance tumor growth.

Teens who may benefit from supplemental tube feedings should meet the following criteria: not end-stage, unable to take adequate nourishment by mouth alone, have minimal gastrointestinal complications, and platelet support is not a concern.[92,93] However, it has been shown that enteral nutrition support may not prevent or correct PEM in those teens receiving intense cancer therapy, especially those malnourished at the time of diagnosis.[4,82,99–102] However, once past the intense treatment, enteral nutrition may help improve nutritional status.[4]

Benefits of tube feeding over total parenteral nutrition (TPN) include a decreased risk of infection, more normal activity, and decreased cost.[91] Nasogastric feedings may be desirable so the tube can be removed during the day, allowing mobilization and minimal interference with oral intake. However, there may be some undesirable psychological effects because of inserting and removing the tube. The side-effects of cancer treatment that may affect absorption and intestinal motility may also be contraindications for tube feeding. If long-term tube feedings are indicated, a gastrostomy may be surgically placed.

The type of tube feeding product must be age- and disease-appropriate (see Table 23.7). Diarrhea and delayed gastric emptying are the most common complications with tube feedings.[103] If the diarrhea occurred prior to initiation of the

Table 23.7 Tube-Feeding Products

Product	Indications/Characteristics
Alitraq	1 kcal/cc; metabolic stress; impaired GI; elemental
Ensure Plus	1.5 kcal/cc; high-energy needs
Glucerna	1 kcal/cc; hyperglycemia; with fiber
Introlite	0.53 kcal/cc; ½ strength
Jevity	1.06 kcal/cc; standard isotonic formula with fiber
Lipisorb	1.35 kcal/cc; fat malabsorption (pancreatitis)
Osmolite HN	1.06 kcal/cc; standard isotonic formula
Pediasure	1 kcal/cc; standard formula for 1–6 yr of age
Perative	1.3 kcal/cc; metabolic stress
Promote	1 kcal/cc; wound healing
Travasorb hepatic	1.1 kcal/cc; high BCAA, hepatic failure
Travasorb renal	1.35 kcal/cc; electrolyte-free, elemental-renal failure
TwoCal HN	2 kcal/cc; volume-restricted, high-protein, cyclic feeding
Promod	28 kcal/scoop; modular protein: 5g/scoop
Polycose	20 kcal/scoop; modular carbohydrate for calories

tube feeding, the cause may have been an infection or medication rather than product intolerance. The risk of diarrhea associated with tube feeding may be minimized by starting with a diluted formula, at a constant infusion, and progressing as tolerated. If long-term tube feeding is indicated, a product containing fiber should be considered to decrease the risk of constipation.

Total parenteral nutrition may be indicated for the patient with severe GI disturbances.[91] It may be used to reverse and/or prevent PEM in patients with certain types of cancer,[4,81,82,99,101,104–106] but this has not been shown to improve survival or response to treatment except in marrow transplant patients.[91,107] Central or peripheral TPN may be chosen depending on nutrient need, duration of support planned, and the availability of peripheral veins. Since many oncology patients receiving chemotherapy have central venous catheters in place, central TPN is often chosen.[91] Important among the adverse effects of TPN in cancer patients are risk of infection and decreased neutrophil function.

Energy composition should be supplied at the desired percentages, e.g., 25–30% fat, 50–60% carbohydrates, and 10–20% protein.[46] If lipids are being provided, triglyceride levels should be monitored weekly to assure normal fat clearance that can be affected by sepsis or cachexia.[108] Other lab values that should be monitored twice a week or at least weekly during parenteral nutrition include electrolytes, calcium, phosphorus, magnesium, renal function, and liver function.[4]

Peripheral TPN is indicated for short-term use (less than 7 d). The limitation with using the peripheral vein alone is that adequate nourishment cannot be provided due to intolerance to hyperosmolar solutions. Dextrose concentrations must be limited to 5–12%, amino acid concentrations to 2–3%, and intravenous lipids to 3.5 g/kg/d.[4,99,109] Central TPN allows hyperosmolar solutions to be provided. Dextrose and amino acid concentrations may be increased to 25–35% and 2–5%, respectively, and the use of IV lipids continued.[4] As long as the gastrointestinal tract is functioning, an oral diet should be provided along with any nutrition support.

Obesity

Obesity in the adolescent oncology patient may be due to genetics, environmental and social factors, and appetite-stimulating medications such as steroids. The issue of obesity is often ignored by the teen, family, and health care professionals because it is not seen as a priority when considering the disease state.

The treatment of adolescent obesity should be approached conservatively (see Chapters 11 and 18). The focus should be placed on modification of behavior, in which the whole family is counseled on healthier eating habits. At least in adult cancer patients receiving chemotherapy, weight gain was attributed to obsessive/compulsive tendencies and introversion.[110] The adolescent should first be assessed to determine if a desire for lower weight exists. After all, the teen's weight is a result of shifting the caloric intake vs. calorie output. To reverse the trend often requires major changes in the patient's lifestyle, which may be relatively easy for a short time, but often difficult on a long-term basis. Such changes deal with many psychosocial and personal trends that often require major determination and persistence on the part of the patient. "Cosmetic" changes resulting in rapid weight loss are usually short-lived, and a periodic fluctuation of weight with losses followed by gains is undesirable. Nutrition intervention includes education on a low-fat balanced diet, with a limitation placed on high-calorie foods and beverages. If activity is not restricted due to illness, it should be emphasized. This decrease in energy intake along with increased energy expenditure should promote a decrease in the rate of weight gain and allow the patient to "grow into" his or her weight.

CASE ILLUSTRATION

Ken, a 14-year-old white male, had experienced abdominal pain, vomiting, and weight loss over a 6-wk interval. The vomiting episodes had gradually increased. Both generalized abdominal pain and vomiting were often associated with oral intakes. Various modalities of therapy, including antiemetics, had been unsuccessful to prevent or treat the vomiting. Ken had been found to have signs of obstruction at the time of his admission. Past family and social histories were recorded to be noncontributory.

On admission to the local hospital, the patient had appeared to be an ill-looking 14-year-old male, who was under no acute distress. Temperature was recorded to be 37.8°C, pulse 100/min, respiration 34/min, blood pressure 113/58, weight 49 kg (10th percentile), and height 160 cm (50th percentile). Reviewing his prior growth chart had revealed a 4 kg weight loss and drop in percentile from 50–10% over the past 2 mo. The positive physical findings had been limited to a distended abdomen, increased bowel sounds, and a "tumor mass" in the right lower quadrant. Ken's complete blood count was reported to be as follows: hemoglobin 13 g%, hematocrit 40%, platelet count 380,000/mm^3, polymorpho-nuclears 58%, eosinophiles 4%, and basophiles 1%. The red cell morphology and indices were recorded to be normal. Urinalysis was reported to be unremarkable. His biochemical profile was significant for increased LDH to 380 units/L, decreased albumin to 2.5 g/dL, proteins to 5.1 g/dL and globulins to 1.5 g/dL. Imaging studies and metastatic workup had been found to be positive for air fluid levels in the flat plate of the abdomen, enlarged mesenteric lymph nodes, and a large ileocecal mass, displacing air-filled bowel in the computerized tomography (CT) scan of the abdomen. Ken underwent surgery, where a 15×12 cm tumor obstructing the ileocecal portion of the bowel was discovered and removed.

The pathology and cell surface phenotyping of the tumor were consistent with lymphocytic lymphoma, stage II.

Ken was referred to a tertiary medical center, where he was placed on allopurinol (to block uric acid formation), sodium bicarbonate containing intravenous (IV) fluids and IV hyperalimentation with a formula containing 8.5% protein, 20% glucose, and 20% lipids. He was also started on a chemotherapy protocol that included vincristine, cyclophosphamide, and doxorubicin. In addition, he received intrathecal chemotherapy with methotrexate, cytosine arabinoside, and hydrocortisone. Ken's course was complicated with episodes of fever and neutropenia (neutrophil count less than $1000/mm^3$) and anticipatory as well as chemotherapy-related vomiting that were poorly controlled by antiemetic therapies and psychological intervention. Unfortunately, he failed to gain weight upon discontinuation of IV hyperalimentation and calorie counts proved his intake to be less than adequate. Ken was then placed on an oral hypercaloric diet. However, due to his newly acquired distaste for meat, this modification provided less protein than required. About 3 mo later, his weight remained steady at 43 kg. His protein was 5.2 g/dL and albumin 3 g/dL. His diet was supplemented with milkshakes, using commercially available hypercaloric products (see Table 23.7). Ken also was given a list of calorie/protein boosters (see Table 23.5). His total calorie intake and diet improved. Ken's weight rose to 48 kg and his total protein globulins and albumin were in the low normal range. When plotted in the growth chart, after a drop prior to his diagnosis and first 6 mo of therapy, his growth and weight gain paralleled those of his prior percentile line, i.e.,50%. He remained in a complete remission. Ken's supplemental diet was discontinued as he resumed his usual balanced diet.

REFERENCES

1. S. S. Donaldson, M. N. Wesley, W. D. de Wys, et al., *AJDC*, **135**, 1107 (1981).

2. P. Carter, D. Carr, J. van Eys, et al., *J. Am. Diet. Assoc.*, **82**, 610 (1983).

3. P. Carter, D. Carr, J. van Eys, et al., *J. Am. Diet. Assoc.*, **82**, 616 (1983).

4. A. M. Mauer, J. B. Burgess, S. S. Donaldson, et al., *J. Parent. Ent. Nutr.*, **14**, 315 (1990).

5. S. S. Donaldson, *Cancer Res.*, **37**, 2407 (1977).

6. T. Ohnuma and J. F. Holland, *Cancer Res.*, **7**, 2395 (1977).

7. K. A. Rickard, V. A. Stallings, J. van Eys, et al., *J. Parent. Ent. Nutr.*, **14**, 315 (1990).

8. V. A. Stallings, N. Vaesman, H. Chan, et al., *Ped. Res.*, **20**, 228A (1986).

9. J. S. Carson and A. Gormican, *J. Am. Diet. Assoc.*, **70**, 361 (1977).

10. W. D. de Wys, *J. Hum. Nutr.*, **32**, 447 (1978).

11. J. V. Pledger, A.D.J. Pearson, A. W. Craft, et al., *Eur. J. Ped.*, **147**, 123 (1988).

12. W. D. de Wys, *Curr. Concepts Nutr.*, **6**, 131 (1977).

13. R. I. Inculet, R. P. Stein, J. L. Peacock, et al., *Cancer Res.*, **47**, 4746 (1987).

14. P.W.T. Pesters and M. R. Brennan, *Ann. Rev. Nutr.*, **10**, 107 (1990).

15. K. A. Rickard, J. L. Grosfeld, T. D. Coates, et al., *J. Am. Diet. Assoc.*, **86**, 1666 (1986).

16. M. R. Rossi and C. Uderzoi, *Rec. Results Cancer Res.*, **108**, 198 (1988).

17. E. Lobato-Mendizábal, G. Ruiz-Argüelles, and A. Marín-López, *Leuk.Res.*, **13**, 899 (1989).

18. C. L. Klein, B. M. Camitta, *Cancer Res.*,**43**, 5586 (1983).

19. J. A. Norton, M. E. Burt, M. F. Brenan, *Cancer*, **45**, 2934 (1980).

20. M. E. Burt, S. F. Lowry, and C. Gorschboth, et al., *Cancer*, **47**, 2138 (1981).

21. J. M. Arbeit, M. E. Burt, I. V. Rubinstein, et al., *Cancer*, **42**, 4936 (1982).

22. K. A. Kern, A. Burnetti, J. A. Norton et al., *J. Nucl. Med*, **29**, 181 (1988).

23. J. T. Goodgame, P. Pizzo, and M. F. Brennan, *Cancer*, **42**, 1800 (1979).

24. E. Eden, S. Edstrom, K. Bennegard, et al., *Surgery* ,**97**, 176 (1985).

25. S. Kitada, E. F. Hays, and J. F. Mead, *Lipids*, **15**, 168 (1980).

26. H. Masumo, N. Yamasaki, and H. Okuda, *Cancer Res.*, **41**, 284 (1981).

27. M. F. Brennan, *N. Engl. J. Med.*, **305**, 375 (1981).

28. W. D. de Wys, *Cancer*, **43**, 2013 (1979).

29. R. Krause, J. H. James, V. Zepara, et al., *Cancer*, **44**, 1003 (1979).

30. M.von Meyenfeldt, W. T. Chance, and J. F. Fischer, *Am. J. Surg.*, **143**, 133 (1982).

31. W. T. Chance, M. von Meyenfeldt, and J. F. Fisher, *Pharmacol. Biochem. Behav.*, **18**, 115 (1983).

32. S. D. Morrison, in *Nutrition and Cancer*, (J. van Eys, B. L. Nichols, and M. S. Seeling, eds.),SP Scientific and Medical Books, New York, p. .31 (1979).

33. H. N. Langstein and J. A. Norton, *Hematol. Oncol. Clin. N. Am.*, **5**, 103 (1991).

34. B. Beutler and A. Cerami, *N. Engl. J. Med.*, **316**, 379 (1987).

35. A. Oliff, D. Defeo-Jones, M.Boyer, et al., *Cell*, **50**, 555 (1987).

36. K. J. Tracey, H. Wei, K. R. Manogue, et al., *J. Exp. Med.*, **167**, 1211 (1988).

37. F. Balkwill, R. Osborne, F. Buke, et al., *Lancet*, **2**, 1229 (1987).

38. S. H. Socher, D. Martinez, J. B.Cray, et al., *JNCI*, **80**, 595 (1988).

39. P. P. Nawroth, I. Bank, J. Cassimeris, *J. Exp. Med.*, **163**, 1363 (1986).

40. C. K. Tebbi and C. Bromberg, *Am. J. Ped. Hematol. Oncol.*, **10**, 185 (1988).

41. I. L. Bernstein, *Science*, **209**, 416 (1980).

42. I. L. Bernstein, M. V. Vilello, and R. A.Sigmundi, *Physiol. Psychol.*, **8**, 51 (1980).

43. I. L. Bernstein, *Cancer Res.*, (suppl.), **42**, 715 (1982).

44. D. R. Copeland, W. H. Freidrich, and J. van Eys, *Cancer Bull.*, **38**, 151 (1986).

45. J. M. Lahorra, M. E. Ginn-Pease, and D. R. King, *Nutr. Cancer,* **12**, 361 (1989).

45a. National Center for Health Statistics, *Monthly Vital Statistics Rep.*, **25**, 1 (1976).

46. K. V. Barale, in *Handbook of Pediatric Nutrition*, (P. M. Queen, and C. E. Lang, eds.), Aspen Publishers, Inc., Gaithersburg, MD, pp. 512–535 (1993).

47. B. K. Harvey, J. Bothe, and G. I. Blackburn, *Cancer*, **43**, 2065 (1979).

48. E. Blichler, *Arch. Otorhinol. Syngol.*, **236**, 115 (1982).

49. C. Coody, C. Carr, J. van Eys, et al., *J. Parent. Enter. Nutr.*, **7**, 151 (1983).

50. M. F. Winkler, S. A. Gerrior, A. Pomp, et al., *J. Am. Diet. Assoc.*, **89**, 684 (1989).

51. L. C. Yu, S. Kuvibidila, R. Ducos, et al., *Med. Ped. Oncol.*, **22**, 73 (1994).

52. R. J. Merritt, M. Kalsch, L. D. Roux, et al., *J. Parent. Enter. Nutr.*, **9**, 303 (1985).

53. J.W.T. Dickerson, *J. Royal Soc. Med.*, **77**, 309 (1984).

54. K. A. Rickard, A. Lopez, B. J. Godshall, et al., *Nutr. Focus*, **6**, 1 (1991).

55. S. O. Ogunshina, M. A. Hussain, *Am. J. Clin. Nutr.*, **33**, 794 (1980).

56. C. M. Pemberton, K. E. Moxness, M. J. German, et al., in *Mayo Clinical Diet Manual, A Handbook of Dietary Practices*, BC Decker, Inc., Burlington, Ontario, pp. 341–343 (1988).

57. I. Ramirez, J. van Eys, D. Carr, et al., *Am. J. Clin. Nutr.*, **41**, 1314 (1985).

58. J. van Eys, *J. Am. Coll. Nutr.*, **8**, 159 (1984).

59. C. G. Neuman, D. B. Telliffe, A. J. Zefras, et al., *Cancer Res.,(suppl.)*, **432**, 699s (1982).

60. N.K.C. Ramsay, in *Principles and Practice of Pediatric Oncology*, (P. A. Pizzo and D. G. Poplack, eds.), J. B. Lippincott, Philadelphia, PA, pp. 971–991 (1989).

61. G. J. Kilpatrick, B. J. Jones, and M. B. Tyers, *Nature*, **330**, 746 (1987).

62. G. J. Kilpatrick, B. J. Jones, and M. B. Tyers, *Eur. J. Pharmacol.*, **159**, 157 (1989).

63. K. R. Brizzee and P. M. Klara, *Fed. Proc.*, **43**, 2944 (1984).

64. H. L. Borison, R. Borison, and L. E. McCarthy, *Fed. Proc.*, **43**, 2955 (1985).

65. O. E. Akawari, *Drugs 25,* (suppl. 1), 18 (1983).

66. H. L. Borison and L. E. McCarthy, *Drugs* **25,** (suppl. 1), 8 (1983)

67. G. A. Higgins, G. J. Kilpatrick, K. T. Bunce, et al., *Br. J. Pharmacol.*, **97**, 247 (1988).

68. P. B. Bradley, G. Engel, W. Feniuk, et al., *Neuropharmacology*, **25**, 563 (1986).

69. M. B. Tyers, *Sem. Oncol.*, **19**, (suppl .1), 1 (1992).

70. S. J. Gunning, R. M. Hagan, M. B. Tyers, *Br. J. Pharmacol.*, **90**, 135P (1987).

71. J. Hawthorn, K. J. Ostler, P.L.R. Andrews, *J. Exp. Phys.*, **73**, 7 (1988).

72. M. Marty, P. Pouillart, S. Scholl, et al., *N. Engl. J. Med.*, **322**, 816 (1990).

73. M. Goodman, *Sem. Oncol. Nurse.*, **3** (suppl. 1), 23 (1987).

74. L. Cubeddu, I. S. Hoffmann, N. T. Fuenmayor, et al., *N. Engl. J. Med.*, **322**, 810 (1990).

75. T. M. Beck, P. J. Hesketh, S. Madajewicz, et al., *J. Clin. Oncol.*, **10**, 1969 (1992).

76. M. V. Relling, R. K. Mulhern, D. Fairclough, et al., *J. Peds.*, **123**, 811 (1993).

77. G. R. Morrow and J. T. Hickok, *Oncology*, **7**, 83 (1993).

78. W. S. Bond, *Am. J. Hosp. Pharm.*, **34**, 479 (1977).

79. D. Osoha, K. Murry, K. Selmon, et al., *Oncology*, **8**, 61 (1994).

80. S. S. Donaldson, *Cancer Res.*, **42** (suppl.), 729s (1982).

81. J. van Eys, E. M. Copeland, A. Cangir, et al., *Med. Ped. Oncol.*, **8**, 63 (1980).

82. K. A. Rickard, J. L. Grosfeld, A. Kirksey, et al., *Ann. Surg.*, **190**, 771 (1979).

83. J. P. Phair, K. S. Riesing, and E. Metzger, *Cancer*, **45**, 2702 (1980).

84. L. Balducci, D. D. Little, N. G. Glover, et al., *Ann. Intern. Med.*, **98**, 610 (1983).

85. R. A. Good, A. West, G. Fernandes, *Fed. Proc.*, **39**, 3098 (1980).

86. M. E. Sherry, S. N. Aker, C. L. Cheney, *Top. Clin. Nutr.*, **2**, 38 (1987).

87. S. A. Bond, A. M. Han, S. A. Wotton, et al., *Arch. Dis. Child.*, **67**, 229 (1992).

88. M.C.G. Stevens, I. W. Booth, D. E. Smith, *Arch. Dis. Child.*, **67**, 1318 (1992).

89. K. A. Rickard, C. M. Detamore, T. D. Coates, et al., *Cancer*, **52**, 587 (1983).

90. W. D. de Wys, C. Begg, P. T. Lavin, et al., *Am. J. Med.*, **69**, 491 (1980).

91. J. A. Norton, J. Peter, in *Principles and Practice of Pediatric Oncology*, (P. A. Pizzo and D. G. Poplack, eds.), J. B. Lippincott, Philadelphia, PA, pp. 869–896 (1989).

92. C. D. Lingard, K. A. Rickard, B. L. Jaeger et al., *TICN*, **2**, 71 (1986).

93. J. N. Lukens, *Am. J. Pediatr. Hematol. Oncol.*, **6**, 261 (1984)

94. P. Reizenstein, *Med. Oncol. Tum. Pharmacol* , **8**, 229 (1991).

95. E. D. Weinberg, *Biol. Trace Element Res.*, **34**, 123 (1992).

96. R. G. Stevens, D. R. Kalkwarf, *Environ. Health Perspec.*, **87**, 291 (1990).

97. K. Forsbeck, K. Bjelkenkrantz, and K. Nilsson, *Scand. J. Haematol.*, **37**, 429 (1986).

98. S. Langard, A. Andersen, and J. Ravnestad, *Brit. J. Ind. Med.*, **47**, 14 (1990).

99. K. A. Rickard, A. Kirksey, R. L.Baehner, et al., *Am. J. Clin. Nutr.*, **33**, 2622 (1980).

100. K. A. Rickard, E. S. Loghmani, J. L. Grosfeld, et al., *Cancer*, **56**, 2881 (1985).

101. D. M. Hays, R. J. Merritt, L. White, et al., *Med. Ped. Oncol.*, **11**, 134 (1983).

102. R. Shepherd, W. G. Cooksley, W. D. Cooke, *J. Peds.*, **97**, 351 (1980).

103. M. Bernard and L. Forlaw, in *Enteral and Tube Feeding*, (I. L. Rombeau and M. D. Caldwell, eds.), W. B. Saunders, Philadelphia, PA, pp. 542–569 (1984).

104. B. A. Cunningham, P. Lenssen, and S. N. Aker, *Nurs. Clin. N. Am.*, **18**, 585 (1983).

105. S. S. Donaldson, M. N. Wesley, F. Ghavimi, et al., *Med. Ped. Oncol.*, **10**, 129 (1982).

106. R. C. Ghavimi, M. E. Shils, B. F. Scott, et al., *J. Peds.*, **101**, 530 (1982).

107. S. A. Weisdorf, J. Lysne, and D. Wind, *Transplantation*, **43**, 833 (1987).

108. J. H. Seashore, *Yale J. Biol. Med.*, **57**, 111 (1984).

109. K. A. Rickard, B. B. Foland, C. M. Detamore, et al., *Am. J. Clin. Nutr.*, **38**, 445 (1983).

110. L. Altman, C. L. Loprinzi, J. R. Kardinal, et al., *Proc. ASCO*, **13**, 61 (1994).

Acquired Immunodeficiency Syndrome

*Carleen Townsend-Akpan, M.S.N.,
C.P.N.P., R.N.C., and
Lawrence J. D'Angelo, M.D., M.P.H.,
F.S.A.M.*

INTRODUCTION

Acquired immune deficiency disease (AIDS) is a profound supression of the immune system caused by the human immunodeficiency virus (HIV) that renders the person susceptible to opportunistic infections and neoplasms. HIV disease is viewed as an increasingly common chronic disease, especially in adolescents and young adults.[1–5] Depending on the degree of immunocompromise present at the time of the diagnosis, HIV-infected individuals may survive up to 15 yr after the diagnosis has been made. As our knowledge of this disease increases, we have had to change our management from one of "reaction" to symptoms to one of "prevention" or "delay" of life-threatening complications.

The human immunodeficiency virus is no longer viewed as the sole cause of progression to AIDS. Investigators have now focused their attention on other probable cofactors in HIV disease progression such as psychological factors, age, genotype, viral strain, sexually transmitted diseases, ilicit drug and alcohol use, and nutrition.[6,7] It is the latter, nutrition, however, that may be a major determinent in disease progression. Nutritional deficiencies, a decline in immune function, involuntary weight loss, generalized protein-energy malnutrition, and opportunistic infections have been documented as factors in the progression of HIV disease.[5,6,8-17] Several nutrition-related factors have been reported to be responsible for the malnutrition and weight loss in progression to AIDS. These factors include increased metabolism, nutrient losses, malabsorption, and an inadequate food intake.[6,8,18] The "wasting" syndrome (the loss of greater than 10% of body weight) seen in HIV-related patients whose disease has progressed significantly, is included as a condition that, when present, allows the diagnosis of AIDS to be made. Approximately 20% of reported cases of AIDS give wasting as the AIDS-defining diagnosis.[4] Once diagnosed with AIDS, an estimated 80% or more of patients will suffer from the effects of this wasting phenomenon.[19] Although an adequate nutritional intake has not been shown to slow the progression of HIV disease, an improved nutritional status has been widely accepted as improving the quality of life for those affected by this disease.[12] Nutritional intervention instituted among AIDS patients is common practice, but rarely is it instituted early in HIV disease. Nutritional deficiencies and increased energy expenditure have been seen during the asymptomatic stages of HIV disease.[9,19-21]

Researchers suggest that malnutrition occurs in the asymptomatic stage of HIV disease long before signs and symptoms are evident.[3] Nutrition is an essential component necessary to maintain a healthy functioning immune system. A compromised immune system coupled with emotional stress, GI symptoms, malabsorption, and side-effects of various treatment regimens place the person with HIV disease at great risk for malnutrition. If we are to be successful in our medical management of this disease, we must address nutrition support from the outset and aggressively intervene as nutitional deficiencies are identified. Adequate and effective nutrition support can improve the quality, if not the length, of life for these patients.[8,22-24]

For adolescents with HIV infection, the management of nutritional support can be both challenging and frustrating. At no other time are nutritional deficits and excesses more evident than during adolescence. Usually, adolescent eating habits are characterized by irregular meal times, fast foods, missed meals, high-calorie snacks, and dieting.[25] The most likely nutrients to be missed or limited in adolescent diets are vitamin A, calcium, and iron. A high intake of saturated fats, cholesterol, and sodium replace the more important nutrients in the typical adolescent diet.[25]

HIV in Adolescence

As of December 31, 1993, 1528 cases of AIDS had been reported in adolescents ages 13–19 yr. The majority of these cases have occurred in minority youth, mainly African American (40.8% of cases) or hispanic (18.1% of cases) adolescents. Adolescent females account for 477 or 31.2% of all cases in this age group, the highest percentage of cases in any age group except children below the age of 5 yr.[15] Prior to the change in the diagnostic criteria that has recently allowed patients to be classified as AIDS on the basis of CD4 lymphocyte counts alone (<200 cells/mm³), the rate of increase in cases in adolescents was doubling in cases every 14 mo.[26] That rate of increase has been accelerated with the new diagnostic criteria and 1993 saw a 65% increase in reported AIDS cases in 13–19-year-olds.

Counting actual cases of AIDS in adolescents underestimates the importance of the problem of HIV infection in this age group. Most teenagers will not proceed in their illness at a sufficiently rapid course to qualify as a reportable case of AIDS during their adolescence. Although the number of adolescents with HIV infection is unknown, several seroprevalence studies done at hospitals; clinics; outpatient facilities; and among job corps, military applicants, and homeless or runaway youths suggest prevalence between 2.9–22/1000.[20,26–28] One study indicated rates as high as 160/1000 adolescents age 18–21 yr encountered at a New York City homeless shelter.[29]

In a study we performed in Washington, D.C., drawn blood samples were tested over a 4-yr period, anonymously from 11,000 adolescents ages 13–19 yr. These data found that 17.53/1000 adolescents tested positive for antibodies to HIV at year 4, up from 4.07/1000 adolescents at year 1. These data are remarkable in one urban area.

Malnutrition and the Immune System

Malnutrition increases a person's risk for infection. Infection may cause some degree of anorexia, result in negative nitrogen balance, and decrease serum vitamins A and C as a result of increased urinary excretion of these vitamins. With negative nitrogen balance, other nutrient losses can occur, including potassium, magnesium, phosphate, zinc, and sulfate. Negative nitrogen balance is also associated with weight loss and the impairment of growth and development.[30] The immunological consequences of the malnutrition that occurs involve secondary immunodeficiency, a reduction in the ability to clear infections, and an occasional increase in inflammatory responses and tissue damage.[31] "Wasting" may be the nutritional consequence of an impairment of the immune response.[30]

Even when this malnourished state lasts a brief time, chemotaxis is affected, leading to abnormalities in monocytes and macrophages.[9] T-helper lymphocytes begin to show a decrease early on, whereas prolonged malnutrition also affects the B lymphocytes. Stress, illness, and infection can further depress the immune system response.[9] In the person with HIV disease, similar changes also occur; there is a decrease in the T4-helper-inducer lymphocytes, a reduction in the excretion of secretory IgA, and abnormalities in B lymphocytes.[9] For the HIV-positive individual who is also malnourished, there may be a marked increase in the incidence and severity of infections, leading to further damage in an already compromised immune system.[9] According to Mascioli,[7] malnutrition in HIV disease is clinically important because it is prognostic. Malnourished patients will die on average by the time they have lost a third of their usual body weight; this is also the point at which half of usual lean body mass (the metabolically active tissue of the body) has been lost. Indeed, several studies have documented this relationship between weight loss and death.[19,32] Although malnutrition may be the ultimate, inescapable result of HIV progression, "early nutritional intervention may reduce susceptibility to or severity of infections, provide some protection to the immune system, and lead to a better quality of life for HIV-related children."[23]

Nutrition and HIV/AIDS

During the course of HIV disease, nutritional deficiencies, anorexia, and progressive weight loss become the norm.[9] In the early stages of the disease, when the teen is asymptomatic, the only evidence of a nutrient deficiency may be a lowering of the serum level of the trace element zinc as well as decreases in the levels of vitamins B-12 and B-6.[19-21] When the adolescent becomes symptomatic, additional nutrient losses coupled with severe weight loss will occur, mainly as a result of gastrointensinal (GI) disturbances and malabsorption.[4,9] In HIV disease, the GI tract, specifically the esophagus, becomes the major target organ for opportunistic infections,[24,33] particularly in patients experiencing a deterioration in their clinical status. A third of patients with AIDS will develop "opportunistic esophagitis," as evidenced by dysphagia and odynophagia.[33] Other estimates predict that 95% of AIDS patients will develop oral and esophageal complications, oral candidiasis being the most common.[24] In addition to fungal involvement, both cytomegalovirus and herpes simplex virus can cause esophageal disease in adolescents and young adults.

Diarrhea is a prominent GI complaint of patients with HIV infection and often one of the first symptoms seen. It may result from drug therapy, opportunistic infections, or malabsorption.[10,30] Over 60% of patients will develop diarrhea during the course of their illness. The list of opportunistic pathogens that can cause diarrhea is long, with bacterial, viral, fungal, and parasitic organisms all possibly involved.

Anorexia with or without nausea and vomiting can be another gastrointestinal problem associated with HIV infection. These symptoms may be the result of oral and/or esophageal infections, fever associated with other infections, an alteration in taste (frequently as a result of medications), or secondary to emotional distress. The later may result from clinical depression or be the result of factors such as economic worries or family concerns. Common medications such as aerosolized pentamidine and trimethoprim-sulfamethoxazole as well as the anti-retroviral drugs can cause nausea and an alteration in taste, resulting in a decreased desire for food.[8] Pentamidine can also induce hypoglycemia.[30]

Early nutritional intervention can possibly prevent the HIV wasting, enhance the drug treatment slowing the progression of disease, and improve the quality of the patient's life.[3,23,24] Researchers suggest the use of the CDC classification for HIV infection (see Table 24.1) as a framework for the identification of those individuals at greatest risk of nutritional deficiencies.[22] Although patients in the earlier stages of HIV/AIDS (groups I-III) may exhibit few if any nutritional problems, once the teen reaches the late stages of this disease (group IV), the consequences of HIV and subsequent treatments may be detrimental.[22] One report examined subjects who were at the stage III disease process; 67% of these patients evidenced a nutrient deficiency, and of these, 36% had multiple deficiencies.[22] These data are supported by another study examining older hemophiliac children with asymptomatic HIV in which 40% were malnourished compared to 4.5% of the noninfected group with hemophilia.[33] McCorkindale et al.[34] monitored the nutritional status in 19-HIV positive patients over the course of 16 mo and found significant decreases in body weight, percentage body fat, and body mass index. These studies suggest that more than nutrient deficiency may be evident early in HIV disease, and indeed, they contend that body weight, percentage of body fat, and body mass index may be the earliest indication of decreased nutritional status in HIV-infected patients. For these reasons, routine nutritional assessments and support should be a part of the HIV-infected individual's medical management.

There is a long list of nutritional deficiencies that may result in depression of the immune system. Of particular importance to the adolescent, however, are vitamins A, C, E, D, B-6 , B-12, folic acid, beta-carotene, iron, calcium, and magnesium. The trace elements zinc and selenium are also important. These nutrients act directly on the lymphoid system and immune cell function, thereby altering the host cell response to invasion by various pathogens.

Table 24.1   Centers for Disease Control Classification System for HIV Infection

Group I:	Acute Infection
Group II:	Asymptomatic Infection
Group III:	Persistent Generalized Lymphadenopathy
Group IV:	Other Disease
	Subgroup A: Constitutional disease
	Subgroup B: Neurologic disease
	Subgroup C: Secondary infectious diseases
	Subgroup D: Secondary cancers
	Subgroup E: Other conditions with HIV

ASSESSMENT

Requirements in HIV-related Adolescent

Among healthy teenagers, the adolescent years are a period of rapid growth and psychosocial development. Because of the rapid growth and tissue deposition that occurs, there are increased demands for energy and nutrients. Fortunately, the nutritional status of most adolescents is good.[35] Other than iron-deficiency anemia, adolescents in the United States are nutritionally healthier than their ancestors. They are essentially free of the many nutritional diseases of the past such as scurvy, kwashiorkor, marasmus, beri-beri, and rickets.[36]

Unfortunately, some subgroups of adolescents in our society still have inadequate dietary intake and/or show evidence of malnutrition. These subgroups include low-income teens, especially minorities; females; drug and alcohol abusers; and the chronically ill, including those who are HIV-positive. For those adolescents with HIV disease, there is a significant alteration in their nutritional requirements that results when either the disease or therapy needed to control the disease places an undo burden on the body.[35]

The rate of progression of HIV disease in the adolescent is unknown. It is assumed that because of adolescents' well-developed immune system, their progression will be similar to that of adults. However, it is believed that the clinical progression is different from that seen in adults. For example, the adult wasting phenomenon is defined by a loss greater than 10%. For adolescents undergoing puberty, when height and weight are increasing rapidly, an arrest of the normal growth process may be significant.[35]

Energy and calories.   Energy from protein, fat and carbohydrates is needed for metabolic maintenance, physical activity, and optimal growth. Its presence or absence will often determine the adequacy of other nutrients in our diet. If energy intake is adequate in the adolescent's diet and properly dispersed between these food groups, it is likely that the other nutrients are also adequate.

During adolescence, a higher intake of nutrients per kilocalorie is required. The number of calories consumed by teens will vary greatly depending on age, body size, and activity level (see Table 24.2). For example, the average daily caloric allowance for boys ages 11–14 yr, is 2500 cal; for ages 15–18, the allowance is 3000 cal. For girls ages 11–18 yr, the average daily allowance is 2200 cal.[31] As one can see, males have a greater need for calories than females.

In HIV infection, anorexia and malabsorption account for most of the weight loss seen in HIV disease. However, studies have shown an increase in resting energy expenditure (REE) in HIV-positive patients.[13,16] Data suggest an REE increase of 11% in HIV-positive patients, 25% in AIDS patients, and in AIDS patients with symptomatology (infections), 29% above a control group.[14] It has

Table 24.2   Caloric Requirements for Normal Adolescents

Category	Age (yr)	Reference Weight (kg)	REE* (cal/kg)	RDA (cal/ kg)	(gm/kg)
MALES					
	11–14	45	32	55	1.0
	15–18	66	27	45	0.9
	19–24	72	25	40	0.8
FEMALES					
	11–14	46	28	47	1.0
	15–18	55	25	40	0.8
	19–24	58	23	38	0.8

* Resting energy expenditure computed from WHO equations.

Adapted from Food and Nutrition Board, National Research Council, in *Recommended Dietary Allowances (RDA), 10th ed.*, National Academy of Sciences, Washington, DC, (1989).

been suggested that the anorexia and rapid weight loss seen in patients with AIDS may be indicative of these infections.[36]

Protein.   Essential for growth and development, and the maintenance of body tissues. About 12–14% of the energy intake comes from proteins.[35] Protein requirements are determined by the adolescents' rate of growth, dietary intake, amino acid composition of the dietary protein, adequate energy intake, and their health and nutritional status. One way to determine the protein needs of the individual teen is to calculate grams of protein per centimeter of height. This method indirectly accounts for the adolescent growth spurt. There is a high correlation between the 1989 Recommended Daily Allowance (RDA) recommendations for protein and grams of protein per centimeter of height. For example, for males and females 11–14 yr, the daily recommendation is 0.29 g/cm of height. Using body weight, boys and girls 11–14 yr require 1 g/kg of body weight, whereas boys 15–18 yr require 0.9g/kg and girls 15–18 yr, 0.8g/kg. Adolescents from low-income families, those who are strict vegetarians, and those who are chronic dieters are subject to protein deficiency.[35] Because growth is a sensitive indicator of protein status,[35] an inadequate intake of protein may impair the teen's growth. Protein deficiency has been shown in animal studies to precipitate the onset of *Pneumocystis carinii* (PCP), an AIDS-defining infection.[37]

Carbohydrates.   A major energy source made up of sugars and starches, as well as the primary source of dietary fiber. Carbohydrates aid in the breakdown of fats and, along with proteins, help to form compounds that are essential for combating infections. No daily requirement for carbohydrates has been established, but most nutritional experts suggest that 50% of total calories in the diet come from carbohydrates. Adolescents often prefer foods high in sugars (soda, candy, or cookies) that tend to be insufficient in nutrients. These "refined" sugars also tend to be high in fat. Complex sugars (starches) found in vegetables, fruits, beans, and grains provide the body with glucose and are a good source of fiber. Because these complex sugars are released more slowly from the stomach than simple sugars, they produce a longer-lasting insulin stimulation that in turn, provides more synthesis of glycogen from glucose.[38] Improved glycogen stores will greatly benefit the HIV-positive adolescent when food intake may be compromised by GI manifestations associated with this disease.

Fats.   Provide more than twice the kilocalories per gram than either proteins or carbohydrates. For this reason, HIV-related adolescents may actually benefit from a higher fat intake than would be usually suggested because these foods are more "calorically dense." Moreover, certain fatty acids, i.e., linoleic, linolenic, and arachidonic acids, cannot be synthesized by the body so they must be supplied directly by our diet. These acids are essential for the production of important chemicals, including hormones that stimulate puberty itself. Fats are also necessary for healthy skin and hair, for body temperature regulation, and to transport certain fat-soluble vitamins (A, D, E, and K) into the body.[39]

There are no RDAs for fat or cholesterol in the diet, although the recommendation is that at least 3% of total energy come from essential fatty acids.[35] Most experts recommend that only 30–40% of our caloric intake be comprised of fat with less than 10% coming from saturated fats. For cholesterol, 300 mg or less/ d is sufficient.[35] There are two types of fats: saturated and unsaturated. Arachidonic acid is the unsaturated fatty acid relevant to immune system functioning. A product of arachidonic acid, prostaglandins, plays a role in immunoregulation such as the proliferation of T cells and the function of natural killer cells. Hence, the adequate intake of fats may be of increased importance for the HIV-related adolescent.

Minerals.   The need for all minerals increases in adolescence. During the adolescent growth spurt, there are two minerals of particular importance: iron and calcium. Additionally, zinc and selenium, trace minerals, are important as they relate to HIV disease.

IRON.   Based on serum ferritin levels, in the healthy noninfected adolescent, iron-deficiency anemia may be seen in up to 20% of girls and 10% of boys. Iron is essential for the expansion of red blood cell volume and tissue growth during this period. Losses of iron in stool and urine, from the skin, and during the menstrual cycle must be balanced by an adequate dietary intake. The National

Research Council (NRC) recommends a daily intake of 12 mg for boys and 15 mg for girls during puberty. The American diet contains 6 mg of iron/1000 cal. Adolescent girls will ingest somewhere between 2000–2400 cal/d, falling short of the RDA requirements from the diet alone. For boys who ingest 3000 cal or more/d, iron intake is likely not problematic.[39]

Anemia is part of the natural progression of HIV disease. It can result from failure of the bone marrow or as a result of destructive cell processes. It can also be caused by bone marrow suppression secondary to drugs such as the antiretroviral drug, zidovudine. Despite iron's overall importance, it is not clear that iron deficiency will be seen in increased frequency in HIV-related adolescents.

CALCIUM.   Alterations in the metabolism of calcium are uncommon in AIDS patients when renal function is normal. However, in the event of lymphoma or with the use of drug therapy, serum calcium may increase or decrease. Hypercalcemia can occur when tumor cells that produce 25-hydroxylase result in the increased hydroxylation of 25-hydroxyvitamin D to dihydroxyvitamin D3. Foscarnet, a drug used in the treatment of CMV retinitis, can impair renal function, leading to an increase or decrease in serum calcium.[40] Calcium is essential during adolescence to ensure bone growth; therefore, it is higher during this period.[7,23]

ZINC.   Essential for synthesizing new skeletal and muscle tissue, as well as adequate sexual maturation. Several studies have shown that pediatric and adult HIV/AIDS patients have a zinc deficiency.[9,23,24,30] Zinc deficiency results in diarrhea, failure to thrive, delayed puberty, serious viral, bacterial, and fungal infections, and a marked reduction in T-helper lymphocytes helper-inducer lymphocytes, and B lymphocytes.[31] Studies reported show a "zinc syndrome" that occurs in pediatric and adult patients.[30] This syndrome involves an eczematous perioral and perianal rash, hair loss, conjunctivitis, chronic diarrhea, bacterial and candida infections concomitantly, stomatitis, growth retardation, and severe immunodeficiency.

SELENIUM.   An "antioxidant," meaning that selenium attaches itself to harmful oxygen molecules called "free radicals," thus providing some protection against disease that may be mediated by these molecules. Selenium plays an important role in production and mobility and may increase immune responses. Selenium deficiency may be related to a decrease in T-helper lymphocytes.[30] Low levels of T-helper numbers were responsive to selenium repletion.[30] Selenium has also been associated with degeneration of the heart muscle and may be related to the cardiomyopathy seen in HIV disease.[24,29,30]

Vitamins.   For optimal functioning of the immune system vitamins and minerals are essential. An adequate diet generally supplies all the essential vitamins and minerals for a healthy body. However, among the HIV-infected, a deficiency of certain vitamins has been documented even when an adequate diet along with supplemental vitamins was consumed.[41] The malabsorption seen in HIV disease is one reason why supplements do not correct vitamin deficiencies. Clinical diagnosis of vitamin deficencies can however, be an early sign of progressive malnutrition and, in turn, disease progression. Clinical examination can reveal severe vitamin deficiency, but in HIV-related individuals, vitamin deficiencies are more likely to be mild and subclinical. During normal adolescence, there is an increased need for vitamins. Of importance are vitamins A, C, D, E; vitamins B-6 and B-12; folate; thiamin; niacin; and riboflavin.

VITAMIN A.   A fat-soluble nutrient, vitamin A plays a role in vision, growth and development, cell differentiation, reproduction, and the integrity of the immune system. A deficiency in vitamin A, seen in HIV-positive individuals, has been associated with an increase in the severity and frequency of bacterial, viral, and parasitic infections.[41] Beta-carotene is an antioxidant, a compound that may protect against disease by the neutralization of unstable oxygen molecules, called free radicals, that form in our bodies.[38] It has been postulated that oxidative stress is a component in the pathogenesis of HIV disease.[38] Lemens and Sterrit[38] define oxidative stress as the net effect of a "deleterious reductive-oxidative (redox) imbalance" that occurs secondary to damage to the immune system from HIV disease. As antioxidant reducing agents are being depleted, oxygen atoms (free radicals) are increasing. The result of this imbalance in HIV disease may be increased viral replication. Beta-carotene is said to bind with these free radicals before they have a chance to cause damage. However, there is no scientific evidence that proves antioxidants like beta-carotene slow down disease progression or improve survival for people with HIV disease.

VITAMIN C.   For adolescents who smoke, studies reveal a lower concentration of ascorbic acid in serum and leukocytes. However, one report found no significant harmful effects on lymphocyte numbers and proliferative responses even in severe vitamin C deficiency.[31]

VITAMIN D.   In only one reported study on vitamin D deficiency in HIV disease, Malcolm et al.[43] found normal levels in all 14 study patients diagnosed with AIDS related complex (ARC) and/or AIDS. Coodley and Girard[44] report a number of in vitro studies that suggest this vitamin may have a strong influence on the immune response, particularly that of T lymphocytes. However, no in vivo studies have been done to date to confirm this suggestion.

VITAMIN E.   Because of an abundance of vitamin E in cereal grains and vegetable oils, a deficiency of this vitamin is highly unlikely.[42] Unfortunately, in HIV this is not the case. Studies show a prevalence of vitamin E deficiency among AIDS patients.[44] The cause of this deficiency is not clear; however, it is thought to be due to the malabsorption seen in the progression of HIV.[45] The "yellow nail syndrome" seen among AIDS patients is associated with Vitamin E deficiency and has been shown to respond to supplementation with vitamin E.[30] Other studies suggest that vitamin E supplements favorably modulate the immune response in HIV disease.[44] Adolescents require more of this vitamin as they form new cells.

FOLIC ACID. Helps prevent anemia and certain birth defects of the spine and brain. It also helps to make DNA. Next to iron-deficiency anemia, folate deficiency is the second leading cause of nutritional anemia. It impairs iron metabolism or iron incorporation into heme. Among adolescents, a rapid growth coupled with an increase in DNA synthesis results in an increase in folic acid. Folic acid deficiency is very common in adolescence. In addition, it may be a common clinical problem in HIV.[44] Malnutrition and malabsorption, along with the widespread use of antifolate drugs in HIV patients, are the reason for this assumption. However, no agreement about the role of folic acid in HIV disease has been reported. Of the studies, either an excess or a deficiency was reported among study populations.[44]

VITAMIN B-6. Although rare within the general population, B-6 deficiency has been reported as a common occurrence in HIV disease.[49] Examination of B-6 deficiency in a group of HIV-positive patients revealed a lower CD4 count, uniformly over a group without B-6 deficiency.[44] These researchers suggest prescribing vitamin B-6 to HIV-positive patients to improve CD4 counts.

VITAMIN B-12. Needed to synthesize DNA and make blood, vitamin B-12 (cobalamin) helps prevent anemia and maintains the nervous system. A deficiency of this vitamin is common in HIV disease and can occur at any stage of the disease. An altered intestinal flora along with malabsorption is said to be the cause of B-12 deficiency.

THIAMIN, NIACIN, AND RIBOFLAVIN. Thiamin is a component of enzymes involved in energy metabolism. It is required for cell reproduction, fatty acid metabolism, and nervous system functions. Data suggest that thiamin deficiency, although associated with malnutrition, is probably not common in HIV disease.[44]

Niacin is involved in energy metabolism and the synthesis of carbohydrates and fats, helps in the functioning of the nervous and digestive systems, and maintains healthy skin. Diarrhea and dementia are seen in patients with niacin deficiency. It has been postulated that this deficiency is responsible for similar symptoms seen in HIV.[44]

Riboflavin helps in the utilization of other B vitamins, carbohydrates, fats, and proteins. Pharyngitis and anemia are commonly found with a deficiency of this vitamin. However, reports completed in asymptomatic HIV-positive patients found no deficiency of this vitamin.[44]

Other Considerations

Cultural. Each culture has a value system that affects behavior and sets norms for the group. Extended families that may not include blood relatives are traditional and should not be overlooked. Nutritional practices and health beliefs of the individual reflect his or her value system.[25] If health care providers are to effectively counsel teens and their families regarding HIV disease and nutrition, they must have a better understanding of group characteristics and dynamics.

African American and hispanic youth are disproportionately affected by this virus. The latest national figures out on AIDS as of 1994, has AIDS as the leading cause of death in African American males aged 24–44 yr. Among members of the hispanic/Latino community, 17% of all reported cases of AIDs were identified even though this group represents only 6% of the population. In addition, this group has a faster rate of disease progression and shorter survival. Flaskerud[37] suggests that the reason for this may be is due to several factors, including a delay in seeking medical care, lower quantity and quality of medical care, poorer health conditions before HIV exposure, and less knowledge of AIDS as well as other risk-taking behaviors.

Pregnacy. There are over 1 million teens who become pregnant each year in the United States, with approximately one-half of these pregnancies culminating in childbirth. Teens of normal weight with appropriate weight gain during pregnancy can expect similar outcomes (specifically birth weight) as adult women.[46] For many adolescents however, impaired fetal as well as maternal growth and development are far more common an outcome (see Chapter 13). For the pregnant adolescent who is HIV-positive, a more complicated picture emerges and morbidity may be compounded.

Pregnancy has been associated with cell-mediated immunity.[47] A significant decrease of T-helper lymphocytes has been shown to occur in normal pregnancy, with a return to normal around the 5th postpartum month. HIV disease, which also causes a decrease in T-helper lymphocytes, has not been demonstrated to lead to higher rates of prematurity, low birth weight, or other poor outcomes associated with pregnancy.[54] Concerns remain regarding the effects of pregnancy on the progression of disease, despite research findings to the contrary.[47] However, a higher risk of serious infections in those women with T-helper lymphocytes fewer than 300/mm3 does occur.[47] Reactivation of latent infections such as herpes simplex virus can lead to higher morbidity. Obviously, infection itself has adverse effects on the immune function and requires a sound nutritional approach for the HIV-positive adolescent.

Nutritional Support Early in HIV Disease

Prevention of malnutrition must be the goal of nutritional care of all those with HIV and AIDS. Optimal nutritional repletion is essential in slowing disease progression. A comprehensive nutritional assessment must be done on all HIV-positive adolescents at the time of diagnosis. Assessment should include the following five components.

Dietary history. Along with an evaluation of the adolescent's nutritional status a dietary history is essential to examine habits, beliefs, or related physical findings that could impact on the nutritional health of the adolescent. The 24–48-h recall is a useful tool to utilize when obtaining a diet history. Assessment of recent weight loss, fever, oral-motor feeding problems, vitamin and mineral supplements, ethnic preferences, lactose intolerance, and recent history of nausea, vomiting, and/or diarrhea should be documented. Timing and meal preparation should also be assessed.

Clinical history. This method relies on an observation of physical signs and symptoms related to nutrient deficiency. However, clinical signs related to nutrient deficiency are often nonspecific for a given nutrient or related to other factors.[48] Symptoms such as pallor, emaciation, edema, or obesity are easily recognized. Used in conjunction with the other methods, a better assessment of nutritional status can be made.

Anthropometric measurement. This technique provides a quantitative measure of nutritional status. It detects inadequate or excessive nutrients compared to an approved standard. One of the best ways to measure nutritional status over time is to look at height and weight. Weight for age is not an appropriate measure because it does not consider differences in height.[48] Besides height and weight, other useful parameters include midarm circumference and triceps skinfold (see Chapter 18). These methods have been useful in the body of research assessing nutrient deficiency in HIV disease.

Biochemical assay. Specific nutrient deficiencies such as hypoproteinemia, iron deficiency, and anemia are identified through biochemical tests that measure their values before these conditions can be picked up clinically.[48] Serum albumin, hemoglobin, hematocrit, mean corpuscular volume, and specific vitamin and mineral levels are the more frequent tests utilized.

Body Image. Should also be assessed by the clinical dietitian (see Chapter 8). In addition to weight loss, hair loss, skin changes, and GI manifestations can be very debilitating to the patient and lead to a loss of self-esteem. For the adolescent, a diagnosis of HIV disease can lead to a very real fear of being rejected by his or her peer group, almost to a greater extent than the fear of dying from this disease.[49] Weaver[49] states that persons with optimal nutritional status report improved body image. This sense of well-being leads to "feelings of hope, purposefulness, and social worth."

MANAGEMENT

Many experts in the field are now recommending nutrition support when the patient is first diagnosed, prior to any symptomatology.[7,9,24,48,50] If initiated early, a baseline can be established from which any changes will be readily seen. Also, early intervention may prevent the wasting seen in disease progression, thereby improving the quality of the adolescent life.[24]

According to Bunce,[50] "the goal of nutritional intervention is to maintain, and, if necessary, replete lean body mass. " The benefits of early intervention include maintenance of weight and prevention of muscle tissue breakdown; optimizing responses to medications and other therapies; improving strength and minimizing fatigue; providing a sense of well-being; and improving quality of life.

Nutrition Support in Early HIV Disease

After the initial assessmnent, education should begin by explaining the importance of nutrition in the management of HIV. One way to achieve this goal is through the use of a "flip chart" that can be viewed by the adolescent during the counseling session. This is an excellent occasion to address the adolescent's image of self, specifically his or her concerns about weight gain and/or weight loss. This is also a good time to discuss the use of oral supplements to enhance caloric intake with a specific discussion of avoiding "megadosing." Other alternative therapies may need to be addressed based on the teen's interest. A nutritional care plan should be initiated and adjusted as the progression of disease becomes evident. As part of the care plan, the recommended diet is high in calories, protein, and fiber, with adequate to upper limits of fat. We also recommend a single multivitamin with iron and minerals that meets the RDA for nutrients (100%).

For the adolescent with asymptomatic disease whose oral intake is found to be two-thirds or more of calculated need, nutritional counseling, supplementation (vitamins, higher caloric solid or liquid supplements), and a focus on nutrients from the five food groups are sufficient. This planning must be done with the teen's involvement and cooperation. As malabsorption and infection become problematic, protein requirements need to be adjusted. As a general rule of thumb, we estimate the protein requirement to be about double the norm.

Nutrition Support in AIDS Patients

Symptoms common to disease progression such as chronic fevers, night sweats, diarrhea, and weight loss significantly increase the need for more protein and calories. In the symptomatic patient, caloric needs may need to be tripled. The Harris and Benedict equations (see Table 24.3) to calculate caloric needs

Table 24.3   Calculating Caloric and Protein Requirements

Weight gain = basal energy expenditure (BEE) $\times$ 1.5
Weight maintenance = BEE + 1.3

To calculate protein requirements for:

Repletion: 1.0–1.2 g of protein daily/kg of body weight
Maintenance: 0.8–1.0 g

Adapted from A. R. Mawson, R. P. Warrier, S. Kuvibidila, R. M.Suskind, in *Textbook of Pediatric Nutrition, 2 ed.,* (R.M. Suskind and L. Lewinter-Suskind, eds.), Raven Press Limited, New York, pp. 447–455 (1993).

can be employed. For the teen who needs to gain weight (when oral intake falls below two-thirds of nutritional requirements), a caloric intake of at least 150% of the RDA is recommended. To prevent continued weight loss and reach a positive nitrogen balance, protein requirements for the patient diagnosed with AIDS are estimated at 2.0–3.0g/kg/d. As long as the patient can tolerate oral feedings, this is the preferable method. By using the GI tract, the integrity of the bowel can be maintained.[24] Small, frequent meals should be encouraged. Because appetite is affected with increased fever, an appetite "stimulant" may need to be utilized. Megestrol acetate (Megace) has been approved by the FDA as an appetite stimulant. Megace increases appetite, leading to weight gain in the patient with AIDS.[7] A dosage of 40 mg orally three times a day is adequate. Side-effects of Megace include venous thrombosis, edema, and impotence.[7] In those with oral manifestions of HIV disease (candidiasis), changes in acidity temperature, texture, consistency, and seasoning of the food can help to maintain oral ingestion of nutrients. For the adolescent with diarrhea, nutritional management is often very difficult. In teens or young adults with "osmotic" diarrhea (associated with hypoalbuminemia and malnutrition), antidiarrheal agents or bowel rest are indicated. Restricting the patient's intake of lactose and fatty foods will also help. If tube feeding is to be initiated, an isotonic formula free of lactose should be given.[30] Patients that develop "cryptosporidiosis" infection end up with "secretory" diarrhea that does not respond to any of the forementioned treatments. Thus, these patients are very difficult to manage.[30] A comprehensive description by Probart[24] suggests that the optimal diet in the presence of symptoms caused by opportunistic infection should "include foods that will not irritate an infected oral cavity considering temperature, texture, and consistency of foods; supply adequate, high quality protein such as glutamine; contribute adequate calories; and provide 100% of the Recommended Dietary Allowances for vitamins and minerals and adequate amounts of trace elements such as selenium and zinc." When oral intake is compromised because of GI tract disturbances (diarrhea, malabsorption, or oral/esophageal lesions), "enteral" formulas may be utilized either orally or via nasogastric tube.[32] An intact-protein, lactose-free formula, low in fat, should be used. Parenteral nutrition is necessary only in severe malnutrition with evidence of lean body mass loss, at which time, the patient is usually hospitalized. This particular therapy may have to be continued when the patient goes home until the wasting syndrome has been reversed.[7]

Alteration of Body Image

For the teen or young adult with AIDS, the effect of malnutrition and severe weight loss on body image may be demoralizing and detrimental.[51] For the adolescent, whose task at this time is to formalize a sense of self, a disorder such as HIV/AIDS can delay or destroy self-image. In working with the adolescent who is HIV-positive, helping him or her to establish a positive sense of self should be a top priority. The importance of weight in the adolescent's identification with health in relationship to this disease should not be overlooked. Most minority youths see unintentional weight loss as a visible sign that he or she has AIDS. In our work with HIV-positive adolescents, it has become apparent that once the diagnosis of HIV infection has been established, the desire to *gain* weight becomes a driving force, especially among adolescent females. Weight gains of 10–35 lb are common. For this reason, nutritional counseling should begin early in HIV disease for adolescents in an effort to prevent unusually *excessive* gains in weight that can occur. Obesity can impair the calculation of optimal drug dosage and cause impairment of the immune system (in the form of a slight impairment of delayed cutaneous hypersensitivity responses, decreased lymphocyte response to mitogens, and reduced bactericidal capacity of neutrophils).[7]

Nutrition and Alternative Therapy

Alternative medical treatments have long been a part of our society and the approach to HIV infection for many patients. Its use in this disease grew out of a frustration with the early lack of conventional treatments that were efficacious. Unconventional, natural, or complementary therapies for AIDS are terms often used to describe these approaches. Alternative therapies focus on a holistic approach rather than on the disease itself.[13] A number of alternative therapies being used with unknown success include traditional Chinese medicine, herbal compounds, physical manipulation techniques, spiritual approaches, and nutritional supplements.[39] Greenberg[39] provides a comprehensive review of these alternative treatments.

Alternative nutrition in HIV disease emphasizes the consumption of raw seasonal fruits, grains, and vegetables. Between 50–200g/d megadoses of vitamin C may be recommended, even though this high amount exceeds a normal person's bowel tolerance. A macrobiotic diet, utilizing *yin* and *yang* to balance foods, will in turn, promote a longer life. Yin foods are acid-forming and yang foods alkaline-forming.

For the adolescent who chooses alternative therapy, we must allow for the discussion to occur in an open, honest manner based on our knowledge of the facts, not personal biases. We must help our patients judge the usefulness of alternative therapy based on cost, safety, effectiveness, and exclusiveness, i.e., all other interventions are discontined in lieu of one. Similiar to other treatments utilized, the risks against the benefits must be carefully examined.[52]

Counseling

Cultural diversity is another area to address in order to provide optimal nutrition support. Dietary planning must include foods chosen from the appropriuate cultural group after discussions with the adolescent and family. Socioeconomic level, diversity in language, culture, and education must be considered to effectively counsel ethnically diverse adolescents. In addition, one must be aware of how health and disease impact each group and what beliefs are held in order to effect change. A survey by Luder[53] suggests that the most effective way to improve the dietary habits of adolescents from diverse groups is to improve the quality of their meals eaten outside the home. For example, replace foods high in fat, sugar, salt, and cholesterol with more nutritious foods like yogurt, fish, fruits, nuts, ethnic breads, high-fiber cereals, juices, and milk. Improvement in the school lunch program to include ethnic choices should be strongly advocated by the clinical dietitian.

As HIV-positive minority youth begin to interface with the medical community for the management and support of their disease, practitioners must begin to individualize care based on cultural understanding. If we do not recognize these differences, noncompliance, poor cooperation, inadequate use of health services, and alienation from health services will prove to be costly for the teen or young adult.[53,54]

Summary

In the coming years, we can expect to see increasing numbers of adolescents who are HIV-infected, some of whom will progress in their disease to fulfill the case definition of AIDS. We will be challenged to provide the best and most comprehensive care possible. This care will by necessity include nutritional support. Ensuring adequate nutrition will give the adolescent who is HIV-infected a better chance to respond to exogenous treatments and give his or her own immune system the best chance to respond to this infection. It is fair to expect that this will result in a longer and better-quality life.

CASE ILLUSTRATION

Mary is a 16-year-old African American female who was diagnosed HIV-positive 10 mo ago. She contracted the HIV disease from heterosexual contact. At the time of diagnosis, her weight was 112 lbs (48.2 kg) and height 5'3" (160 cm). Mary was not referred for nutritional evaluation until her CD4 count began to drop below 500/mm^3 and her appetite decreased. At the time of her appointment with the dietitian, her weight had dropped to 106 lb (48.2 kg). Her appetite had improved slightly, but she has been experiencing watery diarrhea intermittently for the past 2 wk. Anthropometric data were obtained and revealed her weight at 87% index body weight (IBW), indicating stage I, mild acute malnutrition according to Waterlow criteria. Her midarm muscle circumference indicated mildly depleted muscle mass.

Laboratory data obtained consisted of:

ALBUMIN	HEMOGLOBIN
3.2 g/dL	11.1 g/dL
(3.8–5.4)	(12.0–16.0)

HEMATOCRIT	ZINC
35.0%	57 mcg
(36.0–46.0)	(68–94)

Dietary recall indicated limited calories, iron, and calcium. Mary was lactose-intolerant and had routinely avoided most dairy products. A 3-d food record analyzed by computer confirmed that Mary.'s usual intake was providing:

1980 kcal/d	83% goal	(goal=2×REE)
68 g of Protein/d	117% goal	(goal=1.2gm/kg/d)
480 mg of Calcium/d	32% RDA	
10 mg of Iron/d	67% RDA	

Mary appeared receptive to nutritional counseling in order to improve her diet. Her maternal aunt attended the appointments and was committed to helping, even though family resources were limited. Recommendations included a multivitamin with minerals (containing iron and zinc), 8 oz Ensure Plus/d (355 kcal, 13 g of protein); Tums, 1 extra-strength at each meal; and a food record to be kept for 5 d. At her follow-up appointment 5 wk later, Mary reported an improvement in appetite. She had experienced no diarrhea for the past 4 wk. Her weight had increased to 108 lbs (48.3 kg, 89% IBW). She was somewhat compliant with taking her multivitamin and Tums, but had only taken the Ensure Plus for 12 d (the 12-can supply given to her by the clinic) secondary to an improvement in her appetite and because of cost. Her 5-d food record revealed an improvement in the types and amounts of food consumed. Computer analysis showed an intake of 2290 kcal and greater than 100% RDA for vitamins and minerals when the supplements were taken. Mary continues to be monitored closely by her practitioneer and will be reevaluated by the nutritionist in 6 mo. Because Mary's repeat CD4 count was >500/mm^3 1 month after the initial count below 500/mm^3, she was not started on AZT prophylasis.

REFERENCES

1. S. L. Boswell and M. S. Hirsch, in *AIDS: Etiology, Diagnosis, Treatment, and Prevention*, (V. T. DeVita, S. Hellman, and S. A. Rosenberg, eds.), J. B. Lipincott, Philadelphia, PA, pp. 417–433 (1990).

2. *HIV Infection and the Adolescent*, New York State Department of Social Services, New York (1990).

3. C. D. Newman, *AIDS Patient Care*, **4** (suppl1), S6 (1990).

4. M. J. McKinley, J. Goodman-Block, M. L. Lesser, and A. D. Salbe, *J. Am. Diet. Assoc.*, **94**, 1014 (1994).

5. J. C. Melchior, D. Salmon, D. Rigaud, et al., *Am. J. Clin. Nutr.*, **53**, 437 (1991).

6. B. B. Timbo and L. Tollefson, *J. Am. Diet. Assoc.*, **94**, 1019 (1994).

7. E. A. Mascioli, *AIDS Clinical Care*, **5**, 85 (1993).

8. S. S. Resler, *J. Am. Diet. Assoc.*, **88**, 828 (1988).

9. R. J. Andrassy, *AIDS Patient Care*, **4** (suppl.1), S9 (1990).

10. M. B. Heyman, *Personal communication*. (1990)

11. M. S. Singla, S. P. Marcuard, and R. L. Rumley, *AIDS Patient Care*, **7**, 132 (1993).

12. D. C. Macallan, C. Noble, C. Baldwin, et al., *International Conference on AIDS*, June 1993 Abstract no. PO-B36–2373, 9 (Issue 1), p. 531, Toronto, (1993).

13. M. Hommes, J. A. Romijn, E. Endert, and H. P. Sauerwein, *Am. J. Clin. Nutr.*, **54**, 311 (1991).

14. D. Kotler, A. Tierney, J. Wang, and R. Pierson, *Am. J. Clin. Nutr.*, **50**, 444 (1989).

15. D. C. Macallan, C. Noble, C. Baldwin, M. Foskett, T. McManus, and G. E. Griffin, *Am. J. Clin. Nutr.*, **58**, 417 (1993).

16. C. Grunfeld, M. Pang, L. Shimizu, J. K. Shigenaga, P. Jensen, and R. Feingold, *Am. J. Clin. Nutr.*, **55**, 455 (1992).

17. S. J. Sharkey, K. A. Sharkey, L. R. Sutherland, D. L. Church, and GI/HIV Study Group, *J. AIDS*, **11**, 1091 (1992).

18. ADA Reports, *J. Am. Diet. Assoc.*, **94**, 1042 (1994).

19. R. T. Chelebowski, M. B. Grosvenor, N. H. Bernhard, L. S. Morales, and L. M. Bulavage, *Am. J. Gastroenterol.*, **84**, 1288 (1989).

20. S. H. Vermund, K. Hein, H. D. Gayle, J. D. Cary, P. A. Thomas, and E. Drucker, *AJDC*, **143**, 1220 (1989).

21. M. Hambidge, in *Textbook of Pediatric Nutrition, 2nd ed.*, (R. M. Suskind and L. Lewinter-Suskind, eds.), Raven Press Limited, New York, pp. 115–126 (1993).

22. J. K. Keithley and C. L. Kohn, *Oncol. Nurs. Forum*, **17**, 23 (1990).

23. S. W. Nicholas, J. Leung, and I. Fennoy, *J. Peds.*, **119** (suppl.), S59 (1991).

24. C. K. Probart, *J. School Health*, **59**, 170 (1989).

25. Committee on Nutrition American Acadamy of Pediatrics, in *Pediatric Nutrition-Handbook,* American Academy of Pediatrics, Elkgrove Village, IL (1993).

26. M. D. Kipke and K. Hein, *Adol. Med.: State Art Rev.*, **1**, 429 (1990).

27. K. Hein and D. Futterman, *J. Peds.*, **119** (suppl.), 18 (1991).

28. H. D. Gayle and L. J. D'Angelo, in *Pediatric AIDS: The Challenge of HIV Infection in Infants, Children, and Adolescents,* (P. A. Pizza and C. B. Wilfert, eds.), Williams and Wilkins, Baltimore, MD, pp. .38–50 (1991).

29. R. L. Stricof, *Am. J. Pub.Health*, **50**, 232 (1991).

30. A. R. Mawson, R. P. Warrier, S. Kuvibidila, and R. M.Suskind, in *Textbook of Pediatric Nutrition, 2nd ed.*, (R. M. Suskind and L. Lewinter-Suskind, eds.), Raven Press Limited, New York, pp. 447–455 (1993).

31. R. U. Sorensen, L. E. Leiva, and S. Kuvibidila, in *Textbook of Pediatric Nutrition, 2nd ed.,*(R. M. Suskind and L. Lewinter-Suskind, eds.), Raven Press Limited, New York, pp. 141–160 (1993).

32. C. B. Wilcox, *Am. J. Med.*, **92**, 412 (1992).

33. R. U. Sorensen, S. Kuvibidila, and R. M. Suskind, in *Textbook of Pediatric Nutrition, 2nd ed.*, (R. M. Suskind and L. Lewinter-Suskind, eds.), Raven Press Limited, New York, pp. 437–446 (1993).

34. C. McCorkindale, K. Dybevik, A. M. Coulston, and K. P. Sucker, *J. Am. Diet. Assoc.*, **90**, 1236 (1990).

35. J. T. Dwyer, *Adol. Med.: State Art Rev.*, **3**, 377 (1992).

36. M. Story, in *Textbook of Adolescent Medicine*, (E. R. McAnarney, R. E. Kreipe, D. P. Orr, and G. D. Comerci, eds.), W. B. Saunders, Philadelphia, PA, pp. 75–84 (1992).

37. J. H. Flaskerud, in *HIV/AIDS: A Guide to Nursing Care, 2nd Ed.*, (J. H. Flaskerud and P. J. Ungvarski, eds.), W. B. Saunders, Philadelphia, PA, pp. 314–349 (1992).

38. C. Lemens and C. Sterrit, *GMHC Treatment Issues*, **7**, 25 (1993).

39. J. Greenberg, *GMHC Treatment Issues*, **7**, 25 (1993).

40. B. L. Lee, and S. Safin, in *The AIDS Knowledge Base, 2nd ed.*, (P. T. Cohen , ed.), Little, Brown and Company, Boston, MA, pp. 4.6-1- 4.6–18 (1994).

41. D. Link, *GMHC Treatment Issues*, **7**, 15 (1993).

42. R. Wheeler and S. Malone, in *Pediatric Nursing Care*, (G. M. Scipien, M. A. Chard, J. Howe, and M.U. Barnard, eds.), C. V. Mosby, St. Louis, MO, pp. 138–161 (1990).

43. J. A. Malcolm et al., in *Proceedings of the Sixth International Conference on AIDS*, Abstract Th.B 206, **6** (Issue 1), p. 169, San Francisco, CA (1990).

44. G. Coodley and D. E. Girard, *J. Gen. Intern. Med.*, **6**, 472 (1991).

45. R. E. Olson, in *Textbook of Pediatric Nutrition, 2 ed.*, (R. M. Suskind and L. Lewinter-Suskind, eds.), Raven Press Limited, New York, pp. 49–71 (1993).

46. J. M. Rees, and S. A. Lederman, *Adol. Med.: State Art Rev.*,**3**, 439 (1992).

47. K. M. Nokes, in *HIV/AIDS: A Guide to Nursing Care, 2nd Ed.*, (J. H. Flaskerud and P. J. Ungvarski, eds.), W. B. Saunders, Philadelphia, PA, p..396 (1992).

48. R. Figueroa-Colon, T. K. von Almen, and R. M. Suskind, in *Textbook of Pediatric Nutrition, 2 ed.*, (R. M. Suskind and L. Lewinter-Suskind, eds.), Raven Press Limited, New York, pp. .285–293 (1993).

49. K. E. Weaver, in *Gastrointestinal Manifestations of AIDS*, (D. P. Kotler, ed.), Raven Press Limited, New York, pp. 279–292 (1991).

50. L. V. Bunce, *AIDS Clinical Care*, **5**, 88 (1993).

51. A. Smerko, *AIDS Patient Care*, **4** (suppl.1), S17 (1990).

52. G. D. Comerci, K. A. Kilbourne, and G. G. Harrison, in *Adolescent Medicine*, (A.Hofmann and D. Greydanus, eds.), Appleton & Lange, Norwalk, CT, pp. 431–440 (1989).

53. E. Luder, *Adol. Med.: State Art Rev.*, **3**, 405 (1992).

54. H. E. Fox, in *Pediatric AIDS: The Challenge of Infection in Infants, Children, and Adolescents*, (P. A. Pizza and C. B. Wilfert, eds.), Williams and Wilkins, Baltimore, MD, pp. 669–683 (1991).

SURGICAL
PROCEDURES

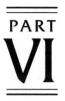

Presurgical Preparation

Michael H. Hart, M.S., M.D.

CHAPTER

25

INTRODUCTION

Organ transplantation in adolescents is an increasingly common occurrence. Although this chapter will focus on liver transplantation, the principles outlined in the presurgical assessment and preparation for transplantation are directly applicable to all adolescent patients undergoing major surgery. This chapter will briefly review various diagnoses that prompted liver transplantation among adolescents. The focus of this chapter is to review those issues that need to be considered in the proper application of nutrition in clinical disease states surrounding possible organ transplantation.

The need for liver transplantation is frequently prompted by an acute (or subacute) decompensation of a preexisting medical condition associated with end-stage liver disease. Alternatively, transplantation may be necessitated by acute hepatic decompensation (referred to as fulminant hepatitis) that results in rapid hepatic failure, with no previous co- or preexisting liver disease. The process prompting liver transplantation determines to a large degree the presurgical preparation and preparedness of the patient, as well as the need for aggressive nutritional intervention and support.

Table 25.1 Cause of End-Stage Liver Disease Requiring Transplantation

Diagnosis	# of Patients
Biliary atresia	121
Metabolic	46
Fulminant hepatic failure	37
Cirrhosis	26
Neonatal hepatitis (includes other)	18
Total	248

Solid Organ Transplantation

Solid organ transplantation, including liver, liver and bowel, bowel, pancreas, and pancreas and kidney, has been performed at the University of Nebraska Medical Center (UNMC) since 1985. Diagnoses resulting in liver transplantation can be divided into acute and chronic conditions. In the newborn period, the acute presentation requiring liver transplantation is often associated with metabolic causes and/or inborn errors of metabolism (tyrosinemia) and neonatal hepatitis/cholestasis, whereas the adolescent will often present acutely as a fulminant hepatic failure associated with a viral infection and/or drug ingestion such as acetaminophen. Alternatively, adolescents may present acutely for transplantation with an acute decompensation of underlying chronic liver disease.

The reasons for liver transplantation and the diagnoses prompting this procedure vary considerably among adults, adolescents, children, and young infants. The diagnoses at UNMC that resulted in liver transplantation in adolescents, children, and infants are shown in Table 25.1. Among adolescents requiring liver transplantation, it is noteworthy to point out the distribution of diagnoses. Diagnoses requiring liver transplantation in adolescents and preadolescents are presented in Table 25.2.

As can be seen, the need for liver transplantation in preadolescents and adolescents can be divided into those patients who develop end-stage liver disease as either a consequence of an acute/fulminant process, or alternatively, as part of a gradual deterioration of a chronic underlying illness. As would be expected, the evaluation process of each teen is different. In addition, the likelihood of associated chronic malnutrition in acute/fulminant hepatic failure would be significantly less than for the teen with chronic illness and acute deterioration.

ASSESSMENT

Medical

The evaluation process developed as part of the pretransplant evaluation has out of necessity required regimentation and a standardized protocol to improve

Table 25.2 Diagnoses for Liver Transplantation Among Adolescents

Diagnosis	# of Patients
Fulminant hepatitis (includes hepatitis A and B)	8
Subacute/chronic hepatitis	4
Cryptogenic cirrhosis	7
Chronic active hepatitis	3
Alpha-1-anti-trypsin	8
Alagille's syndrome	1
Wilson's disease	4
Cystic fibrosis	4
Other metabolic	2
Tumor/malignancy	4
Nonsyndromic bile duct paucity	1

efficiency in the initial patient evaluation. One of the shortcomings of a standardized clinical and laboratory evaluation in all patients anticipating liver transplantation is that the problems which prompt consideration of transplantation are quite variable. For example, adolescents requiring organ transplantation may present as a fulminant presentation of an otherwise healthy individual, or end-stage progression of an underlying chronic process. Obviously, the nutritional status assessment of the otherwise healthy teen may not necessarily warrant the "full work-up." However, it can be argued that since organ transplantation affects a patient's health over his or her life, it is prudent to capture a one-time "crosssection" of an adolescent's nutritional status. Furthermore, many youth who initially present as acute/fulminant hepatitis do not readily have organs available. Thus, they may develop malnutrition during the waiting period of the transplant.

The development of the standardized evaluation does not take into account the variability of the patient diagnoses, but we have developed a standardized "pre-transplant evaluation" that encompasses clinical, radiographic, and biochemical laboratory data, in addition to psychosocial and "environmental" data in anticipation of the transplant. The various tests that are obtained are outlined in Table 25.3. Other tests are ordered as appropriate; however, the above table lists the usual protocol for liver transplantation regardless of specific test outcomes.

Nutrition

Nutritional assessment techniques have become increasingly sophisticated in the last two decades.[1-8] The assessment can be divided into anthropometric measurements (physical examination) and biochemical or laboratory data. Obviously, the history-taking process for dietary intake and the identification of high-risk groups and/or behavioral eating problems need to be considered in the overall evaluation of an adolescent presenting for consideration of surgery. In addition,

Table 25.3   Pretransplant Evaluation (Liver)

1. History and physical examination
     Includes anthropometric data (height, weight, growth percentiles, triceps
       skinfolds, MAC, MAMA)
2. Ancillary staff consultation
     Social work
     Child life services
     Child development
     Finance office
     Psychiatry/psychology
     Dentistry
3. Radiographic testing
     Chest X-ray
     Bone age determination
     Ultrasound (abdomen)
4. Laboratory testing
     Liver function profile
     Electrolytes with urea nitrogen and creatinine
     Nutritional panel (includes Mg, Ca, phosphorus)
     Uric acid
     Prothrombin time and PTT
     CBC (including platelet and reticulocyte counts)
     Cytomegalovirus titers
     Epstein-Barr titers
     Vitamin assays (A, E, 25-OH-D3, 1,25 di-OH-D3)
     Lipid profile
     Alpha-feto-protein
     Coagulation factors (V, VII, and XII)
     HIV antibody screen
     Hepatitis B surface antigen and antibody
     Hepatitis A IgM antibody
     Herpes simplex antibody screen
     Ceruloplasmin
     Ferritin
     Alpha-1-anti-trypsin level and Pi subtyping
     Thyroid-binding prealbumin
     Quantitative immunoglobulins

the developmental physical history is of the utmost importance in evaluating the adolescent to determine whether there is any delay in onset of puberty and/or the pubertal growth spurt, which could be a subtle indication of underlying subclinical disease.[9–15]

The importance of nutritional status in reducing operative morbidity and mortality has been clearly documented. However, there continues to be ongoing difficulty in the development of consistent predictors of changes in surgical outcome based on isolated specific criteria.[16–19] To this end, a number of clinical and biochemical "tools" have been developed in order to try to quantify nutritional assessment.[16–22] Although good normative data exist for normal nutritional status as it pertains to a given population, there are inadequate data to conclude the "abnormal" population of patients relative to all aspects of nutritional status. Moreover, the extrapolation of nutritional data (whether anthropometric, biochemical, or both) leaves much to be desired in drawing conclusions about outcome.

Anthropometric data measure body composition using a wide variety of techniques (see Chapter 18). One of the shortcomings of various body composition measurements is that they tend to be more indicative of chronic, or long-standing, changes in body composition, rather than acute disease processes. Nonetheless, when evaluating adolescents for consideration of transplantation (or other) surgery it is prudent to obtain markers of body composition, i.e., anthropometric data. This is not only helpful to determine whether or not a teen presents with malnutrition, but also provides us with a baseline measurement for future comparisons of treatment and outcome in a dynamic process. Commonly used anthropometric measurements include height, weight, head circumference, weight for height, growth velocity, triceps skinfolds, midarm muscle area, and midarm circumference. These measurements can be compared against normative data for age- and sex-matched individuals, with conclusions in most instances being possible regarding nutritional status for the adolescent. Other techniques are available to determine body composition, including percent of body fat and fat-free body composition. These include, but are not limited to, underwater weighing; total body potassium (lean body mass) measurement using potassium–40; total body water measurement using deuterium-labeled water; use of computer-assisted tomography and magnetic resonance imaging to assess fat stores; in vivo neutron activation to determine lean body mass; bioelectric impedance analysis (BIA); total body electrical conductivity (TOBEC); and bone densitometry (single- and dual-beam photometry).[23–30] The premise for all of these techniques is to measure a given variable that correlates closely with the relative proportion of body masses in the various fat-containing and fat-free compartments.

The biochemical assessment of nutritional status has also been extensively documented.[1,8,16–18,21,22,31–33] Ideally, the biochemical parameter being measured should be reflective of malnutrition only, and not be significantly impacted on by other disease states. Unfortunately, this goal is virtually impossible to meet for any biochemical parameter, as most factors routinely being measured as nutritional markers are affected by a number of variables, in addition to nutritional status. For example, some biochemical markers are too sensitive, whereas others are relatively insensitive. Frequently, biochemical markers change only after prolonged decreased nutrition such as total protein and albumin, whereas some markers that may have implications for nutrition are also elevated as acute-phase reactants or have a "volatile" nature, i.e., ceruloplasmin and transferrin. Useful biochemical factors that have been variably attributed to nutritional status include (1) albumin; (2) retinol-binding protein; (3) transferrin; (4) thyroid-binding prealbumin (transthyretin); (5) insulinlike growth factor-I; (6) 3-methyl-histidine; (7) cholesterol; and (8) triglyceride. Acute-phase reactants, such as ceruloplasmin, C-reactive protein, alpha-1-acid glycoprotein, alpha-1-anti-trypsin may be either elevated or decreased in malnutrition, depending on other factors. Therefore, these markers are not routinely useful in categorization of nutritional assessment of the presurgical teen. However, since acute-phase reactants are hepatically synthesized proteins, we frequently see the increased acute-phase reactants synthesized at the expense of hepatically synthesized visceral proteins. Thus, the increase in acute-phase reactants is usually associated with an increased risk of complication.[34-38]

A number of investigators have attempted to develop prognostic equations that evaluate the potential morbidity associated with nutritional status in hopes of correlating outcomes. Unfortunately, no relationship has been developed for children and adolescents that has withstood limitations in a wide range of clinical situations in patients being considered for surgery, particularly transplantation.

A technique that may be useful in helping to estimate resting energy expenditure is indirect calorimetry.[39-54] This technique utilizes standardized measurements of oxygen consumption and carbon dioxide production, in addition to urinary nitrogen losses, to measure resting energy expenditure at a given moment in the adolescent's clinical presentation. In this fashion, patients' resting energy expenditure can be compared against the predicted energy expenditure from the Harris-Benedict equation[55,56] and nutritional support can be directed from knowing the "actual" patients' caloric requirements; and reducing the "guesswork" in the process. The actual techniques involved in performing indirect calorimetry are straightforward, but it is beyond the scope of this chapter to describe the protocol for indirect calorimetry, as well as the pros and cons of the technique. There are numerous sources readily available to reference this technique, should the reader have additional interest in the topic.[39-54]

MANAGEMENT

By using collected assessment data, adolescents identified to be malnourished need aggressive management. Nutritional support is required to arrest further deterioration of clinical status, as well as return adolescents to optimal condition, if possible.

Teens with acute decompensation of chronic illnesses, as well as progressive deterioration of chronic diseases, are much more likely to have secondary malnutrition when compared to previously healthy patients who develop fulminant hepatic failure following an acute illness or infection, after otherwise being in good health prior to the illness. Although the impact of nutritional assessment and intervention is not to be minimized in the acutely ill patient who enters negative nitrogen balance, frequently patient management is directed toward treatment of fluid and electrolyte disturbances. It is not uncommon for patients presenting with fulminant hepatic failure to require fluid and protein restriction for the prevention and/or treatment of cerebral edema and hyperammonemia such that caloric restriction is a frequent consequence of the treatment. Because patients with fulminant hepatic failure may have difficulty with gluconeogenesis, it is usually necessary to treat patients with hypertonic solutions of dextrose intravenously in the acute management.

A wide range of specialized formulas and parenteral nutrition support techniques have been developed for specialized nutritional needs, such as the child or adolescent presenting for liver transplantation. Much is dependent on presenting nutritional requirements or conditions associated with the pathophysiology of the presenting clinical situation (see Chapter 26).

Practical Considerations

The general health and nutritional problems of adolescents have been well documented.[10-15] However, specific subgroups of adolescents are at high risk for nutritional problems.[10-15] Specifically, poor and rural adolescents have been noted to have a higher than normal prevalence of nutritional disorders. In addition, African American, hispanics, and American Indian groups also have increased risk of nutritional problems in adolescence.[15] Behavioral eating disorders are higher in adolescents than younger or older age groups.[57] Disorders such as anorexia nervosa or bulimia need to be considered in all adolescents, regardless of whether the teen has another underlying health disorder or not. Nutritional problems associated with anorexia nervosa and bulimia nervosa have been well documented in this text and elsewhere.[15,57] Anorexia nervosa patients are typically adolescent females with a variety of nutrition associated problems, including hypoalbuminemia, decreased iron-binding capacity and iron stores, reduced bone density, and occasional hypovitaminosis A with hypocarotenemia. Anorectics often have mild elevations in hepatocellular enzymes levels (AST and ALT), reduced triiodothyronine associated with decreased conversion from thyroxine to tri-iodo-thyronine, elevated serum cortisol, and reduced luteinizing hormone with hypo-estrogenemia. The clinician should always consider the individual presenting for presurgical evaluation as having the possibility of an eating disorder. Dietary history and physical examination should be routinely obtained as part of the preliminary evaluation, with particular attention to abnormal dietary practices that are commonplace among adolescents.[15,57,58]

The largest group of adolescents undergoing liver transplantation at UNMC were those individuals with fulminant hepatitis. Other relatively frequent diagnoses warranting transplantation included cryptogenic cirrhosis, chronic active hepatitis, cystic fibrosis, Wilson's disease, and alpha-1-anti-trypsin deficiency. Patients with fulminant hepatitis may present with hepatitis A, hepatitis B, or other types of infectious hepatitis. Frequently, patients with fulminant hepatitis present following an unidentified "viral" infection with an acute presentation of jaundice and/or clinical hepatic encephalopathy. Often, despite aggressive antibody testing, there is no identifiable cause of the fulminant hepatitis. Patients who present in this fashion are typically healthy prior to their acute illness and also usually in excellent nutritional status. It is this group of patients who are evaluated for "baseline" determination in order to monitor them in a prospective manner through the course of their clinical illness and/or transplant surgery.

Patients with chronic active hepatitis, cystic fibrosis, biliary atresia, and cryptogenic cirrhosis typically present as progressive end-stage liver disease in an insidious fashion. These patients usually are identified long before any anticipated liver transplant is necessary and should have already had prior nutritional assessment and nutrition support performed and instituted, respectively. Patients referred to our transplant center will undergo interval nutritional assessment to determine the present state of malnutrition, as well as identify any other components of nutrition for which supplemental nutritional intervention would be possible, such as vitamin supplementation or TPN. Patients presenting as end-stage decompensation of chronic underlying illnesses will have a much higher prevalence of malnutrition and need to be aggressively managed with nutritional support.

CASE ILLUSTRATION

Case One

Katherine was a 14-year-old white female who was in excellent health until 2 wk prior to being admitted to the hospital for progressive jaundice with a change in mental status. Katherine, in addition to several other family members, developed a "flulike" illness with fever, headache, nausea, and vomiting. She also complained of vague abdominal discomfort. Approximately 1 wk after initial complaints of the flulike illness, Katherine was noted by her parents to be jaundiced. Initial laboratory data obtained by her physician included a CBC that showed mild neutropenia with a normal hemoglobin and differential. AST (aspartate amino transferase/SGOT) and ALT (alanine amino transferase/SGPT) were approximately 20-fold increased over normal values. Serum bilirubin (total) level was noted to be 20.5 mg/dL (milligrams per deciliter), with a direct fraction of 13.0 mg/dL. Initial prothrombin time was 6 sec prolonged over control values, with partial thromboplastin time twice the normal control value. Initial serum ammonia was twice the upper limits of normal. Total protein level was normal at 7.0 gm/dL (grams per deciliter). Serum albumin was also normal at 3.8 gm/dL. Serum prealbumin was borderline low/normal at 20 mg/dL (normal 18–45 mg/dL). Anthropometric data obtained at the time of admission noted normal height for age, weight for age, weight for height, midarm muscle circumference, midarm muscle area, and triceps skinfold assessment.

Katherine was transferred to UNMC due to progressive hepatic encephalopathy, worsening hepatic synthetic function (elevated prothrombin time), and a clinical course of fulminant hepatic failure. The teen's hospital course was significant for clinical deterioration that required orthotopic liver transplantation. Despite extensive diagnostic testing, the cause of the patient's fulminant hepatic failure was not ascertained. Presumably the patient developed fulminant hepatic failure after a viral infection.

The management of this teen was clearly focused on the acute management of hepatic failure, including the prevention and treatment of cerebral edema using standard therapies. This individual was well nourished at the time of her illness; therefore, presurgical preparation was necessarily focused on the treatment of the acute hepatic failure.

Case Two

Cy was a 16-year-old teen with a diagnosis of alpha-1-anti-trypsin deficiency. He was diagnosed in infancy when he was noted to have mild jaundice and hepatocellular enzyme level elevations. Protease inhibitor subtyping noted the patient to have ZZ phenotype. Over the first decade of life, the patient had developed progressive evidence of hepatic cirrhosis with portal hypertension. Subsequently, he developed progressive evidence of declining hepatic synthetic function, with variceal hemorrhage, requiring repetitive endoscopic sclerotherapy treatment sessions. Ultimately, liver transplantation was required for progressive cirrhosis with portal hypertension.

Physical examination of Cy noted anthropometric data quite different from those of Case 1. Height for age was at approximately the 5th percentile prior to transplantation. Furthermore, weight for age percentiles were less than the 5th percentile. Triceps skinfold, midarm muscle area, and midarm circumference were all less than the 5th percentiles for cohort normal values. The teen was noted to have splenomegaly with ascites.

Laboratory data included total protein low at 5.0 gm/dL, with a low albumin value at 2.9 gm/dL. Serum prealbumin was also low at 13.4 mg/dL. Prothrombin time was slightly elevated at 3 sec above normal.

Management of this teen had included aggressive attempts to improve nutritional status in a dual attempt to prolong the quality of life, as well as to try to obtain optimal nutritional status for the anticipated liver transplantation. It was apparent from the patient's clinical course that he had end-stage liver disease that warranted liver transplantation. Cy exhibited evidence of chronic malnutrition with a component of acute malnutrition as well. Other medical problems impacting nutrition included cirrhosis with portal hypertension and ascites. This necessitated the restriction of sodium intake, with diuretic use ultimately being required prior to transplantation. Due to impaired hepatic synthesis and secretion of bile salts, the patient was also at risk for the development of fat-soluble vitamin deficiencies, essential fatty acid deficiency, and impaired intestinal absorption of various nutrients. To this end, the patient received supplemental fat-soluble vitamins. High-calorie feedings were used to provide the teen with supplemental calories to attempt to minimize weight loss. Anorexia frequently accompanies end-stage liver disease and calorie supplements are recommended, either with high caloric foods or specialized formulas. This case illustrates that end-stage liver disease frequently occurs as a progressive process of an underlying illness. These patients need to have their nutritional status monitored as part of a routine medical evaluations. Because these teens are at significant risk for the development of nutritional deficiencies, aggressive attempts at nutritional intervention will improve not only quality of life for the patient, but also improve his or herr operative morbidity and mortality during liver transplantation as well.

REFERENCES

1. K. N. Jeejeehoy, A. S. Detsky, and J. P. Baker, *JPEN*, **14**, 193S (1990).

2. C. L. Johnson, R. Fulwood, S. Abraham, et al., in *Vital and Health Series II, No. 219*, DHHS, PHS, Washington, DC, p. 81 (1981).

3. L. Sann, M. Durand, J. Picard, et al., *Arch. Dis. Child.*, **63**, 265 (1988).

4. D. W. Spady, in *Body Composition Measurements in Infants and Children*, (W. J. Klish and N. Kretchmer, eds.), Ross Laboratories, Columbus, OH, pp. 67–75 (1989).

5. H. H. Sandstead and W. N. Pearson, in *Modern Nutrition in Health and Disease*, (R. S. Goodhart and M. E. Shils, eds.), Lea and Febiger, Philadelphia, PA, pp. 572–592 (1973).

6. R. C. Watson, H. Grossman, and M. A. Meyers, in *Modern Nutrition in Health and Disease*, (R. S. Goodhart and M. E. Shils, eds.), Lea and Febiger, Philadelphia, PA, pp. 547–571 (1973).

7. F. Grande, in *Present Knowledge of Nutrition,* The Nutritional Foundation, Inc., Washington, DC, pp. 7–18 (1984).

8. R. Figueroa-Colon, in *Textbook of Pediatric Ntutrition, 2nd ed.*, (R. M. Suskind and L. Lewinter-Suskind, eds.), Raven Press, New York, pp. 191–205 (1993).

9. R. W. Chesney and B. H. Ault, in *Body Composition Measurements in Infants and Children*, (W. J. Klish and N. Kretchmer, eds.), Ross Laboratories, Columbus, OH, pp. 135–139 (1989).

10. E. J. Burbige, *Pediatrics*, **55**, 866 (1975).

11. P. R. Whittington, *Gastroenterology*, **72**, 1338 (1977).

12. B. S. Kirschner, O. Voincher, and I. H. Rosenber, *Gastoenterology*, **75**, 5048 (1978).

13. F. Daum, in *Pediatric Gastroenterology and Nutrition*, (W. F. Balistreri and J. A. Vanderhoof, eds.), Chapman and Hall, London, pp. 237–243 (1990).

14. E. Siedman, in *Textbook of Pediatric Ntutrition, 2nd ed.*, (R. M. Suskind and L. Lewinter-Suskind, eds.), Raven Press, New York, pp. 341–352 (1993).

15. J. T. Dwyer, in *Textbook of Pediatric Ntutrition, 2nd ed.*, (R. M. Suskind and L. Lewinter-Suskind, eds.), Raven Press, New York, pp. 257–264 (1993).

16. K. L. Vehe, R. O. Brown, D. A. Kuhl, et al., *J. Am. Coll. Nutr.*, **10**, 355 (1991).

17. Y. Ingenbleek and Y. A. Carpentier, *Int. J. Vit. Nutr. Res.*, **55**, 91 (1985).

18. G. P. Buzby, J. L. Mullen, D. C. Matthews, et al., *Am. J. Surg.*, **139**, 160 (1980).

19. G. P. Buzby, *JPEN*, **14**, 197S (1990).

20. W. A. Knaus, E. A. Draper, D. P. Wagner, et al., *Crit. Care Med.*, **13**, 818 (1985).

21. M. B. Tuten, S. Wogt, F. Dasse, et al., *JPEN*, **9**, 709 (1985).

22. P. A. Routledge, W. W. Stargel, and G. S. Wagner, *Ann. Intern. Med.*, **93**, 701 (1980).

23. H. L. Johnson, S.P.S. Virk, A. S. Mayclin, et al., *J. Am. Coll. Nutr.*, **11**, 539 (1992).

24. S. Yasumura, K. Jones, P. Spanne, et al., *J. Nutr.*, **123**, 459 (1993).

25. J. J. Kehayias, *J. Nutr.*, **123**, 454 (1993).

26. R. N. Baumgartner, R. L. Rhyne, P. J. Garry, et al., *J. Nutr.*, **123**, 444 (1993).

27. W. C. Chumlea, S. S. Guo, R. J. Kuczmarski, et al., *J. Nutr.*, **123**, 449 (1993).

28. J. C. Pinella, B. Webster, M. Baetz, et al., *JPEN*, **16**, 408 (1992).

29. D. S. Gray and M. Bauer, *J. Am. Coll. Nutr.*, **10**, 63 (1991).

30. S. B. Heymsfield, Z. Wang, R. N. Baumgartner, et al., *J. Nutr.*, **123**, 432 (1993).

31. T. G. Jensen, *Persp. Prac.*, **84**, 1345 (1984).

32. A. B. Arquitt, B. J. Stoecker, J. S. Jermann, et al., *J. Am. Diet. Assoc.*, **91**, 575 (1991).

33. J. Woo, Y. T. Mak, J. Lau, et al., *Postgrad. Med.*, **68**, 954 (1992).

34. S. D. Deodhar, *Clev. Clin. J. Med.*, **56**, 126 (1989).

35. R. A. Mustard, J.M.A. Bohnen, S. Jaseeb, et al., *Arch. Surg.*, **120**, 187 (1985).

36. W. M. Stahl, *Crit. Care Med.*, **15**, 545 (1987).

37. S. S. Macintyre, D. Schultz, and I. Kushner, *Ann. NY Acad. Sci.*, **389**, 76 1982).

38. G. Sganga, J. H. Siegel, G. Brown, et al., *Arch. Surg.*, **120**, 187 (1985).

39. L. J. Makk, S. A. McClave, P. W. Creech, et al., *Crit. Care Med.*, **18**, 1320 (1990).

40. V. Cortes and L. D. Nelson, *Arch. Surg.*, **124**, 287 (1989).

41. A.M.W.J. Schols, P.F.M. Schoffelen, H. Ceulemans, et al., *JPEN*, **16**, 364 (1992).

42. R. N. Dickerson, K. L. Vehe, J. L. Mullen, et al., *Crit. Care Med.*, **19**, 484 (1991).

43. F. N. Konstantinides, N. N. Konstantinides, J. C. Li, et al., *JPEN*, **15**, 189 (1991).

44. J. J. Cunningham, *JPEN*, **14**, 649 (1990).

45. K. A. Dietrich, M. D. Romero, and S. A. Conrad, *JPEN*, **14**, 408 (1990).

46. C. G. Vermeij, B. W. Feenstra, A. M. Omen et al., *JPEN*, **15**, 421 (1991).

47. E.W.H.M. Fredrix, P. B. Soeters, M. F. von Meyenfeldt, et al., *JPEN*, **15**, 604 (1991).

48. D. Y. Sue and C. Wolff, *JPEN*, **15**, 625 (1991).

49. R. R. Williams and C. R. Fuenning, *JPEN*, **15**, 509 (1991).

50. S. Firouzbakhsh, R. K. Mathis, W. L. Dorchester, et al., *J. Ped. Gastro. Nutr.*, **16**, 136 (1993).

51. B. Just, D. Darmaun, J. Koziet, et al., *JPEN*, **15**, 65 (1991).

52. D. E. Matthews and S. B. Heymsfield, *JPEN*, **15**, 3 (1991).

53. R. A. Forse, *JPEN*, **17**, 388 (1993).

54. M. A. Stokes and G. L. Hill, *JPEN*, **15**, 281 (1991).

55. J. A. Harris and F. G. Benedict, in *A Biometric Study of Basal Metabolism in* Man, Pub. no. 279, Carnegie Institute of Washington, Washington, DC, pp. 1–265 (1919).

56. C. W. van Way, *JPEN*, **16**, 566 (1992).

57. J. J. Pertschuk, in *Textbook of Pediatric Ntutrition, 2nd ed.*, (R. M. Suskind and L. Lewinter-Suskind, eds.), Raven Press, New York, pp. 265–273 (1993).

58. M. H. Hart and D. L. Antonson, in *Pediatric Gastroenterology and Nutrition*, (W. F. Balistreri and J. A. Vanderhoof, eds.), Chapman and Hall, London, pp. 296–308 (1990).

Organ Transplantation

Dean L. Antonson M.D., Mark T. Houser M.D., Bruce G. Gordon M.D., Jean E. Guest R.D., Georgia A. Walter R.D., and David R. Mack M.D.

CHAPTER

26

INTRODUCTION

Transplantation presently offers real hope for the long-term survival of adolescents with severe organ failure. In addition to the important discoveries in immunosuppression that have heralded advancements in transplantation, assurance of an optimal nutritional state for each patient has proven to be one of the most important factors in achieving a successful outcome. This chapter discusses the nutritional assessment strategies for liver, kidney, heart, lung, and bone marrow transplant patients, and details the specific nutritional recommendations for the critical post-transplant period. Issues related to compliance as well as subsequent clinical and nutritional care are also addressed.

Liver

Approximately 100 adolescents between the ages of 11 and 19 yr are currently awaiting liver transplantation according to recent figures compiled by the United Network for Organ Sharing (UNOS) Research Department.[1] In each of the last several years, between 100 and 150 adolescents have undergone liver transplantation. With the exception of patients over 65 yr of age, older children and adolescents comprise the smallest group of liver transplant recipients. Of the 3000 liver transplant recipients in 1991, 5.8% (170) were between the ages of 6–18 yr.[1] In adolescence, the major disorders that result in the need for liver transplantation include fulminant hepatic failure, chronic active hepatitis, acute autoimmune hepatitis, alpha 1-antitrypsin deficiency, Wilson's disease, cystic fibrosis, and toxic ingestion, particularly acetaminophen poisoning.

Prior to 1978, success rates for hepatic transplantation were only 30–50%, using immunosuppressive regimens based primarily on prednisone and imuran.[2] With the introduction of Cyclosporin A, a marked improvement in effective immunosuppression was achieved, resulting in long-term actuarial survival rates that now approach 80% at most centers.[3,4] Furthermore, advances in microsurgical techniques, improved preservation solutions, aggressive management of infections, medical advances in biliary stenting, and improvements in nutritional support have all enhanced survival.

A number of different options are available for the patient in need of liver transplantation. These include cadaveric orthotopic liver transplantation, segmental or split-liver transplantation, augmented segmental liver transplantation, and living-related donor transplantation. To assure adequate hepatic reserve during the stress of transplantation, the mass of the transplanted liver should be at least 1% of the total body weight. In older children and adolescents, therefore, segmental transplantation and living-related donor transplantation become increasingly less available options as age and weight increase. Thus, the majority of adolescents will receive a cadaveric liver transplantation when the need arises. With this procedure, the diseased recipient liver is removed and a cadaveric whole liver graft is transplanted in the orthotopic location with normal anatomic reconstruction. In younger adolescents of less weight, segmental transplantation or transplantation of a left lobe, right lobe, or left lateral segment may be possible. With this operation, the transplanted segment is also placed in the orthotopic position following removal of the diseased organ. For situations of acute liver injury in which hepatic function may ultimately recover, an auxiliary left lobe transplantation may be performed following removal of the native left lobe.[5] If hepatic function recovers, the transplanted segment can then be removed, or immunosuppression withdrawn, allowing for slow resorption of the transplanted segment. Although living-related donor transplantation has significantly improved the availability of organs for younger children,[6] it is rarely applicable for adolescents because of the above-noted size limitations. In the majority of adolescents, hepatic biliary reconstruction is performed in a duct-to-duct manner anastomosing the common bile of the donor organ to the common bile duct of the recipient. Alternatively, if the donor bile duct is small or has been damaged, a duct to small bowel Roux-en-Y anastomosis may be required.

Kidney

Between 800 and 900 new cases of treated pediatric (<20 years of age) end-stage renal disease (ESRD) occur each year in the United States.[7] Although many treatment options exist for these patients, 20% of them receive a renal transplant as their initial therapy,[8] and nearly 50% of them receive a renal transplant in the first year after entering ESRD care.[7] As opposed to adults, nearly 50% of children and adolescents utilize a living-related donor for their first transplant, although only about 25% of repeat transplants will be from living-related donors.[7] Adolescents account for 50–60% of the new pediatric ESRD and renal transplant populations.[7,8]

Heart, Heart-Lung, and Lung

Heart, heart-lung, and lung transplantation are now considered appropriate therapeutic options for adolescents with irreversible severe cardiopulmonary disease.[9–16] Clinical and immunosuppressive advancements through the 1980s have dramatically improved survival rates for these solid organ transplants, paralleling the progress noted for other organ transplantation procedures. Prior to 1980, fewer than five children per year received cardiac transplants, most of these being adolescents.[9] With the introduction of Cyclosporin A and dramatic increase in adult transplantation, pediatric heart transplants increased rapidly.[9] Through January of 1990, out of 12,000 total heart transplants, 874 occurred in pediatric patients.[9] Of these, 58% were performed in children aged 10–18 yr.[9] The primary indication for adolescent heart transplant is cardiomyopathy, followed by congenital heart defects, valvular disease, and retransplantation. Survival rates following heart transplantation are now 74% at 1 yr and about 60% at 5 yr.[15] As with adults, both early and late deaths are primarily related to rejection and infection.[17]

Current experience with heart-lung and lung transplantation is much less extensive, owing to the relatively recent development of these procedures.[9] Fewer than 100 cases of heart-lung transplantation have been recorded through 1991.[9] The major indications for this procedure are primary pulmonary hypertension, complex congenital heart disease with pulmonary vascular disease, and cystic fibrosis. Survival rates as expected are less than with heart transplantation alone, approximating 60% at 1 yr and 40% at 5 yr.[13] Deaths are primarily attributed to rejection and infection, along with the all too frequent development of bronchiolitis obliterans.[9]

Lung transplantation as an independent procedure has only become possible as of 1987, when difficulties involving the tracheal and bronchial anastomosis were resolved.[9] As of 1992, 73 lung transplants have been performed in pediatric patients under 16 yr of age, as recorded by the St. Louis International Registry.[9] The most common indication for lung transplantation is cystic fibrosis, followed by primary pulmonary hypertension, idiopathic pulmonary fibrosis, Eisenmenger's complex, bronchiolitis obliterans, bronchopulmonary dysplasia, and congenital lung abnormalities. One and 2-yr survival rates are 60–70%, whereas 3 yr survival rates fall to 40%, primarily related to the escalating development of bronchiolitis obliterans, along with the problems of chronic rejection and infection.[9]

Surgical techniques for orthotopic heart transplantation have generally followed those detailed by Lower and Shumway.[18] For nonstructural problems such as cardiomyopathy, the transplant operation is relatively simple. For adolescents with complex congenital heart disease who have undergone several palliative repairs, the operation can be difficult and often requires surgical creativity. For cardiac transplantation, the recipient is initially prepared with cardiopulmonary bypass, deep hypothermia, and circulatory arrest.[19] Ductal division, head vessel constriction, and cardiectomy are then performed. The heart is excised first at the atrioventricular junction and then at the ventriculoarterial junction, preserving adequate recipient tissue for anastomosis. The donor heart is then surgically joined, anastomosing first the left and right atria, followed by end-to-end anastomosis of the pulmonary artery and aorta.[19] Construction of an intraatrial baffle or other atrial septal reconstruction is often required for complex lesions, including situs inversus or situs ambiguus.[19] Completion of the surgical procedure is then followed by warming and subsequent discontinuation of cardiopulmonary bypass, with the return of cardiac function being supported by pressor agents and monitored with in-dwelling catheters.

For heart-lung transplantation, recipient heart preparation is similar to that just described, with the obvious exception that pulmonary arterial and pulmonary venous to left atrial donor anatomy is preserved. The lung-heart block in mass along with the trachea is then orthotopically placed and sutured in the correct anatomic position.

For lung transplantation, the present options for adolescents include single or double lung transplantation.[9] Even in the face of severe right heart failure, lung transplantation alone can be accomplished, as normal right ventricular function is almost always recoverable following transplantation.[9] Lobar lung transplantation, either with cadaveric or living-related donor lung tissue, is restricted by size limitations to infants and younger children.

Bone Marrow

High-dose therapy and hematopoietic stem cell transplantation (HSCT), including bone marrow and peripheral blood stem cell transplantation, have become the treatment of choice for a variety of malignant and nonmalignant diseases in children and adolescents. Stem cell transplantation may be curative therapy for children with relapsed acute lymphoblastic leukemia or lymphoma, severe aplastic anemia, or congenital immunodeficiencies, and preliminary data suggest a role for this modality in selected patients with solid tumors (like neuroblastoma or Wilm's tumor) or storage diseases. The 269 transplant centers who form the International Bone Marrow Transplant Registry (IBMTR) reported over 750 children and adolescents undergoing allogeneic bone marrow transplantation in 1990. Of these, 45% were between the ages of 13 and 21 yr[*].

Rescue from the marrow ablative effect of high-dose chemotherapy or chemo-radiotherapy can be achieved by reinfusion of hematopoietic stem cells previously isolated and stored from the patient (autologous bone marrow or peripheral blood stem cell transplantation) or a sibling or other person suitably matched for antigens of the major histocompatibility complex (allogeneic bone marrow transplantation). Patients undergoing allogeneic BMT generally present more complicated clinical and nutritional challenges.

ASSESSMENT

Liver

The patient presenting with end-stage liver disease often has a myriad of attendant medical difficulties that primarily result from the underlying disease process. However, the general medical concerns are quite different between adolescents presenting with acute liver injury compared to those who have had chronic long-standing liver disease. In youth presenting with acute liver injury, such as postviral fulminant hepatic failure or acetaminophen toxicity, the prior medical history is usually normal and patients are often healthy up to the point in time in which the liver injury has occurred. In this group as a whole, additional medical problems are rare. For drug overdoses, the most important considerations are those related to the mental status of individuals whose liver injury has often occurred as a result of a suicide attempt. In patients presenting with chronic liver injury, antecedent problems are expected and numerous. Complications of increased portal pressure and resultant hypersplenism, neutropenia, thrombocyto-penia, and esophageal variceal bleeding frequently necessitate constant medical care. Difficulties with decreased hepatic synthetic function, hypoalbuminemia, ascites, and coagulopathy often require daily support. Patients with chronic inflammatory liver disease, such as chronic active hepatitis, are often on immuno-suppressive medications, including prednisone, and frequently have attendant difficulties with obesity, hyperglycemia, edema, and hypertension. End-stage liver disease in adolescents secondary to primary cholestatic disease processes

---

*Data obtained from the Statistical Center of the International Bone Marrow Transplant Registry. The analysis has not been approved or reviewed by the advisory committee of the IBMTR.

is unusual. Cholestasis as a component of progressive cirrhosis however, is uniformly present and results in elevated cholesterol levels and fat malabsorption including the fat-soluble vitamins. Secondary hyperparathyroidism in association with vitamin D malabsorption causes profound alterations in calcium and phosphorus metabolism. Patients with progressive end-stage liver disease often require intensive support including frequent blood and blood product transfusions, diuretic therapy, fluid and salt restriction, endoscopic or operative procedures for control of variceal hemorrhage, and treatment for drug side-effects as medically required. In patients with acute hepatic failure, cerebral edema and hepatic coma may rapidly develop, requiring acute intensive care with intracranial pressure monitoring and mannitol administration. Rapid transplantation is critical in this patient population, since neurologic outcome is often poor following the onset of acute cerebral edema.[20,21] Because of the devastation that often ensues following the development of cerebral edema, several new techniques are being examined to provide temporary hepatic support and act as a bridge to transplantation. The procedures currently being investigated include extracorporeal liver perfusion,[22] either with a cadaveric or xenograft liver, and hepatic cell perfusion through a extracorporeal capillary device containing hepatoblastoma cell line populations.[23]

The nutritional assessment and support of the adolescent in need of liver transplantation are critical. Nutritional deficiencies and growth failure are quite common. In chronic liver disease, there are numerous causes for decreased nutrient intake, including anorexia, early satiety in association with significant organomegaly and ascites, fat malabsorption secondary to diminished bile flow, and alterations in hepatic metabolism.[4,24] In end-stage liver disease, abnormal amino acid metabolism, fat-soluble vitamin deficiency, and increased energy needs contribute to the development of protein energy malnutrition.[24] Not only is muscle catabolized, but as in other instances of starvation, the organ protein from kidney, gut, and liver is often more significantly affected.[24] In the absence of adequate carbohydrate intake, glucose production will be derived primarily from protein degradation and glycerol formation derived from fat metabolism, resulting in further nutritional compromise.[24] Because poor nutritional status adversely affects long-term survival, an aggressive program for nutritional repletion should uniformly be implemented. Aggressive treatment with strong nutritional and medical support will significantly improve the chances for successful transplantation.[4,25,26]

Nutritional assessment in patients with end-stage liver disease is often difficult as the standard parameters of height, weight, and body composition have all been significantly altered. Weight, often one of the most important parameters for nutritional assessment, is altered by edema, ascites, and diuretic therapy.[26] Because of this, several alternative programs to assess the nutritional status of the patient with end-stage liver disease have been devised including subjective global assessment and the utilization of Z scores.[27,28] No single plan or assessment scale has yet been shown to be uniquely more beneficial than another, and as a consequence, adequate assessment will generally be achieved from a pragmatic summation of available parameters. For the majority of adolescents undergoing hepatic transplantation, these include a dietary history, including assessment of fluid intake, sodium restriction, and fat-soluble vitamin supplementation, a careful physical examination focusing on linear growth rates and anthropometric data including triceps skinfold thickness, midarm circumference, and a calculated midarm muscle area to estimate fat and muscle reserves, biochemical measurements of hepatic synthetic function, and evaluation of immune status.[4,26,28] In combination, these parameters yield as reliably as possible an adequate assessment of the current nutritional state and determine the need for appropriate nutritional corrections.

Treatment includes the administration of sufficient calories to overcome the catabolic state resulting from the underlying liver disease, supplementation of fat-soluble vitamins, treatment of hypoglycemia if present, fluid restriction in the presence of edema or ascites, and supplementation of minerals, particularly calcium, magnesium, and zinc. In spite of diminished hepatic synthetic function, rarely is hepatic metabolic function so diminished that nutritional repletion is unachievable. In severe cases hyperalimentation may be required, particularly if significant fluid restriction and frequent treatment for hypoglycemia are required.

Kidney

General medical considerations relevant to renal transplantation in the adolescent include the patients' primary renal diagnosis (as some diseases reoccur in the transplant); growth and psychosocial development, including an assessment regarding the likelihood of medical noncompliance; the patient's urological status and bladder function; evaluation of the patient's immunologic status; tissue type and prior exposure to herpes family viruses; a thorough search for possible sites of infection; an assessment of the patient's vaccination status (required for all organ transplant patients and includes pneumococcal and Hepatitis B vaccination); an assessment for GI bleeding; and other evaluations as clinically indicated.[29]

Nutritional assessment prior to renal transplantation is a component of an ongoing dietary evaluation and counseling process that begins with the onset of chronic renal insufficiency.[30,31] Growth delay is a common problem in children with chronic renal failure (CRF), and caloric deficiency is only one of many etiologic factors.[30-32] Although energy intake is frequently reduced in patients with CRF, protein intake often exceeds the Recommended Dietary Allowance (RDA) and is usually well tolerated.[30,31,33] The exact dietary recommendations vary, depending on whether the patient is receiving chronic hemodialysis, peritoneal dialysis, or merely has nondialysis-dependent CRF.[34]

The nutritional and growth assessment of adolescents entering renal transplantation include a dietary, biochemical, clinical, and radiographic evaluation. A prospective 3–4-d diet diary is the most useful method of monitoring intake. Assessment of hematological status as well as electrolytes, calcium, phosphorous, bicarbonate, albumin, transferrin, and lipids provides nutritional and metabolic information relevant to the dietary treatment plan.[30,31] Anthropometric measurements including height, weight, weight-for-height index, body mass index, triceps skinfold thickness, and midarm circumference help to assess the patients growth and nutritional status, body fat, and muscle mass.[30,31,34] In addition, the assessment of bone age and pubertal status helps to determine how much growth potential the child has after transplantation.[29,31]

Heart, Heart-Lung, and Lung

End-stage heart and lung disease is often associated with severe problems including multiorgan failure and cardiac cachexia.[35–37] Progressive heart disease often results in severe liver and renal impairment, whereas progressive lung disease causes right heart failure, along with liver and gastrointestinal dysfunction. Patients are uniformly on multiple drugs and medications with frequent attendant side-effects that require careful assessment and thorough knowledge prior to transplantation. Patients with cystic fibrosis are chronically infected, and specific knowledge regarding the colonizing organisms and their sensitivities is required to assist in postoperative antibiotic treatment. Immunizations should all be up to date prior to transplantation if possible. Social, ethical, and psychological factors should all be assessed and addressed.[38]

Malnutrition is again quite commonly present in patients with end-stage cardiac or pulmonary disease.[35–37] Significant weight loss and loss of appetite are almost uniformly reported. Malnutrition results from a variety of causes, including anorexia, hypermetabolism, nutrient losses through urine and stool, and impaired nutrient handling and removal by failing organs.[37] Hypermetabolism often increases energy needs by 20–30%.[35] Right heart failure and the liver involvement result in ascites and intestinal engorgement reducing nutrient absorption. The nutritional status of the patient can significantly affect surgical outcome, length of hospitalization, and mortality.[35–37] In a recent study of adult patients, 10 of 52 patients were noted to be severely compromised nutritionally prior to transplantation.[39] Of these 10 patients, 50% died, whereas only 21% of the less compromised patients expired.[39]

In view of this, adequate nutritional assessment and subsequent nutritional rehabilitation prior to transplantation become of paramount importance. Nutritional assessment parameters should include a review of the past medical history, dietary intake, weight changes, and assessment of medications being utilized. Biochemical parameters of visceral protein status and total lymphocyte count, both of which are decreased in protein energy malnutrition, should be obtained. Physical examination to evaluate for signs of nutritional deficiencies and accurate anthropometric data should be obtained. Based on the above results, specific nutritional recommendations should be made to correct deficiencies and maximize nutritional status prior to transplantation. Patients in heart failure will generally require sodium and fluid restrictions, whereas pulmonary failure patients will require optimal fat-to-calorie ratios to maximize residual pulmonary function.

Bone Marrow

The purpose of pretransplant nutritional assessment is to gauge current status and identify requirements. Patients may come to transplantation with a compromised nutritional status already present.[40,41] This may be due to the effects of prior therapy, increased and unmet caloric requirements, and anorexia and hypophagia, all of which contribute to cancer cachexia. Anthropometric measurements, biochemical data, and nutritional history provide a baseline against which to measure changes following high-dose therapy and identify the need for earlier intervention. In addition, at the time of pretransplant nutritional evaluation, the transplant unit policies with regard to diet and oral care (which intimately affects oral intake) can be discussed with patients and parents.

MANAGEMENT

Liver

The adolescent who has recently undergone orthotopic liver transplantation is faced with a period of severe metabolic and physiologic stress within the first 24–48 h postoperatively. Severe postoperative stress results from the complexity and length of the operation, the amount of blood lost and the need for large amounts of blood products, prolonged anesthesia, and hypothermia.[4,42] Attention during this phase of recovery is primarily directed toward the careful management of fluid and electrolyte problems. During the first 24–48 h postoperatively, significant fluid restriction is required, often limiting fluid intake to one-half of maintenance fluid rates. Carbohydrate is provided with intravenous (IV) fluids of 5 or 10% dextrose, and blood sugar levels are monitored closely. Significant fluid restriction is primarily required to assist in the care of the pulmonary complications occurring postoperatively that include pulmonary edema, atelectasis, and the continued need for increased FIO_2.[42] Most patients remain on the ventilator with an endotracheal tube in place during the first few hours following transplantation. However, within 2 d posttransplant, greater than half of the patients have been extubated.[42] Significant electrolyte problems including hypocalcemia occur in over half of the patients postoperatively, along with diminished levels of magnesium. Almost all patients are hypokalemic and require potassium given as careful bolus infusions during the first 48 h. Liver function studies are monitored carefully, and improving graft function is heralded by improvements in factor levels II, V, and VII, decreasing protime and partial thromboplastin time, decreasing levels of transaminases and bilirubin, and blood glucose stabilization.

Providing nutritional support becomes of paramount importance approximately 2–3 d postoperatively. In the majority of patients, nutritional support in the form of hyperalimentation should be utilized at this time. Calorie requirements are high and have been estimated to be at least 1.5 times basal energy expenditure rates during the first several days following transplantation.[26] A protein intake of 1.3- 2 g/kg of dry weight/d is recommended.[26] In a recent study of adult transplant recipients, caloric requirements increased 36–38% above resting energy expenditure levels in the first few postoperative days.[43] Carbohydrates should be given to supply 50–70% of nonprotein calories, depending on glucose tolerance levels.[26] Fat should be provided by an intravenous fat emulsion solution, providing 30–50% of nonprotein calories, and adjusted depending on serum triglyceride levels.[26] Potassium, magnesium, and phosphorus may need to be supplemented, as several of the medications required post-operatively, particularly cyclosporin A and Lasix, result in altered renal handling of these minerals.

Postoperative ileus generally resolves by the third to fourth day, and in uncomplicated patients, oral feedings may be initiated, beginning with clear liquids and advancing as tolerated.[44] If progression to full oral intake is delayed, either because of postoperative complications or biliary difficulties, alternative enteral routes may be attempted, including continuous nasogastric feedings or jejunal feedings. Parenteral nutrition can be slowly decreased as enteral calories are increased. In the postoperative period, problems of a poor appetite, altered taste sensation, and early satiety are not uncommon.[26] To aid with these problems, supplemental enteral feeding products, especially if volume restriction is also required, may be utilized. Concentrated enteral formulas are available that contain either 1.5 or 2 kcal/mL for this situation. In adolescent patients who have experienced acute liver injury, and whose diet and appetite were normal prior to the transplant, rapid resumption of oral intake is often achievable, with a normal diet being resumed within 7–10d posttransplant.

Once oral nutrition has been reestablished, specific recommendations for continued postoperation nutritional support are then outlined. In order to maintain the adolescent in an anabolic phase, 50–70 cal/kg/day are usually required. Additionally, 1.4–2.0 g of protein/kg/d are needed. Daily calorie counts should be obtained and nutritional parameters followed carefully, including weight, liver function studies, albumin level, electrolytes levels, and mineral status. Cyclosporin A induces retention of potassium, whereas diuretics result in potassium wastage. Accelerated losses of magnesium have also been noted to occur with Cyclosporin A in combination with diuretic therapy. Phosphorus and calcium requirements increase, and not uncommonly patients will require oral supplementation for these minerals. Additionally, cyclosporin A often causes mild renal tubular acidosis that can be corrected with bicarbonate administration.

Although the short-term nutritional goals are to maintain anabolism, the long-term nutritional goals are primarily directed at weight maintenance.[26] Several months following transplantation, nutritional requirements have generally stabilized at approximately 1.2 × basal energy expenditure levels.[26] Protein should be administered as 0.8–1 g/kg/d, and carbohydrate given to supply approximately 60% of total calorie needs. Total fat intake should be at or just below 30% of calories, with < 10% of calories being administered as saturated fat.[26] Maintenance for life on immunosuppressive agents following transplantation, particularly cyclosporin and prednisone, necessitates the encouragement of foods which are rich in the minerals of magnesium, potassium, phosphorus, and calcium. In spite of this, supplemental administration of these minerals is often required for the first few months to 1 yr posttransplant.

Practical considerations. Following liver transplantation, the life of the adolescent is forever changed. In the first several months following transplantation, the need for multiple medications remains significant, and the problems of allograft rejection, infection, and postoperative biliary problems are frequent. Within 1 yr following transplantation, most patients are receiving only Cyclosporin A and prednisone, and have been weaned off blood pressure medications as well as diuretics. However, compliance with taking daily medications remains a significant problem. Additional problems that may also be present include the development of posttransplant obesity, hyperlipidemia, diabetes mellitus, osteoporosis, gingival hyperplasia, dental problems, and delayed growth.[4,26,45] Because steroid medication needs remain high immediately following transplantation, delays in resumption of normal growth rates for adolescents can be expected. However, once steroid therapy has been reduced to an alternate-day schedule, or a markedly lowered daily dose schedule, which is often achieved within the first year, normal resumption of growth rates should occur. Patients should be followed very carefully for this, since resumption of linear growth is not uniformly achieved, with up to 15–59% of patients demonstrating some abnormality in the resumption of linear growth rates.[45] Further adjustments in medication or endocrinologic evaluation and supplementation with growth hormone may be necessary in these patients to further identify and subsequently treat continued growth problems.

Kidney

Although a substantial literature exists regarding the nutritional management of children and adolescents with CRF, including those receiving dialytic therapy,[30,31,33,34] surprisingly little information is available regarding posttransplant dietary management. Nutritional considerations would include the treatment of malnutrition, if present, and thereafter tailoring nutritional goals to minimize the side-effects of immunosuppressive therapy. Corticosteroids, especially in high doses, are well recognized to induce protein catabolism and negative nitrogen balance.[46] In addition, corticosteroids induce carbohydrate intolerance due to impaired glucose metabolism at the cellular level, increased gluconeogenesis, hyperinsulinemia, and increased glucose uptake into fat cells.[47] Cyclosporine also causes carbohydrate intolerance via an alternative mechanism.[48] In addition, hyperlipidemia is a common problem in children receiving dialytic therapy or following renal transplantation,[34,49] and needs to be considered as part of the dietary prescription.

Studies in adult transplant patients have shown that a high-protein diet will prevent the negative nitrogen balance induced by high-dose steroids.[46] Moreover, a diet both high in protein and low in total carbohydrate (1 g/kg) will prevent negative nitrogen balance and significantly moderate cushingoid side-effects.[50] Comparable studies have not been done in adolescents, but total carbohydrate intake this low is impractical for teens and would require increased dietary fat. The latter should be avoided, at least on a chronic basis, as it may exacerbate the hyperlipidemia seen posttransplant.

In view of these considerations, the following recommendations appear reasonable, for the first 6–8 wk following transplant:

1. Protein intake should be at least 3 g/kg to help prevent negative nitrogen balance.[46,50,51]
2. Simple sugars should be eliminated from the diet, although complex carbohydrates should constitute approximately 40% of calories.[51,52]
3. The AHA recommendations regarding total fat, cholesterol, and polyunsaturated fat intake should be followed both early and late following transplantation.[53]
4. Total caloric intake is unrestricted if the patient's body mass index is normal or low, and should be isocaloric or restricted if the body mass index is high. Caloric intake needs to be monitored and tailored to the patient's weight gain.
5. Sodium intake should be restricted to 2 g/day, as the majority of children will be hypertensive posttransplant,[8] and cyclosporine-related hypertension is usually salt-sensitive.[54]
6. Dietary calcium intake is unrestricted and may actually need to be supplemented as steroids frequently promote negative calcium balance. Hypophosphatemia is also not uncommon and may require supplementation if dietary intake is inadequate.[53,54]
7. Hyperkalemia is common in cyclosporine-treated patients[55] and may require dietary moderation.

After the first 6–8 wk posttransplant when steroid doses are reduced, simple sugars can be introduced back into the diet in moderation, and protein intake can be reduced. Dietary fat intake should continue at AHA recommendations, whereas energy intake is dependent on the patient's body mass index. Exercise should be encouraged because of its beneficial effects on carbohydrate metabolism, hyperlipidemia, and muscle anabolism.

Practical considerations. As with all nutritional therapies, compliance is a concern. It is unfortunate that most adolescents approach renal transplantation with the concept that they can eat "anything" after their transplant. Although nutritional recommendations are much less restrictive posttransplant, many teens are reluctant to follow any diet. This is especially true regarding energy intake, due largely to the appetite-stimulating effects of steroids. However, patient education focused on the potential moderation of cushingoid side-effects and weight gain can be helpful to induce dietary compliance, especially among females.

Heart, Heart-Lung, and Lung

Immediately following organ transplantation, patients are in a catabolic state and nutritional requirements are increased. To overcome this, calories for thoracic organ transplantation should be given at 1.5–1.75 times the basal energy expenditure levels, and protein intakes should be 1.2–1.5 g/kg of body weight.[35] This level of nutrient intake can be achieved within the first week post transplantation in most patients. For the initial 48 h following transplantation, IV fluids alone are given, and electrolytes, especially potassium, calcium, and magnesium, are supplemented as needed. Following this initial recovery phase, the diet is generally progressed from clear liquids to full liquids, and ultimately to resumption of full solid food intake. Current recommendations for the post-heart-transplant patient is a diet with 200 mg of cholesterol, low saturated fat, low total fat, high fiber, 4–5 g of sodium, with limited concentrated sweets.[36] The diet should be calculated to supply 45–55% of calories with carbohydrate, 25–35% with protein, and 18–25% with fat.[36] Ten % of the fat should be from monounsaturated fats, 10% or less from saturated fats, and the remainder from polyunsaturated fats.[36] Specific adjustments in calories are also made for each patient, calculated to return the nutritional status to appropriate percentile levels, based on height, weight, and anthropometric data.

Following the acute phase of nutritional rehabilitation, long-term nutritional goals need to be developed. For adolescents, these would include maintenance of adequate weight gain and reestablishment of normal growth rates, moderate restriction of sodium and fat, and supplementation of appropriate vitamins and minerals as needed. Most heart and/or lung recipients are on maintenance doses of immunosuppressive drugs, including cyclosporin, prednisone, and azathioprine. These medications will also necessitate appropriate supplemental dietary support for the associated nutritional side-effects known to occur. Nutritional counseling should be provided to achieve adequate protein status, body cholesterol and lipid levels at 80–100% of those expected for age and gender, desirable body weight and proper proportions of lean body mass to fat, appropriate fluid balance, vitamin and mineral supplementation to appropriate levels, and an overall dietary program that maximizes quality of life.[36]

Compliance, although somewhat more difficult in adolescents, can be maximized with strong nutritional support and education prior to transplantation, and subsequently reinforced throughout the postoperative period.

Practical considerations. Following transplantation for heart and heart-lung recipients, ongoing nutritional assessment should be incorporated into the standard follow-up program, particularly to assure the return of normal growth rates, prevent posttransplantation obesity, and minimize as much as possible the accelerated atherosclerotic coronary artery disease that often occurs in the donor heart.[9,16] Growth rates should return to normal within 6–12 mo following reduction in prednisone dosages to 0.2 mg/kg of weight, or when an alternate-day regimen has been achieved. Posttransplantation obesity is not infrequently present in adults after transplantation and can be anticipated as a problem among adolescents as well.[35-37] A reduction in total caloric intake should be instituted if this occurs. However, of most concern is the need to prevent accelerated atherosclerosis because it frequently jeopardizes long-term graft survival. The causes are not fully known, but several factors are suspected, including atheromatous plaque formation that occurs following immunologic damage from rejection, elevated blood lipid levels associated with posttransplantation weight gain, and altered hepatic synthesis or reduced peripheral catabolism of lipoproteins from cyclosporin therapy.[16,35] Lovastatin may be utilized if cholesterol levels are high without affecting cyclosporin administration and dosages, however, caution to prevent rhabdomyolysis must be taken.[35]

Following lung transplantation, a normal diet can often be rapidly achieved with few attendant difficulties.[9] Again, follow-up as outlined for heart transplantation should be undertaken.

Heart, heart-lung, and lung transplant recipients must be monitored frequently for rejection after transplantation. Frequent myocardial biopsies are required to monitor for cardiac rejection, and more recently, follow-up with coronary artery angiography to monitor for atherosclerosis has been strongly suggested.[16] Lung rejection is followed by frequent pulmonary function studies, as well as endotracheal and bronchial biopsies.[9,56] Side-effects of the immunosuppressive medications should be monitored closely. For cyclosporin, these include hypertension, kidney and liver dysfunction, and increased susceptibility to viral infections and malignancies. For prednisone, these include sodium and fluid retention, diabetes, loss of muscle mass, redistribution of fat, increased appetite, and mood swings. For azathioprine, these include problems with nausea and vomiting along with marrow suppression.

For lung transplant recipients, the most severe problem remains that of the development of bronchiolitis obliterans.[9,13,56] This disease is felt to be the result of repeated episodes of rejection, exacerbated perhaps by recurrent viral infections or aspiration.[9] The prognosis is poor, and the development of this disorder is primarily responsible for the significant fall in long-term survival rates for lung transplantation recipients.[9]

Bone Marrow

High-dose cytoreductive therapy impacts on nutrition through a variety of mechanisms. Oral intake may be reduced by the presence of nausea and vomiting, which may be a direct result of chemotherapy (and to a lesser extent radiotherapy), or due to intestinal dysmotility. Intake is also reduced by the presence of oropharyngeal mucositis and altered taste sensation. Malabsorption occurs due to disruption of the intestinal epithelium by chemotherapy, a situation that may also result in protein and mineral-losing enteropathy. Bacterial overgrowth secondary to antibiotics and narcotics-induced stasis further complicates malabsorption. Diarrhea may occur secondary to malabsorption of fats or water, active secretion due to mucosal damage, or gut infection due to neutropenia and damage to mucosal integrity. Further, tissue breakdown due to high-dose chemotherapy and hypermetabolism secondary to infection may dramatically increase protein and caloric requirements.

Graft vs. host disease (GVHD), a reaction of immunocompetent cells in the marrow graft against recipient tissues (primarily skin, gut, and liver), occurs in a proportion of children and adolescents undergoing allogeneic bone marrow transplantation. Acute GVHD of the gut can involve the entire GI tract from esophagus to rectum, but is most prominent in the ileum and ascending colon. Histopathologic findings associated with GVHD vary from focal crypt cell necrosis to complete denudation. Diarrhea occurs through secretory and malabsorptive mechanisms, and protein loss can be dramatic,[57] leading to profound changes in nitrogen balance. Malabsorption of minerals and zinc loss are also noted. Therapy for GVHD, primarily corticosteroids, complicates the nutritional problem by causing muscle breakdown, negatively impacting on nitrogen balance.

Total parenteral nutrition.   Although the use of total parenteral nutrition (TPN) in undernourished patients undergoing HSCT has become standard practice, the role of prophylactic TPN in well-nourished patients is less clearly defined. It has been suggested that intensive dietary counseling and use of nasogastric feeding make it possible to use the enteral route to support HSCT.[40] However, Weisdorf and colleagues at the University of Minnesota performed a randomized prospective study of prophylactic TPN starting during high-dose chemotherapy.[58] A beneficial effect in terms of duration of hospitalization and overall survival was demonstrated in the group receiving TPN. Other studies have not been this definitive.[59]

Recommended caloric intake is controversial. Although most TPN studies have aimed for caloric intake of 150% or more of basal energy expenditure (BEE), a recent report suggested that use of lower calorie (100% BEE) formulations led to less metabolic complications.[60] Protein requirement is calculated at twice the RDA (1.5–2.0 g/kg of ideal body weight), to compensate for negative nitrogen balance and tissue repair. Lipids may be safely added as an energy source (up to 33% of total calories)[61] and to prevent essential fatty acid deficiency.[62] In addition, the use of fat-free TPN may be complicated by hepatic steatosis. Vitamin and trace elements are added to TPN, generally at RDA, but it has been suggested that requirements of vitamins may be higher than those for nonstressed normometabolic patients. Vitamin A requirements, e.g., are increased in patients with high-protein turnover, and vitamin D requirements may be increased due to the osteoporotic effects of corticosteroid therapy.

Hypokalemia is frequently observed and may be due to the use of furosemide for diuresis, tubular toxicity of various medications (most prominently, amphotericin B), and increased gastrointestinal losses. Profound hypomagnesemia and hypophosphatemia occur and appear to be most severe in patients who have previously received antineoplastic therapy with ifosfamide. Transplant patients therefore require close monitoring of serum electrolytes, and high concentrations of these additives in the TPN are often necessary.

Administration of TPN is not without risks. Catheter-related thrombosis and infection occur, but it is not clear whether the risks of these complications are increased for catheters infusing TPN. Patients receiving TPN are at risk for development of cholestatic jaundice, which may progress to fibrosis, ductular proliferation, and ultimately cirrhosis.[63] Although still controversial, there is some evidence to suggest that the incidence and severity of these changes may be decreased by the use of a TPN-free "window" (i.e., administration of TPN over a 12–18 h period),[64] maintenance of some small enteral intake,[65] or reduction of the nonprotein calorie to nitrogen ratio.[65]

Enteral nutrition. Oral feedings are typically restarted after the stomatitis and other gastrointestinal toxicities of transplantation have resolved. Especially in the pediatric and adolescent patient population, the process of resuming feeding may be very trying for patient, parent, and caretaker alike. Marked food aversion occurs in many cases, particularly in younger patients who recall vividly the transplant-associated mucositis, abdominal pain, and nausea. Taste sensation is altered posttransplant,[66] and previous "favorite foods" may not taste "right." Restrictive diets after transplant further complicate refeeding. Many centers advocate a reduced lactose, fat, or bacteria diet, especially in patients with GVHD,[67,68] but controlled studies demonstrating necessity are lacking.

Early enteral feeding, by nasogastric tube, has been recently advocated by some.[40] Mulder and colleagues have shown that combined enteral and parenteral feedings allow full physiologic support while taking advantage of the mucosal-preserving aspects of enteral alimentation.[69] However, this may not be practical in patients with severe mucositis.

Practical considerations.   As discussed, the resumption of oral feedings after BMT can be difficult and time-consuming. The advent of skilled home health care providers has allowed earlier discharge from the hospital with a continuation of parenteral caloric and protein supplementation. Compliance with special diets (low-fat, low-lactose, low-bacteria) during the immediate postdischarge period has not been studied, but it is expected to be marginal, especially in adolescents. A large proportion of patients will have suboptimal nutrition up to 1 yr after BMT, as seen by continued weight loss or decline in anthropometric indices.[70] This problem is compounded by the presence of chronic graft vs. host disease that continues to adversely affect nutrition status. It is clear that continued monitoring and counseling for months or years are essential in these patients.

CASE ILLUSTRATION

Rose is a 12-year-old white female who was initially admitted initially in August for nutritional rehabilitation and evaluation for combined liver/pancreas transplantation. She was diagnosed with cystic fibrosis at 11 mo of age. At the time of admission, her disease had been complicated by a right middle lobectomy 6 yr earlier, chronic sinusitis with antral window procedures 2 yr earlier, the onset of insulin-dependent diabetes mellitus 1 yr earlier, and the progressive development of cirrhosis with hypersplenism. Although her height and weight parameters had been at the 50% percentile at birth and throughout early childhood, a significant fall-off had been noted over the last several years. On admission, Rose's height was 138 cm, which was less than the 5th percentile, and her weight was 32.5 kg, between the 5th and 10th percentiles. Her height for weight was at the 25th percentile. Anthropometric data demonstrated a midarm circumference of 19.7 cm (10%), triceps skinfold thickness of 8 mm (10%), and MAMA of 23 cm^2 (25%). Dietary analysis over 3 d showed an average caloric intake of 1850 cal/d, and a 72-h fecal fat study demonstrated 14.7% malabsorption, yielding an effective caloric intake of 1200 cal/d. She was absorbing approximately 37–40 cal/kg/d with estimated requirements of 75 cal/kg/d. She was taking 7 Pancrease MT-16 with meals and 4 with snacks, using Lactaid for milk products because of a lactase deficiency and receiving supplements of vitamins A, E, and K. For treatment of her diabetes Rose was requiring 3 U of Ultra Lente and 22 U of regular insulin in divided doses throughout the day with meals. Laboratory studies showed a total protein of 7.2 g % and an albumin that was low at 3.3 g %. A microcytic anemia was also present.

Over the next 7–10 d, supplemental caloric intake was attempted with NG feedings of Isocal HCN. Recurrent sinus difficulties and nausea negated this approach. Following this, Rose was willing to try supplemental Isocal feedings orally and was able to achieve an increased caloric intake of 3500 cal/d. Adjustments in pancreatic enzyme treatment with the addition of Cotazyme and increased amounts of insulin to 65 U of NPH and 120 U of regular insulin were required. She was also found during the hospitalization to have allergic bronchopulmonary aspergillosis as evidenced by a positive skin test to aspergillus and a serum IgE level of 1560, and she was placed on Medrol, 24 mg bid. She was subsequently discharged after having gained 3.7 kg in 2 wk. She was accepted as a candidate for liver/pancreas transplantation.

Over the next 6 mo, she was able to continue on an enteral diet of 3500 cal/d. As her pulmonary function studies improved, her steroid medication was reduced to alternate-day therapy. An increase in linear growth of 1.5 cm and in weight of 4.0 kg was noted during this time.

Rose was subsequently readmitted 5 mo later at 13 yr of age, following two episodes of life-threatening esophageal variceal bleeding. She received sclerotherapy on January 10, 1992, and January 20, 1992, prior to her transfer. Shortly following admission, she experienced a third episode of upper gastrointestinal bleeding, found at endoscopy to be due to an ulcer. To avoid a prolonged period of undernutrition, TPN was initiated. Progression of her liver disease necessitated the daily administration of platelets, fresh frozen plasma, and other blood products, followed by Lasix administration. Fluid restriction requirements then precluded the sole use of enteral nutrition alone, and a continued caloric intake of 3000–3500 cal was provided largely by TPN, limiting her oral intake to 500 cc/d. Over the next 2.5 mo she remained hospitalized, requiring numerous blood products, antibiotics, and maximal medical support, throughout which time Rose continued to receive nutritional support with hyperalimentation, providing calories at 125–150% of the RDA and protein intake at 150% of the RDA. Just prior to transplantation 4 months later, she had gained an additional 4.2 kg and had a midarm circumference of 23.5 cm (50%), triceps skinfold of 17 mm (60%), and MAMA of 26 cm² (45%). Her serum albumin level had increased from 3.3 g to 4.0 g %.

REFERENCES

1. United Network for Organ Sharing, Trends in Organ Transplantation, Part 1, *UNOS Update*, **10**, 4 (1994).

2. S. M. Stewart, R. Uauy, D. A. Waller, B. D. Kennard, M. Benser, and W. S. Andrews, *J. Peds.*, **114**, 574 (1989).

3. S. H. Belle, K. C. Beringer, J. B. Murphy, and K. M. Detre, in *Clinical Transplants 1992*, (P. I. Terasaki and J. M. Cecka, eds.), UCLA Tissue Typing Laboratory, Los Angeles, CA, pp. 17–32 (1992).

4. M. D. Becht, S. H. Pedersen, F. C. Ryckman, and W. F. Balistreri, *Gastroenterol. Clin. N. Am.*, **22**, 367 (1993).

5. B. W. Shaw, Jr., M. Cattral, A. N. Langnas, T. G. Heffron, and I. J. Fox, *Hepatology*, **18**, 66A (1993).

6. C. E. Broelsch, P. F. Whitington, J. C. Emond, T. G. Heffron, J. R. Thistlethwaite, L. Stevens, J. Piper, S. H. Whitington, and J. L. Lichtor, *Ann. Surg.*, **214**, 428 (1991).

7. Dept. of Health and Human Services , USRDS Annual Data Report, Government Printing Office, Bethesda, MD, pp. 59–68 (1991).

8. S. R. Alexander, G. S. Arbus, K. M. H. Butt, S. Conley, R. N. Fine, I. Greifer, A. B. Gruskin, W. E. Harmon, P. T. McEnery, T. E. Nevins, N. Nogueira, O. Salvatierra, Jr., and A. Tejani, *Ped. Nephrol.*, **4**, 542 (1990).

9. D. S. Moodie and P. C. Stillwell, *Clin. Ped.*, **32**, 322 (1993).

10. W. M. Gersony, *J. Peds.*, **116**, 266 (1990).

11. R. E. Michler and E. A. Rose, *Ann. Thorac. Surg.*, **52**, 708 (1991).

12. D. G. Pennington, N. Noedel, L. R. McBride, K. S. Naunheim, and W. S. Ring, *Ann. Thorac. Surg.*, **52**, 710 (1991).

13. V. A. Starnes, S. E. Marshall, N. J. Lewiston, J. Theodore, E. B. Stinson, and N. E. Shumway, *J. Ped. Surg.*, **26**, 434 (1991).

14. L. Benson, R. M. Freedom, W. Gersony, S. R. Gundry, U. Sauer, *J. Heart Lung Transplant.*, **10**, 791 (1991).

15. M. P. Kaye and J. M. Kriett, *J. Heart Lung Transplant.*, **10**, 856 (1991).

16. R. C. Radley-Smith and M. H. Yacoub, *J. Heart Lung Transplant.*, **11**, S277 (1992).

17. D. M. Behrendt, M. E. Billingham, M. M. Boucek, J. M. Marxmiller, and E. A. Rose, *J. Heart Lung Transplant.*, **10**, 841 (1991).

18. R. R. Lower and N. E. Shumway, *Surg. Forum*, **11**, 18 (1960).

19. M. Allard, A. Assaad, L. Bailey, C. Marcelletti, C. Mavroudis, E. Rose, V. Starnes, P. Vouhe, and M. Yacoub, *J. Heart Lung Transplant.*, **10**, 808 (1991).

20. S. Iwatuski, C. O. Esquivel, R. D. Gordon, B. W. Shaw, Jr., T. E. Starzel, R. R. Shade, and D. H. van Thiel, *Sem. Liver Dis.*, **5**, 325 (1985).

21. F. R. Ryckman, R. A. Fisher, and S. H. Pedersen, *Sem. Pediatr. Surg.*, **1**, 162 (1992).

22. I. J. Fox, A. N. Langnas, C. F. Ozaki, J. S. Bynon, J. Vogel, L. Fristoe, J. Merrill, J. Kangas, D. Antonson, D. Schafer, and B. W. Shaw, Jr., *Hepatology*, **16**, 88A (1992).

23. N. L. Sussman, G. T. Gislason, C. A. Conlin, and J. H. Kelly, *Hepatology*, **18**, 65A (1993).

24. J. J. Fath, *Henry Ford Hosp. Med. J.*, **38**, 229 (1990).

25. M. Adler, J. S. Gavaler, R. Duquesnoy, J. J. Fung, G. Svanas, T. E. Starzel, D. H. van Thiel, *Ann. Surg.*, **208**, 196 (1988).

26. J. M. Hasse, *Henry Ford Hosp. Med. J.*, **38**, 235 (1990).

27. A. S. Detsky, J. R. McLaughlin, J. P. Baker, N. Johnston, S. Whittaker, R. A. Mendelson, and K. N. Jeejeebhoy, *JPEN*, **11**, 8 (1987).

28. S. E. Chin, R. W. Shepherd, B. J. Thomas, G. J. Cleghorn, M. K. Patrick, J. A. Wilcox, T. H. Ong, S. V. Lynch, and R. Strong, *Am. J. of Clin. Nutr.*, **56**, 164 (1992).

29. S. M. Mauer, T. E. Nevins, N. Ascher, in *Pediatric Kidney Disease, 2nd ed.*, (C. M. Edelmann Jr., ed.), Little, Brown and Company, Boston/Toronto/London, pp. 941–981 (1992).

30. C. Chantler, in *End Stage Renal Disease in Children*, (R. N. Fine and A. B. Gruskin, eds.), W. B. Saunders Co., Philadelphia/London/Toronto, pp. 193–208 (1984).

31. S. Hellerstein, M. A. Holliday, W. E. Grupe, R. N. Fine, R. S. Fennell, R. W. Chesney, and J. C. M. Chan, *Pediatr. Nephrol.*, **1**, 195 (1987).

32. R. N. Fine, *Kidney Int.*, **42**, 188 (1992).

33. R. A. Weiss, in *Pediatric Kidney Disease, 2nd ed.*, (C. M. Edelmann, Jr., ed.), Little, Brown and Company, Boston/Toronto/London, pp. 815–825 (1992).

34. A. B. Gruskin, H. J. Baluarte, and S. Dabbagh, in *Pediatric Kidney Disease, 2nd ed.*, (C. M. Edelmann, Jr., ed.), Little, Brown and Company, Boston/Toronto/London, pp. 827–916 (1992).

35. C. Moore, Z. Chowdhury, and J. B. Young, *J. Heart Lung Transplant.*, **10**, 50 (1991).

36. D. Ragsdale, *J. Heart Transplant.*, **6**, 223 (1987).

37. K. L. Grady and L. S. Herold, *J. Heart Transplant.*, **7**, 123 (1988).

38. S. Ashwal, A. L. Caplan, W. A. Cheatham, R. W. Evans, and J. L. Peabody, *J. Heart Lung Transplant.*, **10**, 860 (1991).

39. O. H. Frazier, C. T. VanBuren, S. M. Poindexter, and F. Waldenberger, *J. Heart Transplant.*, **4**, 450 (1985).

40. D. J. Szeluga, R. K. Stuart, R. Brookmeyer, V. Untermohlen, G. W. Santos, *Cancer Res.*, **47**, 3309 (1987).

41. S. N. Aker, P. Lenssen, J. Darbinian, C. L. Cheney, and B. Cunningham, *Nutr. Supp. Serv.*, **3**, 22 (1983).

42. A. E. Thompson, *Transplant. Proc.*, **19** (suppl. 3), 34 (1987).

43. B. Delafosse, J. L. Faure, Y. Bouffard, J. P. Viale, J. Goudable, G. Annat, J. Neidecker, O. Bertrand, and J. Motin, *Transplant. Proc.*, **21**, 2453 (1989).

44. A. Grenvik and R. Gordon, *Transplant. Proc.*, **19** (suppl. 3), 26 (1987).

45. S. Sarna, I. Sipila, H. Jalanko, J. Laine, and C. Holmberg, *Transplant. Proc.*, **26**, 161 (1994).

46. M.G. Cogan, J.A. Sargent, S.G. Yarbrough, F. Vincenti, W.J. Amend, *Ann. Intern. Med.*, **95**, 158 (1981).

47. M. McMahon, J. Gerich, and R. Rizza, *Diab. Metab. Rev.*, **4**, 17 (1988).

48. L. S. Dresner, D. K. Andersen, K. U. Kahng, I. A. Munshi, and R. B. Wait, *Surgery*, **106**, 163 (1989).

49. S. van Gool, R. van Damme-Lombaerts, C. Cobbaert, W. Proesmans, and E. Eggermont, *Transplant. Proc.*, **23**, 1375 (1991).

50. F. C. Whittier, D. H. Evans, S. Dutton, G. Ross Jr., A. Luger, K. D. Nolph, J. H. Bauer, C. S. Brooks, and H. Moore, *Am. J. Kid. Dis.*, **VI**, 405 (1985).

51. P. Nelson and J. Stover, in *End Stage Renal Disease in Children*, (R. N. Fine and A. B. Gruskin, eds.), W. B. Saunders Co., Philadelphia/London/Toronto, pp. 209–226 (1984).

52. M. Gammarino, *Dial. Transplant.*, **16**, 497 (1987).

53. National Cholesterol Education Program (NCEP), *Pediatrics*, **89**, 495 (1992).

54. J. J. Curtis, R. G. Luke, P. Jones, and A. G. Diethelm, *Am. J. Med.*, **85**, 134 (1988).

55. K. S. Kamel, J. H. Ethier, S. Quaggin, A. Levin, S. Albert, E.J.F. Carlisle, and M. L. Halperin, *J. Am. Soc. Nephrol.*, **2**, 1279 (1991).

56. D. Metras, B. Kreitmann, H. Shennib, and M. Noirclerc, *J. Heart Lung Transplant.*, **11**, S282 (1992).

57. S. A. Weisdorf, L. M. Salati, J. A. Longsdorf, N. K. Ramsay, and H. L. Sharp, *Gastroenterology*, **85**, 1076 (1983).

58. S. A. Weisdorf, J. Lysne, D. Wind, R. J. Haake, H. L. Sharp, A. Goldman, K. Schissel, P. B. McGlave, N. K. Ramsay, and J. H. Kersey, *Transplantation*, **43**, 833 (1987).

59. S. Weisdorf, C. Hofland, H. L. Sharp, K. Teasley, K. Schissel, P. B. McGlave, N. Ramsay, and J. Kersey, *J. Pediatr. Gastroenterol. Nutr.*, **3**, 95 (1984).

60. A. Taveroff, A. H. McArdle, and W. B. Rybka, *Am. J. Clin. Nutr.*, **54**, 1087 (1991).

61. T. R. Ziegler, L. S. Young, K. Benfell, M. Scheltinga, K. Hortos, R. Bye, F. D. Morrow, D. O. Jacobs, R. J. Smith, J. H. Antin, and D. W. Wilmore, *Ann. Intern. Med.*, **116**, 821 (1992).

62. W. K. Yamanaka, G. Tilmont, and S. N. Aker, *Am. J. Clin. Nutr.*, **39**, 607 (1984).

63. R. J. Merritt, *J. Pediatr. Gastroenterol. Nutr.*, **5**, 9 (1986).

64. M. D. Reed, H. M Lazarus, R. H. Herzig, T. C. Halpin, S. Gross, M. P. Husak, and J. L. Blumer, *Cancer*, **51**, 1563 (1983).

65. R. L. Fisher, *Gastroenterol. Clin. N. Am.*, **18**, 645 (1989).

66. T. Mattsson, K. Arvidson, A. Heimdahl, P. Ljungman, G. Dahllöf, and O. Ringdén, *J. Oral Pathol. Med.*, **21**, 31 (1992).

67. J. M. Gauvreau, P.Lenssen, C. L. Cheney, S. N. Aker, M. L. Hutchinson, and K. V. Barale, *J. Am. Diet Assoc.*, **79**, 673 (1981).

68. S. N. Aker and C. L. Cheney, *JPEN*, **7**, 390 (1983).

69. P. O. Mulder, J. G. Bouman, J. A. Gietema, H. van Rijsbergen, N. H. Mulder, S. van der Geest, and E. G. de Vries, *Cancer*, **64**, 2045 (1989).

70. P. Lenssen, M. E. Sherry, C. L. Cheney, J. W. Nims, K. M. Sullivan, J. M. Stern, G. Moe, and S. N. Aker, *J. Am. Diet. Assoc.*, **90**, 835 (1990).

Vertical Banded Gastroplasty

Edward E. Mason, M.D., Ph. D., F.A.C.S.,
Cornelius Doherty, M.D., F.A.C.S.,
and Joseph Cullen, M.D.

INTRODUCTION

The severely obese adolescent will be defined as a person under 21 yr of age who is at least 100 lb above the estimated ideal weight. The middle value of median-frame size for gender and height in the Metropolitan Life Insurance Tables of 1983 is used as a reference for ideal weight. This requires use of the tables that were developed for adults, but can be used for the severely obese adolescent as a simple way of determining whether the person is sufficiently obese to be considered for surgical treatment. The severely obese adolescent has usually attained the height of an adult.

The weight requirement is a guide, but there are often other reasons for considering operative treatment such as not developing social skills or inability to attend school. A progressive increase in weight is a warning that the individual may develop complications of obesity if the increase is not controlled. When a diagnosis of Prader-Willi syndrome is made, the expectation of continued weight gain and consequent complications of obesity may warrant operative treatment even before severe obesity is present. Prader-Willi syndrome is a genetic disorder identified by weak muscles at birth, underdeveloped gonads and genitalia, low intelligence, and obesity that is progressive and may result in death before adulthood.[1]

There is usually adequate evidence for failure of diet to control weight by the time the patient is considered for surgical treatment, but dietary treatment should be tried if it has not been attempted. Nonsurgical efforts at weight control should not be prolonged once there is evidence of failure. In adults, weight lost by nonsurgical means is usually regained within 5 yr.[2]

If an adolescent is not gaining weight and is able to function, it would seem reasonable to defer a decision regarding surgical treatment in the anticipation that the rapid changes occurring at this time in life might include a decrease to a more normal weight. Clarke and Lauer[3] studied 2631 school children aged 9–18 yr and found that 31% moved from the upper quintile of BMI to a lower level when they became adults, but childhood obesity usually predicted adult obesity. The youngest adults tend to gain the most weight according to Williamson.[4]

Adolescence is a critical period in development, and the decision to use surgery may be much more difficult than for a severely obese adult. Zannolli et al.[5] have suggested that hyperinsulinemic children should be studied more closely as they seem less able to lose weight. Insulin has a lipogenic effect and, in noninsulin-dependent diabetes mellitus, obesity tends to worsen following the institution of insulin therapy according to Fassberg et al.[6] A severely obese adolescent who is gaining more weight in spite of dietary treatment and has recently developed diabetes should be offered surgical treatment without waiting for additional indications. The decision to recommend surgical treatment is difficult and requires the participation of all those who know and care for the patient. The decision will be less difficult if the patient's care providers are aware of surgical choices and the operation recommended is one that is simple, does not change digestion and absorption, and has a low risk of complications.

Etiology

Lay people often ask about abnormal gland function or metabolism as a cause of severe obesity. It is true that overweight occurs in hypothyroidism and Cushing's disease, but these conditions are infrequent and usually diagnosed before the weight is 100 lb in excess of the ideal. Excessive food intake and increasing inability to exercise are the proximate causes of severe obesity. There appear to be both genetic and environmental causes. The only distinctive diagnosis that was found in the 115 patients under age 21 yr who were operated on for severe obesity at UIHC since 1968 was Prader-Willi syndrome diagnosed in 14.

Prognosis

There are children who do not have a cause of obesity that can be identified as genetic and who seem to be normal except for obesity, but who demonstrate a progressive increase in weight that seems to threaten life and longevity. There is no control group of such patients who have been followed without surgery until death or adulthood. Patients with Prader-Willi syndrome often die before adulthood from complications of a progressive increase in weight.

Dietz and Hartung[7] found a decrease in the rate of increase in height in preadolescents during dietary weight reduction. However, most of the adolescents that have been operated on have reached a satisfactory height because of the accelerated growth that occurs in the severely obese person. Deleterious skeletal changes may occur secondary to severe obesity. Henderson[8] found that adolescent tibia vera in his orthopedic practice was seen mainly in severely obese, black males. These patients (27 males and 3 females) averaged 114 kg in weight with a range of 65–163 kg. Early correction of severe obesity should prevent such changes.

Gortmaker et al.[9] found that obesity during adolescence reduces family income in later life and has important social consequences. These overweight adolescents averaged 157% of the ideal for women and 142% for men, so most of them would not have been sufficiently heavy to consider operative treatment.

History of Surgical Treatment

Surgical treatment of the severely obese began at the University of Iowa Hospitals and Clinics (UIHC) in 1955 in adult patients with large hernias or diseased gall bladders who were so heavy that the needed surgical procedure was deferred. Diets were prescribed to prepare patients for the needed operation, but they were ineffective and the only patients who came to operation were those who developed an acute and life-threatening emergency. Of course, the operative mortality of such emergency operations was high and added to the impression that such severely obese patients could not be safely operated on. The history of obesity surgery has been reviewed elsewhere,[10] but a brief description of the operations that are presently used will help understand the recommendations for surgery and the care that is needed. There are two operations with which surgeons have had the most experience: Roux-en-Y gastric bypass (RGB) and vertical banded gastroplasty (VBG).

Roux gastric bypass (RGB).   Gastric bypass, like gastroplasty, divides the stomach into a small food-receiving segment and the rest of the stomach. The small pouch empties into the small bowel in gastric bypass, whereas in gastroplasty, it empties into the larger segment of the stomach. Both gastroplasty and gastric bypass have undergone changes. At the present time, the pouch is usually vertical, located on the lesser curvature, and very small in capacity.

Gastric bypass[11] was originally patterned after an extensive gastric resection, an operation that was used for the treatment of peptic ulcer and had the undesirable effect of producing unwanted weight reduction in patients whose original weight was normal. In the original gastric bypass, a loop of intestine was used for the gastroenterostomy, but this could lead to bile gastritis and esophagitis. To keep bile from the stomach pouch, a Roux-en-Y type of gastroenterostomy was used (see Figure 27.1).

One of the mechanisms of weight reduction after gastric bypass is the dumping syndrome. The pylorus that governs normal emptying of the stomach is bypassed in both gastric resection and gastric bypass. Normally, duodenal and intestinal contents are maintained at the same concentration as body fluids. They are isotonic. After gastric bypass, hypertonic fluids enter the small bowel without control. Hypertonic foods and fluids like ice cream and milkshakes cause many patients to become weak and sweaty from decreased circulating plasma volume and to have cramps from increased peristalsis. When such dumping symptoms are severe, patients may need to lie down until the symptoms subside. There is rapid movement of the ingested food through the entire small bowel even when very little of the bowel has been bypassed. Sudden explosive diarrhea may occur.

Bypass of the duodenum results in poor iron and calcium absorption and may in time produce iron-deficiency anemia and/or metabolic bone disease. More extensive bypass may also cause protein malabsorption and low body proteins. There are certain complications that are peculiar to bypass operations that add to the long-term risk of such operations.

Vertical banded gastroplasty (VBG).   Designed[12] to limit the food intake at any one time (see Figure 27.2), but to allow the food to pass into all of the stomach and the rest of the digestive tract in normal sequence so as to maintain normal digestion and absorption. The pylorus remains in control of emptying of the stomach so that dumping symptons do not occur.

VBG requires the construction of a measured lesser-curvature pouch. The pouch averages 13 mL in volume, measured with a 70-cm head of water pressure during the operation. A partition extends, parallel to the lesser curvature, from the esophagogastric angle of His to the site of the outlet. This provides a narrow pouch with a long intraluminal high-pressure zone and in this way functions not only to reduce food intake, but as an antireflux operation.[13] Heartburn is common in the severely obese, but this is usually relieved after VBG.

The outlet of the pouch is encircled with a 1.5-cm-wide Marlex mesh that is sewn to itself to provide a collar 5.0 cm in circumference. There is a stapled window between the greater and lesser peritoneal cavities through which the collar is placed. This obviates sewing the collar to the stomach wall and avoids contamination from bacteria that might be in the stomach lumen.

VBG is the only operation that is in use at UIHC both as a primary operation and as a revision operation for patients who have had problems with other procedures such as intestinal bypass, horizontal gastroplasty, and gastric bypass. The technique of VBG has not changed at UIHC since 1987.[14] Many of the

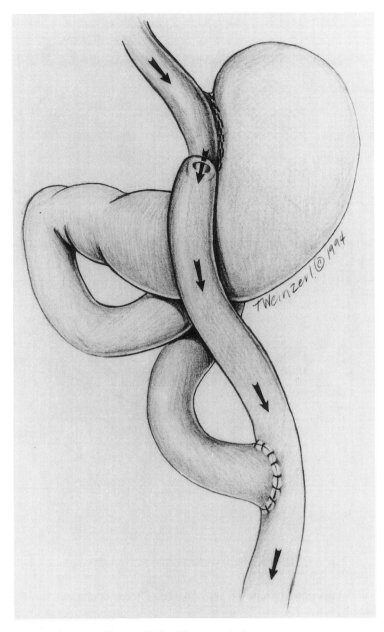

Figure 27-1.   Roux gastric bypass.

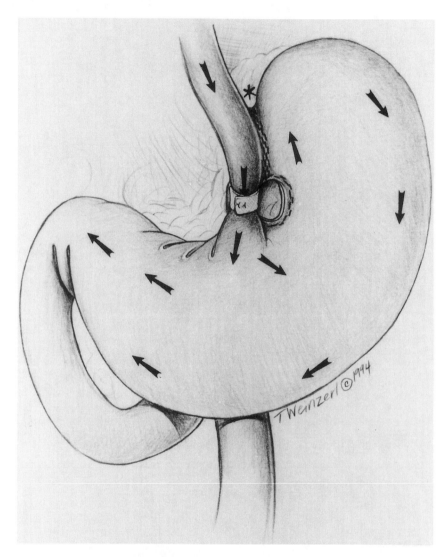

Figure 27-2. Vertical banded gastroplasty.

technical details important in the performance of these operations are reported elsewhere.[15]

Obstruction to the passage of food from the pouch to the greater stomach is not the goal of VBG. In the early experience with the operation, a 5.0-cm circumference collar was found to produce better weight loss than a 5.5-cm collar. When the collar was further reduced to 4.5 cm, the result was not greater weight loss but a change in the diet. The smaller collar led to the use of foods that were not as fibrous and would convert to liquid quickly without mastication. Such foods are easier to eat so that the caloric intake is often increased. The goal of VBG is to reduce the capacity for a meal and allow a normal diet with fibrous foods.

The secret of successful use of a well-constructed VBG is in the chewing. The meal should not be rushed or taken during emotional stress. The meat should be cut in small slices and chewed well. All foods should be chewed to a semifluid consistency before they are swallowed. Proper eating results in excellent digestion after VBG and without regurgitation or distress. The entire stomach can be intubated through the nose or mouth if this is ever needed with VBG, that preserves easy access for radiographic and endoscopic study of the upper gastrointestinal tract. Also, VBG is easily reversed if there is need for a normal stomach at some time later in life.

Biliopancreatic diversion (BPD) and extended gastric bypass. Scopinaro et al.[16] have had extensive experience with an operation called biliopancreatic diversion (Figure 27.3). This operation is similar to a Roux-en-Y gastric bypass, but with much more of the small bowel bypassed. There is a gastroileostomy performed 200 cm proximal to the cecum and jejunoileostomy 50 cm from the ileocecal valve. Because of an increased risk of ulceration at the gastroileostomy stoma with such a reconstruction, a gastric resection is performed by Scopinaro instead of gastric bypass. The stomach pouch is 200–500 mL in volume. The smaller volume pouch is used for patients with the greatest operative weight. After BPD, a patient must eat large amounts of protein to avoid protein malnutrition. Surgeons who use BPD do so because of their desire to bring all patients to normal weight. BPD is not recommended for adolescent patients, although Scopinaro has used it in patients as young as 11 yr of age.

Gastric banding (GB). Another operation that is in use and one that may be more easily performed through the laparoscope since stapling is not involved. In GB, a collar is placed around the stomach near the esophagus so that there is a small upper pouch (Figure 27.4). This operation requires no staples since the entire stomach is gathered together to form the small channel between the pouch and main stomach. Kuzmak[17] has developed a modification of GB called stoma adjustable silicone gastric banding. There is a bladder on the inner surface of the band that is connected by a length of silastic tubing to an injection port placed under the skin on the anterior abdominal wall. It is possible to remove or inject saline into the subcutaneous port using fluoroscopic guidance. This changes the diameter of the channel that empties the pouch. GB with the adjustable band remains under study by a limited group of surgeons, including surgeons at UIHC, but has not yet been approved for general use.

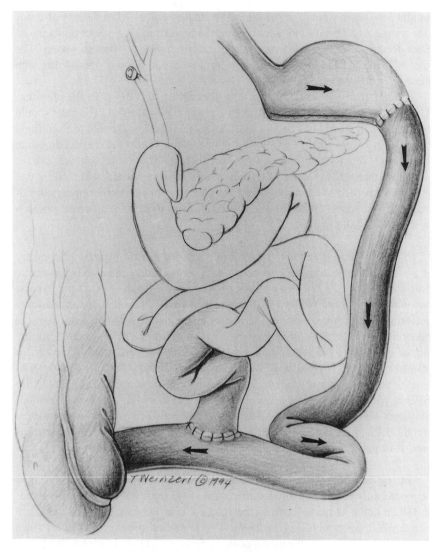

Figure 27-3.   Biliopancreatic diversion.

ASSESSMENT

Once surgical candidacy has been approved, the clinical dietitian seeing the adolescent or young adult before the operation should decide whether the patient's nutrition is adequate. Not all severely obese are well nourished. The determination is based on dietary history. Rarely, will a teen have such an unbalanced diet as

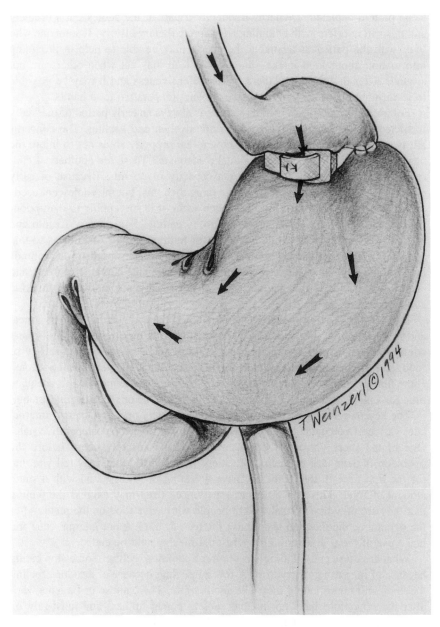

Figure 27-4.   Gastric banding.

to be protein-depleted. Denial is frequently a part of the adolescent's problem and this can interfere with obtaining an accurate dietary history. If someone who lives with the patient is available, he or she may be able to help in providing information about food intake although the teen may eat when others are not around. After the operation, there is less defensiveness and it may be possible to learn more about the current diet and even preoperative food habits.

Following the surgical procedure, there is always an early period of markedly restricted food intake while the tissues are swollen and healing. The concerns are two-fold. Is the patient learning how to eat properly so as not to injure the healing tissues and is the patient's intake adequate? These are antithetical concerns. The average VBG pouch has a capacity of 15 mL. Because of early emptying, the volume of a meal may be more than this, but the adolescent needs to use caution in not overfilling the pouch while it is susceptible to disruption. Adolescents or young adults should begin by eating 15 mL/ every 15 min and gradually increase intake while watching for internal signals of fullness so that they will not regurgitate or become uncomfortable. They need to drink fluids between meals so as to allow room for food. A medicine cup is used to eat and drink from. Eating in this manner while hospitalized keeps the patient thinking about protecting the pouch.

Later, when the teen is seen in the clinic, he or she are eating more at a meal and a wider variety of food. The assessment at this time relates to the young adult's understanding, compliance and comfort with the increasing variety of food, and whether he or she is remembering to cut meat into very small portions, chew fibrous food to a pureed consistency before swallowing, taking adequate time for a meal, and slowing down or quitting before he or she is uncomfortable.

The key to compliance is the recognition of satiety or internal cues. Internal cues vary between patients and between the preoperative and postoperative state. One of the more consistent characteristics of the severely obese before the operation is their lack of feeling of satiety. After VBG, they may tell you that for the first time in their life they have a feeling of fullness and with a small amount of food. This is a welcome experience. They may express the feeling that they are now like normal-weight people who leave food on the plate. After the operation, the dietitian should ask the teen to think about internal cues and make use of them in determining when the meal should be ended.

What are these cues? Fullness is the most common feeling. Some stop eating because of increasing discomfort. A few quit eating because of a sudden feeling that they will regurgitate if they take another bite. There are some patients who, after the operation, have no internal cues to signal fullness and must rely on measuring their food and fluid intake in order to avoid regurgitation. The available internal and external cues for both hunger and satiety determine how the patient can best regulate the amount of food at a meal and the frequency and timing of meals to assure adequate intake without overloading the pouch.

Early after the operation, a patient may feel a need for high-protein liquid supplements or wish to prolong the use of pureed foods to assure an adequate intake. It is preferred for the long-term goal to not recommend these methods of increasing food intake. It is permissible for the young adult to remain in negative nitrogen balance along with the desired negative energy balance during the early months following a restriction operation, provided there is evidence that intake is increasing. Some surgeons like to have the patient remain on a pureed diet for 6 wk at that time the stapled partition will have reached a near-maximum strength. Other surgeons prefer that the patient start early with normal foods so that he or she learns from the beginning how to eat and does not develop the habit of using soft foods, junk foods, and high-calorie liquids. The one common admonition is that nothing should be swallowed that is not of the consistency of pureed food. If the patient will use mastication to prepare the food for swallowing, this is consistent with the life-long behavior that is desired.

There are a few patients who have problems with vomiting. This is usually because they have not followed the recommended pattern of eating. This can occur early or late and may recur because the patient forgets lessons learned, or simply decides to test the operation and make sure it is still working. Occasionally, a patient will forget to chew well enough and a piece of meat or other food will become impacted in the lower end of the pouch. This is usually sudden in onset and the offending food is often the last bite eaten. If this does not respond to a period of abstinence, starting over with clear liquids, and working up to a normal diet, then the patient should come to the clinic for more detailed evaluation and possible admission for intravenous fluids while the diagnosis is made and appropriate treatment provided.

Is the rate of weight loss appropriate for the adolescent's operative weight and for the time following operation? Rapid weight loss is of less concern in a patient who feels well and has no complaints about eating and drinking. However, it may be that the patient is being too cautious and needs to take more by mouth and learn to rely on internal cues instead of restricting intake by measured amounts of food that are inadequate and by eating so infrequently as to have an inadequate intake of fluid and protein.

Weight loss is related to the amount of retained fluid and the amount of fat that is burned from the storage areas. Early weight loss may be at a rate of a pound a day. This should not continue beyond a few weeks unless the patient is extremely heavy. The heavier the patient at operation, the more rapid the weight loss. After a few weeks the loss is a few pounds a week. Most patients lose about 60% of their excess weight in 8 mo. Weight loss is often episodic. There are periods of no weight loss and the teen may become concerned about this. This is the situation in which a patient dieting without the help of an operation would become discouraged and give up. VBG keeps the program going.

Most patients with VBG are aware of the need to chew meat thoroughly. If a patient suddenly discerns that fibrous foods can be eaten with much less chewing and this is associated with a sudden gain in weight, then the patient may need an upper gastrointestinal radiograph to determine if there is disruption of the staple line so that the pouch is no longer limiting the food intake.

Nutritional assessment becomes more complex in patients who have had more complex operations. The dietitian needs to determine whether there has been a change in the patient's eating pattern, bowel habits, abdominal comfort, frequency of feeling nausea, and vomiting. The questions will relate to what the patient has been asked to do about special efforts to obtain additional protein foods and medications and whether this is now possible. Adequate calcium intake may be difficult especially if the patient does not tolerate milk and milk products. The most important question is whether the problem is a simple dietary one that can be worked out with a food diary, or there is need for a medical assessment by the surgeon or a physician.

Assessment of the Presence of VBG

Since there are increasing numbers of patients with operations for obesity, the dietitian can provide great help simply by determining whether a newly admitted patient has had an operation for the treatment of obesity and, if so, the type of operation. The dietitian may then need to educate the other care givers as to the need for caution in the use of a diet for the treatment of such a patient. A commonly used component of treatment for many diseases is an increased intake of food and fluid. Patients with VBG have been given larger than normal meals, with between-meal snacks, and then admonished to eat all of this food. This has resulted in the disruption of the pouch with consequent regain of weight. The assessment of the dietitian in such patients is the key to recognizing that increased oral intake cannot be used. Continuous gavage feeding with a small nasal gastric tube given slowly with a food pump might be considered or parenteral nutrition.

Second generation patients.   We are now seeing severely obese children of patients who have had gastric reduction operations. The response of the parent to gastric reduction surgery may help in predicting the response of the offspring. One multiparous woman was admitted in respiratory failure weighing over 600 lb. She required respiratory support for a month while she lost fluid and some of her stored fat. She had a gastric bypass that was finally converted to a vertical gastroplasty to relieve an intractable iron-deficiency anemia. She had her 10th and 11th pregnancies during the years of gastric bypass. Her weight began at 420% of the ideal, reached a low of 145%, and was 213% of the ideal just before she died. She died after 19 yr of living with gastric reduction operations and fair control of her obesity.

This patient's daughter had a gastric bypass at age 18 yr, when she weighed 388 lb. The daughter had two revisions of her gastric bypass and finally conversion to a VBG. However her weight gradually increased to 418 lb after 20 yr of life with gastric reduction operations. The daughter has had four pregnancies.

There are surgeons who would have used an operation that would create greater malabsorption for such super-obese patients in an attempt to bring them to a normal weight. This would have increased the medical care requirements for these women who had limited resources and rather chaotic family lives. VBG (as a revision) was used to treat postgastric-bypass-iron-deficiency anemia in the mother and to prevent anemia, bone disease and other complications in the daughter.

MANAGEMENT

Preoperative

The fact that an adolescent or young adult is being considered for VBG, has more than 100 lb of stored fat, does not guarantee that nutrition is adequate. If the person is fairly active and not complaining of tiredness and weakness, the protein-dependent muscle mass is likely satisfactory. Serum albumin levels can be misleadingly normal in a patient who has protein malnutrition until after the stress of a major operation, so the dietary history is of greater value than a normal serum albumin. If serum albumin concentration is low, the protein malnutrition should be corrected before the operation. If protein malnutrition is present in an adolescent because of a poor diet, any elective surgical procedure should be deferred until body protein is restored.

When a patient has had an operation for obesity, the dietitian helping to care for that patient will need information about the type of operation performed and any complications that are peculiar to that operation. Iron-deficiency anemia may occur because of bypass of the duodenum, where iron is most actively absorbed. Vitamin B-12 deficiency is more common when the distal stomach is bypassed or removed. Anemia after RGB, or BPD, if there is no distal gastric resection, should raise the question of bleeding from a duodenal ulcer. These are difficult to diagnose when the duodenum has been bypassed because of impaired access for radiographic and endoscopic examination.

Early after VBG, there is such a reduced capacity for food that there may be a temporarily inadequate intake of protein and vitamins. A small multiple-vitamin capsule that will pass through the pouch easily should be routine. High-quality protein foods are emphasized. Meat and other high-fiber foods may be difficult, but if patients take small bites and chew their food until it is of a pureed consistency, they can usually manage all types of food. Eggs are an excellent source of protein. Many adolescents must be taught that it is the white and not the yellow part that contains the protein.

The dietitian's challenge with these patients is to encourage a normal variety of food and discourage the use of highly processed foods that are more easily eaten because they pass through the pouch easily. The goal of the operation is to reduce caloric intake by a reduction in capacity for a meal and provision of a sense of early satiety. The dietitian should help the patient learn healthy eating patterns, with an emphasis on normal foods.`

At UIHC, we have a television presentation that shows patients what to expect and this includes scenes showing the patient using a medicine cup to eat and drink from so that the volumes will not overload the small pouch. This restricted eating is emphasized while the patient is in the hospital and early after he or she returns home.

As the swelling goes down from the operation and patients learn how to eat, they can gradually increase the volume of intake. They may need sips of fluid to help liquiefy dry foods that they eat, but they should drink most of their liquids between meals as there is not pouch capacity to accommodate both liquids and solids during a meal.

Patients are also advised to avoid pregnancy during the early period of rapid weight loss. However, if a patient does become pregnant early after the operation, there is no reason to terminate the pregnancy. Vitamins should be a routine supplement because defects in the embryo, if they occur, may develop before the patient is aware that a pregnancy is present. Developmental defects are rare and the recommendations are based more on theoretical reasons than observed unsatisfactory outcomes of pregnancy. Folic acid is important in the prevention of neural tube defects that develop very early in embryonic development. The dietitian should make sure that adequate amounts of this vitamin are present in food or vitamins if a patient is at risk of pregnancy.

Frequent vomiting is not common after a VBG or any other gastric reduction operation. However, if it develops and lasts more than 2 d, the patient should be encouraged to return to his or her surgeon for diagnosis and treatment. The cause of persistent vomiting must be found and treated before a severe deficiency state develops. Wernicke-Korsakoff syndrome is a result of thiamin deficiency and occurs in patients who are allowed to continue with frequent vomiting for 2 or 3 mo. This is a combined central and peripheral neuropathy that is rapidly progressive, often irreversible, and rapidly lethal if not treated. Severe protein malnutrition may develop in a patient with uncorrected vomiting. These are rare complications, but the dietitian may at times be in a position to direct the patient to needed care and the prevention of such complications.

Clinical Experience

During the first 13 yr of experience with VBG at UIHC, there were 45 patients under 21 yr of age (31 females and 14 males).[18] Sixteen were 20 yr of age, five

19, ten 18, four in each of the ages 15, 16, and 17, and two were 14. There were no operative deaths and no instances of a leak with peritonitis. There were no patients with pneumonia and no wound infections. The days of hospitalization following the operation ranged from 3–10 with an average of 5.2 d and mode of 6 d. Thirteen patients went home on the 4th postoperative day. The operation is therefore safe, although the teen and family are warned about the possibility of peritonitis, wound infection, hernia, pulmonary embolism and death. During this time, the operative mortality rate for over 1000 adult patients was 0.4% and complications serious enough to result in a hospital stay of 1 or 2 d more occurred in less than 1% of patients.

Information is available for 25 (74%) of the 34 of patients eligible for a 5 yr follow-up. Their initial weights averaged 138 kg at operation and 103.6 kg at 5 yr. Body mass index was 48.1 at operation and 36.2 at 5 yr. The average 5 yr excess weight loss was 45.6%. One revision was required within the first 5 yr and this was to restaple a disrupted staple line.

At 10 yr after VBG there are 14 patients who have been contacted out of the 19 eligible for contact for a 74% follow-up. The average weight at operation was 135.8 kg and at 10 yr this was 107.6 kg. The body mass index was 49.6 at operation and 39.2 at 10 yr. The figures for the five males were 168.6 kg at operation and 129.6 kg at ten years with the BMI changing from 55.7 to 42.4. For the nine women the operative weight averaged 159.3 at operation and 95.3 at 10 yr with a change in BMI from 46.2 to 37.3. There were two additional revisions between 5 and 10 yr, and both of these were to correct pouches that were too large. This had caused weight gain in one patient and there had developed poor emptying with reflux, heartburn, and vomiting. These problems were corrected by a revision in which the pouch was reduced in size. The other patient had not lost as much weight as she desired. The pouch was enlarged by upper gastrointestinal radiographic study. Revision to a smaller pouch caused only temporary weight reduction, but perhaps the small pouch will prevent future enlargement to a size that might create problems with emptying. Both of these patients had pouches measured at their primary operation that were over twice the volume that we now recommend. Both had pouches reduced to 15 mL at the revision, that is the average size we have used in all VBGs performed since 1987.

Most of the operations that are in use today for the treatment of obesity have been described in order that dietitians will have a better understanding of these operations. VBG is recommended for a severely obese adolescent whose weight is more than 100 lb above the estimated ideal and especially if there is a progressive increase in weight. VBG is simple, well standardized, and will control the weight in most adolescents. It seldom will bring the adolescent or young adult to a normal weight, but it does not have the potential for malnutrition and late complications that follow bypass operations, especially those that include an extensive intestinal bypass.

CASE ILLUSTRATION

The first adolescent who underwent VBG, in 1981, was an 18-year-old male who had a lifelong history of increasing obesity, unresponsive to diet. Mike was unable to sleep because of heavy breathing and a cough so severe that it caused him to gag. He weighed 178 kg before VBG, 129 kg at 5 yr after operation, and 105 kg at 12 yr. He weighed 280% of the ideal preoperatively, 203% at 5 yr and 165% at 13 yr. Thirteen yr after his operation, Mike still forgets to chew his food to a semisolid consistency when he comes home with excessive hunger after a day of heavy physical work. As a consequence he has epigastric discomfort from failure of the food to pass. He can relieve this by regurgitation and then, by eating properly can retain the meal in comfort. This is an abnormal eating pattern and unusual. It illustrates that the underlying disease remains, even though the operation controls his weight at a safe level. It also illustrates the type of counseling that a dietitian must provide for patients with VBG. Mike does not need a special diet. He has had instruction in eating and has learned to take small bites, chew his food well, and stop eating before he is uncomfortably full. Although he has learned how to eat, he is frequently unable to follow this pattern, especially if he is very hungry. Mike has not missed a day's work in 13 yr. He feels well and is living a full life. It is reasonable to believe that had he not had the operation, weight gain would have continued and he would have been unable to work. He might not even be alive now, 13 yr after his operation.

REFERENCES

1. H. Zellweger and H. J. Schneider, *AJDC*, **115**, 588 (1968).
2. NIH Technology Assessment Conference Panel, *Ann. Intern. Med.*, **119**, 764 (1993).
3. W. E. Clarke and R. M. Lauer, *Crit. Rev. Food Sc. Nutr.*, **33**, 423 (1993).
4. D. F. Williamson, *Ann. Intern. Med.*, **119**, 646 (1993).
5. R. Zannolli, A. Rebeggiani, R. Chiarelli, and G. Morgese, *AJDC*, **147**, 837 (1993).
6. J. Fassberg, W. L. Toffler, S. A. Fields, and L. D. Loriaux, *J. Fam. Prac.*, **37**, 837 (1993).
7. W. H. Dietz and R. Hartung, *AJDC*, **139**, 705 (1985).
8. R. C. Henderson, *J. Peds.*, **121**, 482 (1992).
9. S. I. Gortmaker, A. Must, J. M. Perrin, A. M. Soboi, and W. H. Dietz, *N. Engl. J. Med.*, **329**, 1008 (1993).
10. E. E. Mason, *Surgical Treatment of Obesity*, W. B. Saunders Co., Philadelphia, PA (1981).
11. E. E. Mason and D. Ito, *Surg. Clin. N. Am.*, **47**, 1345 (1967).
12. E. E. Mason, *Arch. Surg.*, **117**, 701 (1982).

13. M. Deitel and I. Riivo, *Prob. in Gen. Surg.*, **9**, 390 (1992).

14. E. E. Mason, *Surg. Clin. N. Am.*, **67**, 521 (1987).

15. E. E. Mason and C. Doherty, in *Surgery of the Upper Gastrointestinal Tract*, (G. G. Jamieson and H. T. Debas, eds.), Chapman and Hall, New York, pp. 548–560 (1994).

16. N. Scopinaro, E. Gianetta, D. Friedman, E. Traverso, G. F. Adami, B. Vitale, G. Marinari, S. Cuneo, F. Ballari, M. Colombini, and V. Bachi, *Prob. in Gen. Surg.*, **9**, 362 (1992).

17. L. I. Kuzmak, *Prob. in Gen. Surg.*, **9**, 298 (1992).

18. E. E. Mason, D.H. Scott, C. Doherty, J. J. Cullen, E. M. Rodriguez, J. W. Maher, and R. T. Soper, *Obesity Surg.*, **5**, 23 (1995).

CHAPTER

28

Plastic and Reconstructive Surgery

Susan Porter Levy, Psy.D., and
Laurie Macleod, R. N.

INTRODUCTION

Issues of nutrition are particularly relevant to adolescents undergoing orthognathic surgery for correction of significant malocclusion, craniofacial deformity, and reconstruction or repair following trauma. The timing of orthognathic surgery is carefully planned (except in cases of trauma) and it is frequently performed during adolescence, once the bones have reached maturity and significant growth is no longer expected. The process of orthognathic surgery requires that one or both of the jaws be surgically broken, moved, and fixed into a more appropriate alignment with plates and wires or elastic bands. The external fixation process lasts from 2 to 10 wk, depending on the surgical technique. During that time, the patient's diet is restricted to liquid or soft foods, again, depending on the specific type of fixation used. Immediately following surgery, adequate fluid intake is necessary to prevent dehydration, and during recovery, proper nutrition is essential to wound healing and prevention of infection.

There are many issues that influence a patient's decision to have reconstructive craniofacial surgery. Much of the important social, academic, and emotional functioning of the adolescent is dependent on oral-motor functioning. Activities such as telephone conversations, eating, giving a school book report, as well as expressing feelings, are central to adolescent life. The surgery may be considered primarily to change the appearance, but frequently (32–78%) is sought to improve the function of the face and mouth.[1] The social standards for beauty and the stigma associated with being "different" are especially important to teens who have profound facial deformity.[2] Unfortunately, a dental or facial disproportion is considered ugly in our society. Unattractive individuals, solely as a result of their appearance, are more likely to receive negative social reactions from others. Consequently, they have less peer involvement and also tend to display more aggressive, impulsive, or withdrawn behaviors.[3] In contrast, attractive people are seen as kinder, brighter, more likable, and more successful.[4] The work of the attractive person tends to be judged more favorably, whereas the errors of the unattractive are judged more harshly.[5] Thus, the teen with a craniofacial deformity is likely to suffer from a cumulative assault, resulting in lowered self-esteem, poor body image, and poor peer relationships, and possibly, lowered academic performance.

Left uncorrected, craniofacial malformations are associated in adolescence and adulthood with measurable disturbances in mood, self-concept, and socialization.[6] There is also evidence to suggest that treatment regimens that improve facial appearance appear to have concomitant improvements in aesthetic self-satisfaction and body image.[7] Unfortunately, patients also often expect surgery to fulfill certain psychosocial needs, including increased popularity, improved speech, better looks, less teasing about appearance, and more friends. Although surgery can contribute to improved self-esteem and potentially lead to those positive psychosocial results, the procedure, in and of itself, does not create magical personality or behavioral changes. Before the surgery is performed, it is essential that the teen's expectations of results be explored. If the patient or family's expectations of results are unrealistic, they will inevitably be dissatisfied with the results of surgery. The adolescent patient must personally identify with the treatment and develop an appreciation for the functional and aesthetic goals of therapy.

ASSESSMENT

There are myriad factors that influence the adolescent's ability and willingness to participate in his or her own postoperative recovery and to gain adequate nutrition following surgery. Among these factors are developmental, family, and psychosocial issues; common and idiopathic emotional responses; fund of knowledge and information about the procedure and recovery; and degrees of practice and preparation. A dietitian might be called to consult on a teen who is refusing to drink or eat following orthognathic surgery.

Immediately following surgery, patients may refuse to drink liquids. As mentioned, it is essential that the adolescent drink after the surgical procedure to liquify secretions and facilitate the healing process. The teen's emotional state, fear, nausea, pain experience, and nasal congestion can all inhibit his or her willingness to take liquids immediately following surgery.

The orthognathic surgery procedure can potentially have a significant impact on a teen's emotional well-being.[8] Studies of the mood states of patients undergoing this procedure suggest that the anticipation of surgery results in considerable tension and anxiety. The days immediately following surgery are characterized by fatigue, loss of vigor, moderate levels of tension and anxiety, and some depression. The adolescent often wakes from surgery to see frightened, terrified, and anxious parents hovering over the bed. Feelings of helplessness to ease the teen's fears or pain tend to accelerate the anxiety experienced by the parents. This anxiety is readily transferred to teens who tend to take their cues about how to respond to the experience from those around them. The parents who are prepared to see their teen immediately postoperatively will likely wear less of a pained, worried expression and be a more calming emotional resource.

Immediately following surgery, especially in the first 24–48 h after surgery as edema peaks, patients often report feelings of claustrophobia and fears of vomiting, suffocation, and death. They are primarily motivated to protect their airway and resist actions (such as drinking) that might jeopardize their ability to breathe. The adolescent may also need to be encouraged to swallow his or her own saliva. The realization that fluids can pass through the wires or bands and not cause choking or suffocation is often of great relief to the oral surgery patient. These fears often persist and inhibit the teen's willingness to drink well into the recovery period. In addition, anesthesia, narcotics, analgesics, swallowed blood, and some antibiotics can cause stomach upset or nausea. They need to be assured that liquids can pass through the wires and shown how to self-suction, how to turn their heads, or spit.

Adolescents will experience a certain degree of pain or discomfort following the procedure. The problem with pain is that it, too, interferes with the teen's willingness to take fluids necessary to hydrate his or her secretions. Adolescents should not be told that they won't hurt, but instead, convinced that people will hear and respond if they are in pain. Adolescent males, in particular, may need to be given permission to admit when they are in pain. There should be adequate trust established between patient and provider so that pain control will be achieved. However, it is very easy to overmedicate these adolescents to calm their fears and ease their pain. However, sedated teenagers don't drink. The degree of discomfort is related to the surgical technique employed. For example, if bone has been harvested from a rib or pelvis, greater pain is expected and the patient may not feel like drinking. The teen may have a sore throat from an intubation tube and feel that swallowing may further irritate his or her throat.

Initially, there is also likely a great deal of nasal congestion and drainage that further serves to decrease appetite and change the taste of food. If the adolescent is reassured that this will diminish over time, he or she is less likely to believe that it is a permanent result of surgery.

The dietitian may also be called to consult on a teen who is refusing to eat during the initial recovery phase after surgery. Swelling, emotional responses, instructions to perform uncomfortable or painful mouth care, and a desire to lose weight quickly and effortlessly can each negatively influence the maintenance of an adequate nutritional status.

Swelling makes eating difficult because there is not much room into that to insert nourishment, and the lips don't work very well. We believe that it is humiliating to the adolescent to be fed by parents or staff. Further, feeding the teen encourages him or her to regress emotionally and forestalls the healing process. We encourage parents to adopt an expectant attitude that their teen will recover and not to tolerate behaviors such as tantrums or disrespect that they find unacceptable at home. If the adolescent is encouraged to talk, even though it is difficult to make him- or herself understood, the increased mobility of the lips and lower face helps decrease the edema more quickly. In the past, we encouraged the writing of requests, but discovered that notes perpetuated the edema. We have found that encouraging a rapid return to normal activity facilitates a prompt recovery. The more quickly the teen sits up, gets out of bed, and wears regular clothes, the faster he or she seems to recover. A lengthy acute postoperative period may facilitate the "sick role."

Most adolescents are shocked with the amount of swelling and their frightful postoperative appearance. It may appear that their preoperative fear of "looking worse than they started" has come true. They need to be convinced of the transient nature of the swelling and bruising, as well as educated about the importance of diet, oral care and pain management. They should be convinced that *everything* they do affects the long-term result of their appearance. If they are noncompliant with oral care, an infection could adversely affect the surgical outcome. Although the research suggests that adolescent females are most critical of their appearance, studies also indicate that adolescent males have a more difficult time accepting a change in appearance.[9] These findings may suggest that males have a more difficult time with postoperative change. Both genders often are reluctant to look in a mirror postoperative. If the adolescent has nasal trumpets to maintain a patent airway, these are often removed by the second day. The removal of the trumpets may act as proof of how quickly his or her appearance can change. Photographs taken at the peak of swelling may also prove to be useful to demonstrate improvement to the doubting adolescent as recovery progresses.

Physicians recommend that the patient complete mouth care following each episode of eating food or drinking. The solutions used are often either peroxide and saline mouthwash, or Peridex® (an antiseptic rinse), both of them are noxious. Unfortunately, Peridex® also temporarily yellows the teeth. Teens will often avoid eating because it means that they will have to complete oral care. They may be instructed to use the Water Pik®, but the use of this device is clearly a learned skill. Immediately after surgery, its use may be painful, especially if used incorrectly. Water Pik® technique is also somewhat awkward and messy, even if one is accustomed to using it without swollen lips and clenched teeth. Our experience has been that when the parent hovers while the teen learns, conflict ensues. The most helpful approach is for the parent to initially supervise in a "consultant" role and adopt a supportive stance, "you will master this." The more the adolescent is encouraged to Water Pik® independently, the more successful, and less stressful, the experience will be for everyone. Also, once oral care is mastered, the adolescent may feel more like eating.

Adolescents are frequently told by their surgeons that they "can expect" to lose between 10–15 lb during the fixation process. This is often seen as a boon, especially to the adolescent female, who is sees this as her opportunity to lose weight by consuming nothing but diet drinks. These patients need to be convinced that inadequate nutrition will interfere with proper tissue healing and not help their bodies fight off infection. In addition, the trauma of surgery results in various degrees of hypermetabolism.[10] Again, these teens should be reminded that everything they do will affect the long-term result of their appearance. Educating the adolescent about the daily caloric intake that is essential for wound healing is critical. This information may give adolescents a tool they can use in their own recovery and something that they can control. Seashore[11] has published guidelines for calculating energy requirements in hospitalized children based on the basal metabolic rate, that includes an adjustment for activity, severity of illness, and growth. The *Mayo Clinic Diet Manual*[10] states that protein requirements are increased by severe trauma or illness. The initial response of the body to illness or stress is the mobilization of protein for the synthesis of proteins associated with the immune response. Protein requirements during the recovery phase may nearly double to 11% or more of the total calories.

MANAGEMENT

Nutritional management of the adolescent following orthognathic surgery may require that the clinician be sensitive to a variety of psychological issues. Because reconstructive jaw surgery takes place at the end of the growth period, adolescents often have much time to anticipate the procedure. Given that the primary task of adolescence is to establish independence, they should be allowed to participate in decision making whenever possible. Allowing the adolescent to dictate the timing of surgery will substantially increase the likelihood of compliance and ability to assume responsibility for postoperative care. Orthognathic surgeries are frequently planned during times that coincide with breaks from school, such as summer and Christmas holidays. Social activities occur during both of these times that are usually very important to the adolescent. Summer surgeries mean that there will be no swimming, soccer camp, and the like. Winter surgeries may necessitate school absences, resulting in social isolation or school attendance with fixation appliances. Problem-solving experiences that involve determining the adolescent's priorities for future events, anticipating potential consequences of different timing decisions, and decision making can all be valuable learning tools. Future planning will also be beneficial because the adolescent will have the opportunity to schedule alternative summer or holiday activities to occupy time during the postoperative fixation phase of treatment. It needs to be recognized that surgery is a major event in a teen's life. We strongly believe that the adolescent is much more capable of cooperating and participating in the postoperative process when he or she is specifically informed about what to expect and has the opportunity to master the requisite skills.

Preparation and practice for fixation will substantially reduce many postoperative fears and problems that interfere with healing. It is essential that the adolescent be given the opportunity to express his or her expectations for surgery relative to appearance and perceived effort required. An interview with an experienced psychologist or other mental health provider to determine the teen's current understanding and knowledge base regarding the surgery is a good first step. A frank discussion of the surgical and immediate postoperative experience should be initiated at a level appropriate to the individual teen. This conversation needs to include both honest descriptions of the experience and postoperative appearance, as well as an acknowledgment of common fears. With each topic broached, the teen should be given some concrete tool or information that can used to influence recovery. The goal of this discussion is to decrease the knowledge deficit and diminish fears, thus allowing teens to anticipate and master some of their own reactions in order to put them in control of their own recovery.

A tour of the hospital unit(s) where he or she will be staying, with an opportunity to ask questions about the surgical process and equipment, is extremely useful. If this is not possible, the teen should be walked through the surgical experience verbally. Fears about pain should not be downplayed or dismissed; instead, the usual progression of pain medications from IV or IM to oral analgesics should be outlined. The adolescent needs to trust that his or her subjective analysis of personal pain will be respected and discomfort adequately managed.

Postoperative edema and bruising must be described honestly. The teen can be given responsibility for its rapid resolution by describing positions and activities he or she can assume to help, such as elevating the head of the bed and frequent, early ambulation. The teen should be made aware of the possibility of postoperative nausea and vomiting due to swallowed blood, anesthetic agents, or narcotics and the common fear of suffocation this creates. Simple skills like self-suctioning and turning the head to allow secretions to drain are easily learned. It is important to demonstrate that when vomiting does occur, even with a wired jaw, the liquid can pass through the wires without compromising the airway.

Since dehydration can delay wound healing and increase the risk of bleeding, the importance of drinking fluids after surgery needs to be stressed with the teen. He or she needs to understand that the intravenous (IV) line will give full fluid support initially after surgery, but then he or she will be expected to drink increasing amounts so that the IV can be removed. The sore throat from the endotracheal tube coupled with edema make drinking difficult and uncomfortable. The teen can be taught techniques such as tipping the head back or using a syringe to take fluids during the immediate postoperative period. He or she can set goals for total intake by frequently taking small amounts.

Speaking immediately after the procedure is frustrating, embarrassing, painful and awkward. The teen often doesn't want friends to see him or her until this behavior has been mastered. The few weeks before surgery are a good time to practice talking with clenched teeth in order to be understood. This may take hours of practice, but will definitely increase the likelihood that he or she will verbally communicate after surgery. Also, since the telephone is the lifeline for the social adolescent, practice in speaking through clenched teeth may decrease postoperative social isolation.

The importance of mouth care should be stressed before surgery as a means of preventing infection. The use of a Water Pik® is frequently recommended. It is a noisy, often messy procedure that requires experience to master. The adolescent should learn this skill well before the surgery takes place. Mastery of Water Pik® technique will assist him or her in assuming more responsibility at an early stage of postoperative care, and lessen the likelihood of infection or struggles with parents.

The adolescent should also be educated in advance of surgery about the caloric requirements for wound healing and the real risk of poor nutrition during healing. He or she should be focused on the long-term goal of improved appearance and function as well as reminded that everything he or she does affects subsequent appearance. A useful preparation activity before surgery is to "stockup" on appealing liquid foods. The teen and his or her parents can be encouraged to shop for samples of liquid supplements (Enrich, Ensure, or Sustacal) or instant breakfasts (which are far less "medicinal") in different flavors for "taste tests." Nearly any food can be reduced to liquid form using a blender or food processor. Although some teens have managed to liquify pizza by adding sauce, others think this is terribly unappealing. It can be helpful for the teen to try several recipes for pureed or liquid foods in order to experiment with tastes, temperatures, and textures for postsurgical diets. Then, several meals can be prepared in advance so the adolescent will be able to make choices when he or she returns home from the hospital and not be stuck with bouillon and jello.

When preparing the teen for responsibilities during the immediate postoperative period, it is also necessary to prepare him or her for discharge. It may be helpful to acknowledge that food, it's preparation, and mealtime may dominate his or her thinking for the next several weeks. Once the teen returns home from the hospital, new fears can emerge in terms of diet because the choices are not dictated by a clinical dietitian or hospital menu. Basically, the adolescent should be encouraged to select foods that are appealing and eat frequent, but small meals. It is extremely useful if the adolescent has mastered the operation of the blender and has tried a few recipes before surgery. It is important for the parent to recognize that the more involved the adolescent is in food selection and preparation, the more control is exercised and, therefore, compliance is enhanced. Experimenting with temperature, texture, seasoning, and presentation of foods can make the "no chew" eating more enjoyable. The teen can be encouraged to buy "Dixie" cups for the first few days at home. These cups are available in graduated sizes such as 3, 5, or 7 oz. Small amounts of food can be poured easily into the mouth by molding a spout for pouring. The teen can practice this skill before surgery in private, with a mirror for guidance.

The swelling after surgery takes a couple of weeks to resolve, but the adolescent may feel well enough to resume his or her social activities long before. Drinking and eating while edema persists are messy and potentially embarrassing activities. For many teens, drinking and eating are also core social activities. Having a "fun food" available that is universally enjoyed (such as ice cream sundaes) may help decrease the adolescent's feelings of isolation and difference from peers.

The emotional reactions the teen may have should be openly discussed. Research suggests that emotional responses of anger and hostility peak 4–6 wk after surgery. This may represent the increased frustration and helplessness in these patients just before fixation wires or bands are removed. Some teens report an increase in resentful feelings because they are not allowed to eat their favorite foods, or what others are eating. Some become overly focused on the foods they are denied while it bothers others very little. The teen may find it helpful to make a special presentation of meals during the fixation process. The addition of a flower or colorful paper plates, napkins, or placemats can increase the appeal of the food that has become boring. He might get pleasure from planning his "unwiring meal," the specific food or restaurant where he will have the first meal after the appliances are removed.

CASE ILLUSTRATION

Jessica is a 17-year-old Caucasian female who presented for the final stage in treatment of her right unilateral cleft lip and palate. She had undergone a number of previous surgeries, including lip and palate repair and revisions. Hearing was normal and speech judged to be excellent on evaluation. Social history demonstrated an intelligent, reasonably well-adjusted teenager who did well in school and reported that she had many friends. She was an only child in an intact family, living in a fairly small rural community.

After preparatory orthodontics, Jessica underwent a Lefort I maxillary advancement. Miniplates were used for internal fixation of the osteotomy sites, so the jaws were not wired postoperative. Orthodontic elastics were in use to train the muscles in the new occlusion. Surgery was without incident, and Jessica was returned to the pediatric intensive care unit extubated, for overnight monitoring of her airway. A nasal trumpet was maintained in the left nare for airway protection, with bedside suction to keep it patent. She was started on sips of clear fluids via syringe when fully awake, but took very little. Oral care beyond saline rinses was not yet initiated. Pain was controlled with intravenous morphine.

Early the next morning, Jessica's condition was stable and she was transferred to the pediatric floor to continue her recovery. Both her parents were in attendance. On arrival to the floor, Jessica was visibly anxious and tearful. She cried openly when she caught a glimpse of her face in the bathroom mirror. Her facial edema was moderately severe, especially to the lower face and lips. The nasal trumpet remained in place, and she was receiving fluids intravenously. She found it difficult to talk or swallow her secretions and reached continuously for the Yankeurs suction at her bedside. She refused all oral fluids and oral care. She nodded affirmatively when asked if she were in pain, but refused PO analgesia, pointing instead to the IV. The staff's attempts to encourage ambulation met with resistance from both patient and parents, and she remained huddled under her blankets. Her parents hovered protectively; her mother stated, "None of us realized it would be this bad!" and began to cry.

Since the surgeon's expectations were that Jessica would wean quickly from parenteral fluids, progress to a full liquid diet by mouth, complete independent oral care with a Water Pik®, and mobilize, the staff caring for her had an enormous challenge. Jessica and her parents had received minimal preoperative preparation; much of their understanding came from discussions with the surgeon and did not focus on the *practical* aspects of the postoperative recovery period. There were no local friends or relatives to offer emotional support. Both Jessica and her parents admitted to being exhausted and overwhelmed. In addition, the family had traveled a great distance for care and the insurance company had refused to authorize a preoperative night. Consequently, Jessica was admitted the day of her operation, allowing very little time to prepare her for the experience.

A plan was designed and implemented by the staff caring for Jessica and her family. The goals were basic: to educate Jessica about the recovery period, giving her the tools she needed to regain some control and independence, and achieve a positive long-term outcome.

After careful assessment, the first step taken was to minimize Jessica's pain and allow the entire family a period of uninterrupted rest. She was medicated parenterally, and her room was darkened. This one action had the immediate effect of gaining Jessica's and her parent's trust. Later, all three were much more receptive to intervention. Jessica was assured that her request for analgesia would be respected, and she was encouraged to ask for medication before the pain became too great. The staff also agreed to premedicate Jessica prior to any potentially painful procedures, and suggestions were made to the parents to provide nonpharmaceutical interventions, such as a backrub, to help their daughter relax and become more comfortable. The usual progression from IV to PO analgesia was detailed to the family, and Jessica was quickly weaned from IV and PO narcotics without incident.

Jessica's distorted appearance postoperative had startled and alarmed both her and her parents. Staff described the usual course of postoperative edema to the family and suggested practical ways to influence a more rapid return to a normal appearance. Jessica was encouraged to keep the head of her bed elevated and sleep on two pillows. The role of early ambulation in limiting edema and influencing its early resolution was explained to the family, and Jessica became much more willing to get out of bed and walk in the halls when she understood she could positively influence her appearance. Jessica's parents were encouraged to bring her street clothes from their hotel room and adopt the attitude with her that she was not sick, merely recovering from surgery. When the unattractive nasal trumpet was removed later in the day and Jessica was wearing her own clothes, she became even more active. Jessica's difficulty communicating persisted due to the edema of her lips, but her parents and the staff encouraged her to talk rather than gesture or write her needs. She gradually became less frustrated as the edema resolved.

Encouraging Jessica to drink presented a major challenge. Her throat was extremely sore and the generalized edema made swallowing difficult. She expressed a fear that she would "drown" if she took too much fluid at once. Adequate pain management was imperative in gaining her cooperation, and the use of special tools helped as well. The first day after surgery, Jessica found it almost impossible to drink from a cup without spilling, due to the edema of her lips, but was successful when given a 30-cc syringe equipped with a small piece of extension tubing. With experimentation, Jessica found she could position the tubing into her cheek pouch, tip her head back a little, and slowly depress the syringe plunger as she swallowed. This gave her a means to control the amount and flow rate of oral fluids, and she seemed pleased to have mastered the skill. She soon became much more interested in drinking. By the second postoperative day, the edema had resolved enough that Jessica could drink from a medicine cup, pinching the edges slightly to form a spout. From there she progressed rapidly to Dixie cups. It became clear quickly that the large amounts of fluids Jessica needed to drink to maintain hydration overwhelmed her, so the parents were enlisted to offer small, frequent amounts.

Jessica had never used a Water Pik® oral irrigator before, and she was initially very fearful it would hurt her fresh oral incisions. She was also repulsed by the mess it created while in use. This became problematic because she deliberately began to refuse fluids in order to avoid having to complete oral care. The staff was prepared for this response and much effort was expended to teach Jessica to master the Water Pik®. A demonstration of correct technique was given to Jessica and her parents, initially with the machine turned off, and each was given the opportunity to handle the Water Pik® and ask questions. Then a staff member repeated the demonstration, using Jessica as the model. Much humor was employed in the sessions, as she drenched the bathroom and her parents in her first efforts. Jessica's parents were encouraged to allow her to master the technique with their supervision, and to monitor that oral care was being done frequently. As Jessica became more skilled and competent with the Water Pik®, her avoidance of nourishment decreased.

The staff was concerned that Jessica regarded weight loss during her recovery period as inevitable and even desirable. So, they chose to emphasize the need for adequate nutrition to prevent wound infection and aid healing. The thought of repeating the surgery was not something the family wanted to consider, and they all became eager for suggestions for nutritious meal planning. A dietary consultation was arranged prior to discharge, and the dietitian reinforced the importance of sound nutritional practices during the recovery phase. Since Jessica's surgeon wanted her to follow a "no chew" diet for several weeks after surgery, the dietitian explored the possibilities available. She provided Jessica with recipes for blender meals and samples of various nutritional supplements she could try. Jessica became very interested in planning her own meals and presented her parents with a shopping list on discharge from the hospital.

On follow-up several weeks later, Jessica demonstrated excellent wound healing and oral care. She was pleased with the surgical result and appeared confident and comfortable when discussing her hospital experience. She had not lost weight since surgery and was eagerly planning her first "real" meal. Her parents reported that Jessica had assumed almost total responsibility for her own meals during her recovery period and had spent much time experimenting with different blender recipes.

REFERENCES

1. R. C. Sather and M. C. Hollen, in *Psychological Aspects of Facial Form*, (G. W. Lucker, K. A. Ribbens, and J. A. McNamara, eds.), Center for Human Growth and Development, Ann Arbor, MI, pp. 161–170 (1980).

2. T. Pruzinsky and T. F. Cash, in *The Promotion of Social Competence in Adolescence*, (T. P. Gullotta, ed.), Sage, Beverly Hills, CA (1990).

3. M. L. Belfer, A. M. Harrison, F. C. Pillemer, and J. D. Murray, *Clinics in Plastic Surgery*, **9**, 307 (1982).

4. K. K. Dion, E. Berscheid, and E. Walters, *J. Person. Soc. Psychol.*, **24**, 285 (1972).

5. D. Landy and H. Sigall, *J. Person. Soc. Psychol.*, **29**, 299 (1974).

6. M. J. Pertschuk and L. A. Whitaker, *Clin. Plast. Surg.*, **14**, 163 (1987).

7. L. W. Graber, in *Psychological Aspects of Facial Form*, (G. W. Lucker, K. A. Ribbens, and J. A. McNamara, eds.), Center for Human Growth and Development, Ann Arbor, MI, pp. 81–117 (1980).

8. H. A. Kiyak, R. W. McNeill, and R. A. West, *Am. J. Orthod.*, **88**, 224 (1985).

9. S. Fisher, in *Development and Structure of the Body Image (Vol. 1 and 2)*, Lawrence Erlbaum, Hillsdale, NJ (1986).

10. J. K. Nelson, K. E. Moxness, M.D. Jenson, and C. F. Gastineau, in *Mayo Clinic Diet Manuel: A Handbook of Nutrition Practices, VII ed.,* The C. V. Mosby Co., St. Louis, MO (1988).

11. J. H. Seashore, *Yale J. Biol. Med.*, **57**, 111 (1984).

FUTURE DIRECTIONS

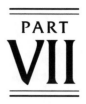

Training and Education: Building the Nutritional Team

Lucy B. Adams, M.S.

INTRODUCTION

The preceding chapters have addressed diverse aspects of adolescent nutrition, from normal growth and development to eating disorders and chronic illness. The professionals that address these issues with adolescents are just as diverse. In addition to clinical nutritionists and dietitians, they include professionals from the fields of medicine, nursing, psychology, social work, and others (see Table 29.1). However, these providers often are inadequately trained in nutritional evaluation and care[1] and reluctant to provide these services,[2] especially to adolescents.[3] Primary health care providers often agree that dietary change is important, yet they lack sufficient confidence in their own skills or their patient's ability to make changes.[4–7]

A TEAM APPROACH

The concept of a "nutrition team" presents a way to enhance the services offered to patients by filling gaps where primary providers may have insufficient time

593

Table 29.1   Who Provides Nutritional Support Services to Adolescents

Nursing	Nurse Practitioner or Registered Nurse
Nutrition	Nutritionist/Registered Dietitian
	Food-service director and staff
	Dietetic Technician
Pharmacy	Pharmacist
Physical Therapy	Physical Therapist
Medicine	*Primary Care Physicians*
	Pediatrician
	Adolescent medicine specialist
	Family practitioner
	Physician Subspecialist
	Endocrinologist
	MedicineGastroenterologist
	Gynecologist/obstetrician
	Hematology/oncology specialist
	Psychiatrist
	Pulmonary specialist
	Rheumatologist
	Surgeon
	Medical students
Psychology	Psychologist
School Personnel	Coach
	Teacher
Social Work	Social Worker

or skills. Such teams have been frequently employed in adult and pediatric populations in a variety of situations, including eating disorders and diabetes mellitus.[8] This approach fits well into managed health care with the team's focus on prevention, accountability, and nonduplication of essential services.[9] With major reorganization planned for the health care industry, there is more emphasis on cost-effectiveness and a shift toward preventive care. Nutrition and dietetics enjoy a greater preventive emphasis since the relationships between dietary behavior and chronic diseases have been elucidated.[10]

The period of adolescence is the ultimate interdisciplinary experience requiring little justification for team involvement. Table 29.2 highlights the major developmental changes that occur during adolescence and the related nutrition issues that can arise. Nutritional requirements and dietary behavior change dramatically during this time, creating a nutritionally vulnerable population. In addition, more youth than ever before are homeless, live in poverty, lack health insurance, are largely unsupervised, and may be responsible for their own food purchasing and preparation.[11,12] These adolescents are at even greater nutritional risk and have

Table 29.2   Association of Nutrition with Major Physiological and Psychological Changes During

Adolescence	Adolescent Development Potential Nutrition Issues
The body becomes that of an adult.	Nutrition-related delay in normal growth/ development.
There are major changes in body composition, especially body fat and muscle mass.	Body-image concerns or eating disorders in response to increased body fat in females or late-developing male with less muscle mass.
The adolescent becomes physiologically able to parent a child.	Contraception, adolescent pregnancy and related complications/issues, AIDS and nutritional factors.
Cognitive development nearly complete, moving beyond concrete thought into formal operations.	Adjustment of nutrition: counseling approach, depending on the level of cognitive development.
Experimentation with new behaviors occurs as a means to establish autonomy and self-identity.	Increased vulnerability to fad diets, nutritional supplements, dieting, etc.
Peers occupy a greater sphere of influence and source of identification.	Poor eating habits. Adolescents on therapeutic diet need assistance in maintaining compliance and peer relationships.

multiple medical, psychosocial, or legal constraints, that make them difficult to reach by conventional nutritional approaches.[13] Thus, adolescents are in need of an integrated, interdisciplinary, and culturally sensitive approach to their care.

There has been increasing recognition that an interdisciplinary approach is preferable, when working with children and adolescents.[11,14] Such an approach can help direct interventions that are tailored to the individual, within the constraints of cost containment and the need to demonstrate cost-effectiveness. Examples of the major opportunities for adolescent nutrition teams in both inpatient and outpatient settings are presented in Table 29.3. Major advantages to a nutrition team include improved time utilization, cost-effectiveness, and more comprehensive care for the patient (see Table 29.4).

NUTRITION TEAMS

Many nutrition teams "come together" informally, in response to the multiple needs of a patient or client, and may become integral to the institution. Some may never become cohesive, but consist of several individuals separately providing some degree of patient care that is nutrition-related.[15] There are existing

Table 29.3   Opportunities for Nutrition Team Building

Inpatient	Outpatient
AIDS	AIDS, HIV+
Burns	Alcohol abuse
Cancer, chemotherapy	Anemias, nutritional
Cystic fibrosis	Cancer
Diabetes mellitus	Cystic fibrosis
Eating disorders	Diabetes mellitus
Enteral or parenteral nutrition	Eating disorders and body-image concerns
GI disease	Growth concerns, hunger, and malnutrition
Iatrogenic malnutrition	Homeless, runaway, detained
Inborn errors of metabolism	Hypertension, hyperlipidemia
Liver disease	Multiple-medication regimen
Morbid obesity	Obesity and weight management
Multiple-medication regimen	Pregnancy and lactation
Renal disease	Preventive guidance: cancer, cardiovascular risk factors, osteoporosis, etc.
Surgery	
Transplantation	Renal disease
Trauma	Sports nutrition

models that integrate the dietitian into the inpatient health care team, such as the areas of enteral and total parenteral nutrition.[16] Some examples and their relevance to adolescent nutrition are discussed below.

Cardiovascular Disease Prevention

In the late 1970s, the Multiple Risk Factor Intervention Trial (MRFIT) was funded by the National Heart, Lung, and Blood Institute to alter the risk of heart disease by changing multiple behaviors over time in adult men at risk of developing heart disease.[10] Nutritionists and dietitians were brought together in this trial with nurses, physicians, and psychologists, working closely as case managers and cocounselors. More recently, the recommendations of the Expert Panel on Blood Cholesterol Levels in Children and Adolescents of the National Cholesterol Education Program and other investigators advocate a team approach to cholesterol reduction.[17–18]

Nutrition Support

The nutrition support team (NST) or metabolic support team (MST) (including medicine/gastroenterology, nursing, pharmacy, social work, and nutrition) has

Table 29.4   Potential Advantages of Nutrition Team

Comprehensive and cost-effective care
Consistent message to patient
Enhanced skill level of all team members
Improved patient outcome, i.e., faster recovery time
Diagnosis facilitated by unique contributions from team members
Improved nutritional status and/or fewer complications

been well integrated into the inpatient care of patients unable to tolerate oral feedings.[19] The primary roles of the dietitian on these teams are the identification of patients appropriate for nutrition support, implementation, and monitoring of total parenteral nutrition (TPN) and enteral nutrition (EN). The involvement of the nutrition consultant has been shown to be cost-effective and aids the physician provider in maintaining nutrition adequacy for the patient. In comparison to patients not cared for by a comprehensive team, patients managed by a parenteral nutrition support team had fewer complications.[16]

Insulin-Dependent Diabetes Mellitus

Insulin-dependent diabetes mellitur (IDDM) is often diagnosed during adolescence and extensive patient and family education is required. Nutrition professionals have long been integral members of the diabetes team,[20] along with providers from nursing, social work, and medicine (endocrinology). They develop meal plans that bridge patient acceptance and glycemic control without sacrificing nutritional status, growth, and development.[21] Their input is considered when diabetic adolescents are hospitalized for complications such as ketoacidosis. Demonstration of reduced pharmacy costs with nutrition counseling for diabetes has been cited as an example of how reimbursement for outpatient nutrition services can be enhanced.[22]

Eating Disorders

The team approach to eating disorders is considered essential in the management of these challenging patients.[23] Inpatient and outpatient team members treating patients with bulimia nervosa and anorexia nervosa typically include the disciplines of nutrition, nursing, psychology, social work, and medicine (adolescent medicine, psychiatry, gastroenterology).[24] The dietitian evaluates their nutrition adequacy,[8] makes recommendations regarding refeeding in anorexia nervosa, encourages patients' transition to making appropriate food choices, and supports the behavioral-psychological care plan around body image and self-esteem issues. This team could also facilitate the identification of patients at risk of eating disorders in a general adolescent clinical population. McClain et al.[25] cited the unique contributions of nutritionists, along with psychiatrists and gastroenterologists, in diagnosing eating disorders among patients with gastrointestinal complaints.

Weight Management

Obesity is one of the most prevalent nutritional issues affecting adolescents and an area that health professionals often feel ill-equipped to address. The Expert Committee on Clinical Guidelines for Adolescent Preventive Services (GAPS) recently recommended criteria for screening for overweightness.[26,27] It will be essential for the medical team to have the input from skilled nutrition professionals to implement these screening recommendations and assist in weight management for obese adolescents. The outpatient approaches to adolescent obesity that have shown effectiveness utilize an interdisciplinary team, usually consisting of a physician or nurse, an exercise physiologist, a nutritionist, and a mental health provider.[28,29] The dietitian working in a hospital setting may encounter adolescents with morbid obesity for evaluation and treatment of various medical complications.

Adolescent Pregnancy

Comprehensive recommendations are available for integrating nutrition counseling into most clinical settings serving pregnant teens to optimize the pregnancy outcome and provide anticipatory guidance around infant feeding choices and other postpartum nutrition issues.[30,31] Nutrition counseling is provided primarily by nurses or dietitians. Clinical settings offering the Women, Infant, and Children Program (WIC) provide medical care as well as supplemental foods and nutrition counseling. These sites serve many adolescents and WIC participation has been associated with improved dietary intake.[32]

Adolescents with Special Needs

Adolescents with special health care needs, including those with developmental disabilities, present unique challenges that demand input from various disciplines. The nutrition-related issues include feeding difficulties, poor growth, dental disease, gastrointestinal illness, and obesity (see Chapter 13–15). In addition to the disciplines already discussed, this team might also include a pharmacist, dentist, exercise physiologist, or a speech, occupational or physical therapist.[33]

Nutritional Roles

The specific tasks of the adolescent nutrition team member will vary considerably based on the type of setting (inpatient versus outpatient), age of the teen, medical severity, and psychosocial concerns. Table 29.5 outlines some of the roles that this team member plays. Assessment and counseling interactions make up a majority of the patient-oriented activities. Team-oriented activities, such as developing a nutrition protocol for adolescents with HIV disease, provide direct input to other team members. Updating other team members on patient status is another important role, especially if there are urgent or emergent issues. Also, patients may reveal data to one team member (such as reporting a drug allergy or recent medical symptoms to the dietitian) that is most relevant to the physician or another team member. These point to the need for good communication between team members.

There are situations where a nutrition consultation to the team involves little or no contact with the patient. One example is an adolescent hospitalized with anorexia nervosa who may focus on the dietitian as an ally in achieving menu modifications to lower the caloric value of the meals. The dietitian can make a valuable team contribution by channeling her or his limited time into developing a patient care plan that incorporates appropriate dietary guidelines and strategies, but is implemented by other team members.

These examples are helpful in framing the concept of the adolescent nutrition team (ANT) as part of an existing adolescent health team, and defining probable roles for the dietitian. However, the above teams emerged in response to patients presenting with a specific nutrition problem. In the nutrition support team, the team responds to patients unable to tolerate oral feedings, with the need for

Table 29.5   Nutrition's Role Within Adolescent Health Team

Patient-oriented activities

Comprehensive nutrition assessment; development and implementation of nutrition care plan

Documentation, emphasizing cost savings from nutrition care

Identify patients at nutritional risk

Implement/monitor TPN/EN

Individual counseling with adolescent or family to translate dietary prescriptions into food habits

Group patient education: cooking classes, consumer skills

Develop adolescent-appropriate patient educational materials

Team-oriented activities

Dietary, exercise, and nutrition support recommendations

Develop protocols for nutrition care

Provide consultation to other team members

Liason to food-service department

Update other team members regarding patients

Participant or presenter: rounds, case conferences, journal clubs, or staff inservices nutrition intervention implicit in the diagnosis. In contrast, the need for nutrition intervention with an adolescent may not always be apparent unless nutrition-screening protocols and nutritionally savvy primary providers are in place to identify adolescents at risk. For example, homeless or runaway youth are often seen and treated for specific acute medical conditions only, yet they are likely to be at increased nutritional risk.[13] Unfortunately, the homeless youth may fail to return for recommended comprehensive follow-up or nutrition appointments. An adolescent health team might approach such a young person addressing the adolescent's chief complaint first, but screening for other concerns while the patient is available. The physician or nurse could assure that available time was made for a nutrition and psychosocial assessment. The team would confer briefly on short- and long-term goals, and recommendations would be made for laboratory evaluations and other referrals.

TEAM DEVELOPMENT

Interdisciplinary health care teams often emerge after dealing with a complicated patient, with the realization that there must be a more efficient and rewarding way to deal with such challenging patients. Team building requires one member's initiative to communicate to prospective members and to enable obstacles to be overcome[15]; this is often the dietitian.[33,34]

Despite the benefits that adolescent nutrition teams offer, few formal groups exist. Table 29.6 reviews some common barriers to building a cohesive, adolescent nutrition team. The most common difficulties in developing any team revolve around issues of resources (staff time, costs, and reimbursement), other provider's attitudes and perceptions, role delineation, and competing priorities of complicated patients.[15] These obstacles may be overcome if changes are made in the following areas: communication, visability, and accountability. Table 29.7 outlines suggestions for addressing these concerns and encouraging collaboration. *Communication* lets prospective team members know that a nutrition professional is available (also increasing visibility) and informs others of the depth of a clinical dietitian's background, possibly changing their attitude toward the profession. Gaare et al.[34] cited the need for more effective communication about role perceptions among team members. If other team members have had limited contact with nutrition professionals, they may still be seen as linked solely with food service and inpatient tray delivery tasks.[35] Communication with administrators is equally important because of their control over institutional staffing and funding decisions. They may understand administrative dietitians, whose value can be expressed by the number of meals served or employees supervised.[36] But, if they have not had an opportunity to talk to clinical dietitians, it may be harder for them to appreciate the qualitative aspects of their contribution and support them.

Team formation will also be enhanced by finding opportunities to increase

Table 29.6   Barriers to Adolescent Nutrition Team Building

Institutional
Lack of protected time to meet
Inadequate physical space
Limited reimbursement for nutrition intervention
Competing patient priorities (multiple diagnoses, regimens)
Institutional bias toward unidisciplinary care
Communication, especially about urgent issues, hampered by team members housed at
    different locations

Interprofessional
Conflicting goals of care plan
Nutrition not viewed as "essential" component of care
Provider doubt of efficacy of nutritional intervention
Role disparity and interprofessional conflict
Gap in perceived status of team members
Poor communication between team members
Team member(s) with low level of self-confidence in skills
Inadequate experience in negotiation and problem-solving

Table 29.7   Enhancing Team Collaboration

Communication
Regular communication between team members and with others
Set and periodically reassess team priorities and goals
Discussions about nutriton as part of sound medical management of adolescents
Acknowledgment of other team members' contributions
Share historical perspectives of each discipline to gain insight into unique contributions
    team members make
Clearly define roles for team members (e.g., case-management responsibility)

Visibility
Include team members on patient rounds, case conferences, or patient management
    meetings
Host a monthly journal club or case conference open to interested professionals
Availability of team for patient consultations

Accountability
Concise chart documentation
Promote and document cost-effectiveness of treatment modalities
Consistency in plan implementation

dietitian *visibility* and the interest of other team members in nutrition consultation and collaboration. Most of inpatient dietitians' available time is devoted to patient assessment, counseling, and documentation. There are few opportunities to attend patient-management meetings, rounds, or other settings where prospective team members are likely to congregate. Dietitians working in outpatient settings are often in different locations and may rarely see the health providers referring these teens. Increased visibility is essential to adolescent nutrition team building.

Accountability can support requests for caseload reduction, increases in nutrition staffing, and justify delegation of appropriate tasks to diet technicians or administrative dietitians. The dietitian must document data relating to cost savings as a result of nutrition input or the initiation of an adolescent nutrition team. For example, since hospital-associated or iatrogenic malnutrition has been identified in over a third of pediatric patients surveyed,[37] the incorporation of nutrition training of providers and additional direct nutritional care has the potential of significant cost savings.[38]

As with any organization, adolescent nutrition team members need to be clear about team goals and patient priorities in order to ensure that these do not conflict with individual team members' goals. It is important for the team to systematically overcome identified obstacles and implement strategies that will maintain communication, increase visibility, and provide accountability. Existing patient rounds and conferences should be reassessed and expanded to assure interdisciplinary focus and attendance. Channels of communication about patient management should be clarified. Even if dietary intervention is the first line of treatment, such as in dyslipoproteinemias, drug treatment may be initiated before a sufficient trial of dietary intervention, even though it is more expensive and associated with more side-effects. Each team member needs to contribute to policy decisions and plans for accountability. There is some suggestion that comprehensive dietary recommendations inserted in the medical chart by the dietitian may be skimmed or not read at all.[35] This undermines the ability to be accountable, negates the effort made by the nutrition professional, and may compromise the patient's nutritional status. Admittedly, some comprehensive nutrition evaluations are several pages long; the entire team benefits from concise chart notes. In addition, a phone message for the primary provider or note stuck to the front of the chart *would* be noticed and could summarize the recommended actions that need to be taken. There are situations when these recommendations are not followed, which medically- and legally is the attending physician's prerogative.

TRAINING NEEDS

Interdisciplinary Health Professional Training

Individual team members may form more collaborative relationships with others and have greater recognition of the role of the nutritionist if they have

9.9   Interdisciplinary Skills Seminar: Sample Topics

roles: How do we know who does what?
tion: How to provide it and when to request it
nd fatness assessment skills
ntation: What to include and what to leave out? Or avoiding chart note chaos
e reimbursement and nutrition services
feud": Which team member will talk to the family?
computers for team member communication
assurance issues
and acronyms: What they really mean?
club

---

s concern that introducing interdisciplinary training before professional
fidence is strong may limit the benefits from collaboration. For example,
nced dietitians had more input in TPN decisions than those with less than
service.[40] Most interaction of adolescent health professionals occurs
lly, usually in clinical settings, [such as the pediatric intensive care unit
, eating disorders units], patient rounds, or case-management conferences.
the framework of the AHTP, practicing health professionals may choose
cipate in continuing education experiences, intended to expand their
e in adolescent health. Other opportunities for interdisciplinary training
community involvement in volunteer activities, such as the American
ssociation (AHA) or the American Cancer Society (ACS) where many
vorking committees are multidisciplinary.
ough collaboration is important as a way to enhance adolescent nutritional
e importance of unidisciplinary interaction and training should not be
zed. The confidence professionals need to "hold their own" within the
ay be primarily derived from the support and feedback from within one's
ne.[40]

ILLUSTRATION

e described below provides many opportunities for an interdisciplinary nu-
eam. Denise is a 13 ½-year-old obese Caucasian female seen in the Ado-
Clinic of the University of California at San Francisco with her mother. She
the clinic with a chief complaint of weight gain and request for a checkup
with losing weight. She was seen by a pediatrician/adolescent medicine
in consultation with an adolescent nutritionist, who outlined Denise's op-
weight management. With the adolescent's input, a plan was developed
ise to have a comprehensive nutrition evaluation and be considered for
DOWN, an interdisciplinary weight management program.

Table 29.8   Adolescent Nutrition Team: Opportunities

Health Professional Students	Healtl
Formal Training	
Core curriculum in adolescent health	Continuing
Fellowship or traineeship in adolescent health (i.e., AHTP)	Conferenc(
Interdisciplinary skills seminar	Interdiscip
Informal Training	
Inpatient rounds	Inpatient r(
Case-management conferences	Case-mana
Receiving clinical consultation	Providing
Cocounseling with other disciplines	Faculty m(
Attend conference on nutrition or adolescent health	Attend con
Alternate sites: school-based clinic; weight-management program	Volunteer

experienced that collaboration in their own trainin
the Adolescent Health Training Program (AHTP)
Child Health Bureau (MCHB) within the Public F
representation and training reflect at least five disci
ogy, nutrition, nursing, and medicine. Other discip
some of these training programs and include anth
policy, and education. Each of the seven AHTP pr
training curriculum that is stratified to meet the nee
stages of training within the five different discipl
variety of clinical, research, and policy experience
adolescent health that is cotaught by faculty repres
medicine, endocrinology, obstetrics and gynecology
tion, social work, and psychology. The major nutriti
include nutrition in pubertal growth and developr
disease prevention, eating disorders, and obesity.

MCHB also sponsors University Affiliated Prog
country to train nurses, nutritionists, physicians, psy(
physical, and speech therapists in collaborating to
and adolescents with developmental disabilities. Ta
portunities for training for health professional stud(

Team Building for Practicing Health Professionals

Training efforts in nutrition team building are
health professionals with firmly established roles ar

Upon evaluation, endogenous obesity was ruled out and Denise was recommended as an excellent candidate for SHAPEDOWN, based on her motivation, support from her mother, and her realistic expectations regarding the weight-management process. At the time of assessment, the major contributors to the obesity appeared to be genetic, family food patterns and food choices available at home, physical inactivity, and a possibility of binge eating. At that time, the Shapedown group leaders included graduate students from nursing, nutrition, and social work as well as an adolescent medicine physician fellow. The group leaders were supervised by the faculty nutritionist from the Division of Adolescent Medicine. Some of the assessment information is as follows:

Weight History	86 lb weight gain in past year and report of being overweight since age 10; denied any previous attempts at weight loss, including diet pills
Family history	Obesity, insulin-dependent diabetes mellitus, premature cardiovascular disease
Eating habits:	2 meals/d; vegetarian past 2 yr; denied snacking, binge eating, or purging; many family activities involve food
Dietary recall:	1000 cal/d; "light" food choices
Physical activity:	No regular aerobic activity
Psychosocial:	Moved from rural area last year; teased considerably by new "friends"; father brings home high-fat snacks; father discourages Denise's weight management; mother obese, but supportive of Denise; frustrated by weight gain, but is motivated
Physical Exam:	normal exam; blood pressure within normal limits; weight, 107 kg (236 lb); he ight, 162.5 cm (64 in.); body mass index = 40.5 (> 95th percentile); felative body weight (RBW)=200%; Tanner III ; menarche had started at 11 yr

Denise's weight management plan involved changes in four arenas: *dietary* (lighter food choices without the exclusion of favorite foods; 3–4 meals/d; monitor overeating situations and risk for eating disorder), *exercise* (start regular aerobic activity), *psychosocial* (improve family communication and support; improve assertiveness; consider referral for individual or family therapy), and *medical* (monitor elevated serum cholesterol and other risk factors for early CVD). Barriers to her participation included geographic distance from home to clinic and SHAPEDOWN program; father's lack of support for her weight management efforts; and the possibility of emotion-associated binge eating. Denise participated in SHAPEDOWN and mother attended all of the SHAPEDOWN parent meetings, and at follow-up, she showed the following changes: *dietary* (improved food choices; 12-lb weight loss), *exercise* (established a regular aerobic exercise regimen), *psychosocial* (improved family support from mother; increase in personal responsibility for her own food choices and exercise behavior; improved self-esteem; increase in assertiveness skills and self-efficacy) and *medical* (reduction in serum cholesterol). At this same time, the parents separated and Denise was looking forward to moving with mother to a more rural area. Referrals were made in their new community to support Denise continuing progress with weight management and the other issues in her life.

As it happens with other adolescents, Denise's entry into the health care system for one issue, led to the exploration of many others, and the resolution of some. She came into the clinic because of her obesity, but the health care professionals considered a much larger constellation of concerns because of the myriad of disciplines that were represented. Medical concerns included evaluating endogenous obesity, eating disorders, menstrual irregularities, and surgical approaches to morbid obesity. Behavioral specialists evaluated family functioning, Denise's school performance, and her psychosocial development. The nutritionist evaluated body image, reported eating and exercise behaviors, family attitudes and food-related behaviors (binging and the use of diet pills), and physical activity as well as objective growth and anthropometric data. The whole adolescent health and nutrition team is much more than a sum of its individual practitioner parts.

A unified team approach presents real potential in efforts toward early identification and prevention of adolescent health problems. The challenge will be demonstrating measurable savings and cost-effectiveness at the same time as attending to the main objective of cohesive team building: optimal care of the adolescent.

REFERENCES

1. K. Lazarus, R. L. Weinsier, and J. R. Boker, *Am. J. Clin. Nutr.*, **58**, 319 (1993).
2. C. T. Orleans, L. K. George, J. L. Houpt, and K. H. Brodie, *Prev. Med.*, **14**, 636 (1985).
3. M. Story and M. D. Resnick, *J. Nutr. Ed.*, **18**, 188 (1986).
4. S.Y.S. Kimm, G. H. Payne, E. Lakatos, *AJDC*, **144**, 967 (1990).
5. P. R. Nader, H. L. Taras, J. F. Sallis, and T. L. Patterson, *Pediatrics*, **79**, 843 (1987).
6. R. W. Blum and L. H. Bearinger, *J. Adol. Health Care*, **11**, 289 (1990).
7. J. H. Price, S. M. Desmond, R. A. Krol, F. F. Snyder, and J. K. O'Connell, *Am. J. Prev. Med.*, **3**, 339 (1987).
8. R. E. Kreipe and M. Uphoff, *Adol. Med.: State Art Rev.*, **3**, 519 (1992).
9. K. M. Fiedler, *J. Am. Diet. Assoc.*, **93**, 1111 (1993).
10. M. E. Farrand and L. Mojonnier, *J. Am. Diet. Assoc.*, **76**, 347 (1980).

11. American Dietetic Association, *J. Am. Diet. Assoc.*, **93**, 334 (1993).

12. C. L. Perry, S. H. Kelder, K. A. Komro, in *Promoting the Health of Adolescents: New directions for the Twenty-First Century*, (S. G. Millstein, A. C. Petersen, and E. O. Nightingale, eds.), Oxford University Press, New York, pp. 73–96 (1993).

13. J. T. Dwyer, *Adol. Med.: State Art Rev.*, **3**, 377 (1992).

14. L. H. Bearinger and J. Gephart, *J. Ped. Child Health*, **29 (suppl. 1)**, S10 (1993).

15. F. Nason, *Soc. Work Health Care*, **9**, 25 (1983).

16. A. E. Nehme, *JAMA*, **243**, 1906 (1980).

17. National Cholesterol Education Program, *Report of the Expert Panel on Blood Cholesterol Levels in Children and Adolescents*, NIH Pub. No. 91–2732, USDHHS, Bethesda, MD (1991).

18. G. C. Frank, *JACC*, **12**, 1098 (1988).

19. R. G. Glassman, *Top. Clin. Nutr.*, **1**, 16 (1986).

20. M. Franz, *J. Am. Diet. Assoc.*, **81**, 302 (1981).

21. J. E. Connell and D. Thomas-Doberson, *J. Am. Diet. Assoc.*, **91**, 1556 (1991).

22. N. J. Weese, J. Jones, and M. A. Miller, *J. Am. Diet. Assoc.* , **93**, 458 (1993).

23. M. Eckstein-Harmon, *J. Am. Diet. Assoc.*, **93**, 1039 (1993).

24. J. Schebendach and M. P. Nussbaum, *Top. Clin. Nutr.*, **3**, 541 (1992).

25. C. J. McClain, L. L. Humphries, K. K. Hill, and N. J. Nicki, *J. Am. Coll. Nutr.*, **12**, 466 (1993).

26. J. H. Himes and W. H. Dietz, *Am. J. Clin. Nutr.*, **59**, 307 (1994).

27. American Medical Association, in *AMA Guidelines for Adolescent Preventive Services (GAPS)—Recommendations and Rationale*, (A. B. Elster and N. J. Kuznets, eds.), Williams & Wilkins, Baltimore, MD, pp. 41–57 (1994).

28. L. M. Mellin, *Dir. Appl. Nutr.*, **1**, 1 (1987).

29. S.L.M. Hoerr, R. A. Nelson , and D. Essex-Sorlie, *J. Adol. Health Care*, **9**, 28 (1988).

30. M. Story, in *Nutrition Management of the Pregnant Adolescent: A Practical Reference Guide*, (M. Story, ed.), Maternal and Child Health Bureau, U. S. Department of Health and Human Services and March of Dimes, Washington, DC, (1990).

31. L. B. Adams, in *Nutrition Management of the Pregnant Adolescent: A Practical Reference Guide*, (M. Story, ed.), Maternal and Child Health Bureau, U. S. Department of Health and Human Services and March of Dimes, Washington, DC, (1990).

32. E. S. Farrior and C. H. Ruwe, *Nutr. Res.*, **7**, 451 (1987).

33. L. A. Wodarski, *J. Am. Diet. Assoc.*, **85**, 218 (1985).

34. J. Gaare, J. O'Sullivan Maillet, D. King, and J. A. Gilbride, *J. Am. Diet. Assoc.*, **90**, 54 (1990).

35. O. Rosen, N. J. Downes, K. P. Sucher, and B. Shifflett, *J. Am. Diet. Assoc.*, **91**, 1074 (1991).

36. P. L. Pierce, in *Primary and Team Health Care Education*, (T. L. Thompson and R. L. Byyny, eds.), Praeger, Menlo Park, CA, pp. 189–193 (1983).

37. R. J. Merritt and R. M. Suskind, *Am. J. Clin. Nutr.*, **32**, 1320 (1979).
38. R. L. Weinsier, J. A. Bacon, C. E. Butterworth, *Ala. J. Med. Sci.*, **19**, 402 (1982).
39. S. G. Millstein, E. O. Nightingale, A. C. Petersen, A. M. Mortimer, and D. A. Hamburg, *JAMA*, **269**, 1413 (1993).
40. A. J. Ducanis and A. K. Golin, *The Interdisciplinary Health Care Team*, Aspen Systems Corporation, London, pp. 153–166 (1979).

Research: Current and Future

Ella H. Haddad, Dr.P.H., R.D., and
Patricia K. Johnston, Dr.P.H., M.S., R.D.

INTRODUCTION

Adolescence represents a period of rapid physiological, social, emotional, and hormonal change. Heald[1] first called attention to the remarkable fact that adolescence is the only time following birth when the rate of growth actually increases. Unlike the adult who has reached maturity and nutritional stability, the teenager undergoes complex biologic and cognitive alterations. These changes create special nutritional needs with lifelong implications on health and wellness.

At a conference on nutrient requirements in adolescence in 1973, it was stated that "we know little of the nutrient requirements [during adolescence], and we are also uncertain about which body measurements would provide us with the best criteria of optimal nutrition for the adolescent."[2] A similar statement can be made today over two decades later. Although much has been learned, our knowledge in these areas remains sketchy and inadequate.

NUTRITION AND GROWTH

Indicators of Growth and Development

Nutrient requirements are strongly influenced by patterns of growth and development and much attention has focused on the pubertal growth spurt that occurs

609

in early adolescence.[3-9] It has been estimated that pubertal growth accounts for almost 50% of the ideal adult weight, 20–25% of the final adult height, and 45% of peak skeletal mass.[4] An important feature of adolescent growth is the great variability that exists in the timing and magnitude of the growth spurt both between genders and among individuals.[7,8] In 95% of cases, girls experience the most rapid increase in growth between ages 9.7 and 13.3 yr; the growth spurt of boys occurs about 2 yr later, between 11.7 and 15.3 yr.[7]

The pubertal growth spurt usually occurs in tandem with the emergence of the secondary sex characteristics (external genitalia, breasts, and pubic hair). These indicators have been grouped into a series of stages and rated by Tanner,[7,8] and these "Tanner stages" are widely used to evaluate sexual maturity. The wide variations in timing in pubertal processes among individual adolescents make chronological age a poor indicator of growth status and biological maturity. With both males and females, early maturers typically have larger peak height velocities than late maturers. The final mean adult height is the same because late maturers are usually taller when the growth spurt begins.[4] In girls with early puberty, menarche may occur at the same time or slightly before peak height velocity; in middle maturers, menarche occurs on the descending limb of the height velocity curve; and those with delayed adolescence have menarche later on the descending limb when growth has nearly ceased.[9] In boys, genital and pubic hair development is nearly complete by the time they reach their maximal pubertal growth rate.[4]

Developmental considerations are most important in the nutritional care of the individual adolescent. Growth assessment, body weight evaluation, and the estimation of energy and nutrient needs must be considered in the context of the adolescent's developmental stage. Skeletal age assessed by roentgenograms most accurately reflects development, but its use is limited by cost and inconvenience.[5] Although relatively easy to obtain, height and weight measurements are subject to complexities of interpretation during adolescence and must be coupled to indicators of sexual maturation.

The cross-sectional growth charts compiled by the National Center for Health Statistics[10] provide percentiles based on a large national probability sample. Because of the variability in timing of the growth spurt, the cross-sectional data are often inaccurate when applied to individual children during puberty. For late and early maturers, the discrepancy for height attained is exaggerated.[11] Weight and height velocity charts that incorporate both longitudinal and cross-sectional growth data for North American children were published by Tanner and Davis[7] in 1985 and are appropriate for repeated measurements in a given individual. Also valuable for height and weight evaluations are the adolescent growth charts developed by Wilson et al.[12] which include corrections for sexual maturity ratings, provide percentiles, and estimate expected adult height.

Health professionals working with youth must be able to interpret both growth and maturational parameters. Adolescents are most concerned about their changing bodies and ask questions related to these issues. The inclusion of the maturational indexes in assessment will help determine whether a teen is growing normally or as expected. Clinicians must assess the stages of sexual maturation yearly and record these ratings along with height and weight. These ratings may be based on the adolescent's own self-assessment. Questionnaires for the self-assessment of pubertal stage have been developed by Duke et al.[13] and these tools have been tested and validated. Adolescent's self-assessment correlates highly with physician ratings and is independent of level of fatness.[14]

Future research must be directed toward further evaluation and validation of growth curves and sexual maturity ratings. Are these instruments applicable to all ethnic groups within the population? How do these measures correlate with final growth and nutritional status?

Nutrition and Hormonal Influences

For both males and females, normal pubertal growth involves an interaction between the neuroendocrine and skeletal systems and the individual's nutritional status. Hormonal regulation of somatic and sexual maturation is influenced by critical body weight or fat, nutrition, heredity, race, climate and season.[5] Many of the body's hormones that promote growth are modulated to a great extent by nutritional factors. These hormones include growth hormone, thyroxin, insulin, corticosteroid, parathyroid hormone, 1,25-dihydroxyvitamin D, and calcitonin.[3] It has been shown that overnutrition accelerates growth and undernutrition retards it.[13] Growth hormone is the key hormone and its effects are mediated through the insulinlike growth factors (IGFs) or somatomedins. In man, two IGFs have been described: IGF-I and IGF-II. Of the two, IGF-I is the peptide that is tightly regulated by growth hormone and by nutrition. It is reduced in fasting and various states of restricted-energy intake.[3]

Steroid hormones mediate sexual maturation and the partition of nutrients during growth. In females, estrogen and progesterone promote the deposition of proportionately more fat than muscle tissue. Under the influence of testosterone and the anabolic adrenal androgens, boys gain proportionately more muscle mass than fat.[3] It has been shown that lean body mass decreases in girls during adolescence from 80–75%, whereas in boys, it increases from 80- 90%.[4] Girls enter puberty with 15.7% mean body fat and by adulthood reach 26.7%. In contrast, boys enter puberty with 4.3% body fat, increase to 11.2% in early puberty, and then remain constant until adulthood.[15]

Influence of Nutrition on Adolescent Growth

It has been documented that successive generations in many countries are taller and have attained puberty at younger ages.[7,16] For example, age at menarche has decreased in most developed countries.[17] These secular trends are attributed to better nutrition and health during childhood. The influence of nutrition on the timing of puberty and linear growth is established early in life. In a prospective study of diet and growth in 78 boys followed from age 6 mo to 14 yr, heavier weight during infancy and childhood was associated with early maturation and greater adult height.[18]

Longitudinal growth data on children who developed obesity during childhood reveal a distinct tendency for height gain to accelerate coincident with, or after the onset of, excessive weight gain.[19] In recent study evaluating the food intake and rate of biological maturation of 200 boys and girls during adolescence, early maturers of both genders were fatter, but consumed less energy per kilogram of body weight and were less physically active than late maturers. Late maturation seems to coincide with an energy intake appropriate to activity pattern and significantly lower body fat mass.[20]

The association of body fat and menarche remains a controversial topic. Frisch and McArthur[21] postulated that the amount of body fat modulates the timing of the growth spurt and onset of menarche. Current data do not substantiate that a specific level of fatness is critical for menarche and variations exist in the percentage at which menarche is attained.[22] Although the "body fat-age of menarche" hypothesis remains controversial, it is often invoked to explain the events of puberty. Recent research suggests that the distribution of body fat, rather than its mass, is related to the plasma concentration of sex steroids in girls in early puberty.[23] The importance of this finding stems from epidemiological associations that suggest early menarche and the composition of diet during puberty may be related to increased risk of breast cancer later in life.[24]

Assessment of Obesity and Fatness

Issues relating to body weight and fatness are of great concern to adolescents and a challenge to dietitians and health counselors. On the one hand, inadequate intake may result in growth retardation and stunting, whereas overfeeding has implications for lifelong fatness and obesity. What may seem like overweight or subcutaneous fatness be associated with maturational status. Although it is imperative that careful evaluations be made and hasty diagnoses avoided, adequate tools that have been duly validated do not exist. Being incorrectly labeled as overweight or obese may have serious consequences on teenagers' psychological and socioemotional health.

In addition to clinical care, the definition of adolescent overweight is vital to preventive services and impacts the study of fatness and obesity trends in the population over time. Of the several methods that may be used to assess body fat, hydrostatic weighing is the most accurate, but not practical for most survey and practice settings. Body mass index (BMI) is calculated as the ratio of weight (in kilograms) to height (in meters) squared. It is highly correlated with densitometrically estimated percent of body fat and total body fat in children and adolescents.[25-27] Future investigations must be designed to include the evaluation of this measure as a research tool.

The establishment of appropriate guidelines for defining overweight during adolescence is undergoing much discussion at present. The national health objectives, *Healthy People 2000,* define cutoff points for obesity in adolescence as greater than the age- and sex-specific 85th percentiles of BMI derived from the second National Health and Nutrition Examination Survey.[28] In a recent report,[29] the Expert Committee on Clinical Guidelines for Overweight in Adolescent Preventive Services established an alternate set of criteria to define overweight or obesity for use in the routine annual preventive screening of adolescents in clinical settings. The committee recommended that two categories of BMI be used. First, adolescents whose BMIs are ≥95th percentile for age and sex, or whose BMIs are >30 (whichever is smaller), are considered overweight for screening purposes and referred for comprehensive medical evaluation to determine underlying medical problems and needed intervention. Adolescents whose BMIs are >85th percentile, but <95th percentile or equal to 30 (whichever is smaller), are considered at risk of overweight and should be referred for a second level of screening. They suggested that the second-level screening include family history, blood pressure, total cholesterol, large recent change in BMI, and concern about weight. They also recommended that the only appropriate reference data for use nationally are those provided by Must et al.[30,31]

Adolescent obesity is often implicated as a risk factor for obesity in adulthood. The prediction of overweight in middle age from childhood obesity seems to be more reliable for males than females.[32] Regardless, evidence from longitudinal studies shows that fatness during adolescence does increase both present and later mortality and morbidity.[33]

Although health professionals have been concerned about the effects of adolescent growth patterns and weight status on adult weight and health, there remains much controversy about the most appropriate growth measurements and reference data. Unfortunately, data from adolescent surveys have been difficult to interpret. What is needed are better growth curves that differentiate early and late maturers, and better age- and sex-specific cutoff points to define overweight. Also, growth curves derived from national probability sampling may not be applicable to all race and ethnic groups. Research indicates variations do exist in growth patterns, body proportions, and body fat distribution in groups such as American Indians, Mexican Americans, and African Americans when compared to Caucasians.[34-36] Another important area that requires examination is whether the degree of excess body fat at which increased health risks occur is similar across various racial groups.

Further research is needed to determine the impact of early vs. late maturation on diseases later in life. What factors account for the variations observed? Longitudinal studies are needed to examine whether rapid and early maturation does, in fact, increase the risk for certain conditions. If so, what are the food and dietary factors that influence these maturational parameters?

NUTRIENT REQUIREMENTS DURING ADOLESCENCE

The dramatic growth and increased activity level that characterize adolescence greatly increase nutrient needs and influence nutritional status. Teenagers, however, often follow unusual and irregular eating habits. Although most adolescents in the United States are adequately nourished, subtle deficiencies and excesses are prevalent and, if not corrected, may lead to serious health problems.

The nutrient needs of adolescents must be related to the timing and intensity of their physiological growth and maturation rather than chronological age. However, for practical reasons, the Recommended Dietary Allowances (RDAs) of the Food and Nutrition Board of the National Research Council are given in terms of age-gender categories.[37] Table 30.1 lists selected RDAs that apply to the adolescent years. As noted by the Food and Nutrition Board,[37] the RDAs for youth are estimates of intakes associated with good health and growth, extrapolation from animal research, or interpolation from studies using children and adults.

Data in Tables 30.2 and 30.3 review nutrient intake trends over the past 20 yr based on information collected from the first and second National Health and Nutrition Examination Survey (NHANES I, 1971–74; NHANES II, 1976–80), the Nationwide Food Consumption Survey (NFCS, 1977–78, and NFCS, 1987–88),[39] and recently released data from the third National Health and Nutrition Examination Survey (NHANES III, 1989–94).[40] Comparing mean daily intake with the RDAs shows that, on the average, diets of teens may be low in vitamin E, vitamin B-6, folate, calcium, magnesium, and zinc.

The 1987–88 Nationwide Food Consumption Survey data were subjected to further analyses by Johnson et al.[41] It was determined that vitamin A, vitamin E, calcium, magnesium, and zinc were nutrients adolescents most often consumed below the recommended levels. Results indicated that for the most part, diet quality did not vary with income level, but did with gender and race.[41]

Energy

The energy requirement of adolescents is a subject of much debate, but there is little objective research on which to base an accurate expression of teen's individual needs. Early research emphasized the importance of relating energy needs to height.[41] Actual energy needs vary with physical activity and must be adjusted to balance energy expenditure. The current RDAs for energy are derived

Table 30.1 Recommended Dietary Allowances (RDA) for Selected Nutrients During Adolescent Years

	Females		Males	
	11–14 yr	15–18 yr	11–14 yr	15–18 yr
Energy (kcal)	2200	2200	2500	3000
Protein (g)	46	44	45	59
Thiamin (mg)	1.1	1.1	1.3	1.5
Riboflavin (mg)	1.3	1.3	1.5	1.8
Niacin (mg NE)	15	15	17	20
Vitamin B-6 (mg)	1.4	1.5	1.7	2.0
Folate (mcg)	150	180	150	200
Vitamin B-12 (μg)	2.0	2.0	2.0	2.0
Vitamin C (mg)	50	60	50	60
Vitamin A (μg RE)	800	1000	800	1000
Vitamin D (μg)	10	10	10	10
Vitamin E (mg a-T)	8	10	8	10
Vitamin K (μg)	45	55	45	65
Calcium (mg)	1200	1200	1200	1200
Phosphorus (mg)	1200	1200	1200	1200
Magnesium (mg)	280	270	300	400
Iron (mg)	15	15	12	12
Zinc (mg)	12	12	15	15

From Food and Nutrition Board, National Research Council, *Recommended Dietary Allowances,X ed.*, National Academy Press, Washington,DC, (1989). Reprinted with permission.

from equations published by international agencies and adjusted to reflect typical activity patterns in the United States. Reference points for height and weight are the medians of data collected by the National Center for Health Statistics (NCHS).[37] Studies of actual energy intakes of adolescents in the United States demonstrate that girls appear to consume their peak caloric intake at about the time of menarche. In boys, the caloric intake appears to parallel the adolescent growth spurt, increasing until age 16 yr and decreasing thereafter.[42]

Recent data from the third National Health and Nutrition Examination Survey (NHANES III) are consistent with earlier survey results (Table 30.2) and suggest that mean energy intake based on reported food consumption has remained relatively stable over time. Although the national survey results and the RDA lists do not employ similar age-gender categories to allow for direct comparison, mean energy intakes for girls seem to fall substantially below the RDAs. The lower than recommended reported energy intakes of female teens may reflect the concerns frequently expressed by adolescents about weight. Increased physical activity allows greater energy consumption without increasing weight. Appro-

Table 30.2 Mean Daily Intake of Energy, Protein, Fat, % of Energy from Fat, % of Energy from Saturated Fat

	Sex/Age	NHANES I 1971–74	NCFS 1977–78	NHANES II 1976–80	NCFS 1987–88	NHANES III 1988–94
Energy (kcal)	Female 12–15	1910	1870	1821	1744	1838
	16–19	2626	2431	2490	2152	2578
	Male 12–15	1735	1720	1687	1618	1958
	16–19	3010	2629	3048	2406	3097
Protein (g)	Female 12–15	73	72	66	66	—
	16–19	97	94	92	83	—
	Male 12–15	67	69	63	62	—
	16–19	118	106	122	93	—
Fat (g)	Female 12–15	80	83	76	71	69
	16–19	108	108	102	88	95
	Male 12–15	72	77	69	66	75
	16–19	127	120	126	99	119
% Energy from fat	Female 12–15	38	39	37	36	34
	16–19	37	39	37	37	33
	Male 12–15	37	40	37	36	34
	16–19	38	40	38	37	35
% Energy from saturated fat	Female 12–15	14	—	13	14	12
	16–19	14	—	14	14	12
	Male 12–15	13	—	13	14	12
	16–19	14	—	14	14	13

Adapted from National Health and Nutrition Examination Survey (NHANES I), 1971–74; Nationwide Food Consumption Survey (NCFS), 1977–78; Second National Health and Nutrition Examination Survey (NHANES II), 1976–80; Nationwide Food Consumption Survey (NCFS), 1987–88; and, Third National Health Nutrition Examination Survey (NHANES III),1988–94.[38-40]

priate food choices to supply the energy will also provide greater intake of essential nutrients. Thus, it is important to encourage physical activity not just for improved fitness, but as a means to support adequate nutrient consumption. Further research is needed to examine the relationships between actual energy intake, activity, and growth, and to quantify the interactions between them.

Protein

Protein needs during adolescence are largely influenced by the velocity of growth of the individual.[43] Due to gaps in experimental data, the protein RDAs were based on the modified factorial approach used by the World Health Organization (WHO).[44] For 11–14-year-old and 15–18-year-old females, the RDAs are 1.0 and 0.8 g/kg of body weight, respectively. For 11–14-year-old and 15–18-year-old males, the RDAs are 1.0 and 0.9 g/kg of body weight, respectively.

ments are based on energy intake and are as follows: thiamin 0.5 mg/1000 kcal, riboflavin 0.5 mg/1000 kcal, and 6.6 niacin equivalent/1000 kcal.[37] Survey data show that the dietary intake of these nutrients is generally adequate due to enriched breads and cereals. However, a recent small survey showed that 7% of a healthy urban adolescent population had marginal riboflavin status when biochemical indices were used. This emphasizes the importance of functional assessments in addition to dietary intake and the need for continued study.[52]

Vitamin B-6.   These coenzymes function primarily in the metabolic transformations of amino acids and the requirement for the vitamin increase as the intake of protein increases. The RDA for adolescents is similar to that of children and based on 0.02 mg of the vitamin/g of protein in the diet.[37] A number of studies have indicated that the intake and nutritional status of teenagers may be marginal for vitamin B-6. Kirksey et al.[54] reported a calculated mean intake of 1.24 ± 0.7 mg (89% of the RDA) for 12–14-year-old females. The most recent National Food Consumption Survey (1987–88)[39] reported a mean intake of 1.2 + 0.6 mg (80% of the RDA) for 16–19-year-old female. In a study of Caucasian and African American adolescent females, 12, 14, and 16 years of age, about half of the subjects reported consuming less than 55% of the RDA for vitamin B-6.[55] Approximately 20% of the girls had marginal and 13% had deficient status as assessed by biochemical indicators.[55] In general, males have higher average intakes of B-6 as well as other vitamins and minerals due to their higher energy intake.

Although vitamin B-6 is widely distributed in food, substantial losses of the vitamin occur through processing and cooking. Also, the bioavailability of the vitamin varies among foods and impacts nutritional status. Important sources of the vitamin include foods that are not popular among teens such as whole grains, beans, nuts, and some fruits.

Biotin and pantothenic acid.   The lack of definitive studies of biotin and pantothenic acid requirements in all age groups prompted the Food and Nutrition Board to cite "insufficient evidence" as a reason for not establishing an RDA.[37] It has, however, determined a daily intake of 4–7 mg for pantothenic acid and 30–100 μg for biotin as an estimated safe and adequate level for adolescents and adults.[37] Studies have determined dietary intakes and evaluated pantothenic acid levels in urine and blood of adolescents.[56–58] Although dietary intakes of the vitamin were low, especially in the adolescent female, average blood levels were in the normal range relative to other populations.[58]

Biotin is synthesized by intestinal microorganisms, but the extent of its availability for absorption is not established. Little is known about the needs and status of adolescents in regard to this vitamin and more research is indicated.

Folate.   Adolescents are at high nutritional risk for inadequate folate intake because of increased needs for growth and sexual maturation. The folate requirement increases as de novo cell synthesis increases during rapid growth and development. The RDA for folate is accepted to be approximately 3 µg/kg body weight for men; nonpregnant, nonlactating women; and adolescents.[59]

Although clinical evidence of folate deficiency in adolescents is rare, the 1987–88 NFCS survey data indicate that folate intakes are frequently below the recommended level in both male and female teens.[41] There is some evidence that low serum and/or erythrocyte folate levels are common and folacin status may be less than adequate,[60–64] especially for low-income and female youth. In a recent evaluation of the folate status of a biracial sample of 164 adolescents 12–15 yr old, 13% of the boys and 40% of the girls were folate-deficient as judged by the amount of erythrocyte folate. Supplementation of 400 µg folic acid daily for 2 mo resulted in significant increases in serum folate, erythrocyte folate, and hemoglobin values and a decrease in mean corpuscular volume.[64] These same investigators found positive correlations between blood folate levels and grade point average in adolescents.[64]

Attention has recently focused on the importance of folic acid in the prevention of neural tube defects.[65] This vitamin is particularly important before conception and in the early weeks of pregnancy. The Centers for Disease Control and Prevention recommended 400 µg for all females of childbearing age.[66] Due to the unplanned nature of many teen pregnancies and their increased needs for growth, it is especially important that an adequate intake be encouraged and assured.

Folate is rapidly destroyed by heat such as through canning and prolonged cooking. The consumption of fresh fruits and vegetables is low in adolescents and must be encouraged to ensure against marginal folate intake.[65]

Vitamin B-12.   Needed along with folate for rapid cell growth. Little is known about the vitamin B-12 status of adolescents. The 1987–88 NFCS survey suggests that dietary intakes are probably adequate except for those following diets devoid of all animal products.[41]

Vitamin C.   Important in collagen formation, neurotransmitter synthesis, antioxidant defense and leukocyte function. Very little is known about the requirements of vitamin C for adolescent growth and immunocompetence. Smoking seems to increase demands since smokers show reduced blood levels.[67,68] The impact of smoking on vitamin C status in the adolescent has not been assessed, and because smoking continues to increase among this population, such a relationship requires careful examination.

Vitamin A.   Essential for vision, growth, cellular differentiation, reproduction, and the integrity of the immune system. The body's need for vitamin A can be met by the dietary intake of preformed retinoids or from the consumption of carotenoid precursors such as beta-carotene. Presently, there is considerable interest in the vitamin because of epidemiological observations and clinical trials linking vitamin A intake to reduced childhood morbidity and mortality, and carotenoid intake to reduced cancer risk.

Recent findings have shown a rise in plasma retinol and retinol-binding protein in both males and females at puberty. Plasma retinol concentration is positively related to plasma cholesterol and triglyceride levels, sexual maturation, and body fat. Beta-carotene in blood is related to plasma cholesterol and dietary intake.[69]

Recommended intakes during the adolescent years are similar to those for adults and data analyses from national surveys show a high prevalence of low dietary intake among adolescents, especially in the South.[41,70,71] Low vitamin A and carotenoid intake may be associated with an increased risk of cancer later in life.

Vitamin D. The function of vitamin D is to maintain serum calcium and phosphorus concentrations in a range that supports cellular processes, neuromuscular function, and bone mineralization. The difficulty in establishing a requirement is due to the variability of exposure to sunlight in meeting vitamin D needs. In situations where teenagers are not exposed to or avoid the sun for long periods of time, exogenous sources of vitamin D may need to be increased.

Vitamin E. Substances with vitamin E activity function chemically as antioxidants and prevent the oxidation of polyunsaturated fatty acids by trapping peroxyl-free radicals. Oxidation of lipids causes cell damage. In a small survey of adolescent females, about 12% had marginal to low plasma total tocopherol, and about 12% consumed less than two-thirds of the RDA.[72] Plasma alpha-tocopherol levels in adolescents were positively related to cholesterol levels and dietary intake and negatively associated with the sexual-maturation index.[69]

The dietary intake of vitamin E among teens may be marginal.[73] In the 1987–88 NFCS, mean intakes were approximately 80% of the RDA for younger male and female adolescents. About 76% of both male and female adolescents had intakes below the RDAs.[41] Recently, much attention has focused on vitamin E and other antioxidants. Research is needed to elucidate the relationship between adolescent intake and long-term health effects.

Vitamin K. Essential for the formation of at least three proteins involved in blood clotting, as well as other proteins found in plasma, bone, and kidney. It is provided from both the diet and from endogenous bacterial synthesis, presumably in roughly equal measure. There are no data on vitamin K status in adolescents.

Minerals

Calcium. Dietary calcium has been identified as a nutrient of great potential concern for adolescents. It is needed along with other dietary minerals (phosphorus, magnesium, fluoride) for bone mineralization. Achieving a high peak bone mass at skeletal maturity is thought to protect against bone loss and the development of osteoporosis later in life. Little is known about mechanisms for increasing peak bone mass other than factors known to influence body stature. Peak bone mass is the result of age, gender, genetically determined factors, and nutritional intake. The importance of genetic factors is suggested by twin studies and family-resemblance studies between mothers and their daughters.[74–76]

The acquisition of bone mineral density proceeds rapidly during adolescence. The period of puberty and early adolescence (ages 9–14 yr) appears to be critical for the achievement of peak bone mass, especially for girls. During this time, the gain is 7–8%/yr. By age 14 yr, bone size, bone mass, and bone density of adolescent girls seem to approach trabecular and cortical peak bone mass. Although bone density also increases substantially in adolescent boys, the increase appears to extend over a longer period.[77] Female adolescents may be at increased risk for the development of skeletal inadequacy due to an imbalance between calcium intake and high requirements for calcium during this period of bone modeling and skeletal consolidation.[78,79]

The effect of activity on bone mass must also be considered. For example, exercise is known to increase bone mass. However, intensive exercise has been shown to lead to menstrual irregularities and stress fractures.[80]

Recent data (Table 30.3) suggest the mean dietary calcium intakes among adolescents to be approximately 70% of the RDA for females 12–15 yr old, and 60% of the RDA for those 16–19 yr old. The 1987–88 NFCS data indicate that a high proportion (86%) of adolescent females have intakes below the RDAs.[41] Longitudinal studies are needed to further clarify the timing of peak bone mass development, especially among females, as well as the long-term implications of calcium intake under varying conditions.

Phosphorus.   Another important component of bone is phosphorus. For both calcium and phosphorus an RDA of 1200 mg is recommended for both genders from ages 11–24 yr. The relationship between dietary calcium and phosphorus is complex. Dietary phosphorus seems to increase the absorption of calcium; however, an excess of phosphorus, i.e., a calcium-to-phosphorus ratio lower than 1:2, has been shown in several species of animals to lower the blood calcium level and cause secondary hyperparathyroidism with resorption and loss of bone.[81] It is presently accepted that a 1:1 ratio of calcium to phosphorus is ideal for most age groups. It has been suggested that carbonated soft drinks, which have been replacing milk in the diet of teens, contain significant amounts of phosphate and may have an impact on bone mineralization at this critical age.[82] Further, the influence of a low Ca:P ratio in the diet has never been satisfactorily determined among teens.

Magnesium.   Results of the 1987–8 NFCS have identified magnesium as a nutrient frequently low in the diets of many adolescents.[41] As mentioned above, low intakes of calcium and magnesium are associated with osteoporosis and poor bone health. Investigations are needed to determine the long-term implications of low magnesium intake in this population.

Iron.   Adolescents require iron, to not only maintain hemoglobin concentrations, but also increase their total iron for the expansion of blood volume and muscle mass during the period of growth. Data from the second National Health and Nutrition Examination Survey (NHANES II, 1976–80) demonstrated that the prevalence of impaired iron status among males ages 11–14 yr was 4–12%, and among females ages 15–44 was 5–14% depending on the assessment model used.[70] The survey also found adolescent females to be at increased risk for iron-deficiency anemia. The prevalence may be higher in certain ethnic and socioeconomic groups.[83–85] The increased risk of iron-deficiency anemia in the adolescent female has been attributed to rapid growth, menstrual losses, and dietary habits. However, oral contraceptive use was associated with improved iron status.[85]

Current discussion focuses on factors implicated in the excessive loss of body iron noted among athletes. Athletes with adequate iron intake and sufficient pretraining stores may adapt to changes in iron metabolism. This is not the case in individuals with low iron reserves and marginal dietary iron intake. The gastrointestinal tract is the major avenue of iron excretion in males and nonmenstruating females. Research suggests that GI bleeding occurs with prolonged exercise and is probably mediated by visceral ischemia. Although the quantity of blood and iron lost through the GI tract may be small, iron loss in an athlete, already in negative iron balance, will accelerate the depletion of iron stores.[86] Moreover, iron losses in endurance-trained athletes are greater than in normal individuals.[87] Thus, iron deficiency in adolescent athletes may be due to initially decreased iron stores and the gastrointestinal bleeding associated with exercise.[88]

Zinc.   Essential for growth, as well as sexual maturation during puberty. A number of studies have shown that zinc status may not be adequate in some teenagers.[89–92] A study of adolescent girls showed they consumed 75% of RDA for zinc, and 3% of those assessed had serum zinc below 70 μg/dL (normal range = 75–120 μg/dL).[91] In a study of Southern adolescent girls, 11 of the 59 participants had low-to-marginal levels of plasma zinc. Plasma zinc values were significantly lower in girls below the 25th percentile for height for age and race.[93] The 1987–88 NFCS demonstrated that 75% of adolescent males and 81% of adolescent females had dietary intakes below the RDA.

In the area of nutrient needs and requirements, additional research is needed to establish levels of intake critical to improved health and physiological outcomes. These issues must address whether the RDAs for nutrients as presently recommended are appropriate for adolescents. Research is needed to determine the optimum nutrient intake patterns that alter the risk of disease.

DIETARY PATTERNS

Despite low intake of some nutrients, the nutritional status of adolescents as a group generally appears adequate. However, their eating patterns as individuals may put them at risk of developing disease later in life. Adolescents frequently skip meals, eat unstructured meals, and eat too many snacks. As fewer and fewer meals are eaten together with the family, sources of food for teens have become fast-food outlets and convenience products. Such foods are usually highly processed, low in fiber, have a low nutrient density and contain high amounts of fat, saturated fat, cholesterol, sugar, and sodium.[94-96]

Concern about the "unhealthy" dietary practices of adolescents has prompted researchers to examine the prevalence of this problem. The National Adolescent Students Health Survey (NASHS)[97] conducted in 1987 provides a national profile of adolescent students' health-related knowledge, beliefs, and behaviors. Of those surveyed, 35% scored low on knowledge about the fat content of food, 40% ate fried foods more than four times a week, and more than 80% ate butter or margarine with bread. In the NASHS survey, 91% had eaten at least one snack on the previous day and 61% reported consuming "junk food" items such as chips, soda, candy, ice cream, and cake for a snack.[97] Although snacks do make a contribution toward meeting the nutrient intake needs of teenagers, they tend to displace foods not usually consumed as snacks.[98] Teenagers frequently skip meals and the meal most frequently omitted by teens is breakfast. The NASHS data showed that 32% percent of the boys and 48% of the girls reported having eaten breakfast two times or less during the week before the survey.[99]

As shown in Table 30.2, the proportion of fat and saturated fat in the diets of young people is above the target level of 30% of total energy from fat, with no more than 10% of energy from saturated fat recommended by the "Year 2000 Objectives." What are the major sources of fat and saturated fat in the diets of adolescents? Studies have identified three food groups to be the primary sources of fat and saturated fat in the diets of teens: dairy foods; meat, fish, poultry, eggs; and baked products.[100,101] In one report, the combination of dairy foods, bakery products, and snack-type foods contributed approximately 55% of the total fat and 58% of the saturated fat in the diets of adolescent girls.[101]

Similar to the adult population, adolescents in the United States tend to consume too few servings of fruits and vegetables. The Centers for Disease Control's Youth Risk Behavior Surveillance System has compiled data from the national, state and local youth risk behavior surveys conducted in 1991. Students were asked about foods they had consumed the day preceding the survey, including fruit, fruit juice, green salad, and cooked vegetables. Only 13% reported eating the recommended five or more servings of fruits and vegetables. Fruits and vegetables provide the nutrients which are usually low in the diets of adolescents. They may be the most important dietary groups which contribute to a reduction of risk for chronic conditions such as heart disease and cancer.

The excessive consumption of soft drinks may also be problematic. Studies have shown that these beverages have been substituted for milk, and there is a negative correlation between soft drink consumption and the adequacy of calcium intake, especially among girls.[102] Trends such as these may have a significant impact on bone health later in life.

The factors that influence adolescent dietary patterns are complex. Teenagers are often searching for independence and self-identity and have a strong need for peer acceptability. At the same time, teenagers often have considerable freedom to make personal decisions and the purchasing power to obtain meals, snacks, and beverages. Future research should focus on those factors that influence the eating behaviors of teens and how to effect positive changes in these patterns. Very little is known about the eating patterns in early adolescence as compared to late adolescence. Ideally, research must determine the optimum food and nutrition intake patterns that alter the risk of chronic disease.

PROBLEM AREAS OF ADOLESCENT NUTRITION

Although much remains to be learned about nutrient needs and requirements during adolescence, the major focus of future research must be directed toward problem areas where needs are greatest and interventions most effective.

Overweight and Obesity

Obesity during adolescence is a serious health problem with consequences that extend beyond the teenage years. Although difficult to quantify, obesity may be increasing among adolescents ages 12–17 yr.[103] Overweight or fatness during adolescence is associated with risk factors for chronic disease similar to those found among adults. Recent studies document that a majority of obese adolescents have the following risk factors: elevated serum triglyceride levels, decreased high-density lipoprotein cholesterol levels, increased total cholesterol level, elevated systolic or diastolic blood pressure, a diminished maximum work capacity, and a strong family history of coronary heart disease.[104–106] Longitudinal studies have shown that being overweight during adolescence may predict later elevated health risks and increased adult morbidity and mortality.[107–110] Overweight during adolescence has also been associated with an increased risk for cancer.[111]

It is important to note that changes in obesity during childhood are effective in reducing serum lipids and other risk factors.[104,112] Effective interventions included both dietary change and increased exercise and activity.[104] Health promotion efforts should be directed toward identifying adolescents with risk factors and implementing appropriate interventions such as those outlined by the National Cholesterol Education Program.[113]

The impact of obesity during adolescence goes far beyond physiological health.[114] It also influences psychosocial health. Obesity in adolescence has been associated with decreased peer acceptance, discrimination by significant adults, and poor body-image and lowered self-esteem. Obesity in adolescence has also been related to depression, problems in family relations, and poor school performance.[115]

Obesity risk factors are multifactorial and include familial, developmental, dietary, lifestyle, and psychosocial components. Future research on adolescent obesity must be broad and encompass a complex array of factors. How do psychosocial factors such as peer relations, self-esteem, and self-efficacy influence eating in adolescence? How do familial factors such as socioeconomic status, parental obesity and attitudes, and dietary practices in the home impact the condition? How do lifestyle factors such as physical inactivity, fat intake, and energy intake interact to increase risk? What interventions are most effective during adolescence and how should they be implemented?

There is a great need for new and innovative ways with which to approach the problem of overweight during adolescence. Is it possible that the development of self-esteem, self-efficacy, and self-worth during adolescence is a consequence of the acquisition of certain skills? If so, what are those skills? In addition to sports, games, music, dance, art, and technical skills, it is imperative for teens to become proficient in the art and science of preparing attractive and "healthy" food.

Dieting

At the same time that obesity poses a health risk for adolescents, undernutrition from inappropriate weight-loss practices may also be a problem. Adolescents may practice potentially dangerous weight-control strategies, including low-calorie and unbalanced diets, diet pills, diuretics, laxatives, and self-induced vomiting.[116,117] The pressures for thinness are pervasive and many normal weight teens are dissatisfied with their weight or body size and would like to be thinner. Adolescents diet mainly by restricting food on their own toward self-identified and sometimes unrealistic weight-loss goals.

The prevalence of dieting behavior during adolescence is difficult to assess.

Various studies have suggested that almost two-thirds of adolescent females in some population groups are dieting for weight loss, regardless of their body weight, possibly because of body image and size misperceptions.[118–120] Recent data from the Youth Risk Behavior Surveillance System (1990) and Behavioral Risk Factor Surveillance System (1989) are representative of the national picture.[121] Among high school students, 44% of female students and 15% of male students reported that they were trying to lose weight. Students reported that they had used the following weight-control methods in the seven days preceding the survey: exercise (51% of female students and 30% of male students); skipping meals (49and 18%, respectively); taking diet pills (4 and 2%, respectively); and vomiting (3 and 1%, respectively).[121]

High levels of dieting pose a significant threat to adolescents' nutritional status. In early adolescence dieting may lead to growth retardation and pubertal delay.[122] Overemphasis on thinness during adolescence may also contribute to the increasing incidence of anorexia nervosa and bulimia nervosa. Adolescent females are at risk for the development of these two health problems and compose 90–95% of individuals with these disorders.[116,123]

Research must be directed toward developing evaluation tools that may be used to identify adolescents with disturbed eating attitudes and behaviors. More needs to be learned about the development of healthy eating habits and attitudes.

Pregnancy and Lactation

The pregnant adolescent is another cohort at increased nutritional risk. Nutrients that are usually low in the diets of many teens become crucial at this time due to the demands of both the growing fetus and mother. Current research has been directed toward determining nutrient needs and the effect of energy intake on birth outcome. What remains unexamined is the impact of teenage pregnancy on growth and long-term nutritional status of the young person. Maternal growth during adolescent pregnancy has been a source of controversy because of the difficulties of quantifying growth. Recent research suggests that continued maternal growth occurs in both primiparas and multiparas during adolescent pregnancy and this results in diminished infant birth weight.[124,125] Does the apparent competition between maternal and fetal needs result in diminished stature in the mother? What are the consequences of adolescent pregnancy on skeletal maturation, bone health, and the risk of osteoporosis later in life? Is adolescent pregnancy a risk factor for reduced stature, diminished growth, or other conditions?

Little is known about the effect of adolescent lactation on the teenager's long-term health. To determine the calcium and bone mineral status of lactating adolescents, investigators compared the bone mineral content of lactating adolescents to that of nonlactating adolescents, nonlactating adults and nulliparous adolescents over time.[126] After 16 wk of lactation, the bone mineral content of the lactating adolescents was significantly lower than that of the other groups. In another study, lactating adolescents who consumed 1600 mg of dietary calcium did not show a significant change in their bone mineral content.[127] Such results underscore the physiological demands of reproduction in the teenage years. More research is needed on how early reproductive experiences impact the physiological and psychosocial health of the teenager.

Groups at Risk

Research efforts should also be directed toward meeting the needs of selected population groups that are at greater risk for nutrient deficits and imbalances. Data from surveys suggest the greater prevalence of low vitamin and mineral intake and status among certain ethnic and socioeconomic groups, especially those from urban low-income households, native American reservations, and economically depressed rural areas.[128-134] The 1987–88 NFCS identified African Americans as having higher cholesterol and salt intakes and Asian Americans as consuming more salt.[41] Research is needed to identify ways to simplify and streamline assessment measures and identify the intervention most likely to accomplish change.

Smoking, Alcohol Abuse, and Drug Abuse

Smoking, alcohol abuse, and drug abuse among adolescents are a national problem of great significance. Little is known about the nutritional impact of these addictive substances in young individuals or the influence of abuse on dietary practices and habits.[135-137] A recent study suggested that Caucasian female adolescents may use smoking as a weight-control strategy.[137]

Some may argue that the consequences of aberrant eating styles in teens pale when compared to the consequences of smoking, alcohol and drug abuse, indiscriminate sex, and risk-taking. It is possible that all these behaviors have common determinants in the adolescents' quest for independence, self-identity, and self-esteem. Although these psychological constructs are difficult to evaluate, recent studies suggest a relationship between self-concept and the dietary quality of adolescent girls.[138,139] Further research is needed to determine how self-perceptions interact with behavior during the critical developmental years.

What motivates adolescents to make healthy food choices? Contento et al.[140] identified a number of orientations among teenagers including health-motivated ones. The science of foods and nutrition is an integrating field that may involve many different disciplines. Research in nutritional science must be coordinated with behavioral sciences and epidemiology to help solve the problems of the adolescent. Efforts must be directed toward factors that encourage teenagers to follow healthy lifestyles.

REFERENCES

1. F. P. Heald, *Med. Clin. N. Am.*, **59**, 1329 (1975).

2. J. I. McKigney and H. N. Munro, in *Nutrient Requirements in Adolescence*, (J. I. McKigney and H. N. Munro, eds.), MIT Press, Cambridge, MA, pp. 147–171 (1976).

3. R. E. Kreipe, O.J.Z. Sahler, in *The Health of Adolescents*, (W. R. Hendee, ed., Jossey-Bass, San Francisco, CA, pp. 21–57 (1991).

4. L. S. Neinstein and F. R. Kaufman, in *Adolescent Health Care: A Practical Guide,* 2nd ed., (L. S. Neistein, ed.), Urban & Schwarzenberg, Baltimore, MD, pp. 3–37 (1991).

5. G. B. Slap, *J. Adol. Health Care*, **7**, 13S, (1986).

6. E. J. Gong and B. A. Spear, *J. Nutr. Ed.*, **20**, 273 (1988).

7. J. M. Tanner and P.S.W. Davis, *J. Peds.*, **107**, 317 (1985).

8. J. M. Tanner, *J. Adol. Health Care*, **8**, 470 (1987).

9. W. R. Harlan, E. A. Harlan, and G. P. Grillo, *J. Peds.*, **96**, 1074 (1980).

10. National Center for Health Statistics, in *Height and Weights of Youths 12–17 Years, United States, Vital and Health Statistics*, Series 11, no. 124, Government Printing Office, Washington,DC, pp. 1–81 (1973).

11. B. R. Carruth, *J. Nutr. Ed.*,**20**, 280 (1988).

12. D. M. Wilson, H. C. Kraemer, P. L. Ritter, and L. D. Hammer, *AJDC*, **141**, 565 (1987).

13. P. M. Duke, I. F. Litt, and R. T. Gross, *Pediatrics*, **66**, 918 (1980).

14. R. L. Williams, K. L. Cheyne, L. K. Houtkooper, and T. G. Lohman, *J. Adol. Health Care*, **9**, 480 (1988).

15. S. M. Garn and D. C. Clark, *Pediatrics*, **57**, 443 (1976).

16. P. B. Eveleth and J. M. Tanner, (ed.), *Worldwide Variation in Human Growth, 2nd ed.*, Cambridge University Press, Cambridge, MA, pp. 191–208 (1990).

17. G. Wyshak and R. E. Frisch, *N. Engl. J. Med.*, **306**, 1033 (1982).

18. J. L. Mills, P. H. Shiono, L. R. Shapiro, P. B. Crawford, G. G. Rhoades, *J. Peds.*, **109**, 543 (1986).

19. G. B. Forbes, *J. Peds.*, **91**, 40 (1977).

20. G. B. Post and H. C. Kemper, *Eur. J. Clin. Nutr.*, **47**, 400 (1993).

21. R. E. Frisch and J. McArthur, *Science*, **185**, 949 (1974).

22. E. C. Scott and F. E. Johnston, *J. Adol. Health Care*, **2**, 249 (1982).

23. C. M. de Ridder, P. F. Bruning, M. L. Zonderland et al., *J. Clin. Endocrinol. Metab.*, **70**, 888 (1990).

24. M. Pryor, M. L. Slattery, L. M. Robinson, and M. Egger, *Cancer Res.*, **49**, 2161 (1989).

25. A. F. Roche, R. M. Siervogel, W. C. Chumlea, and P. Webb, *Am. J. Clin. Nutr.*, **34**, 2831 (1981).

26. L. G. Bandini and W. H. Dietz, *J. Am. Diet.Assoc.*, **87**, 1344 (1987).

27. J. D. Marshall, C. B. Hazlett, D. W. Spady, and H. A. Quinney, *Am. J. Clin. Nutr.*, **51**, 22 (1990).

28. U. S. Public Health Service, *Healthy People 2000, National Health Promotion and Disease Prevention Objectives*, DHHS (PHS) Pub. no. 91–50212, Government Printing Office, Washington, DC, (1991).

29. J. H. Himes and W. H. Dietz, *Am. J. Clin. Nutr.*, **59**, 307 (1994).

30. A. Must, G. E. Dallal, and W. H. Dietz, *Am. J. Clin. Nutr.*, **53**, 839 (1991).

31. A. Must, G. E. Dallal, and W. H.Dietz, *Am. J. Clin. Nutr.*, **54**, 773 (1991).

32. V. A. Casey, J. T. Dwyer, K. A. Coleman, and I. Valadian, *Am. J. Clin. Nutr.*, **56**, 14 (1992).

33. A. Must. P. F. Jacques, G. E. Dallal, C. L. Bajema, and W. H. Dietz, *N. Engl. J. Med.*, **327**, 1350 (1992).

34. D. W. Harsha, R. R. Rerichs, and G. S. Berenson, *Hum. Biol.*, **50**, 261 (1978).

35. A. F. Roche, S. Guo, R. N. Baumgartner, W. C. Chumlea, A. S. Ryan, and R. J. Kuczmarski, *Am. J. Clin. Nutr.*, **51**, 917S (1990).

36. M. Y. Jackson, *J. Am. Diet. Assoc.*, **93**, 1136 (1993).

37. Food and Nutrition Board, National Research Council, *Recommended Dietary Allowances*,X ed., National Academy Press, Washington, DC (1989).

38. Life Sciences Research Office, Federation of American Societies for Experimental Biology, *Nutrition Monitoring in the United States—An Update Report on Nutrition Monitoring*, DHHS (PHS) Pub. no. 89–1255, Government Printing Office, Washington, DC (1989).

39. H. S. Wright, H. A. Guthrie, M. Q. Wang, and V. Bernardo, *Nutr. Today*, **26**, 21 (1991).

40. C. Lenfant and N. Ernst, *MMWR*, **43**, 116 (1994).

41. R. K. Johnson, D. G. Johnson, M. Q. Wang, H. S. Wright, and H. A.Gurthrie, *J. Adol. Health Care*, **15**, 149 (1994).

42. B. Waite, R. Blair, and L. Roberts, *Am. J. Clin. Nutr.*, **22**, 1279 (1969).

43. E. J. Gong and F. P. Heald, in *Diet, Nutrition, and Adolescence*, VIII ed., (M. E. Shils, J. A. Olson and M. Shike, eds.), Lea & Febiger, Philadelphia, PA, pp.759–769 (1993).

44. World Health Organization (WHO), *Energy and Protein Requirements,* Report of a Joint FAO/WHO/UNU Expert Consultation, Technical Report Series 724, World Health Organization, Geneva, (1985).

45. B. Wait, *Am. J. Clin. Nutr.*, **26**, 1303 (1973).

46. V. Gattas, G. A. Barrera, J. S. Riumallo, and R. Uauy, *Am. J. Clin. Nutr.*, **56**,499 (1992).

47. E. C. Dick, S. D. Chen, M. Bert, and J. M. Smith, *J. Nutr.*, **66**, 173 (1958).

48. M. Hart and M. S. Reynold, *J. Home Econ.*, **49**, 35 (1957).

49. L. G. Warnock, G. E. Nichoalds, and V. J. Burkhalter, *Am. J. Clin Nutr.*, **27**, 905 (1973).

50. H. E. Sauberlich, J. H. Judd, G. E. Nichoalds, H. P. Broquist, and W. J. Darby, *Am. J. Clin. Nutr.*, **25**, 756 (1972).

51. R. Lopez, J. V. Schwartz, and J. M. Cooperman, *Am. J. Clin. Nutr.*, **33**, 1283 (1980).

52. B. Cromer, S. D. Thomas, L. D. Padilla, and V. M. Vivian, *J. Adol. Health Care*, **10**, 382 (1989).

53. R. A. Jacob, M. E. Swendseid, R. W. McKee, C. S. Fu, and R. A. Clemens, *J. Nutr.*, **119**, 591 (1989).

54. A. Kirksey, K. Keaton, R. P. Abernathy, and J. L. Greger, *Am. J. Clin. Nutr.*, **31**, 946 (1978).

55. J. A. Driskell, A. J. Clark, T. L. Bazzarre, L. F. Chopin, H. McCoy, M. A. Denney, and S. W. Meak, *J. Am. Diet. Assoc.*, **85**, 46 (1985).

56. S. H. Cohenour and D. H. Calloway, *Am. J. Clin. Nutr.*, **25**, 512 (1972).

57. J. V. Kathman and C. Kies, *Nutr. Res.*, **4**, 245 (1984).

58. B. R. Eissenstat, B. W. Wyse, and R. G. Hansen, *Am. J. Clin. Nutr.*, **44**, 931 (1986).

59. V. Herbert, *Am. J. Clin Nutr.*, **45**, 661 (1987).

60. W. A. Daniel, E. G. Gaines, and D. L. Bennett, *Am. J. Clin. Nutr.*, **28**, 363 (1975).

61. L. B. Bailey, P. A. Wagner, G. J. Christakis, C. G. Davis, H. Appledorf, P. E. Araujo, E. Dorsey, and J. S. Dinning, *Am. J. Clin. Nutr.*, **35**, 1023 (1982).

62. A. J. Clark, S. Mossholder, and R. Gates, *Am. J. Clin. Nutr.*, **46**, 302 (1987).

63. L. A. Reiter, L. M. Boylan, J. Driskell, and S. Meak, *J. Am. Diet. Assoc.*, **87**, 1065 (1987).

64. J. C. Tsui and J. W. Nordstrom, *J. Am. Diet. Assoc.*, **90**, 1551 (1990).

65. L. G. Bailey, *J. Am. Diet. Assoc.*, **92**, 463 (1992).

66. Centers for Disease Control and Prevention, *MMWR*, **41**, 1 (1992).

67. J. S. Smith and R. E. Hodges, *Ann. N. Y. Acad. Sci.*, **144**, 498 (1987).

68. G. Schectman, J. C. Byrd, and H. W. Gruchow, *Am. J. Pub. Health*, **79**, 158 (1989).

69. B. Herbeth, Y. Spycherelle, and J. P. Deschamps, *Am. J. Clin. Nutr.*, **54**, 884 (1991).

70. S. A. Pilch, *J. Nutr.*, **117**, 636 (1987).

71. G. Lockitch, A. C. Halstead, L. Wadsworth, G. Quigley, L. Reston, and B. Jacobson, *Clin. Chem.*, **34**, 1625 (1988).

72. L. R. Sutker and J.A. Driskell, *J. Am. Diet. Assoc.*, **83**, 678 (1983).

73. A. C. Looker, B. A. Underwood, J. Wiley, R. Fulwood, and C. T. Sempos, *Am. J. Clin. Nutr.*, **50**, 491 (1989).

74. N. A. Pocock, J. A. Eisman, J. L. Hopper, M. G. Yeates, and P. N. Sambrook, S. Eberl, *J. Clin. Invest.*, **90**, 706 (1987).

75. J. Lutz, *Am. J. Clin. Nutr.*, **44**, 99 (1986).

76. E. Seeman, J. L. Hopper, L. A. Back, et al., *N. Engl. J. Med.*, **320**, 554 (1989).

77. V. Matkovic, D. Fontana, C. Tominac, P. Goel, and C. H. Chesnut, *Am. J. Clin. Nutr.*, **52**, 878 (1990).

78. L. Halioua and J.J.B. Anderson, *Am. J. Clin. Nutr.*, **49**, 534 (1989).

79. A. M. Fehily, R. J. Coles, W. D. Evans, and P. C. Elwood, *Am. J. Clin. Nutr.*, **56**, 579 (1992).

80. G. W. Barrow and S. Saha, *Am. J. Sports. Med.*, **16**, 209 (1988).

81. M. B. Zemel and H. M. Linkswiler, *J. Nutr.*, **111**, 315 (1981).

82. R. B. Sandler, C. W. Slemenda, R. E. La Porte, J. A. Cauley, M. M. Schramm, M. L. Bresi, and A. M. Kriska, *Am. J. Clin. Nutr.*, **42**, 270 (1985).

83. E. G. Gaines and W. A. Daniel, *J. Am. Diet. Assoc.* 65, 275(1974).

84. M. Liebman, M. A. Kenney, W. Billon, A. J. Clark, G. W. Disney, E. G. Ercanli, E. Glover, H. Lewis, S. W. Moak, J. H. McCoy, P. Schilling, F. Thye, and T. Wakefield, *Am. J. Clin. Nutr.*, **38**, 109 (1983).

85. S. B. Fitzpatrick, M. R. Chacko, and F. P. Heald, *J. Adol. Health. Care*, **5**, 71 (1984).

86. R. J. Moore, K. E. Friedl, R. T. Tulley, and E. W. Askew, *Am. J. Clin. Nutr.*, **58**, 923 (1993).

87. C. M. Weaver and S. Rajaram, *J. Nutr.*, **122**, 782 (1992).

88. H. J. Nickerson, M. C. Holubets, B. R. Weiler, R. G. Haas, S. Schwartz, and M. E. Ellefson, *J. Peds.*, **114**, 657 (1989).

89. J. L. Greger, M. M. Higgins, R. P. Abernathy, A. Kirksey, M. B. DeCorso, and P. Baligar, *Am. J. Clin. Nutr.*, **31**, 269 (1978).

90. J. L. Greger, S. C. Zaikis, R. P. Abernathy, O. A. Bennett, and J. Huffman, *J. Nutr.*, **108**, 1449 (1978)

91. M. A. Kenney, S. J. Ritchey. P. Culley, W. Sandoval, S. Moak, and P. Schilling, *Am. J. Clin. Nutr.*, **39**, 446 (1984).

92. B. A. Sloane, C. C. Gibbons, and M. Hegsted, *Am. J. Clin. Nutr.*, **42**, 235 (1985).

93. P. Thompson, R. Roseborough, E. Russek, M. Jacobson, and P. B. Moser, *J. Am. Diet. Assoc.*, **86**, 892 (1986)

94. A. S. Truswell and I. Darnton-Hill, *Nutr. Rev.*, **39**, 73 (1981).

95. M. Story and M. D. Resnick, *J. Nutr. Ed.*, **18**, 188 (1986).

96. M. C. Farthing, *Nutr. Today*, **26**, 35 (1991).

97. B. Portnoy and G. M. Christenson, *J. School Health*, **59**, 218 (1989).

98. S. Bigler-Doughton and R. M. Jenkins, *J. Am. Diet. Assoc.*, **87**, 1678 (1987).

99. Centers for Disease Control and Prevention, *MMWR*, **38**, 147 (1989).

100. R. Kuczmarski, E. Brewer, F. Cronin. B. Dennis, K. Graves, and S. Haynes, *Ped. Res.*, **20**, 309 (1986).

101. J. C. Witschi, A. L. Capper, and R. C. Ellison, *J. Am. Diet. Assoc.*, **90**, 1429 (1990).

102. P. M. Guenther, *J. Am. Diet. Assoc.*, **86**, 493 (1986).

103. S. L. Gortmaker, W. H. Dietz, A. M. Sobol, and C. A. Wehler, *AJDC*, **141**, 535 (1984).

104. M. D. Becque, V. L. Katch, A. P. Rocchinni, C. R. Marks, and C. Moorehead, *Pediatrics*, **81**, 605 (1988).

105. C. G. Smoak, G. L Burke, L. S. Webber, D. W. Harsha, S. R. Srinivasan, and G. S. Berenson, *Am. J. Epidemiol.*, **125**, 364 (1987).

106. R. N. Baumgartner, R. M. Siervogel, W. C. Chumlea, and A. F. Roche, *Int. J. Obes.*, **13**, 31 (1989)

107. R. M. Lauer, and W. R. Clarke, *JAMA*, **264**, 3034 (1990).

108. L. S. Webber, S. R. Srinivasan, W. A. Wattigney, and G. S. Berenson, *Am. J. Epidemiol.*, **133**, 884 (1991).

109. A. Must, P. F. Jacques, G. E. Dallal, C. J. Bajema, and W. H. Dietz, *N. Engl. J. Med.*, **327**, 1350 (1992)

110. F. J. Nieto, M. Szklo,and G. W. Comstock, *Am. J. Epidemiol.*, **136**, 201 (1992)

111. L. Garfinkel, *Ann. Intern. Med.*, **103**, 1034 (1985).

112. D. S. Freedman, G. L. Burke, D. W Harsha, S. R. Srinivasan, J. L. Cresanta, L. S. Webber, and G. S. Berenson, *JAMA*, **254**, 515 (1985).

113. National Cholesterol Education Program, National Institutes of Health, *Report of the Expert Panel of Blood Cholesterol Levels in Children and Adolescents*, NIH publ., Washington, DC (1991).

114. K. D. Bronwell, *J. Am. Diet. Assoc.*, **84**,406 (1984).

115. K. M. Kaplan and A. T. Wadden, *Beh. Ped.*, **109**, 367 (1986).

116. J. D. Killen, C. Hayward, I. Litt, et al., *AJDC*, **146**, 323 (1992).

117. W. Feldman, P. McGrath, and M. O'Shaughessy, *AJDC*, **140**, 249 (1986).

118. D. Moore, *AJDC*, **77**, 561(1988).

119. N. Moses, M. M. Banilivy, and F. Lifshitz, *Pediatrics*, **83**, 393 (1989).

120. R. C. Casper and D. Offer, *Pediatrics*, **86**, 384 (1990).

121. M. K. Serdula, E. Collins, D. F. Williamson, R. F. Anda, E. Pamuk, and T. E. Byers, *Ann. Intern. Med.*, **119**, 667 (1993).

122. H. T. Pugliese, F. Lifschitz, G. Grad, P. Fort, and M. Marks-Katz, *New Engl. J. Med.*, **309**, 513 (1983).

123. D. Herzog and P. Copeland, *N. Engl. J. Med.*, **313**,295 (1985).

124. T. O. Scholl, M. L. Hediger, and I. G. Ances, *Am. J. Clin. Nutr.*, **51**, 790 (1991).

125. T. O. Scholl and M. L. Hediger, *J. Am. Coll. Nutr.*, **12**, 101 (1993).

126. G. M. Chan, N. Roland, P. Slater, J. Hollis, and M. R. Thomas, *J. Peds.*, **101**, 767 (1982).

127. G. M. Chan, M. McMurry, K. Westover, K. E. Fenton, and M. R. Thomas, *Am. J. Clin. Nutr.*, **46**, 319 (1987).

128. L. B. Bailey, P. A. Wagner, G. J. Christakis, C. G. Davis, H. Appledorf, P. E. Araujo, E. Dorsey, and J. S. Dinning, *Am. J. Clin. Nutr.*, **35**, 1023 (1982).

129. M. Liebman, M. A. Kenney, W. Bilton, A. J. Clark, G. W. Disney, E. G. Ercanli, E. Glover, H. Lewis, S. W.Moak, J. H. McCoy, P. Schilling, F. Thye, and T. Wakefield, *Am. J. Clin. Nutr.* **38**, 109 (1983).

130. S. B. Fitzpatrick, M. R. Chacko, F. P. Heald, *J. Adol. Health Care*, **5**, 71 (1984).

131. H. McCoy, M. A. Kenney, A. Kirby, G. Disney, F. G. Ercanli, E. Glover, M. Korslund, H. Levis, M. Liebman, and E. Levant, *J. Am. Diet. Assoc.*, **84**, 1453 (1984).

132. J. D. Skinner, N. N. Salvetti, J. M. Exell, M. P. Penfield, and C. A. Costell. *J. Am. Diet. Assoc.*, **85**, 1093 (1985).

133. M. Story and P.V.Z. York, *J. Am. Diet. Assoc.*, **87**, 1680 (1987).

134. L. A. Reiter, L. M. Boylan, J. Driskell, and S. Meak, *J. Am. Diet. Assoc.*, **87**, 1065 (1987).

135. M. E. Mohs, R. R.Watson, and T. Leonard-Green, *J. Am. Diet. Assoc.*, **90**, 1261 (1990).

136. J. A. Farrow, J. M. Rees, B. S. Worthington-Roberts, *Pediatrics*, **79**, 218 (1987).

137. D. E. Camp, R. C. Klesges, and G. Relyea, *Health Psychol.*, **12**, 24 (1993).

138. D. J. Witte, J. B. Skinner, B. R. Carruth, *J. Am. Diet. Assoc.*, **91**, 1068 (1991).

139. G. K. Newell, C. L. Hammig, A. P. Jurich, and D. E. Johnson, *Adolescence*, **25**, 117 (1990).

140. I. R. Contento, J. L. Michela, and C. J. Goldberg, *J. Nutr. Ed.*, **20**, 289 (1988).

APPENDICES

Vegetarian Diets

Appendix A.1 Percent of Total Calories as Protein in Typical Foods

Category	Item	%
Fruits	Pear	3
	Grape	4
	Orange	8
Grains	Corn	8
	Rice	8
	Whole wheat	15
	Oats	16
Vegetables	Yam	5
	Potato	8
	Bell pepper	13
	Tomato	17
	Green pea	26
	Mushroom	30
	Broccoli	40
	Spinach	45
	Mustard green	48

continued on next page

Appendix A.1   *Continued*

Category	Item	%
Legumes	Garbanzo bean	22
	Pinto bean	24
	Lentil	30
	Black-eyed pea	31
	Soybean	38
	Tofu	43
Milk and dairy products	Whole milk	21
	Nonfat milk (skim)	40
	Cheddar cheese	25
	Cottage cheese (low-fat)	60
	Egg	31
	Egg white	85
Meats	Chuck roast	26
	Ground beef, hamburger	33
	Chicken without skin	60
Nuts and seeds	Almond	14
	Walnut	16
	Peanut (a legume)	18
	Pumpkin/squash seed	18

P. K. Johnston, E. Haddad, and J. Sabate, in *Adol. Med.: State Art Rev.*, **3**, 417 (1992). Reprinted with permission.

Appendix A.2   Total Calories and Grams of Protein in Selected Foods

	Serving Size	Energy (kcal)	Protein (g)
Grains and cereals			
Bread, whole wheat	1 slice	60	2.5
Bulgar, cooked	1 cup	150	4.2
Cereal, ready to eat	1 cup	150	3.5
Cornbread, 2 in. square	1 piece	130	3.0
English muffin	1	135	4.5
Oatmeal, cooked	1 cup	155	4.5
Pita pocket, 6 in.	1	105	4.0
Spagetti, cooked	1 cup	160	5.2
Vegetables			
Artichoke	1 medium	55	2.8
Baby limas, cooked	½ cup	95	6.0
Broccoli, cooked	½ cup	25	2.3
Corn kernals, cooked	½ cup	70	2.5
Green peas, cooked	½ cup	65	4.0
Potato, baked with skin	1 large	220	4.6
Tomato, raw	1 medium	25	1.0
Dry Beans, peas, and soy products			
Beans, cooked	½ cup	115	7.5
Lentils, cooked	½ cup	115	10.0
Soybeans, cooked	½ cup	150	14.3
Soy milk	1 cup	80	6.6
Tofu, regular	½ cup	95	10.0
Nuts and seeds			
Almonds	1 oz	165	5.7
Peanut butter	1 tbsp	95	4.6
Pumpkin or squash seeds	1 oz	155	7.0
Milk and dairy products			
Cheddar cheese	1 oz	115	7.1
Collage cheese, low-fat	½ cup	100	15.5
Egg	1 medium	80	6.0
Milk, low-fat (2%)	1 cup	125	8.5
Yogurt, nonfat	1 cup	145	12.0

P. K. Johnston, E. Haddad, and J. Sabate, in *Adol. Med.: State Art Rev.*, **3**, 417 (1992).
Reprinted with permission.

Appendix A.3   Sources of Calcium

	Serving Size	μg
Milk and dairy products		
Yogurt, low-fat	1 cup	415
Skim milk powder	¼ cup	400
Ricotta (skim milk)	½ cup	335
Milk, low-fat (2%)	1 cup	315
Mozzarella cheese (part skim)	1 oz	260
Cheddar cheese	1 oz	205
Cottage cheese (low-fat)	½ cup	75
Green Vegetables		
Turnip greens, cooked	1 cup	250
Broccoli, cooked	1 cup	180
Collards, cooked	1 cup	150
Dandelion greens, cooked	1 cup	145
Spinach, cooked	1 cup	145
Mustard greens, cooked	1 cup	100
Okra, cooked	1 cup	100
Legumes and Soy Products		
Soymilk (fortified)	1 cup	300
Tofu, firm	½ cup	260
Soybean nuts, dry roasted	½ cup	230
Garbanzo beans, cooked	1 cup	80
Kidney beans, cooked	1 cup	60
Miscellaneous		
Blackstrap molasses	1 tbsp	135
Figs, dried	5	135
Sesame butter (tahini)	2 tbsp	130
Almonds	1 oz (24 nuts)	75

P. K. Johnston, E. Haddad, and J. Sabate, in *Adol. Med.: State Art Rev.*,**3**, 417 (1992). Reprinted with permission.

Appendix A.4   Sources of Iron and Zinc

Food Source	Serving Size	Iron (mg)	Zinc (mg)
Dry beans and peas			
Black-eyed peas, cooked	½ cup	2.2	1.1
Garbanzo beans, cooked	½ cup	2.4	1.3
Kidney beans, cooked	½ cup	2.6	0.9
Lentils, cooked	½ cup	3.3	1.3
Pinto beans, cooked	½ cup	2.2	0.9
Soybeans and products			
Soybean nuts	1 oz	1.3	1.0
Soybeans, cooked	½ cup	4.4	1.0
Soy milk	1 cup	1.4	0.5
Tempeh	½ cup	1.9	1.5
Tofu, regular	½ cup	6.7	1.0
Breads, grains, and cereals			
Bagel	1	1.5	0.3
Cereals, cooked (fortified)	¾ cup	4.0-9.0	0.3-1.3
Cereals, dry (fortified)	1 oz	4.0-8.0	1.0-3.7
Corn tortilla (enriched)	1 6 in.	2.7	0.4
Pita pocket	1 6 in.	0.9	0.3
Spaghetti (enriched)	1 cup	2.2	0.7
Wheat bran	2 tbsp	0.7	0.5
Wheat germ, toasted	¼ cup	2.6	4.7
White bread	1 slice	0.7	0.1
Whole wheat bread	1 slice	0.9	0.4
Vegetables			
Artichoke	1 medium	1.6	0.4
Broccoli, cooked	½ cup	0.9	0.1
Green beans	½ cup	0.8	0.2
Green peas	½	1.2	1.0
Mushrooms, cooked	½ cup	1.4	0.7
Potato, baked with skin	1 large	2.8	0.7
Spincach, cooked	½ cup	3.2	0.7
Tomatoes, cooked	½ cup	0.7	0.2
Turnip greens, cooked	½ cup	1.6	0.3
Fruits and Fruit Juice			
Apricots	6 medium	1.2	0.7
Avocado	½ medium	1.0	0.4
Dates, dried	10 dates	1.0	0.2
Figs,	5 medium	2.1	0.5

continued on next page

Appendix A.4   *Continued*

Food Source	Serving Size	Iron (mg)	Zinc (mg)
Fruits and Fruit Juice, continued			
Pear	1 medium	0.4	0.2
Prune juice, canned	½ cup	1.5	0.25
Raisins	⅓ cup	1.3	0.1
Strawberries	1 cup	0.6	0.2
Tomato juice cocktail, canned	1 cup	2.2	0.3
Nuts and Seeds			
Almonds	1 oz	1.0	0.8
Cashews	1 oz	1.7	1.6
Peanut butter	2 tbsp	0.6	0.9
Pumpkin or squash seeds	1 oz	4.3	2.1
Sesame butter (tahini)	2 tbsp	2.7	1.4
Sunflower seeds	1 oz	1.9	1.4
Milk and Dairy Products			
Cottage cheese (low-fat)	½ cup	0.2	0.5
Egg	1 large	1.0	0.7
Milk, low-fat (2%)	1 cup	0.1	1.0

P. K. Johnston, E. Haddad, and J. Sabate, in *Adol. Med.: State Art Rev.*,**3**, 417 (1992).
Reprinted with permission.

VEGETARIAN FOOD GROUP DESCRIPTION
Breads, Grains, and Cereals

The nutrient contribution of this groups was based on 50% whole-grain products and 50% enriched products. Wheat, rice, corn, millet, oats, and other grains are the staple foods for most of the world's population and they form the foundation of vegetarian eating. Foods from this group are important sources of complex carbohydrates, fiber, the B vitamins, and minerals. The importance of whole grain breads cannot be overemphasized. The phytate present in whole grains is reduced by yeast fermentation during bread making, thus increasing the availability of the minerals present. Fortified breakfast cereals can provide substantial amounts of B vitamins, iron, and zinc for the adolescent.

Legumes

There are many varieties of dried seeds, commonly called legumes. These include kidney beans, navy beans, lima beans, black beans, garbanzo beans, peas, black-eyed peas, and lentils. These foods are important sources of protein, calcium, iron, zinc, and vitamin B-6. Soybeans and soy products are also included in this group and are excellent sources of these same nutrients. LOV must include at least one serving from this group in their diet every day, whereas vegan adolescents, to obtain enough zinc, must include at least two servings from this group.[1]

Vegetables

The nutrient contribution of this group was calculated on the basis of one-third starchy vegetables, one-third other commonly eaten vegetables, and one-third salad greens and salad vegetables.[2] The dark green and leafy vegetables are especially important for the calcium they supply. Fiber and vitamins A and C are also important contributions from this group.

Fruits

This group as well as the vegetable group is important for the vitamin C and fiber that it contributes. As noted, vegetarians should be sure to include good sources of iron and vitamin C at each meal in order to ensure adequate iron status.

Nuts and Seeds

This group is particularly important for its contribution of magnesium, zinc, iron, and niacin. It includes the many different kinds of nuts and seeds and the nut butters or spreads. It is preferable to use those that are not fried in oil or highly salted.

Milk, Yogurt, and Cheese

The major contribution of calcium to the diet comes from this group. It is also a good source of protein and vitamin B-12. Although calcium is found in all plant foods, it is difficult to obtain the RDA of 1200 mg needed by adolescents only from plant food sources.[2]

Milk Alternates and Tofu

Vegans must include at least three servings of calcium-fortified soymilk or calcium-containing tofu in their daily diet. There are many new soy-based drinks available in the market place, however only a few are fortified with calcium and vitamin B-12. Some are very low in protein. It is important that consumers read labels to determine the nutrient content and assure adequate intake of those nutrients usually obtained from animal foods.

Eggs

Eggs have been listed in a separate category in this vegetarian food guide. They may be deleted from the diet without greatly influencing the nutritional contribution of the guide as a whole.[2]

Fats and Oils

Fats and oils provide essential fatty acids. They can help meet the energy requirements of physically active adolescents. Total vegetarians may need to increase foods from this group in order to meet their energy needs from a plant-based diet that has low caloric density. It is, however, important for vegetarians, just as for omnivores, to limit the total fat in their diet to 30% of calories or less.

Sugar and Sweets

Sugars include not only table sugar, but also brown sugar, honey, syrup, and high-fructose corn syrup. Foods containing a high proportion of sugar and other nutritive sweeteners such as soft, drinks, candies, and desserts contribute few nutrients other than calories and should be eaten in moderation.

REFERENCES

1. P. K. Johnston, E. Haddad, and J. Sabate, *Adol. Med.:State Art Rev.* **3**, 417, (1992).
2. E. H. Haddad, *Am. J. Clin. Nutr.*, **59**, 1248S (1994).

Appendix A.6 Suggested Pattern for Lacto-ovovegetarian Adolescents

	2200 kcal	2800 kcal
	Daily Number of Servings	
Dietary pattern		
Bread, grains and cereals*	9	11
Legumes and plant proteins	2	3
Vegetables	4	5
Fruits	3	4
Nuts and seeds	1	1
Milk, yogurt, and cheese	3	3
Eggs	½	½
Added fats and oils (tsp)†	4	6
Added sugar (tsp)‡	6	9
Approximate composition		
Protein (g)	88	103
Fat (g)	62	74
% kcal as fat	25	24
Saturated fat (g)	18	20
% kcal as saturated fat	7	6

* At least half the servings from whole-grain breads and cereals.

† Fat added to food during food preparation and/or used as spreads and dressings.

‡ Sugar and other coloric sweeteners (syrup, honey, etc.) added to food and bakery items during food preparation and used in drinks, beverages, and desserts.

Adapted from E. H. Haddad, *Am. J. Clin. Nutr.*, **59**, 1248S (1994). Reprinted with permission.

Appendix A.7   Suggested Pattern for Total Vegetarian Adolescents

	2200 kcal	2800 kcal
	Daily Number of Servings	
Dietary pattern		
Bread, grains and cereals*	10	12
Legumes and plant proteins	2	3
Vegetables	3	4
Dark green leafy vegetables	2	2
Fruits	4	6
Nuts and seeds	1	1
Fortified soy drinks and tofu†	3	3
Added fats and oils (tsp)‡	4	6
Added sugar (tsp)**	6	9
Approximate composition		
Protein (g)	76	95
Fat (g)	58	78
% kcal as fat	24	25
Saturated fat (g)	10	12
% kcal as saturated fat	4	4

* At least half the servings from whole-grain breads and cereals.

† Milk alternates fortified with calcium, vitamin D, and vitamin B-12 and/or multivitamin and mineral supplements.

‡ Fat added to food during food preparation and/or used as spreads and dressings.

** Sugar and other coloric sweeteners (syrup, honey, etc.) added to food and bakery items during food preparation and used in drinks, beverages, and desserts.

Adapted from E. H. Haddad, *Am. J. Clin. Nutr.*, **59**, 1248S (1994). Reprinted with permission.

Anorexia Nervosa

Appendix B.1 Symptoms

In the last 6 months, have you had any of the following symptoms? If yes, circle the number that best describes how often each occurs.

	No	Yes	Less than once a week	Once a week	2–6 × a week	Once a day	More than once a day, or all the time
Headache	☐	☐	1	2	3	4	5
Dizziness	☐	☐	1	2	3	4	5
Fainting	☐	☐	1	2	3	4	5
Cold hands/feet	☐	☐	1	2	3	4	5
Puffiness or fluid buildup	☐	☐	1	2	3	4	5
Trouble with teeth or gums	☐	☐	1	2	3	4	5
Hair loss	☐	☐	1	2	3	4	5
Hair growth	☐	☐	1	2	3	4	5
Heat or cold intolerance	☐	☐	1	2	3	4	5
Constipation	☐	☐	1	2	3	4	5

Diarrhea	☐	☐	1	2	3	4	5
Painful urination	☐	☐	1	2	3	4	5
Frequent urination	☐	☐	1	2	3	4	5
Stomach pains	☐	☐	1	2	3	4	5
Muscle cramps	☐	☐	1	2	3	4	5
Chest pain	☐	☐	1	2	3	4	5
Breast discharge	☐	☐	1	2	3	4	5
Trouble breathing	☐	☐	1	2	3	4	5
Numbness or tingling	☐	☐	1	2	3	4	5
Bone pain	☐	☐	1	2	3	4	5
Joint pain	☐	☐	1	2	3	4	5
Nausea	☐	☐	1	2	3	4	5
Bloating or fullness	☐	☐	1	2	3	4	5
Being tired	☐	☐	1	2	3	4	5
Loss of appetite	☐	☐	1	2	3	4	5
Weakness	☐	☐	1	2	3	4	5
Feeling irritable	☐	☐	1	2	3	4	5
Feeling anxious	☐	☐	1	2	3	4	5
Feeling depressed	☐	☐	1	2	3	4	5
Trouble sleeping	☐	☐	1	2	3	4	5
Being afraid that I won't be able to stop eating	☐	☐	1	2	3	4	5
Thinking about food	☐	☐	1	2	3	4	5
Difficulty concentrating	☐	☐	1	2	3	4	5
Difficulty making decisions	☐	☐	1	2	3	4	5
Difficulty getting along with friends	☐	☐	1	2	3	4	5
Difficulty getting along with family members	☐	☐	1	2	3	4	5
Feeling bad about myself	☐	☐	1	2	3	4	5
Eating	☐	☐	1	2	3	4	5
Other symptoms (specify) _____	☐	☐	1	2	3	4	5

Have you ever had **treatment** for any symptoms listed above? No ☐ Yes ☐
If yes, when and by whom were you treated? _____

_____

If yes, have you ever been hospitalized or taken medication as part of the treatment?

_____

Appendix B.2   Weight-Change History

This information will help us to understand how your weight has changed. Please answer each item as best you as you can; don't worry about being exact.

1. Approximate weight now _____ 6 months ago _____ 1 year ago _____ 2 years ago _____ 3 years ago _____

2. Height _____ (ft) _____ (in.)

3. Do you think that your *body frame* is small ☐, medium ☐, or large ☐?

4. What is the *most* you have ever weighed? _____
   When did you *first* reach that weight? Month _____ Year _____
   When were you *last* at that weight? Month _____ Year _____
   What is the longest period of time you *stayed* at that weight? _____ (months)

5. Since childhood, what is the *least* you have ever weighed? _____
   When did you *first* reach that weight? Month _____ Year _____
   When were you *last* at that weight? Month _____ Year _____
   What is the longest period of time you *stayed* at that weight? _____ (months)

6. What is a *normal* weight for someone your height and body frame? _____

7. What would you *like* to weight? _____

8. Are you involved in *activities* that require you to control your weight?
   ☐ No ☐ Yes
   If yes, check all the reasons that apply:

Work	Sport	Dance	Other (specify)
☐	☐	☐	☐ _____

9. How often do you *weigh* yourself?

Less than once a week	Once a week	2–6 times a week	Once a day	More than once a day
☐	☐	☐	☐	☐

10. Does your weight often go *up and down* from day to day? ☐ No ☐ Yes
    If yes, how many pounds does it typically fluctuate? _____

11. If I *gained* (or lost) 2 pounds, I would feel

	Very bad	Bad	No different	Good	Very good
Gained	☐	☐	☐	☐	☐
Lost	☐	☐	☐	☐	☐

12. How did you *feel* in grades 1-4, and how do you feel now?

	Very thin	Thin	Normal weight	Fat	Very fat
Grades 1–4	☐	☐	☐	☐	☐
Now	☐	☐	☐	☐	☐

Appendix B.3 Eating History

This information will help us to understand your eating habits. Please choose the *one* answer that best describes a typical day or week.

1. On a scale of 0–5, how much do you now eat at each of the following times in a typical day?

Nothing	Snack	Small meal	Meal	Large meal	Binge
0	1	2	3	4	5

At		*Between*		*After*	
Breakfast	————	Breakfast and lunch	————	Going to bed	————
Lunch	————	Lunch and dinner	————	Something upsetting	————
Dinner	————	Dinner and bedtime	————	Other (specify)	————————

2. How many times of week do you eat the following meals?

Breakfast	0	1	2	3	4	5	6	7
Lunch	0	1	2	3	4	5	6	7
Dinner	0	1	2	3	4	5	6	7

3. How many times a week do you eat the following meals with your family?

Breakfast	0	1	2	3	4	5	6	7
Lunch	0	1	2	3	4	5	6	7
Dinner	0	1	2	3	4	5	6	7

4. Please rate your preference for eating the following food groups. Look over the choices in the list before you start to answer.

	Extreme dislike	Dislike	Take it or leave it	Favorite Like	food
Bread/cereal/pasta	1	2	3	4	5
Cookies/cake/pie	1	2	3	4	5
"Fast food"	1	2	3	4	5
Fish	1	2	3	4	5
Fruit	1	2	3	4	5
Milk/cheese/yogurt	1	2	3	4	5
Poultry	1	2	3	4	5
Red meat	1	2	3	4	5
Snack foods, (e.g., popcorn, chips)	1	2	3	4	5
Sweets/candy	1	2	3	4	5
Vegetables	1	2	3	4	5
Other (specify)					
————————	—	—	—	4	5
————————	—	—	—	4	5

continued on next page

5. How well do the following words describe your food choices and eating habits now? (Please circle one choice for each word.)

	Extremely	Very much	Somewhat	Slightly	Not at all
Impulsive	1	2	3	4	5
Monotonous/boring	1	2	3	4	5
Well-planned	1	2	3	4	5
Fattening	1	2	3	4	5
Nutritious	1	2	3	4	5
Flexible	1	2	3	4	5

6. Please record what you typically eat and drink at breakfast:

	Description	Amount
B	_____	_____
K	_____	_____
F	_____	_____
S	_____	_____
T	_____	_____

7. Please record what you typically eat and drink at lunch:

	Description	Amount
L	_____	_____
U	_____	_____
N	_____	_____
C	_____	_____
H	_____	_____

8. Please record what you typically eat and drink at dinner:

	Description	Amount
D	_____	_____
I	_____	_____
N	_____	_____
N	_____	_____
E	_____	_____
R	_____	_____

Appendix B.4   Weight Control Activity

1. In the last year, have you used any of the following methods to control your
   weight, or used them for other reasons? If yes, circle how often you used each
   method, on the average, approximately 6 months ago and mark with an "X" how
   often you used each method, on the average, over the past 3 months.

	No	Yes	Less than once a week	Once a week	2–6 × a week	Once a day	More than once a day
Limiting food intake	☐	☐	1	2	3	4	5
Exercising	☐	☐	1	2	3	4	5
Vomiting	☐	☐	1	2	3	4	5
Ipecac	☐	☐	1	2	3	4	5
Laxatives	☐	☐	1	2	3	4	5
Diuretics (water pills)	☐	☐	1	2	3	4	5
Diet pills	☐	☐	1	2	3	4	5

If you answered No to *all* of the above, then you do not have more questions to
answer on this form. Please answer 2–6 for any item that was marked Yes.

2. Limiting food intake (dieting) to lose weight:
      When did you *first* begin to diet? Month _____Year _____
      What was your height and weight at that time? Height _____ Weight _____
      What is the *longest* you've stayed on a diet? _____ (months)

3. Exercising:

	No	Yes	Hours/Week
Walking	☐	☐	_____
Running or jogging	☐	☐	_____
Aerobics or calisthenics	☐	☐	_____
Weight-lifting/nautilus	☐	☐	_____
Dancing or ballet	☐	☐	_____
Swimming	☐	☐	_____
Gymnastics	☐	☐	_____
Team sports	☐	☐	_____

   Other (specify)   _____
   How long do you exercise at a time?   _____ (minutes)
   How many times a week do you exercise?   _____
   When did you begin your exercise program?   _____ (month) _____ (year)
   Has your exercise pattern changed in the last 24 months? No ☐ Yes ☐
      If yes, how _____

4. Vomiting:

  Vomit after eating small amounts ☐, large amounts ☐, or both ☐?

  Vomit how son after finishing eating? _____ (minutes)

  How do you make yourself throw up? (Check all that apply.)

Stick something in my throat	Take ipecac	Put pressure on stomach	"It just happens"	Other
☐	☐	☐	☐	☐

  How did you first get the idea to vomit? (Check all that apply.)

Read about it	TV/radio	Friend	Family member	Thought of it myself	Other
☐	☐	☐	☐	☐	☐

5. Medications or drugs in the past month to lose weight:

  (Please list the type, amount and frequency of use.)

	No	Yes	Amount per dose	Doses per month
Ipecac	☐	☐	_____	_____
Laxatives	☐	☐	_____	_____
Diuretics	☐	☐	_____	_____
Diet pills	☐	☐	_____	_____

6. Rate on a scale of 1-5 how other people and things have influenced your weight control? If a category has more than one possible answer, e.g., if you have two sisters or have read several different diet books, pick the most influential person or thing in that category.

Strongly influenced weight loss	Influenced weight loss	Neutral or no influence	Influenced weight gain	Strongly influenced weight gain	Does not apply
1	2	3	4	5	6

Sister	_____	Brother	_____	Coach	_____
Mother	_____	Father	_____	Doctor/nurse	_____
Girlfriend	_____	Boyfriend	_____	Other person (specify)	_____

T.V.	_____	Book	_____	Other thing	_____
Radio	_____	Magazine	_____	(specify)	_____
Movie	_____	Advertisement	_____		

Hypertension

Appendix C.1   Typical Food Intake Screening

Obtain the following information for the meals and/or snacks listed below:
1. Approximate time and place(s) for each meal and snack eaten:
2. Describe the variety of the types of food and drink selected:
3. Frequency of meal skipping:
4. Eating out pattern:
    a) Participation in school breakfast and/or lunch program.
    b) Use of "take-out" food from a restaurant that's eaten at home.
    c) Frequency and types of food/drink eaten out at a fast-food or full-service restaurants.
    d) Frequency of meals or snacks eaten at a relative's or friend's home.
    e) Meals/snacks bought from vending machines or local convenience stores (e.g. mini-mart, drugstore, gas station, etc.).

Breakfast: _____

_____

_____

_____

Lunch: _____

_____

_____

_____

Dinner: _____

_____

_____

_____

Snacks: (Morning) _____

(Afternoon) _____

(Evening) _____

Weekend differences: (e.g., timing, place, types of food/drink consumed, meal
                       skipping):

_____

_____

_____

Consumption of foods high in potassium and low in sodium:
   How often do you eat fruits or drink fruit juices? (Describe type and amount.)

_____

   How often do you eat fresh or frozen vegetables? (Describe type and amount.)

_____

   How often do you drink milk or eat yogurt? (Describe type and amount.)

_____

Other factors affecting food intake and nutritional status

Vitamin/mineral supplement use: ☐ Yes ☐ No
   If yes, describe (what kind, frequency, and reason):

_____

continued on next page

Appendix C.1   *Continued*

Food allergies/intolerances or abstentions for religious or other reasons:

_____

Member(s) of household responsible for food purchasing and meal preparation for the home:

_____

Economic status:
1. Participation in food assistance programs:
    ☐ Food stamps   ☐ WIC   ☐ School lunch   ☐ School breakfast

2. Appliances in the home and in good working order:
    ☐ Refrigerator   ☐ Stove   ☐ Oven   ☐ Microwave oven

Meal atmosphere (who is with you when meal is eaten; other activities done while meal is eaten, e.g., watching TV, reading, listening to music, etc.; extent of interaction with family member(s) or peers present):

At home: _____

_____

At school: _____

_____

Alcohol intake:
1. Do any of your friends drink alcohol? ☐ Yes ☐ No (Circle one.)
    If yes, describe (where, when, type, amount, frequency, etc.):

_____

_____

2. Have you ever had beer, wine, a wine cooler or hard liquor to drink?
    ☐ Yes ☐ No
    If yes, describe (where, when, with whom, type, amount, frequency, etc.):

_____

_____

Cigarette smoking:
Do you smoke cigarettes? ☐ Yes ☐ No
If yes, describe (when, name brand, amount, frequency, duration):

_____

Appendix C.2 Selected Food Item from Fastfood Resturants with High-Sodium Contents*

Food Item	Sodium (mg)
Arby's	
Ham 'n cheese	1350
Roast chicken club	1500
Burger King	
Scrambled egg platter with sausage	1271
Chicken aandwich	1417
Whopper with cheese sandwich	1177
Hardee's	
Big country ham breakfast	2870
Hot ham & cheese	1420
Turkey club	1280
Long John Silver's	
Crispy breaded fish sandwich	1220
3-Piece fish dinner	1890
McDonald's	
Biscuit with sausage & egg	1250
Quarter pounder with cheese	1150
Pizza Hut	
Thin and crispy supreme: 2 slices, medium	1328
Personal pan pizza	1335
Subway	
Spicy Italian sub (Italian roll)	3020
Subway club sub (regular)	2717
Turkey breast sub (Italian roll)	2460
Taco Bell	
Enchirito - with red sauce	1243
Beef burrito	1051

*Food items listed provide approximately one-half or more of the recommended intake of sodium (1500–2500 mg/d) for hypertensive youth.

Appendix C.3 Food Frequency Checklist for Salt and Sodium

Please indicate in the following tables how often you eat the foods listed by checking the appropriate box. The definitions for the categories given are as follows:

Regularly: Eaten 4–7 times/week
Frequently: Eaten 1–3 times/week
Occasionally: Eaten 1–3 times/ month
Never: Not eaten at all

Circle those items you consider to be your favorite foods.

Meat, poultry, fish

Food Item	Regularly 4–7 ×/Week	Frequently 1–3 ×/Week	Occasionally 1–3 ×/Month	Never
Ham				
Bacon				
Sausage				
Hot dogs				
Luncheon meats (bologna, salami, turkey loaf, smoked beef)				
Fish sticks (or other pre-fried and pre-breaded fish products)				
Tuna fish (canned in oil)				

Meat substitutes

Food Item	Regularly 4–7 ×/Week	Frequently 1–3 ×/Week	Occasionally 1–3 ×/Month	Never
Canned beans (pinto, kidney, navy, garbanzo, chick peas)				
Nuts, salted (peanuts, cashews, almonds, pistachios, mixed nuts, etc.)				
Sunflower seeds, salted				

Vegetables

Food Item	Regularly 4–7 ×/Week	Frequently 1–3 ×/Week	Occasionally 1–3 ×/Month	Never
Canned vegetables (peas, corn, grean beans, etc.)				
Pickles				
Vegetable juices (tomato juice, V-8)				

continued on next page

Appendix C.3   *Continued*

Main dish items

Food Item	Regularly 4–7 ×/Week	Frequently 1–3 ×/Week	Occasionally 1–3 ×/Month	Never
Chicken or turkey pot pie (frozen)				
TV dinners (frozen)				
Pizza (frozen or restaurant)				
Mexican food: tacos, enchiladas, burritos (Frozen or Restaurant)				
Soups (canned or instant)				
Canned meat products (chili, meat stew, pork and beans, etc.)				
Boxed main dish item (hamburger or Tuna Helper)				
Canned/frozen Italian food (meatballs and spaghetti, ravioli, lasagne)				

Dairy Products

Food Item	Regularly 4–7 ×/Week	Frequently 1–3 ×/Week	Occasionally 1–3 ×/Month	Never
Cheese: American, Swiss, cheddar				
Cheese spread				
Cottage cheese Buttermilk				
Butter (not margarine)				
Instant cocoa mixes				

Bread, potatoes, or other starches

Food Item	Regularly 4–7 ×/Week	Frequently 1–3 ×/Week	Occasionally 1–3 ×/Month	Never
Biscuits				
Waffles or pancakes (frozen or boxed mix)				
Potato chips or other snack chips				
Pretzels, salted				
Popcorn, salted				
Crackers				
French fries, salted				
Potato side dishes (boxed or frozen)				
Pasta or rice side dishes (boxed or frozen with a sauce)				
Bread stuffing (boxed or frozen)				

continued on next page

Appendix C.3 *Continued*

Miscellaneous

Food Item	Regularly 4–7 ×/Week	Frequently 1–3 ×/Week	Occasionally 1–3 ×/Month	Never
Ketchup or chili sauce				
Mustard				
Olives				
Gravy				
Steak or barbeque sauce				
Soy sauce				
Tartar sauce				
Seasoning salts (garlic, onion, celery)				
Salad dressings (commercially packaged)				

Answer the following questions:
1. Do you add salt to your food
   - At the table?   ☐ Yes ☐ No
   - Before tasting it?   ☐ Yes ☐ No
   - During cooking?   ☐ Yes ☐ No

2. Do other family members add salt to the foods they prepare for you?
   ☐ Yes   ☐ No   ☐ I don't know.

   If yes, specify which family member(s) (mother, father, aunt, grandparent, sister, brother, etc.):

Appendix C.4   Selected Foods with a High-Potassium and Low-Natural-Sal Content

	Potassium Content (mg)
Fruit Juices	
Apple juice (1 cup)	249
Apricot nectar (¾ cup)	279
Grape juice, bottled (¾ cup)	209
Orange juice, freshor canned (½ cup)	250
Pineapple juice, canned (¾ cup)	284
Prune juice (¾ cup)	423
Fruits	
Apricots	
Fresh (2–3 medium)	281
Dried (8 large halves)	461
Canned, juice packed (3 medium halves)	362
Banana (1 small, 6 in.)	370
Dates	
Fresh (5 medium, pitted)	324
Dried (½ cup, cut)	575
Melons, fresh	
Cantaloupe (¼ melon, 5 in. diameter)	251
Honeydew (¼ melon, 5 in. diameter)	251
Watermelon (1 slice, 6 in. diameter × 1 ½ in. thick)	600
Nectarines, fresh (2 medium)	294
Orange, fresh (1 medium)	311
Peaches	
Fresh (1 medium)	202
Canned, juice packed (2 medium halves with 2 tbsp. of juice)	205
Plums, fresh (2 medium)	299
Prunes, dried (5 large)	347
Milk and Milk products	
Milk (1 cup)	
Skim	408
Low-fat (1%)	381
Low-fat (2%)	374
Yogurt (1 cup)	
Nonfat, plain	579
Low-fat, fruit-flavored	442
Meats and meat substitutes	
Hamburger (1 medium patty)	382
Pot roast, rump (3 oz)	464
Chicken, roasted (3 oz)	321

continued on next page

Appendix C.4 *Continued*

	Potassium Content (mg)
Meats and meat substitutes, continued	
Turkey, roasted (3 oz)	341
Pork tenderloin, roasted (3 oz)	436
Dried beans, cooked	
White (½ cup)	416
Red kidney (½ cup)	425
Tuna, canned in water (½ cup)	279
Flounder or sole, baked (3 oz)	587
Vegetables	
Broccoli	
Raw, fresh (1 stalk, 5 ½ in. long)	382
Cooked, fresh (2/3 cup)	267
Cooked, frozen (3 ½ oz)	212
Brussel Sprouts	
Cooked, fresh (6-7)	273
Cooked, frozen (3 ½ oz)	295
Cabbage, raw (1 cup shredded)	233
Carrots, fresh	
Raw (1 large)	344
Cooked (2/3 cup)	222
Cauliflower, fresh	
Raw (1 cup of flower pieces)	295
Collard Greens, cooked (½ cup)	234
Green Pepper, fresh, raw (1 large shell)	213
Kale, cooked (¾ cup)	318
Lima beans	
Cooked, fresh (½ cup)	338
Cooked, frozen (½ cup)	341
Mushrooms,fresh, raw (10 small or 4 large)	414
Mustard greens, cooked (½ cup)	220
Peas, fresh, cooked (2/3 cup)	196
Potato,fresh	
Baked (2 ½ in. diameter)	503
French fried, no added salt (10 pieces)	427
Spinach	
Cooked, fresh (½ cup)	291
Cooked, frozen (½ cup)	333
Sweet potato, fresh, baked (1 large)	540
Tomato, fresh, raw (1 medium)	366

*High potassium > 200 mg/serving.

Adapted from *Bowes & Church's Food Values of Portions Commonly Used,* XIII ed., Revised, (J.A.T. Pennington and H. N. Church, eds.), Lippincott Company, Philadelphia, PA, (1980).

Appendix C.5   Food Frequency Checklist for Dietary Fat

Please indicate in the following tables how often you eat the foods listed by checking the appropriate box. The definitions for the categories given are as follows:

Regularly: Eaten 4–7 times/week
Frequently: Eaten 1–3 times/week
Occasionally: Eaten 1–3 times/month
Never: Not eaten at all

Circle those items you consider to be your favorite foods.

Meat, poultry, fish

Food Item	Regularly 4–7 ×/Week	Frequently 1–3 ×/Week	Occasionally 1–3 ×/Month	Never
Hamburger				
Steak				
Roast beef				
Fried fish				
Tuna salad				
Fried chicken				
Chicken eaten with skin on (baked, boiled, or roasted)				

Meat substitutes

Food Item	Regularly 4–7 ×/Week	Frequently 1–3 ×/Week	Occasionally 1–3 ×/Month	Never
Peanut butter				
Nuts				
Sunflower seeds				
Egg salad				
Fried or scrambled eggs				

continued on next page

Appendix C.5 *Continued*

Vegetables

Food Item	Regularly 4–7 ×/Week	Frequently 1–3 ×/Week	Occasionally 1–3 ×/Month	Never
Onion rings (fried)				
Cole slaw				
Avocado				

Bread, potatoes , or other starches

Food Item	Regularly 4–7 ×/Week	Frequently 1–3 ×/Week	Occasionally 1–3 ×/Month	Never
Croissant rolls				
French fries				
Hash browns				
Potato salad				

Baked goods

Food Item	Regularly 4–7 ×/Week	Frequently 1–3 ×/Week	Occasionally 1–3 ×/Month	Never
Doughnuts				
Cake				
Pie				
Brownies				
Muffins				
Cookies				
Sweet rolls or Danish				

Dairy products

Food Item	Regularly 4–7 ×/Week	Frequently 1–3 ×/Week	Occasionally 1–3 ×/Month	Never
Whole milk				
Chocolate milk				
Ice cream				
Milk shakes				
Cream cheese				
Sour cream†				
Margarine‡				

†Sour cream as used in dips, added to baked potatoes, or as a topping with Mexican food.
‡Margarine use includes what is added to potatoes, rice, pasta, and cooked vegetables, or spread on bread, rolls, or crackers.

Miscellaneous

Food Item	Regularly 4–7 ×/Week	Frequently 1–3 ×/Week	Occasionally 1–3 ×/Month	Never
Mayonnaise or Miracle Whip**				
Candy bars				

**Mayonnaise or Miracle Whip used as spread on bread with sandwiches.

Appendix C.6   Contract for Promoting Nutritional Health

Date: _____

I, _____, agree to make the following change(s) for the
next_____:

(Participant's Name)   (Length of time)

_____

_____

_____

_____

_____

I, _____, agree to make the following change(s) for the
next_____:

(Participant's Parent/Guardian)   (Length of time)

_____

_____

_____

_____

_____

Participant's Signature

_____

Parent/Guardian's Signature

_____

Clinician/Nutritionist

Appendix C.7   Physical Activity Screening

1. When in school, I participate in physical education class (check one):
   ___ For 1 quarter or 1 semester   ___ For 3 quarters
   ___ For 2 quarters or 2 semesters   ___ Throughout the school year
   ___ I do *not* participate in physical education classes.
      If not, explain: _____

2. When physical education class is offered at school, I attend (check one):
   ___ Once a week   ___ Three to four times a week
   ___ Twice a week   ___ Every day
   ___ I do *not* attend physical education classes in school

3. Physical activities done during after-school hours, on weekends, and/or summer vacation in the past year (check all that apply; *circle* those activities you enjoy the most):

___ Soccer	___ Basketball	___ Brisk walking
___ Football	___ Cross-country	___ Track and field
___ Aerobics	___ Bicycling	___ Roller skating
___ Baseball	___ Dancing	___ Weightlifting
___ Tennis	___ Gymnastics	___ Jogging
___ Swimming	___ Wrestling	___ Roller blading
___ Ice skating	___ Karate	___ Volleyball
___ Other (specify)	___ I don't like to do any of the activities listed.	

4. The amount of television (TV) I watch is (check one):
   ___ Too much   ___ Just right
   ___ Too little   ___ I don't watch television at all

5. At home, I can watch as much TV as I want to (check one):
   ___ Yes
   ___ No
      If you checked "No," explain why: _____
      _____

   ___ I don't watch TV.

Appendix C.8 Follow-Up Physical Activity Screening

Physical activity

List activities checked from the physical activity screening and determine their frequency, duration, and setting:

Activity	Frequency	Duration	Setting

Inactivity
Television viewing time: List hours of TV watched for each time segment.

Weekdays

Mornings (before school): ___ × ___ (# of weekdays) = ___
Afternoons (after school): ___ × ___ (# of weekdays) = ___
Evenings (during/after dinner): ___ × ___ (# of weekdays) = ___
Total hours of TV watched on weekdays = ___

Weekends

Saturday: ___
Sunday: ___
Total hours of TV watached on weekdays: ___
Total (Hours/week): ___

Index